D1571822

Oxford Medical Publications

Higher-order motor disorders

Higher-order motor disorders

From neuroanatomy and neurobiology to clinical neurology

Edited by

Hans-Joachim Freund

Professor of Neurology, Heinrich-Heine-Universität
Düsseldorf, Germany

Marc Jeannerod

Professor in Physiology, University of Lyon
Lyon, France

Mark Hallett

Chief, Chief, Human Motor Control Section,
National Institute of Neurological Disorders and Stroke,
National Institute of Health, Bethesda MD, USA

Ramón Leiguarda

Professor of Neurology, University of Buenos Aires
and Chairman, Department of Neurology
Institute of Neurological Research FLENI
Buenos Aires, Argentina

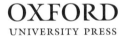

OXFORD

UNIVERSITY PRESS

OXFORD
UNIVERSITY PRESS

Great Clarendon Street, Oxford OX2 6DP

Oxford University Press is a department of the University of Oxford.
It furthers the University's objective of excellence in research, scholarship,
and education by publishing worldwide in

Oxford New York

Auckland Cape Town Dar es Salaam Hong Kong Karachi
Kuala Lumpur Madrid Melbourne Mexico City Nairobi
New Delhi Shanghai Taipei Toronto

With offices in

Argentina Austria Brazil Chile Czech Republic France Greece
Guatemala Hungary Italy Japan Poland Portugal Singapore
South Korea Switzerland Thailand Turkey Ukraine Vietnam

Oxford is a registered trade mark of Oxford University Press
in the UK and in certain other countries

Published in the United States
by Oxford University Press Inc., New York

© Oxford University Press, 2005

A catalogue record for this title is available from the British Library

Library of Congress Cataloging in Publication Data (attached)

Higher-order motor disorders : from neuroanatomy and neurobiology to clinical neurology /
editors Hans-J. Freund (et al.).

Includes bibliographical references and index.
1. Psychomotor disorders. [DNLM: 1. Movement Disorders–physiopathology.
2. Motor Cortex–physiology. 3. Motor Cortex–physiopathology.
4. Psychomotor Disorders–physiopathology. WL 390 H638 2005] I. Freund, H.-J.
RC 376.5.H54.2005   616.8′3-dc22   2004029454

Typeset by Newgen Imaging Systems (P) Ltd., Chennai, India
Printed in Great Britain
on acid-free paper by
Biddles Ltd., King's Lynn

ISBN 0-19-852576-1 (Hbk: alk. paper)   978-0-19-852576-9 (Hbk)

10 9 8 7 6 5 4 3 2 1

Preface

Most movements that humans make are complex. Execution and control of motor behaviour depends on the intricate interleaving of operations that occur at multiple neural levels. The control of an action involves volition, planning, selection, programming, and execution of movements. The ensemble of covert steps that precede execution make up the representation of the action: incoming sensory stimuli as well as cognitive and motivational factors intervene to determine its goal; the action is then planned with respect to the behavioural context and to external constraints; finally, a programme is constructed to generate the specific movement parameters in relation to the physical state of the organism and to trigger automatic motor performance. Thus the representation of a given action operates at several levels, each of which is subserved by a specific neural system. Disruption of either of these systems will be responsible for selective behavioural deficits. In this volume we will consider higher-order motor disorders, understood as disturbances resulting from damage to areas upstream of the primary motor cortex. These disturbances cover a wide range of disorders, including apraxias and sensorimotor transformation deficits, motor neglect, anarchic hand syndrome, and action motivational and action monitoring disorders.

Whereas approaches to movement disorders have undergone revolutionary changes over the last decades, the impact of neuroscience on higher-order motor disorders has been less dramatic. However, in recent years the investigation of processes at the interface between action and cognition has been plentiful and the field of higher-order motor control or cognitive-motor control has expanded enormously. Novel views on cortical organization emanating from experimental work and neuro-imaging have begun to change our picture of the complex motor disorders. The modular cortical organization was revealed in non-human primates by neurophysiological and neuroanatomical studies and also by the complementary approach of probing function by focal chemical inactivation. In humans, the high resolution of clinical neuro-imaging has made it possible to examine small purely cortical lesions and to establish structure–function relationships by combining this information with meticulous behavioural analysis. The advantage of this approach is that functional deficits can be analysed for all those facets of behaviour that can be investigated so uniquely in humans. Against this background, lesion studies continue to contribute to a better understanding of human brain function and specify nodal points in a given functional network. Therefore refined lesion analysis, together with functional activation studies after brain injury, represents a strategy complementary to experimental work and to functional activation studies in normal subjects.

This book attempts to offer a comprehensive overview and a useful reference source that we hope will stimulate research and new insight into higher-order or cognitive motor disorders. The first part deals with the neuroanatomical, neurobiological, and cognitive basis of motor behaviour. In the second part we approach the clinical features of higher-order motor disorders, including abnormalities of bimanual coordination and speech motor disorders, as well as imitation and utilization behaviour. It is aimed at a wide readership within the neurosciences and beyond, comprising clinicians and researchers in neurology, neuropsychology, and cognitive psychology, as well as in rehabilitation medicine.

The contributors and editors of this book are distinguished basic and clinical investigators in their respective fields, who work at the forefront of current research.

Hans-Joachim Freund
Mark Hallett
Marc Jeannerod
Ramón Leiguarda

Contents

List of contributors

Pierre Baraduc
INSERM U483
9 quai Saint-Bernard
Paris, France

Alexandra Battaglia-Mayer
Dipartimento di Fisiologia Umana e
  Farmacologia
Università di Roma 'La Sapienza'
Piazzale Aldo Moro
Rome, Italy

Sarah-Jayne Blakemore
Institute of Cognitive
  Neuroscience
University College London
17 Queen Square
London, UK

Driss Boussaoud
Institut des Sciences Cognitives
CNRS UMR 5015
67 Boulevard Pinel
Bron, France

Yves Burnod
Institut des Sciences Cognitives
67 Boulevard Pinel
Bron, France

Roberto Caminiti
Dipartimento di Fisiologia Umana e
  Farmacologia
Università di Roma 'La Sapienza'
Piazzale Aldo Moro
Rome, Italy

Pablo A. Celnik
Human Cortical Physiology
  Section
National Institute of Neurological
  Disorders and Stroke
National Institutes of Health
Bethesda, MD, USA and Department of
Physical Medicine and Rehabilitation
Johns Hopkins University
Baltimore, MD, USA

Robert Chen
Movement Disorders Clinic
Toronto Western Hospital
399 Bathurst Street
Toronto, Ontario
Canada

Leonardo G. Cohen
Human Cortical Physiology
  Section
National Institute of Neurological
  Disorders and Stroke
National Institutes of Health
Bethesda, MD, USA

Elena Daprati
IRCCS Fondazione Santa Lucia
Rome, Italy

Sergio Della Sala
Neuropsychology Research Group
Department of Psychology
University of Aberdeen
Aberdeen, UK

Michel Desmurget
INSERM U534
16 avenue du Doyen Lépine
Bron, France

Bruno Dubois
INSERM U610 and Fédération de
Neurologie
Hôpital de la Salpêtrière
Paris, France

Luciano Fadiga
Dipartimento di Scienze Biomediche e
  Terapie Avanzate
Sezione di Fisiologia Umana
Università di Ferrara
Ferrara, Italy

Stefano Ferraina
Dipartimento di Fisiologia Umana e
  Farmacologia
Università di Roma 'La Sapienza'
Piazzale Aldo Moro
Rome, Italy

Gereon R. Fink
Department of Neurology
University Hospital
RWTH Aachen
Aachen, Germany
and Institute of Medicine
Research Centre Jülich
Jülich, Germany

Hans-Joachim Freund
Institute of Medicine
Research Centre Jülich
Jülich, Germany

Christoph Fromm
Department of Neurology
University Hospital
RWTH Aachen
Aachen, Germany

Stefan Geyer
C. and O. Vogt Brain Research Institute
Heinrich Heine University
Düsseldorf, Germany

Georg Goldenberg
Neuropsychologische Abteilung
Krankenhaus München Bogenhausen
Englschalkingerstrasse 77
München, Germany

Emmanuel Guigon
INSERM U483
9 quai Saint-Bernard
Paris, France

Patrick Haggard
Institute of Cognitive
  Neuroscience
University College London
17 Queen Square
London, UK

Mark Hallett
Human Motor Control Section
NINDS, NIH
Bethesda, MD, USA

Joseph Jankovic
Parkinson's Disease Center and
Movement Disorders Clinic
Department of Neurology
Baylor College of Medicine
Houston, TX, USA

Marc Jeannerod
Institut des Sciences Cognitives
67 Boulevard Pinel
Bron, France

Ray D. Kent
University of Wisconsin-Madison
Madison, WI, USA

Günther Knoblich
Max Planck Institute for Psychological
    Research
Amalienstrasse 33
Munich, Germany

Anthony Lang
Movement Disorders Clinic
Toronto Western Hospital
399 Bathurst Street
Toronto, Ontario
Canada

Ramón Leiguarda
Department of Neurology
FLENI, Montañeses 2325 (C 1428 AQK)
Buenos Aires, Argentina

Facundo Manes
Department of Cognitive Neurology
FLENI, Montañeses 2325
    (C 1428 AQK)
Buenos Aires, Argentina

Clelia Marchetti
Neuropsychology Unit
Division of Neurology
Salvatore Maugeri Foundation IRCCS
Scientific Institute of Veruno (NO)
Veruno, Italy

John C. Marshall
University Department of Clinical
Neurology
Radcliffe Infirmary
Oxford, UK

Massimo Mascaro
Dipartimento di Fisiologia Umana e
    Farmacologia
Università di Roma 'La Sapienza'
Piazzale Aldo Moro
Rome, Italy

Johannes Noth
Department of Neurology
University Hospital
RWTH Aachen
Aachen, Germany

John G.Nutt
Departments of Neurology,
    Pharmacology & Physiology
Oregon Health & Science University
3181 SW Sam Jackson Park Road
Portland, OR, USA

Bernard Pillon
INSERM E 007 and Fédération de
    Neurologie
Hôpital de la Salpêtrière
Paris, France

Tamara Pringsheim
Movement Disorders Clinic
Toronto Western Hospital
399 Bathurst Street
Toronto, Ontario
Canada

Wolfgang Prinz
Max Planck Institute for Psychological
    Research
Amalienstrasse 33
Munich, Germany

Giacomo Rizzolatti
Dipartimento di Neuroscienze
Sezione di Fisiologia Umana
Università di Parma
Parma, Italy

Gilles Rode
Espace et Action
Institut National de la Santé et de la
    Recherche Médicale
Unité 534, 16 avenue Lépine
Bron, France

Yves Rossetti
Espace et Action
Institut National de la Santé et de la
    Recherche Médicale
Unité 534, 16 avenue Lépine
Bron, France

Jeremy D. Schmahmann
Department of Neurology
Massachusetts General Hospital
Harvard Medical School
Boston, MA, USA

Deborah J. Serrien
Sobell Department of Motor
    Neuroscience and Movement
    Disorders
Institute of Neurology
Queen Square
London, UK

Angela Sirigu
Institut des Sciences Cognitives
67 Boulevard Pinel
Bron, France

Mario Wiesendanger
Department of Neurology
Laboratory of Motor Systems
University of Berne
Berne, Switzerland

Daniel M. Wolpert
Sobell Department of Motor
    Neuroscience and Movement
    Disorders
Institute of Neurology
University College London
Queen Square
London, UK

Karl Zilles
C. and O. Vogt Brain Research
    Institute
Heinrich Heine University
    Düsseldorf
and Institute of Medicine
Research Center Jülich
Jülich, Germany

Introduction

Hans-Joachim Freund, Mark Hallett, Marc Jeannerod, and Ramón Leiguarda

In his selected writings Hughlings Jackson (1931), predicted that one day three levels of functional differentiation would be demonstrated in the central nervous system. The lowest level, he said, was to be found in the spinal cord, medulla, and pons where the different portions of the body have representation as units. The middle level would lie, according to him, in the pre-Rolandic primary motor and primary sensory cortices, not of body portions but of functions, i.e. coordinated movements and differentiation of sensation. Such differentiating activity is what Pavlov called analysing and what Sherrington termed integration. In turn, the highest level of integration would be the final sensory and motor rearrangement which might form the neuronal substrate of consciousness, which, Jackson suggested, might be found in the frontal regions. In Jackson's view of the organization of the motor cortex, the 'highest level' of motor integration or the final representation of 'educated skills' (the function of eupraxia, as Walshe called it in 1948), was to be found within the frontal cortex anterior to the excitable motor cortex.

Whereas the physiological basis of the middle level was extensively investigated and strongly influenced neurological thought during the twentieth century, it was not until recently that the concept of the highest level of motor integration could be approached through the field of motor cognition and the introduction of neuroimaging techniques. What Sherrington replied to Walshe when he mentioned his proposal to study the role of the pyramidal system in willed movements, 'You chose a hard question, and one which the bedside is a far better place to solve than is the laboratory', is no longer so. The situation is now rapidly changing. New concepts emerging from basic neurosciences have impacted the field of cognitive motor control and opened a new era in the study and understanding of higher-order motor disorders far beyond the traditional field of topological diagnosis.

On the experimental side, deactivation studies have established quasi-'clinical' models of focal brain damage and shown that virtually every aspect of modular cortical functions can be compromised. The respective disturbances can selectively interfere with a wide range of sensorimotor tasks including the coordinate transformations elaborating the appropriate reference frames of the upcoming motor act.

Human studies are complementary as they can assess the more complex aspects of motor behaviour, including motor cognition, which can barely be studied in non-human primates. As emphasized by Ettlinger (1969), there is no animal model of apraxia representing a disorder of motor concept formation. The disturbances of the identification and selection of the goal of an action, of the motivational, affective, and cognitive aspects of motor behaviour, provide information that cannot be gained from experimental approaches.

The meticulous clinical analysis of these complex dysfunctions established the basis of our knowledge about motor disorders such as apraxia, motor neglect, and other higher-order motor disorders. The disadvantage of the human studies lay in their methodological limitations. Following the classical period of clinical–pathological correlations, lesion studies gained a new dimension by the advent of *in vivo* imaging techniques. Initially, however, straightforward structure–function relationships were hampered by the fact that most of the lesion data were derived from larger and often poorly defined lesions. In addition, the attribution of the deficits to the cortical versus subcortical extent of the lesion was difficult. Further, the clinical description of the observed motor disturbances did not always facilitate comparisons with experimental or functional imaging studies.

High-resolution structural imaging of small lesions and the selective analysis of cortical versus subcortical damage changed this situation and opened new avenues for the study of structure–function relationships. In conjunction with functional imaging this provides an investigational repertoire that offers direct links to experimental research. Comparing the effects of lesions with functional activation studies revealed that specific dysfunctions resulting from brain damage are often mirrored by neuroimaging data in normal subjects evidencing activations in those tasks that reflect a positive image of the deficits seen after lesions. However, functional imaging adds another important aspect by disclosing how the respective activations are nested in widely distributed functional networks. Thus the comparison of deficits imposed by focal brain lesions and of functional activations by comparable tasks in normal subjects provides a powerful tool for the investigation of motor behaviour and its disorders.

Advances in the functional analysis of disturbed motor behaviour complemented the progress made possible by imaging techniques. Kinematic movement recordings and transcranial magnetic stimulation provided new insights into the functional organization of motor behaviour. They disclosed alterations of the spatial and temporal characteristics already present at the level of simple movements that are not clinically apparent, and revealed how their cumulative effects compromise the production of more complex motor behaviours. Further, they allowed researchers to perturb ongoing cortical processing and to trace lesion-induced excitability changes underlying reorganization. On the conceptual side, motor cognition has opened a new dimension to understanding motor behaviour and its disorders. The novel methodology of considering mental states as real entities and the concept of motor representations set the scene for neuroimaging studies of covert mental states. Thus the functional anatomy of motor cognition could be elaborated. These studies showed that imagination, observation, imitation, and the performance of movement all activate a similar network. This led to new vistas regarding the role of action observation and its neural representations for the recognition of the meaning of others. The investigation of the first- versus third-person perspective was a powerful tool for identifying the neural circuitries involved in the distinction between self and others, an important issue to bridge the gap to psychiatry. In the early 1990s, the concept of motor imagery put forward by Jeannerod found its experimental counterpart in the discovery of the mirror neuron concept by Rizzolatti. The capacity of the mirror system to code the observation and performance of the same gesture even by the same neurons provided a new perspective for understanding the neural basis of imitation and gestural communication.

The aim of this book is to relate the theoretical background for this approach to the discussion of higher-order motor distrubances rather than to dwell on terminological debates. We had originally thought that we would make firm definitions for various terms and insist that all the authors use them consistently. However, the more we worked at it, the more difficult this task became. Hence we do not want to be dogmatic, but a brief introduction to some concepts and terminology here may be of value.

The concept of goal-directed behaviour (GDB) is crucial to understand the focus of the book, because it seeks to integrate cognitive, motivational, emotional, and motor processes served by diverse neuronal systems, to provide a meaningful description of how the brain controls voluntary action. It is particularly useful for rendering functional a broad spectrum of purposeful actions and their determinants, from a simple reaching and grasping movement, to the most complex pattern of behaviour, providing a framework for bridging the neurobiology and clinical manifestations of many higher-order motor disorders.

GDB is construed as a set of related processes by which an internal state (derived from an internal or external event) is translated, through action, into the attainment of a goal (Brown and Pluck 2000). The process of the act appears to be directed by its goal, which thus defines the act as distinct from the action and constitutes behaviour of movement. It may be immediate and physical, such as relieving hunger, or long-term and abstract such as being successful at a job (Dickinson and Balleine 1994). By 'directed' it is meant that the action is mediated by a representation of the goal and that there should be some knowledge within the system of the contingency between the action and the desired outcome.

Purposeful behaviour may be driven by intention to act, motivations, and emotions and/or environmental stimuli, including verbal and social information; thus a conscious wish/desire, urge or need, or an external stimulus may trigger a willed (intentional) action or a mainly automatic or routine one. The internal determinants are drives or motivational states. The motivational state is dependent on at least two factors: immediate biological needs, or long-term goals. Thus motivational properties may be innate or learned through experience, as well as being labelled emotionally.

To pursue a GDB, the subject must have an internal representation of the goal, together with knowledge (though not necessarily conscious awareness) of a causal relationship between a particular course of action and its outcome (Dickinson and Balleine 1994). A routine action such as 'prepare breakfast' usually unfolds without wilful control in an automatic manner when triggered by internal needs and/or external cues, or occurs in the context of habitual tasks. The 'motor schemas' (or elementary units), which are predetermined sets of commands that interact for controlling motor output when assembled with other schemas, give rise to a 'coordinated control programme' (a higher-order schema) which in turn can be assembled with others, and so on. Motor schemas are activated by perceptual schemas that encode visual attributes of objects. Thus, during visually guided prehension the perceptual schemas activate the corresponding motor schemas for the subactions of 'reach', 'preshape', 'orient', and 'enclose'. The 'reach' and 'grasp' schemas are temporally coordinated by an additional schema, which receives from each of the constituent schemas a structure of the time it needs to move its current state to the desired final state (Hoff and Arbib 1993). Thus, the proposal of Arbib and colleagues regarding 'coordinated control programmes' or motor representations updates the classical concept of 'motor programmes'. When used in this book, the term motor programme will refer to 'a set of muscle commands that are structured before a movement sequence begins, and that follow the entire sequence to be carried out' (Keele 1968). Accordingly, the term programme is reserved for lower-level forms of motor preparation generally considered to occur without conscious awareness and directly leading to motor activity. Programmes are dependent on past motor learning of useful synergies and the ability to learn new synergies.

The time-based coordination of the interacting reach and grasp schemas results in a coordinated control programme or a higher-order schema for a prehensive movement such as reach and grasp a jar of coffee. This schema is assembled with other schemas to give rise to a 'component schema' like 'make coffee'. In turn, this higher schema interacts with others to finally generate a 'source-schema' like 'prepare breakfast'. The source-schemas are structures that control complex actions, not simple movements. The schemas (or elements of action) have been learned and stored (memorized) and are then activated by the action planning process.

Thus an action plan represents an ensemble of actions that converge to a single goal. The function of action planning is to select and activate the cooperative schemas, which implies inhibiting the non-desirable or competing ones, associating them with the proper external and internal cues, organizing them into an adequate sequence, and checking goal achievement (Jeannerod 1997). The mechanism through which planning operates and directly controls routine actions has been called 'contention scheduling' by Norman and Shallice (1980). A novel, partially learned, or non-routine action requires an additional conscious mechanism for drawing up a new plan or modifying an ongoing plan [called the supervisory intentional system by Shallice and colleagues or the 'goal-based search process' by Duncan (1986)]. Thus intentional (willed) action may need redirection of attention, working memory, and decision-making, among other cognitive processes for specifying the goal of the action and developing an action plan. We define intention (prior intention) as the conscious desire to perform a movement or an action without direct relation to the movement or action itself (consciousness = awareness). Intention in a broader sense implies free will as well as the recognition of the action as being self-generated. However, we realize that the feeling of intentionality, which is the basis of the sense of agency/ownership, in a freely voluntary act may arise during the performance of a repetitive (or) act and not prior to it (so-called intention in action), meaning that it is implicitly and not consciously generated. Motor intention is another term that deserves to be clarified; it is used as synonymous with motor preparation, neurophysiologically referring to the act of establishing a state of readiness to make a specific movement, and neuropsychologically encompassing any of the cognitive processes preceding the initiation of movements (e.g. motor planning). Finally, attention to action is defined as the specific attention towards the goal of the primary motor task 'to think about the next move', which may transiently improve movement, whereas motor attention (motor awareness) refers to attentional processes (preparation or redirection) that are associated with a particular arm/hand movement (Rushworth *et al.* 1997).

When an action is initiated, it needs to be properly controlled and efficiently executed. Control and maintenance of the planning action requires it to adapt to the behavioural context and external constraints, which is achieved through on-line evaluation of goal outcome against goal representation (comparison process). Output from this comparator will maintain or stop the ongoing action and may influence the on-line modification of the action according to situational demands. Where the goal is distant, the action can be sustained by the motivating properties of the goal representation. Outcome is associated with a change in motivational state and with the emotional and hedonistic response. Goal achievement and its subsequent reward produce positive responses, whereas failure to achieve the envisaged goal causes a negative response, leading to the implementation of an alternative plan (Brown and Pluck 2000).

The impact of this framework on observations on patients with higher-order motor disorders and activation studies performed in normal subjects are beginning to bridge the gap with the experimental data. They also demonstrate that special test procedures are becoming increasingly valuable as they complement the analysis of clinical observations. This approach strengthens hypothesis-driven research and the application of investigational tools suitable for tracing the modular functional organization of the cortex and of its connectivity maps. Here, new methods such as diffusion-weighted tensor imaging and new algorithms testing functional connectivity of functional imaging data hold the promise of disentangling the effects of cortical dysfunctions and those implied by the disturbed connectivity.

How the new concepts evolving from the field of motor cognition will be nested in traditional clinical thinking and terminology will emerge from novel data and better understanding of the pathophysiology. We hope that those aspects discussed in this book will assist along that way.

References

Brown R, Pluck G (2001). Negative symptoms: the 'pathology' of motivation and goal-directed behaviour. *Trends Neurosci*, **23**, 412–17.

Dickinson A, Balleine B (1994). Motivational control of goal-directed action. *Anim Learn Behav*, **22**, 1–18.

Duncan J (1986). Disorganization of behaviour after frontal lobe damage. *Cogn Neuropsychol*, **3**, 271–90.

Ettlinger G (1969). Apraxia considered as a disorder of movements that are language-dependent: evidence from cases of brain bisection. *Cortex*, **5**, 285–9.

Hoff B, Arbib MA (1993). Models of trajectory formation and temporal interaction of reach and grasp. *J Mot Behav*, **25**, 175–92.

Jackson HJ (1931). *Selected Writings*. London: Hodder and Stoughton.

Jeannerod M (1997). *The Cognitive Neuroscience of Action*. Cambridge, MA: Blackwell.

Keele SW (1968). Movement control in skilled motor performance. *Psychol Bull*, **70**, 387–404.

Norman DA, Shallice T (1980). Attention to action: willed and automatic control of behaviour. In: GE Schwartz, D Schapiro, (ed.) *Conciousness and Self-regulation*. New York: Plenum Press.

Rushworth MF, Nixon PD, Penowden S, Wade DT, Passingham PE (1997). The left parietal cortex and motor attention. *Neuropsychologia*, **35**, 1261–73.

Walshe FMR (1948). *Clinical Studies in Neurology*. Edinburgh: Livingston.

Part 1

Neuroanatomical, neurobiological, and cognitive basis

Chapter 1

Functional neuroanatomy of the human motor cortex*

Stefan Geyer and Karl Zilles

The cortical motor system in macaques: lessons from nonhuman primates

Until the second half of the twentieth century, it was widely believed that the cortical motor system of humans could be subdivided into three regions: the primary motor cortex (area 4) in the caudal wall and on the vertex of the precentral gyrus, the supplementary motor area further rostral on the mesial aspect of the frontal lobe (mesial part of area 6), and the premotor cortex on the lateral aspect of the frontal lobe (lateral part of area 6).

In recent years, however, data from nonhuman primates (especially macaques) have shown that this relatively simple view is no longer adequate: instead of three functional entities, the macaque cortical motor system is a mosaic of areas, each processing different aspects of motor behavior. Most investigators agree that the primary motor cortex [area 4 or F1 according to Matelli *et al.* (1985, 1991)] is homogeneous, whereas the rostrally adjoining area 6 can be subdivided into three groups of areas: (i) the supplementary motor areas SMA proper (area F3) and pre-SMA (area F6) on the mesial cortical surface; (ii) the dorsal premotor cortex (PMd) (areas F2 and F7) on the dorsolateral convexity; (iii) the ventral premotor cortex (PMv) (areas F4 and F5) on the ventrolateral convexity (Fig. 1.1(a) and (b)). Similarly to the motor cortex, a mosaic of areas has been defined in the posterior parietal cortex (including the intraparietal sulcus), each analyzing particular aspects of sensory (somatosensory, visual, and auditory) information. Posterior parietal and frontal motor areas are connected in a specific way. These connections provide the anatomical framework for several parietofrontal circuits that operate in parallel and perform sensory–motor transformations as a prerequisite for goal-directed actions (see Chapter 2, this volume).

In addition, motor responses have also been found in the cingulate cortex of the macaque. Unfortunately, the interpretation of the data is more complicated, since

* We would like to dedicate this chapter to Professor Massimo Matelli (Institute of Human Physiology, University of Parma, Italy), an enthusiastic researcher and our close friend, who died unexpectedly in August 2003 at the age of only 51. We grieve for his tragic loss, but we know that his eminent contributions to neuroscience will live on.

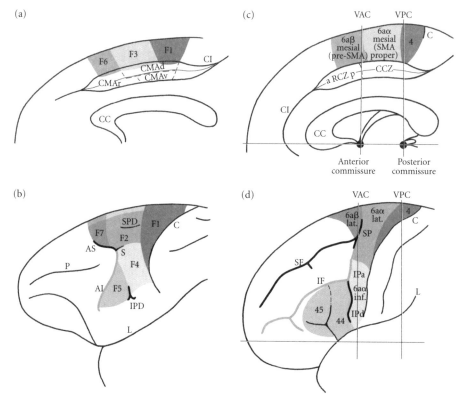

Fig. 1.1 (a) Mesial and (b) lateral views of the macaque frontal lobe with areas F1–F7 according to Matelli *et al.* (1985, 1991). Cingulate areas CMAr, CMAd, and CMAv according to Dum and Strick (1991) are depicted in an unfolded view of the cingulate sulcus (CI; thin line indicates fundus). (c) Mesial and (d) lateral views of the human frontal lobe with areas 4, $6a\alpha$, $6a\beta$, 44 and 45 according to Brodmann (1909) and Vogt and Vogt (1919). Cingulate areas RCZa, RCZp, and CCZ according to Picard and Strick (1996) are depicted in an unfolded view of the cingulate sulcus (CI; thin line indicates fundus). Identical gray values in (a) and (c) and in (b) and (d) indicate areas and sulci considered to be homologous. See text for further details. AI, inferior arcuate sulcus; AS, superior arcuate sulcus; C, central sulcus; CC, corpus callosum; IF, inferior frontal sulcus; IPa, inferior precentral sulcus (ascending branch); IPd, inferior precentral sulcus (descending branch); IPD, inferior precentral dimple; L, lateral sulcus; P, principal sulcus; S, spur of the arcuate sulcus; SF, superior frontal sulcus; SP, superior precentral sulcus; SPD, superior precentral dimple; VAC, vertical anterior commissure line; VPC, vertical posterior commissure line.

different investigators have proposed different anatomical maps of the dorsal and ventral banks of the cingulate sulcus and the free surface of the cingulate gyrus. Most widespread are the parcellations of Matelli and coworkers and Strick and coworkers. Matelli *et al.* (1991) followed Brodmann's (1909) nomenclature and subdivided the cingulate region into a rostral part (areas 24a, 24b, 24c, and 24d) and a caudal part (areas 23, 29, and 30). A different parcellation was proposed by Dum and Strick (1991): a rostral cingulate motor area (CMAr) in the anterior part of the cingulate sulcus (both the dorsal and the ventral bank) and two areas in the posterior part (ventral cingulate motor area (CMAv) in the ventral bank, and dorsal cingulate motor area (CMAd) in the dorsal bank) (Fig. 1.1(a)).

It is beyond the scope of this chapter to describe the cortical motor system of the macaque in more detail. Further information can be found in the literature (Picard and Strick 1996; Wise *et al.* 1997; Caminiti *et al.* 1998; Geyer *et al.* 2000; Rizzolatti *et al.* 1998; Rizzolatti and Luppino 2001; Dum and Strick 2002). However, recent data have shown that striking similarities exist between the cortical motor systems of humans and macaques.

The cortical motor system in humans

The data on the motor system in macaques are based on the elementary biological concept that differences in structure (in this context the microstructure of the motor cortex) should reflect differences in function and vice versa. In other words, neurons with similar electrophysiological properties should lie within the same cortical area and, conversely, the properties of neurons should change across a microstructural border. This can be tested in a straightforward and **direct** way in laboratory animals, since upon completion of the electrophysiological experiments the brain can be sectioned, sections can be cell-stained, and penetration sites can be **directly** correlated with the microstructural (e.g. cytoarchitectonic) pattern. This correlation has been demonstrated many times in macaques and has led to a very elaborate view of the cortical motor system in this primate species.

In humans, however, ethical constraints limit the use of invasive approaches, functional *in vivo* and anatomical post-mortem studies cannot be performed in the same brain, and many anatomical techniques yield poorer results than in the macaque (e.g. immunohistochemistry) or cannot be used at all (e.g. *in vivo* tract tracing techniques). Hence, our knowledge of the structure and function of the human cortical motor system is not as detailed as that for the macaque. We start with some remarks on the structure of the primary motor cortex, followed by the cingulate cortex, the supplementary motor areas SMA proper and the pre-SMA, and the dorsal and ventral premotor cortex (Fig. 1.1(c) and (d)). At the end of the chapter, some functional data are presented and interpreted in the light of this structural framework.

Structural organization

Primary motor cortex

Low cell density, poor lamination, absence of layer IV, a diffuse border between layer VI and the underlying white matter, and giant pyramidal or Betz cells in layer V differentiate the primary motor cortex (Brodmann's area 4) from the caudally adjoining primary somatosensory cortex. The border lies in the depth of the central sulcus close to its fundus. Scattered or absent giant pyramidal cells and large, elongated, and densely packed pyramids in lower layer III characterize the nonprimary motor cortex (Brodmann's area 6) that abuts rostrally on area 4. Dorsomedially (towards the midline), the rostral border of area 4 lies on the exposed cortical surface, i.e. on the vertex of the precentral gyrus. Ventrolaterally (towards the Sylvian fissure), the rostral border of area 4 recedes in a caudal direction and in most cases disappears in the central sulcus. The mesial part of area 4 occupies parts of the paracentral lobule (Fig. 1.1(c) and (d)).

Recently, human area 4 has been subdivided into a caudal (area '4 posterior' or 4p) and a rostral (area '4 anterior' or 4a) region based on differences in cytoarchitecture and neurotransmitter binding sites (Geyer *et al.* 1996). These two areas are two parallel bands within area 4 running mediolaterally from the midline to the Sylvian fissure. Clear-cut changes in the laminar binding patterns, especially of muscarinic cholinergic (revealed with [^{3}H]oxotremorine-M) (Fig. 1.2) and serotoninergic (revealed with [^{3}H]ketanserine) binding sites, closely match the cytoarchitectonic borders. Lower-layer III pyramidal cells are small and loosely aggregated in area 4p (Fig. 1.3(a)), larger and more densely packed in area 4a (Fig. 1.3(b)), and even larger, more elongated, and sometimes arranged in several parallel rows like a phalanx in area 6 (Fig. 1.3(c)). There are no obvious differences in size, packing density, or arrangement of giant pyramidal (or Betz) cells between areas 4a and 4p. Mean regional binding densities of many

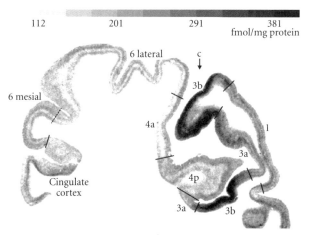

Fig. 1.2 Contrast-enhanced autoradiograph of [^{3}H]oxotremorine-M binding sites (predominantly muscarinic cholinergic M$_2$ receptors) in a coronal section of the human frontal lobe. Light gray shading indicates low densities of binding sites, and dark gray indicates high densities (cf bar). B_{max} values are in fmol/mg protein. Changes in the laminar binding pattern that coincide with cytoarchitectonically defined borders in an adjacent cell-stained section are marked. Average binding densities are high in somatosensory areas 3a, 3b, and 1, but are considerably lower in primary motor areas 4a and 4p, mesial and lateral areas 6, and the cingulate cortex. C, central sulcus.

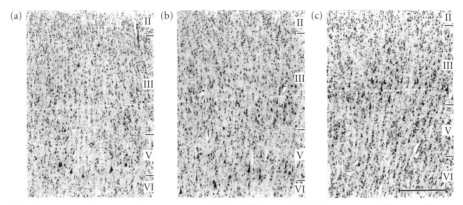

Fig. 1.3 Cytoarchitecture of human areas (a) 4p, (b) 4a, and (c) 6. Lower layer III pyramids are small and loosely aggregated in area 4p, larger and more densely packed in area 4a, and even larger, more elongated, and sometimes arranged in several parallel rows in area 6. Roman numerals indicate cortical layers. Scale bar, 500 μm (a–c). Reproduced from Geyer *et al.* (2000). *Anat Embryol*, **202**, 443–74.

neurotransmitter binding sites tend to be higher in area 4p than in area 4a (Geyer *et al.* 1997) (Fig. 1.2). Hence there is a clear neurochemical dichotomy within area 4. At the moment, it is unclear whether there is any homology between human areas 4a and 4p and areas M1r and M1c that have been described in the primary motor cortex of the New World owl monkey (*Aotus trivirgatus*) (Stepniewska *et al.* 1993). The topography of areas 4a/4p and M1r/M1c is comparable in both species, but the cytoarchitectonic criteria differ between *Homo sapiens* and *A.trivirgatus*.

Cingulate cortex

The human cingulate cortex can be subdivided into an anterior and a posterior part (Brodmann 1909; Vogt *et al.* 1995) with the border approximately in the middle between the VAC line (which traverses the anterior commissure vertically to a line passing through the anterior and posterior commissure) and the VPC line (which traverses the posterior commissure vertically to a line passing through both commissures).

The anterior cingulate cortex is agranular (i.e. layer IV is missing) and in most instances has a prominent layer V. Areas 25 and 33 are the two least differentiated areas in the anterior cingulate region. They are poorly laminated and abut the corpus callosum. Area 24 consists of three bands running parallel to each other in a rostrocaudal direction: area 24a is adjacent to area 33 and partially within the callosal sulcus, area 24b is on the free surface of the cingulate gyrus, and area 24c is in the ventral bank of the cingulate sulcus. Each region is cytoarchitectonically nonuniform in its rostrocaudal extent: the rostral part (areas 24a, 24b, and 24c) differs from the caudal part (areas 24a', 24b', and 24'c). Caudal to area 24c' lies area 24c'g, or the primitive gigantopyramidal area of Braak (1976), with very large pyramidal neurons in layer V. Area 32 is a cingulofrontal transition area between area 24 and the frontal cortex. It lies predominantly in the dorsal bank of the cingulate sulcus. Area 32 is also nonuniform in its rostrocaudal extent: area 32 (rostrally) differs from area 32' (caudally) (Vogt *et al.* 1995).

The posterior cingulate cortex is granular (i.e. layer IV is present). Areas 29 and 30 are the two least differentiated areas in the posterior cingulate region. They abut the corpus callosum. Area 23 consists of three parallel bands with rostrocaudal orientation: area 23a is adjacent to area 30 and partially within the callosal sulcus, area 23b is on the free surface of the cingulate gyrus, and area 23c is in the depth of the cingulate sulcus. Each region is cytoarchitectonically uniform in its rostrocaudal extent. Area 31 is a cinguloparietal transition area between area 23 and the parietal cortex (Vogt *et al.* 1995).

Based on investigations in macaques (see above) and functional imaging data in humans, Strick and coworkers subdivided the human cingulate sulcus region into two zones, separated by the VAC line: the caudal cingulate zone (CCZ) and the rostral cingulate zone (RCZ). The CCZ overlaps with the posterior part of area 24 and probably also with the gigantopyramidal field of Braak (1976). It may be homologous with the CMAd in the macaque. The RCZ overlaps with the anterior part of area 24 and with area 32. A detailed analysis of functional imaging studies (see below) has shown that the RCZ may split up into an anterior (RCZa) and a posterior (RCZp) part. Several lines of evidence indicate that the RCZa and RCZp may be homologous with the macaque CMAr and CMAv, respectively (Picard and Strick 1996) (Fig. 1.1A and C).

Supplementary motor areas SMA proper and pre-SMA

Two microanatomical studies (Zilles *et al.* 1995, 1996) found striking architectonic similarities between macaque areas F3 and F6 and the mesial parts of areas $6a\alpha$ and $6a\beta$ [nomenclature of Vogt and Vogt (1919)], respectively, in humans. Area F3 and mesial area $6a\alpha$ are characterized by increased cell density in lower layer III and layer V. Both areas are well demarcated on the cortical convexity from area F2 and from lateral area $6a\alpha$, respectively. Area F6 and mesial area $6a\beta$ are clearly laminated and are characterized by a prominent layer V, well separated from layers III and VI. Both areas are well demarcated on the cortical convexity from area F7 and from lateral area $6a\beta$, respectively. Additional similarities have been found on a neurochemical basis (Zilles *et al.* 1995, 1996; Geyer *et al.* 1998). For example, [^{3}H]kainate binding sites are mainly concentrated in the deep layers in both areas in macaques and humans. The mean binding density in area F3/mesial $6a\alpha$ is higher than in the primary motor cortex and lateral premotor cortex in both species. [^{3}H]Oxotremorine-M binding sites show a superficial and deep cortical band of maximal binding densities in both species (Fig. 1.2). Mean binding densities increase in a caudorostral direction from the primary motor cortex to area F6 in macaques and to mesial area $6a\beta$ in humans. The authors concluded that human mesial areas $6a\alpha$ and $6a\beta$ are possibly homologous to macaque areas F3 (SMA proper) and F6 (pre-SMA), respectively.

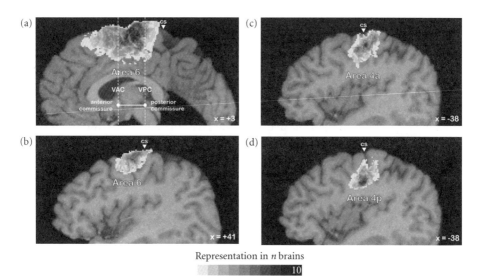

Representation in *n* brains

10

Fig. 1.4 Cytoarchitectonic population map of (a, b) area 6, (c) area 4a, and (d) area 4p. The sagittal section in (a) intersects the right hemisphere 3 mm lateral ($x = +3$), and the section in (b) intersects it 41 mm lateral ($x = +41$) to the midline. The sections in (c) and (d) intersect the left hemisphere 38 mm lateral ($x = -38$) to the midline. In each voxel, the number of brains ($1 \leqslant n \leqslant 10$) that have a representation of area 6, 4a, or 4p is coded as a gray value (cf bar). The reference brain from the computerized atlas is shown in the background. CS, central sulcus; VAC, vertical anterior commissure line; VPC, vertical posterior commissure line. (a) and (b) are reproduced from Geyer (2004) *The Microstructural Border Between the Motor and the Cognitive Domain in the Human Cerebral Cortex*, Berlin: Springer.

In humans, the border between the primary motor cortex and mesial area 6aα (possibly SMA proper) coincides approximately with the VPC line (Figs 1.1c and 1.4A). The border between mesial area 6aα and mesial area 6aβ (possibly pre-SMA) coincides approximately with the VAC line (Zilles *et al.* 1996) (Fig. 1.1c). The coincidence of the borders between the primary motor cortex–SMA proper and the SMA proper–pre-SMA with the VPC and VAC lines, respectively, has also been shown by Vorobiev *et al.* (1998). In the latter study, human SMA proper was further subdivided into a caudal (SMAc) and a rostral (SMAr) part. Whether these two subdivisions reflect somatotopy or a more fine-grained functional differentiation within human SMA proper is an unresolved issue.

In a recent study (Grosbras *et al.* 1999), a macroanatomical landmark was sought that indicates the position of the human supplementary eye field (SEF). Such a landmark was indeed found, namely the upper part of the paracentral sulcus on the mesial cortical surface 'in the anterior part of the region usually described as the SMA-proper, and posterior to the VAC line, which is usually considered as being the posterior limit of the pre-SMA' (Grosbras *et al.* 1999, p. 710). This position of the human SEF on the mesial cortical surface is at clear variance with the position of its monkey homolog on the dorsolateral convexity in area F7. There is no straightforward explanation of this discrepancy. Some clues can be gained from a functional imaging study (Fink *et al.* 1997) that detected an arm and a leg representation in the human mesial nonprimary motor cortex that was confined to the **caudal** half of the region between the VPC and VAC line (which could correspond to area SMAc). Macaque area F3 (SMA proper) contains a representation of the arm, leg, and face (the latter was not tested in the imaging study). Hence it is possible that only area SMAc is the human homolog of macaque area F3 and area SMAr contains the human SEF.

Dorsal and ventral premotor cortex

On the cortical convexity of the macaque, a conspicuous macroanatomical landmark, the arcuate sulcus, separates the agranular frontal from the granular prefrontal cortex, and the border between them looks like a horizontally reflected 'C'. A comparable sulcus does not exist in the human brain, but the spatial distribution of the agranular cortex (Brodmann's areas 4 and 6 plus dysgranular area 44; see below for further discussion of areas 44 and 45) is strikingly similar. Its rostral border also bears some resemblance to a horizontally reflected 'C'. In both species the prefrontal cortex extends caudally in the middle of the dorsolateral convexity as if pushing back the agranular cortex, and conversely recedes rostrally in the dorsomedial and ventrolateral parts of the convexity.

In a recent review article (Rizzolatti *et al.* 1998) an attempt was made to define homologies between the human and macaque dorsal and ventral premotor cortex (Fig. 1.1(b) and (d)). Macaque data were compared with data obtained in humans from cytoarchitectonic parcellation (Vogt and Vogt 1919), motor representations as determined with electrical stimulation (Förster 1936), sulcal ontogeny (Turner 1948), and the putative location of the human frontal eye field in functional imaging studies (Paus 1996). It was proposed that the superior frontal and superior precentral sulcus (black in Fig. 1.1(d)) represent the human homolog of the macaque superior arcuate sulcus (black in Fig. 1.1(b)). Accordingly, the lateral part of area 6aα of Vogt and Vogt (1919) might correspond to macaque area F2, and the lateral part of area 6aβ of Vogt and Vogt (1919) to macaque area F7. The inferior frontal sulcus and the ascending branch of the inferior precentral sulcus (gray in Fig. 1.1(d)) correspond to the macaque inferior arcuate sulcus (gray in Fig. 1.1(b)). The descending branch of the inferior precentral sulcus (black in Fig. 1.1(d)) corresponds to the inferior precentral dimple of the macaque monkey (black in Fig. 1.1(b)). Accordingly, the inferior part of area 6aα of Vogt and Vogt (1919) might be homologous to macaque area F4, and Brodmann's (1909) area 44 might be homologous to macaque area F5. An open issue is the macaque homolog of Brodmann's (1909) area 45. Walker (1940) described an area 45 in the macaque that lies in the rostral bank of the inferior arcuate sulcus and is related to eye movements (Suzuki and Azuma 1983; Bruce *et al.* 1985). However, human area 45 (together with area 44) is the cytoarchitectonic correlate of Broca's speech region (Aboitiz and Garcia 1997), and there are no reports in the literature that human area 45 might be involved in eye movements. On the other hand, when one considers the cytoarchitectonic similarities between human areas 44 and 45 and their similar myelinization onset (Vogt and Vogt 1919), an alternative interpretation would be that human areas 44 and 45 evolved from one and the same area in the macaque, namely area F5.

Functional organization

Functional evidence from neuroimaging studies indicates that human motor cortices share several general organizational principles with macaque motor cortices. One important aspect is that multiple representations of body movements also exist in humans. For example, simple flexion and extension movements of the fingers induce several independent activations in the primary motor cortex, SMA proper, dorsal premotor cortex, frontal operculum, and cingulate motor areas (Fink *et al.* 1997). In addition to the primary (SI) and secondary (SII) somatosensory area, two further arm and finger representations are located in the superior and inferior parietal lobule (Fink *et al.* 1997). These observations fit well with the notion that multiple motor representations are also present in the posterior parietal cortex. Further evidence in favor of the existence of multiple representations of body movements in the frontal and posterior parietal cortex comes from studies of motor imagery (Jeannerod and Decety 1995). A recent study in which motor imagery was compared with motor execution suggests that largely overlapping neural substrates in the frontal and parietal cortex are involved in both aspects of motor control (Gerardin *et al.* 2000). However, whether or not the primary motor cortex is involved in motor imagery remains an open question. Several studies have shown that the precentral gyrus is activated during imagined movements, although to a lesser extent than during executed movements (Porro *et al.* 1996; Roth *et al.* 1996; Gerardin *et al.* 2000). Since these studies related the activations to macroanatomical landmarks (precentral gyrus) and not to cytoarchitectonically defined areas (4 and 6), one can only speculate to what extent the primary motor cortex (area 4) has been involved. The activation of a network of parietal and frontal areas during motor imagery and execution suggests that the parietofrontal circuits described above in macaques are also key functional units in humans. Their topography in humans has recently been elucidated in greater detail using experimental paradigms comparable to those applied in macaques. Binkofski *et al.* (1999) and Grefkes *et al.* (2002) asked subjects to manipulate complex three-dimensional objects with their hands and fingers. They found activations in the intraparietal sulcus [possibly the human homolog of the macaque anterior intraparietal (AIP) area] and the ventral premotor cortex [possibly area 44 due to an activation of the human homolog of the 'AIP–area F5 bank' circuit in the macaque (Rizzolatti *et al.* 1998; Rizzolatti and Luppino 2001)]. Bremmer *et al.* (2001) stimulated subjects with moving visual, tactile, and auditory stimuli and found activations in all three modalities in the depth of the intraparietal sulcus [possibly the human homolog of the macaque ventral intraparietal (VIP) area] and the ventral premotor cortex [possibly the human homolog of macaque area F4 due to an activation of the 'VIP–area F4' circuit (Rizzolatti *et al.* 1998; Rizzolatti and Luppino 2001)].

Primary motor cortex

The most complete functional map of the human precentral cortex was provided by Penfield between the 1930s and 1950s (Penfield and Boldrey 1937; Penfield and Rasmussen 1952). The results, summarized in the famous cartoon of the 'motor homunculus', showed a somatotopic organization of the human precentral region that replicated Woolsey's findings in nonhuman primates. In this respect it is important to note that surface electrical stimulation reveals mainly the cortical origin of the descending corticospinal tract which, in the macaque, is not restricted to the primary motor cortex (area 4). Since the free surface of the precentral gyrus in humans is mostly occupied by area 6 (especially close to the Sylvian fissure), it is reasonable to conclude that a significant part of Penfield's homunculus belongs to the nonprimary motor cortex (area 6). The somatotopic organization of the precentral region has been replicated in recent years using functional imaging techniques [e.g. positron emission tomography (PET)] in single subjects (Fink *et al.* 1997). Despite an orderly representation of the body's periphery in each subject, topographical variability between individuals has been detected (Fink *et al.* 1997). Nonetheless, a macroanatomical landmark which reliably indicates the hand area has been identified, namely a knob-like structure in the precentral gyrus which looks like an Ω in the axial plane and corresponds to the 'middle knee' of the central sulcus in post-mortem brains (Yousry *et al.* 1997). As in macaques, somatotopic organization should not be over-interpreted. Also in humans, individual finger movements are represented as multiple and spatially overlapping activation sites (Sanes *et al.* 1995).

Activations in the caudal bank of the precentral gyrus (or rostral bank of the central sulcus) have been detected in many PET and functional magnetic resonance (fMRI) studies with a wide variety of different motor paradigms. Since the foci of activation were related to macroanatomical landmarks and not to cytoarchitectonic areas, none of these studies could exclude extension of the foci (at least to some extent) into the rostrally adjoining area 6. The technique of microstructural–functional correlation with a computerized brain atlas overcomes this dilemma. In such a study, PET foci were correlated with the population maps of primary motor areas 4a and 4p (Geyer *et al.* 1996) (Fig. 1.4(c) and (d)). Roughness discrimination of two cylinders with different microprofiles with the right thumb and index finger activated area 4p significantly more than did a control condition of self-generated movements without object interaction. This could mean that a voluntary motor act that is closely modulated by somatosensory feedback (i.e. scanning the surface texture of an object) leads to a stronger activation of area 4p.

Cingulate cortex

Since population maps of the cingulate areas are not yet available, the functional interpretation of this cortical sector is based on the 'traditional' approach, namely comparing functional activation sites with macroanatomical landmarks of the cortex. However, the variability in the geometry of the cingulate sulcus (Ono *et al.* 1990) introduces a great degree of uncertainty and makes this approach problematic.

In a review of the neuroimaging literature, Picard and Strick (1996) studied the sites of activation depending on the complexity of movements. They classified as 'simple' those tasks that required the most basic spatial or temporal organization of movements or tasks that were over-learned and highly practiced (e.g. moving a joystick in a fixed direction upon an auditory trigger signal). 'Complex' tasks were characterized by additional motor or cognitive demands such as the selection of a motor response (e.g. moving a joystick in a random self-selected direction upon an auditory signal) or the acquisition of a conditional association that determined the motor response. 'Complex' tasks activated the cingulate sulcus rostral to the VAC line (in the RCZ); 'simple' tasks activated the cingulate sulcus caudal to the VAC line (in the CCZ). Simple tasks also activated the SMA proper (see below). However, the activations in the CCZ were consistently separable from those in the SMA proper, indicating that the CCZ and SMA proper are functionally independent entities despite their proximity and their tendency to be coactivated during manual tasks (Koski and Paus 2000). It will be a challenge for the future to elucidate differences in function between the CCZ and the SMA proper.

What are the differences between the RCZa and the RCZp ? Picard and Strick (2001) proposed that the RCZa is involved in conflict monitoring and the RCZp in selection for action. In a series of imaging studies which carefully controlled conflict monitoring (Botvinick *et al.* 1999; Barch *et al.* 2000; Carter *et al.* 2000; Casey *et al.* 2000), the activation sites were located 24 ± 7 mm (mean $\pm$ standard deviation) rostral to the VAC line (in the RCZa). In contrast, when a similar paradigm was used which did not specifically dissociate conflict monitoring from response selection (MacDonald *et al.* 2000), the response-related activation was located 1 mm rostral to the VAC line (in the RCZp). Another imaging study analyzed different versions of Go/NoGo and Stop tasks (Rubia *et al.* 2001). In the Go/NoGo task, a motor response had to be selectively executed or inhibited depending on whether a Go or a NoGo cue was presented. One cue was always associated with a single response that the subject had to select according to a fixed rule without any interfering conflict situation. The anterior cingulate activation was located at $x = -3$, $y = 0$, $z = 42$ (in the RCZp). In the Stop task, the motor response to a Go signal had to be retracted if a Stop signal was presented unexpectedly shortly (250 ms) after the Go signal. This situation introduced a significant conflict by requiring the subject to discard a selected motor plan suddenly and switch over to a new one. The anterior cingulate activation was located at $x = 6$, $y = 25$, $z = 37$ (in the RCZa).

Supplementary motor areas SMA proper and pre-SMA

The role of the SMA in human motor control has been a matter of debate for a long time. Electrical stimulation studies, clinical observations of deficits caused by vascular lesions or surgical ablations, recordings of cortical potentials during the execution of motor tasks, and early functional imaging studies provided conflicting results (reviewed by Freund 1996). On the one hand, the high electrical excitability of the SMA and its activation during the execution of simple aimless movements were taken as evidence for an 'executive' role in motor control. On the other hand, the presence of global akinesia without paralysis and the observation of slow negative potential shifts long before the execution of a motor task, as well as its activation when subjects were requested to rehearse mentally a series of digit movements, led to the concept of a 'supramotor' function of the SMA. However, none of these studies attempted a precise identification of the anatomical location of the stimulated or damaged cortex, mainly because of the assumption that the SMA is a structurally and functionally homogeneous entity. The discovery, in nonhuman primates, that the mesial agranular cortex consists of two different structural and functional areas led to a re-evaluation of these apparently conflicting data in humans.

As mentioned above, there is increasing evidence that the human SMA also consists of two areas, namely SMA proper and pre-SMA. The border between the two areas does not coincide with any macroanatomical landmark; it is thought to correspond approximately to the VAC line. Owing to similarities in cytoarchitecture and neurochemistry, human SMA proper and pre-SMA are possibly homologous to macaque areas F3 and F6, respectively (Zilles *et al.* 1995, 1996).

When functional data are correlated with the location of the VAC line, it becomes obvious that the two areas caudal and rostral to it are also functionally distinct and their roles in motor control are in many ways comparable to those proposed for macaque areas F3 (SMA proper) and F6 (pre-SMA). At first glance, the results of electrical stimulation studies of the human mesial frontal cortex do not seem to be consistent with this proposed homology, since stimulating cortical sites on either side of the VAC line evokes relatively low-threshold movements. However, by using chronically implanted subdural electrodes and better stimulation parameters, a somatotopic organization of the SMA proper comparable with that in the macaque could also be demonstrated in humans (Fried 1996; Lim *et al.* 1996). In contrast, electrically stimulating a region spanning about 3 cm rostral to the region where movements can be elicited more frequently (i.e. SMA proper) induced 'negative symptoms' (e.g. transient speech arrest) or more complex effects [e.g. an 'urge' to move or the feeling of an impending movement (Fried 1996)]. These results led Fried to consider the caudal 'motor excitable' zone to be comparable to macaque SMA proper (area F3) and the rostral 'negative motor' or 'motor arrest' zone to be comparable to macaque pre-SMA (area F6).

The classification of motor tasks as 'simple' and 'complex', as introduced by Picard and Strick (1996), also showed a functional segregation along the mesial wall of the frontal lobe: 'simple' tasks typically activated regions caudal to the VAC line (in the

SMA proper); 'complex' tasks activated regions rostral to it (in the pre-SMA). Functional imaging data on motor sequence learning corroborate this dichotomy: SMA proper plays a role in the execution of well-learned 'automatic' motor sequences, whereas pre-SMA is crucial for learning new 'unfamiliar' sequences. Sergent *et al.* (1992) demonstrated this difference in a study of professional pianists. SMA proper was activated when the subjects were playing scales (i.e. a highly automatic movement sequence), whereas pre-SMA became active when the same subjects were playing an unfamiliar piece of music. When subjects were studied at different stages of learning motor sequences, the activation shifted from pre-SMA to SMA proper as the task became more routine and eventually 'automatic' (Grafton *et al.* 1992a; Seitz and Roland 1992; Jenkins *et al.* 1994; Schlaug *et al.* 1994). Finally, Hikosaka *et al.* (1999) showed that pre-SMA was involved in learning motor sequences by trial and error, while executing a learned sequence activated SMA proper.

More recent imaging studies have shifted the view of pre-SMA 'function' towards a more cognitive or 'supramotor' role. In a study by Sakai *et al.* (1999) subjects had to learn visuomotor association sequences. Activation in the pre-SMA was found to be related to establishing or retrieving visuomotor associations but not to motor sequence learning *per se*. The contribution of the pre-SMA to sensory–motor associations seems to be independent of the input modality [pre-SMA activity was also found in associations based on auditory stimuli (Kurata *et al.* 2000)] and of the output modality [similar regions in the pre-SMA were activated in conditional hand motor tasks (Kurata *et al.* 2000) and oculomotor tasks (Merriam *et al.* 2001)]. Other recent studies have shown that pre-SMA is more closely involved in maintaining or processing relevant sensory information than in response selection or production. For example, sustained activity in the pre-SMA was found during both spatial and visual working memory delays (Petit *et al.* 1998) and during attention shifts between object features (color or shape) in a card-sorting task (Nagahama *et al.* 1999). Finally, when subjects directed their attention to object-specific, spatial, or temporal properties of the same sensory event (i.e. moving objects), pre-SMA was activated independently of the attended stimulus property, but most intensively during object-related attention (Schubotz and von Cramon 2001).

Dorsal premotor cortex

Electrophysiological, clinical, and neuroimaging evidence suggests that there are also similarities between the human dorsal premotor cortex and its putative homolog in the monkey. Stimulation studies in humans showed that the electrically excitable cortex extends approximately 2–3 cm rostral from the central sulcus into the caudal sector of area 6 (Uematsu *et al.* 1992). This finding suggests that, as in the monkey, the caudal region of the human dorsal premotor cortex is the origin of a corticospinal projection. Lesion studies indicated an involvement of the dorsal premotor cortex in both preparation and execution of motor acts and motor learning. Unilateral damage of the dorsal premotor cortex caused an inability to perform arm or leg movements requiring temporal coordination of proximal muscles, whereas the performance of distal skilled movements was normal (Freund and Hummelsheim 1985). PET data provided further evidence for an involvement of the dorsal premotor cortex in the motor control of arm and leg movements (Fink *et al.* 1997). With regard to arm movements, Colebatch *et al.* (1991) found activation in the superior frontal gyrus associated with the execution of simple movements involving proximal and distal joints. The mean regional cerebral blood flow increase associated with shoulder movements was significantly higher than with distal movements, suggesting that in this region, as in the monkey dorsal premotor cortex, there is an extensive representation of proximal movements. In agreement with these data, several neuroimaging studies showed that this cortical region was activated during tasks involving proximal and/or distal arm movements (Deiber *et al.* 1991; Grafton *et al.* 1992b, 1996b; Seitz *et al.* 1997). As in the monkey, the human dorsal premotor cortex is involved in movement preparation (Kawashima *et al.* 1994) and in movement selection according to arbitrary rules. Learning complicated finger-movement sequences (Seitz and Roland 1992), acquiring new key-press sequences on the basis of trial and error (Jenkins *et al.* 1994), and performing reaching and pointing movements according to the internal representation of targets (Kawashima *et al.* 1995) all activated the superior frontal gyrus. Involvement of the human dorsal premotor cortex in movement selection according to arbitrary rules was demonstrated in two PET studies: activations were detected as subjects learned to make an association between a cue and the direction of a movement (Deiber *et al.* 1997) and when subjects had to select more complex movements (e.g. a precision or power grip) based on arbitrary cues (Grafton *et al.* 1998). This particular role of the dorsal premotor cortex had already been identified in an earlier clinical study showing that patients with lesions of this cortical region (but **not** with parietal or primary motor cortex lesions) failed to associate hand movements with arbitrary sensory cues (Halsband and Freund 1990).

A possible rostrocaudal segregation within the dorsal premotor cortex was proposed by Picard and Strick (2001). A meta-analysis of functional imaging studies revealed that movement-related processes (e.g. movement preparation or execution) activated more caudal portions of the dorsal premotor cortex, whereas higher-order processes (e.g. conditional visuomotor associations, response selection or motor imagery) engaged more rostral portions. According to Picard and Strick (2001), these differences are comparable to those that generate the subdivision of the SMA into SMA proper and pre-SMA. By analogy with this nomenclature, the caudal sector of the dorsal premotor cortex (PMd) was termed 'PMd proper' and the rostral sector 'pre-PMd'. Whether 'PMd proper' and 'pre-PMd' are homologous to macaque areas F2 and F7, respectively, remains to be determined in the future.

Ventral premotor cortex

Early neuroimaging studies of subjects performing grasp movements failed to identify activation in the ventral premotor cortex. First evidence for a hand representation in this region came from studies of learning finger-movement sequences (Seitz and Roland 1992), mental imagery of grasping (Decety *et al.* 1994; Grafton *et al.* 1996a), and preparation of finger movements on the basis of copied movements (Krams *et al.* 1998). More direct evidence that the ventral premotor cortex contains a hand representation came from a recent study by Binkofski *et al.* (1999). These authors found that manipulating complex objects with the hand and fingers resulted in an activation of presumed area 44, while covertly naming the manipulated objects led to an additional activation more rostrally in presumed area 45. One interesting result of this study was that manipulating objects also activated parietal areas, one of them lying in the anterior part of the lateral bank of the intraparietal sulcus (possibly the human homolog of macaque area AIP). It seems that the parietofrontal circuits for object manipulation described in macaques also exist in humans, and the data of Binkofski *et al.* (1999) suggest an activation of the human homolog of the 'AIP–area F5 bank' circuit.

Several lines of evidence indicate that the action recognition or 'mirror' system described in macaque area F5 (Gallese *et al.* 1996) also exists in the human brain. First, experiments with transcranial magnetic stimulation showed that observation of hand actions facilitated the motor cortex of the observer, as shown by an increase in the amplitude of the motor-evoked potential in those hand muscles of the observer that matched the activated muscles in the observed hand (Fadiga *et al.* 1995; Strafella and Paus 2000). Secondly, electrophysiological studies demonstrated that observing hand actions desynchronized the motor cortex of the observer similarly to actually performing hand actions (Hari *et al.* 1998; Cochin *et al.* 1999). Finally, brain imaging studies showed that observing hand actions activated a region in the ventral premotor cortex that seemed to correspond to Broca's area (Grafton *et al.* 1996a; Rizzolatti *et al.* 1996; Decety *et al.* 1997; Grezes *et al.* 1998; Iacoboni *et al.* 1999). The possibility that the activation of Broca's area during action observation was due to internal verbalization rather than a mirror mechanism was ruled out in a recent study by Buccino *et al.* (2001).

These data suggest that in Broca's area (as in macaque area F5) there is both a mouth representation and a representation of hand movements. At first glance, it may seem surprising that, despite its pre-eminent role as a motor speech area in humans, this cortical region is also important for internally representing and thus 'understanding' motor events. It is beyond the scope of this chapter to discuss theories of human language evolution that are based on this 'mirror neuron' concept. However, the results support the theory that parts of Broca's area in humans and area F5 in macaques may be homologous entities.

Concluding remarks

More than a century after John Hughlings Jackson's revolutionary proposal that the human motor system is organized in a hierarchical manner with the motor cortex representing the top level, the data accumulated ever since still support this view.

Although our knowledge of the detailed organization of the cortical motor system is still fragmentary, the definition of parietofrontal circuits suggests that, in addition to a hierarchical component, there are also parallel pathways that influence cortical motor control.

In recent years, numerous studies have provided new insights into the structural and functional organization of human motor cortices. The data presented here indicate that striking similarities have been found between humans and nonhuman primates. However, in contrast with laboratory animals, ethical constraints greatly limit the use of invasive techniques in humans. This is why our knowledge of the human motor cortices is still fragmentary compared with that of macaques. Thus it will be important to establish a more detailed architectonic map of the human motor cortices in the future, especially since new neurochemical techniques are now available. Given the important role played by monkey studies in the investigation of human cortical functions, a special effort should be made to extend our knowledge of the comparative anatomy of the motor cortices of humans and nonhuman primates.

Acknowledgements

We would like to thank Ursula Blohm and Nadine Ivens for excellent histological and autoradiographic processing of human brain tissue, and Christine Opfermann-Rüngeler for expert help with the artwork. This work was supported by grants from the Human Brain Project (jointly funded by the National Institute of Mental Health, National Institute of Neurological Disorders and Stroke, National Institute on Drug Abuse, and National Cancer Institute) and the European Commission under the Fifth Framework Programme (Contract QLG3-CT-2002–00746).

References

Aboitiz F, Garcia VR (1997). The evolutionary origin of the language areas in the human brain. A neuroanatomical perspective. *Brain Res Rev*, **25**, 381–96.

Barch DM, Braver TS, Sabb FW, Noll DC (2000). Anterior cingulate and the monitoring of response conflict: evidence from an fMRI study of overt verb generation. *J Cogn Neurosci*, **12**, 298–309.

Binkofski F, Buccino G, Posse S, Seitz RJ, Rizzolatti G, Freund HJ (1999). A fronto-parietal circuit for object manipulation in man: evidence from an fMRI-study. *Eur J Neurosci*, **11**, 3276–86.

Botvinick M, Nystrom LE, Fissell K, Carter CS, Cohen JD (1999). Conflict monitoring versus selection-for-action in anterior cingulate cortex. *Nature*, **402**, 179–81.

Braak H (1976). A primitive gigantopyramidal field buried in the depth of the cingulate sulcus of the human brain. *Brain Res*, **109**, 219–33.

Bremmer F, Schlack A, Shah NJ, Zafiris O, Kubischik M, Hoffmann K, *et al.* (2001). Polymodal motion processing in posterior parietal and premotor cortex: a human fMRI study strongly implies equivalencies between humans and monkeys. *Neuron*, **29**, 287–96.

Brodmann K (1909). *Vergleichende Lokalisationslehre der Großhirnrinde*. Barth, Leipzig.

Bruce CJ, Goldberg ME, Bushnell MC, Stanton GB (1985). Primate frontal eye fields. II. Physiological and anatomical correlates of electrically evoked eye movements. *J Neurophysiol*, **54**, 714–34.

Buccino G, Binkofski F, Fink GR, Fadiga L, Fogani L, Gallese V, *et al.* (2001). Action observation activates premotor and parietal areas in a somatotopic manner: an fMRI study. *Eur J Neurosci*, **13**, 400–4.

Caminiti R, Ferraina S, Battaglia-Mayer A (1998). Visuomotor transformations: early cortical mechanisms of reaching. *Curr Opin Neurobiol*, **8**, 753–61.

Carter CS, Macdonald AM, Botvinick M, Ross LL, Stenger VA, Noll D, *et al.* (2000). Parsing executive processes: strategic vs. evaluative functions of the anterior cingulate cortex. *Proc Natl Acad Sci USA*, **97**, 1944–8.

Casey BJ, Thomas KM, Welsh TF, Badgaiyan RD, Eccard CH, Jennings JR, *et al.* (2000). Dissociation of response conflict, attentional selection, and expectancy with functional magnetic resonance imaging. *Proc Natl Acad Sci USA*, **97**, 8728–33.

Cochin S, Barthelemy C, Roux S, Martineau J (1999). Observation and execution of movement: similarities demonstrated by quantified electroencephalography. *Eur J Neurosci*, **11**, 1839–42.

Colebatch JG, Deiber MP, Passingham RE, Friston KJ, Frackowiak RSJ (1991). Regional cerebral blood flow during voluntary arm and hand movements in human subjects. *J Neurophysiol*, **65**, 1392–401.

Decety J, Perani D, Jeannerod M, Bettinardi V, Tadary B, Woods R, *et al.* (1994). Mapping motor representations with positron emission tomography. *Nature*, **371**, 600–2.

Decety J, Grezes J, Costes N, Perani D, Jeannerod M, Procyk E, *et al.* (1997). Brain activity during observation of actions—influence of action content and subject's strategy. *Brain*, **120**, 1763–77.

Deiber MP, Passingham RE, Colebatch JG, Friston KJ, Nixon PD, Frackowiak RSJ (1991). Cortical areas and the selection of movement: a study with positron emission tomography. *Exp Brain Res*, **84**, 393–402.

Deiber MP, Wise SP, Honda M, Catalan MJ, Grafman J, Hallett M (1997). Frontal and parietal networks for conditional motor learning: a positron emission tomography study. *J Neurophysiol*, **78**, 977–91.

Dum RP, Strick PL (1991). The origin of corticospinal projections from the premotor areas in the frontal lobe. *J Neurosci*, **11**, 667–89.

Dum RP, Strick PL (2002). Motor areas in the frontal lobe of the primate. *Physiol Behav*, **77**, 677–82.

Fadiga L, Fogassi L, Pavesi G, Rizzolatti G (1995). Motor facilitation during action observation: a magnetic stimulation study. *J Neurophysiol*, **73**, 2608–11.

Fink GR, Frackowiak RSJ, Pietrzyk U, Passingham RE (1997). Multiple nonprimary motor areas in the human cortex. *J Neurophysiol*, **77**, 2164–74.

Förster O (1936). Motorische Felder und Bahnen. In O Bumke, O Förster, (ed.) *Handbuch der Neurologie*, pp. 1–357. Berlin: Springer.

Freund HJ (1996). Historical overview. In HO Lüders, (ed.) *Supplementary Sensorimotor Area*, pp. 17–27. Philadelphia, PA: Lippincott–Raven.

Freund HJ, Hummelsheim H (1985). Lesions of premotor cortex in man. *Brain*, **108**, 697–733.

Fried I (1996). Electrical stimulation of the supplementary sensorimotor area. In HO Lüders, (ed.) *Supplementary Sensorimotor Area*, pp. 177–85. Philadelphia, PA: Lippincott–Raven.

Gallese V, Fadiga L, Fogassi L, Rizzolatti G (1996). Action recognition in the premotor cortex. *Brain*, **119**, 593–609.

Gerardin E, Sirigu A, Lehericy S, Poline JB, Gaymard B, Marsault C, *et al.* (2000). Partially overlapping neural networks for real and imagined hand movements. *Cereb Cortex*, **10**, 1093–1104.

Geyer S (2004). *The Microstructural Border Between the Motor and the Cognitive Domain in the Human Cerebral Cortex.* Advances in Anatomy Embryology and Cell Biology, vol. 174. Berlin: Springer.

Geyer S, Ledberg A, Schleicher A, Kinomura S, Schormann T, Burgel U, *et al.* (1996). Two different areas within the primary motor cortex of man. *Nature*, **382**, 805–7.

Geyer S, Schleicher A, Zilles K (1997). The somatosensory cortex of human: cytoarchitecture and regional distributions of receptor-binding sites. *Neuroimage*, **6**, 27–45.

Geyer S, Matelli M, Luppino G, Schleicher A, Jansen Y, Palomero-Gallagher N, *et al.* (1998). Receptor autoradiographic mapping of the mesial motor and premotor cortex of the macaque monkey. *J Comp Neurol*, **397**, 231–50.

Geyer S, Matelli M, Luppino G, Zilles K (2000). Functional neuroanatomy of the primate isocortical motor system. *Anat Embryol (Berl)*, **202**, 443–74.

Grafton ST, Mazziotta JC, Presty S, Friston KJ, Frackowiak RSJ, Phelps ME (1992a). Functional anatomy of human procedural learning determined with regional cerebral blood flow and PET. *J Neurosci*, **12**, 2542–8.

Grafton ST, Mazziotta JC, Woods RP, Phelps ME (1992b). Human functional anatomy of visually guided finger movements. *Brain*, **115**, 565–87.

Grafton ST, Arbib MA, Fadiga L, Rizzolatti G (1996a). Localization of grasp representations in humans by positron emission tomography. 2. Observation compared with imagination. *Exp Brain Res*, **112**, 103–11.

Grafton ST, Fagg AH, Woods RP, Arbib MA (1996b). Functional anatomy of pointing and grasping in humans. *Cereb Cortex*, **6**, 226–37.

Grafton ST, Fagg AH, Arbib MA (1998). Dorsal premotor cortex and conditional movement selection: a PET functional mapping study. *J Neurophysiol*, **79**, 1092–7.

Grefkes C, Weiss PH, Zilles K, Fink GR (2002). Crossmodal processing of object features in human anterior intraparietal cortex: an fMRI study implies equivalencies between humans and monkeys. *Neuron*, **35**, 173–84.

Grezes J, Costes N, Decety J (1998). Top down effect of strategy on the perception of human biological motion: a PET investigation. *Cogn Neuropsychol*, **15**, 553–82.

Grosbras MH, Lobel E, van de Moortele PF, Le Bihan D, Berthoz A (1999). An anatomical landmark for the supplementary eye fields in human revealed with functional magnetic resonance imaging. *Cereb Cortex*, **9**, 705–11.

Halsband U, Freund HJ (1990). Premotor cortex and conditional motor learning in man. *Brain*, **113**, 207–22.

Hari R, Forss N, Avikainen S, Kirveskari E, Salenius S, Rizzolatti G (1998). Activation of human primary motor cortex during action observation: a neuromagnetic study. *Proc Natl Acad Sci USA*, **95**, 15061–5.

Hikosaka O, Sakai K, Nakahara H, *et al.* (1999). Neural mechanisms for learning of sequential procedures. In MS Gazzaniga, (ed.) *The New Cognitive Neurosciences*, pp. 553–72. Cambridge, MA: MIT Press.

Iacoboni M, Woods RP, Brass M, Bekkering H, Mazziotta JC, Rizzolatti G (1999). Cortical mechanisms of human imitation. *Science*, **286**, 2526–8.

Jeannerod M, Decety J (1995). Mental motor imagery: a window into the representational stages of action. *Curr Opin Neurobiol*, **5**, 727–32.

Jenkins IH, Brooks DJ, Nixon PD, Frackowiak RSJ, Passingham RE (1994). Motor sequence learning: a study with positron emission tomography. *J Neurosci*, **14**, 3775–90.

Kawashima R, Roland PE, O'Sullivan BT (1994). Fields in human motor areas involved in preparation for reaching, actual reaching, and visuomotor learning: a positron emission tomography study. *J Neurosci*, **14**, 3462–74.

Kawashima R, Roland PE, O'Sullivan BT (1995). Functional anatomy of reaching and visuomotor learning: a positron emission tomography study. *Cereb Cortex*, **5**, 111–22.

Koski L, Paus T (2000). Functional connectivity of the anterior cingulate cortex within the human frontal lobe: a brain-mapping meta-analysis. *Exp Brain Res*, **133**, 55–65.

Krams M, Rushworth MFS, Deiber MP, Frackowiak RSJ, Passingham RE (1998). The preparation, execution and suppression of copied movements in the human brain. *Exp Brain Res*, **120**, 386–98.

Kurata K, Tsuji T, Naraki S, Seino M, Abe Y (2000). Activation of the dorsal premotor cortex and pre-supplementary motor area of humans during an auditory conditional motor task. *J Neurophysiol*, **84**, 1667–72.

Lim SH, Dinner DS, Lüders HO (1996). Cortical stimulation of the supplementary sensorimotor area. In HO Lüders, (ed.) *Supplementary Sensorimotor Area*, pp. 187–97. Philadelphia, PA: Lippincott–Raven.

MacDonald AW, Cohen JD, Stenger VA, Carter CS (2000). Dissociating the role of the dorsolateral prefrontal and anterior cingulate cortex in cognitive control. *Science*, **288**, 1835–8.

Matelli M, Luppino G, Rizzolatti G (1985). Patterns of cytochrome oxidase activity in the frontal agranular cortex of the macaque monkey. *Behavioural Brain Res*, **18**, 125–36.

Matelli M, Luppino G, Rizzolatti G (1991). Architecture of superior and mesial area 6 and the adjacent cingulate cortex in the macaque monkey. *J Comp Neurol*, **311**, 445–62.

Merriam EP, Colby CL, Thulborn KR, Luna B, Olson CR, Sweeney JA (2001). Stimulus-response incompatibility activates cortex proximate to three eye fields. *Neuroimage*, **13**, 794–800.

Nagahama Y, Okada T, Katsumi Y, Hayashi T, Yamauchi H, Sawamoto N, *et al*. (1999). Transient neural activity in the medial superior frontal gyrus and precuneus time locked with attention shift between object features. *Neuroimage*, **10**, 193–9.

Ono M, Kubik S, Abernathey CD (1990). *Atlas of the Cerebral Sulci*. Stuttgart: Thieme.

Paus T (1996). Location and function of the human frontal eye-field: a selective review. *Neuropsychologia*, **34**, 475–83.

Penfield W, Boldrey E (1937). Somatic motor and sensory representation in the cerebral cortex of man as studied by electrical stimulation. *Brain*, **60**, 389–443.

Penfield W, Rasmussen T (1952). *The Cerebral Cortex of Man*. New York: Macmillan.

Petit L, Courtney SM, Ungerleider LG, Haxby JV (1998). Sustained activity in the medial wall during working memory delays. *J Neurosci*, **18**, 9429–37.

Picard N, Strick PL (1996). Motor areas of the medial wall: a review of their location and functional activation. *Cereb Cortex*, **6**, 342–53.

Picard N, Strick PL (2001). Imaging the premotor areas. *Curr Opin Neurobiol*, **11**, 663–72.

Porro CA, Francescato MP, Cettolo V, Diamond ME, Baraldi P, Zuiani C, *et al*. (1996). Primary motor and sensory cortex activation during motor performance and motor imagery: a functional magnetic resonance imaging study. *J Neurosci*, **16**, 7688–98.

Rizzolatti G, Luppino G (2001). The cortical motor system. *Neuron*, **31**, 889–901.

Rizzolatti G, Fadiga L, Matelli M, Bettinardi V, Paulesu E, Perani D, *et al*. (1996). Localization of grasp representations in humans by PET: 1. Observation versus execution. *Exp Brain Res*, **111**, 246–52.

Rizzolatti G, Luppino G, Matelli M (1998). The organization of the cortical motor system: new concepts. *Electroencephalogr Clin Neurophysiol*, **106**, 283–96.

Roth M, Decety J, Raybaudi M, Massarelli R, Delon-Martin C, Segebarth C, *et al*. (1996). Possible involvement of primary motor cortex in mentally simulated movement: a functional magnetic resonance imaging study. *Neuroreport*, **7**, 1280–4.

Rubia K, Russell T, Overmeyer S, Brammer MJ, Bullmore EJ, Sharma T, *et al*. (2001). Mapping motor inhibition: conjunctive brain activations across different versions of go/no-go and stop tasks. *Neuroimage*, **13**, 250–61.

Sakai K, Hikosaka O, Miyauchi S, Sasaki Y, Fujimaki N, Pütz B (1999). Presupplementary motor area activation during sequence learning reflects visuo-motor association. *J Neurosci*, **19** (RC 1), 1–6.

Sanes JN, Donoghue JP, Thangaraj V, Edelman RR, Warach S (1995). Shared neural substrates controlling hand movements in human motor cortex. *Science*, **268**, 1775–7.

Schlaug G, Knorr U, Seitz RJ (1994). Inter-subject variability of cerebral activations in acquiring a motor skill: a study with positron emission tomography. *Exp Brain Res*, **98**, 523–34.

Schubotz RI, von Cramon DY (2001). Functional organization of the lateral premotor cortex: fMRI reveals different regions activated by anticipation of object properties, location and speed. *Cogn Brain Res*, **11**, 97–112.

Seitz RJ, Roland PE (1992). Learning of sequential finger movements in man: a combined kinematic and positron emission tomography (PET) study. *Eur J Neurosci*, **4**, 154–65.

Seitz RJ, Canavan AGM, Yágüez L, Herzog H, Tellmann L, Knorr U, *et al.* (1997). Representations of graphomotor trajectories in the human parietal cortex: evidence for controlled processing and automatic performance. *Eur J Neurosci*, **9**, 378–89.

Sergent J, Zuck E, Terriah S, MacDonald B (1992). Distributed neural network underlying musical sight-reading and keyboard performance. *Science*, **257**, 106–9.

Stepniewska I, Preuss TM, Kaas JH (1993). Architectonics, somatotopic organization, and ipsilateral cortical connections of the primary motor area (M1) of owl monkeys. *J Comp Neurol*, **330**, 238–71.

Strafella AP, Paus T (2000). Modulation of cortical excitability during action observation: a transcranial magnetic stimulation study. *Neuroreport*, **11**, 2289–92.

Suzuki H, Azuma M (1983). Topographic studies on visual neurons in the dorsolateral prefrontal cortex of the monkey. *Exp Brain Res*, **53**, 47–58.

Turner OA (1948). Growth and development of the cerebral cortical pattern in man. *Arch Neurol Psychiatr*, **59**, 1–12.

Uematsu S, Lesser R, Fisher RS, Gordon B, Hara K, Krauss GL, *et al.* (1992). Motor and sensory cortex in humans: topography studied with chronic subdural stimulation. *Neurosurgery*, **31**, 59–71.

Vogt BA, Nimchinsky EA, Vogt LJ, Hof PR (1995). Human cingulate cortex: surface features, flat maps, and cytoarchitecture. *J Comp Neurol*, **359**, 490–506.

Vogt C, Vogt O (1919). Allgemeinere Ergebnisse unserer Hirnforschung. *J Psychol Neurol*, **25**, 279–461.

Vorobiev V, Govoni P, Rizzolatti G, Matelli M, Luppino G (1998). Parcellation of human mesial area 6: cytoarchitectonic evidence for three separate areas. *Eur J Neurosci*, **10**, 2199–203.

Walker AE (1940). A cytoarchitectural study of the prefrontal area of the macaque monkey. *J Comp Neurol*, **73**, 59–86.

Wise SP, Boussaoud D, Johnson PB, Caminiti R (1997). Premotor and parietal cortex: corticocortical connectivity and combinatorial computations. *Annual Review of Neuroscience*, **20**, 25–42.

Yousry TA, Schmid UD, Alkadhi H, Schmidt D, Peraud A, Buettner A, *et al.* (1997). Localization of the motor hand area to a knob on the precentral gyrus. A new landmark. *Brain*, **120**, 141–57.

Zilles K, Schlaug G, Matelli M, Luppino G, Schleicher A, Qu M, *et al.* (1995). Mapping of human and macaque sensorimotor areas by integrating architectonic, transmitter receptor, MRI and PET data. *J Anat*, **187**, 515–37.

Zilles K, Schlaug G, Geyer S, Luppino G, Matelli M, Qu M, *et al.* (1996). Anatomy and transmitter receptors of the supplementary motor areas in the human and nonhuman primate brain. In HO Lüders, (ed.) *Supplementary Sensorimotor Area*, pp. 29–43. Philadelphia, PA: Lippincott–Raven.

Chapter 2

Parallel parietofrontal circuits for sensorimotor transformations

Roberto Caminiti, Stefano Ferraina, Alexandra Battaglia-Mayer, Massimo Mascaro, and Yves Burnod

Introduction

The functional interplay between the parietal and frontal lobes is based on the operations of a continuum of cortical areas linked by reciprocal association connections. Some of these are very selective, since they connect a specific parietal area to only one specific frontal area. However, these private routes are rather uncommon. In most instances, any given parietal area is linked to a discrete number of frontal areas, and vice versa, in a gradient-like fashion. This pattern of connectivity sculpts different corticocortical systems in the brain with varying degrees of parallelism (Caminiti *et al.* 1996; Johnson *et al.* 1996; Wise *et al.* 1997; Matelli *et al.* 1998; Marconi *et al.* 2001; Tanné-Gariépy *et al.* 2002). The question arises as to whether each of these pathways subserves a specific coordinate transformation, or whether they are part of a distributed network that operates on a multiplicity of signals, selectively combined on the basis of task demands. The analysis of coordinated eye–hand movements, such as those underlying reaching, offers an excellent model for answering this question.

In this chapter we will discuss recent developments concerning the relationships between the organization of the parietofrontal pathways and information processing at the early stages of the composition of motor plans for eye and hand movement in the parietal cortex. We will then illustrate the outcome of different network models of parietal operations concerning early combinatorial mechanisms, and conclude with a hypothesis on optic ataxia, a common higher-order visuomotor disorder that follows parietal lesions.

Coding eye and hand movement within the distributed parietofrontal network

Cortical coding of eye and hand movements occurs within a distributed network including different parietal and frontal areas, selectively linked by reciprocal association connections (Fig. 2.1; see also Chapter 4, this volume). The cortical areas of the parieto-occipital

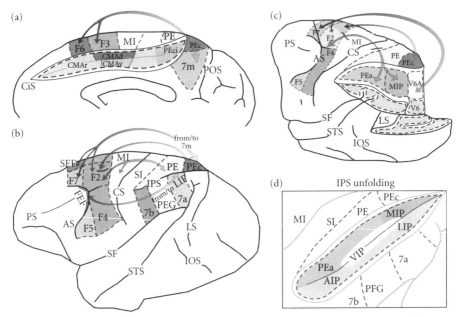

Fig. 2.1 Diagrams of monkey brain showing some of the corticocortical connections linking different parietal and the frontal areas, as discussed in the text. (a) Mesial view of the hemisphere with the cingulate sulcus opened (grey shading) to show the location of the cingulate motor areas (Picard and Strick, 1996). (b) Lateral view of the hemisphere. (c) Parts of the parietal and occipital lobe have been 'removed' (Galletti *et al.* 1996) to show the location of the areas buried in the medial bank of the intraparietal sulcus and in the rostral bank of the parieto-occipital sulcus. (d) Unfolding of the parietal region flanking the intraparietal sulcus to show the location of the areas buried in its medial and lateral banks (Caminiti *et al.* 1996). PS, AS, CS, IPS, SF, STS, LS, IOS, POS indicate the principal, arcuate, central, intraparietal, Sylvian, superior temporal, lateral, inferio-occipital, and parieto-occipital sulci, respectively.

junction, and those of the mesial wall of the parietal lobe, are believed to play a special role since they are the first recipient of visual input from the occipital lobe, and project to the premotor cortex and/or to other parietal areas which in turn project to the frontal lobe. Thus, these parietal regions can be regarded as an interface between vision and movement.

Anatomical layout

The parieto-occipital cortex consists mainly of the rostral bank of the parieto-occipital sulcus (Figs. 2.1(a)–(c)). This region, originally labeled area PO (Gattas *et al.* 1985), has been redefined by Colby *et al.* (1988), and more recently by Galletti *et al.* (1996). These last authors have identified a ventral visual area (V6) and a dorsomedial area (V6A) with more complex functional properties. Area V6A (Fig. 2.1(c)) receives visual inputs from different extrastriate areas such as V3/V3A, V5, and V6 (Shipp and Zeki

1995), and is connected to parietal areas V5A/MST, 7a, 7m, MIP and VIP (Matelli *et al.* 1998; Shipp *et al.* 1998; Marconi *et al.* 2001). Frontal projections of V6A (Fig. 2.1(c)) are addressed to the lateral part of the dorsocaudal premotor cortex (PMdc/F2) and to the dorsorostral premotor cortex (PMdr/F7) (Johnson *et al.* 1993, 1996; Tanné *et al.* 1995; Matelli *et al.* 1998; Shipp and Zeki 1998; Marconi *et al.* 2001; Tanné-Gariépy *et al.* 2002). These projections are reciprocal (Marconi *et al.* 2001).

Dorsally, the parieto-occipital cortex continues into area PEc (Figs. 2.1(a)–(c)), while in the medial wall of the hemisphere it merges into area 7m (Fig. 2.1(a)). Area PEc receives from a variety of visuomotor areas, mostly PEa, MIP, PEci (Marconi *et al.* 2001), and projects to the premotor cortex (PMdc/F2) in the precentral-dimple region (Figs. 2.1(b) and (c)) (Matelli *et al.* 1998; Marconi *et al.* 2001), which in turn is linked to the motor cortex.

Area 7m (Fig. 2.1(a)) is largely coextensive with area PGm (Pandya and Seltzer 1982), and has reciprocal corticocortical relationships with portions of V2, V6A, PEc, and LIP, the visual motion sensitive areas of the superior temporal sulcus MT/MST, area 7a, and MIP (Cavada and Goldman-Rakic 1989a,b). Area 7m is also connected to area 23c in the posterior part of the cingulate sulcus, and to area 24c (Petrides and Pandya 1984; Cavada and Goldman-Rakic 1989a,b). It remains to be determined whether these mesial projections are addressed to that part of cingulate cortex including the caudoventral (CMAv) and rostrocingulate (CMAr) motor areas (Dum and Strick 1991a,b; He *et al.* 1995; Picard and Strick 1996). Of interest to the subject of this review are the outputs that 7m (Cavada and Goldman-Rakic 1989a,b) addresses to MIP and, within the frontal lobe (Figs. 2.1(a) and (b)), to the reaching-related zone of PMdc/F2 (Johnson *et al.* 1993, 1996; Tanné *et al.* 1995; Matelli *et al.* 1998; Marconi *et al.* 2001; Tanné-Gariépy *et al.* 2002), to PMdr/F7 (Johnson *et al.* 1993, 1996; Tanné *et al.* 1995; Matelli *et al.* 1998; Marconi *et al.* 2001; Tanné-Gariépy *et al.* 2002), and to pre-SMA, SMA, and the supplementary eye fields (SEFs) Schlag and Schlag-Rey 1987). Reciprocal connections of 7m with the prefrontal cortex mostly concern the caudal part of the dorsal bank of the principal sulcus (Cavada and Goldman-Rakic 1989a,b).

Areas MIP (medial intraparietal) and PEa lie in the medial bank of the IPS (Fig. 2.1(c) and (d)). They both project to the post-arcuate zone of F2 (Johnson *et al.* 1996). Finally, area PE occupies the exposed rostral part of the posterior parietal cortex and projects directly to the primary motor cortex (Johnson *et al.* 1996).

There are at least three important features of the organization of parietofrontal connections that emerge from the scenario described above. First, all these connections are reciprocal, which suggests that, in the information-processing flow leading from vision to movement, recursive signaling could play a crucial role in the composition of motor commands. Secondly, in most instances each individual parietal area is linked not to a unique frontal area, but to a constellation of them, although with different strengths (Johnson *et al.* 1996; Matelli *et al.* 1998; Marconi *et al.* 2001; Tanné-Gariépy *et al.* 2002). Thirdly, a rich set of local connections links different cortical areas within the parietal and frontal lobes. Therefore the parietofrontal system can be regarded as a network of networks characterized by a gradient-like architecture, where local computations participate in shaping plans for movement.

Physiological properties

Area V6A contains a representation of both central and peripheral vision (Colby *et al.* 1988; Galletti *et al.* 1999; Battaglia-Mayer *et al.* 2000, 2001) characterized by a coarse topography of the visual field. Visual topography has not yet been found in PEc (Battaglia-Mayer *et al.* 2001; Squatrito *et al.* 2001; Raffi *et al.* 2002). In both V6A and PEc, visual neurons have rather large receptive fields, and are sensitive to the orientation and direction of motion of visual stimuli. In PEc, neural activity is also influenced by optic flow fields (Battaglia-Mayer *et al.* 2001; Raffi *et al.* 2002), with selectivity for the position of the focus of expansion relative to the fovea. This property could depend, at least in part, on inputs from MST (Marconi *et al.* 2001); in turn, PEc could be the source of optic flow information to the motor cortex (Merchant *et al.* 2001) via PMdc/F2 (Matelli *et al.* 1998; Marconi *et al.* 2001).

In most of the cells of V6A, visual activity is dependent on the angle of gaze, but in a minority it displays gaze-independent spatial tuning (Galletti *et al.* 1991, 1993). Neurons in V6A, PEc, and 7m are also tuned to the direction of reaching and to the position of the hand in space (Ferraina *et al.* 1997a,b; Johnson *et al.* 1997; Lacquaniti and Caminiti 1998; Battaglia-Mayer *et al.* 2000, 2001). Limb-movement-related activity in V6A has also been observed during simple stereotyped wrist movements (Galletti *et al.* 1997). The activity related to preparation for arm movements in V6A (Johnson *et al.* 1997; Lacquaniti and Caminiti 1998; Battaglia-Mayer *et al.* 2000, 2001; Fattori *et al.* 2001), PEc (Battaglia-Mayer *et al.* 2001), and 7m (Ferraina *et al.* 1997a,b) displays a differential light–dark sensitivity (Ferraina *et al.* 1997a,b; Battaglia-Mayer *et al.* 2000, 2001), suggesting a role in the visual control of hand movement trajectory and position in space. Finally, a significant relationship between cell activity and both eye position and movement direction has been described in V6A (Galletti *et al.* 1991; Nakamura *et al.* 1999; Battaglia-Mayer *et al.* 2000, 2001; Kutz *et al.* 2003), in 7m (Ferraina *et al.* 1997a,b), and in PEc (Battaglia-Mayer *et al.* 2001).

A general property of parieto-occipital neurons, i.e. the power to integrate different reaching-related variables, emerges from this brief overview. The way that individual parietal neurons combine retinal, eye, and hand signals is suggested by studies in which monkeys performed eye and hand movements to visual targets under a variety of task conditions requiring different types of eye–hand coordination (Ferraina *et al.* 1997a,b, 2001; Battaglia-Mayer *et al.* 2000, 2001). Three main results were described. First, neural activity is directionally tuned to different types of information, such as position and direction of motion of visual stimuli (see also Squatrito *et al.* 2001), eye position and movement direction, hand position and movement direction, preparation for hand movement, and signals about monitoring hand position and trajectory in the

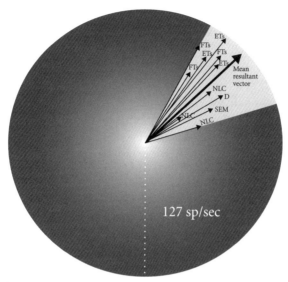

Fig. 2.2 The global tuning field of superior parietal neurons. Macaque monkeys made arm and/or eye movements in eight different directions, starting from a common central origin, in different task conditions. Preferred directions (PDs) (arrows) of cell activity were computed during different epochs of different tasks requiring various forms of eye–hand coordination:reaching to foveated targets (FTs), reaching to extrafoveal targets (ETs), saccadic eye movement (SEM), and instructed-delay reaching in normal light conditions (NLC) and darkness (D). The circle displays the orientation of the PDs of a typical parietal cell across different task epochs. The length of each vector is proportional to the firing rate of the cell in that particular task epoch. The radius of the circle is normalized to the vector of maximum length. The length of the mean resultant vector (thick arrow) is proportional to the amount of clustering of the PDs. In clockwise direction, PDs vectors refer to signals about eye-hand position, hand reaction time when reaching to foveated targets (FTs), hand movement to extrafoveal target (ETs), hand reaction-time to extrafoveal target (ETs), hand movement to foveated targets (FTs), hand position (ETs), eye reaction-time and eye movement-time in the delayed reaching under visual feed-back (NLC), preparation for hand movement to foveated targets in darkness (D), eye position (SEM), preparation for hand movement to foveated targets in light conditions (NLC). All PDs cluster withina a restricted part of the workspace, referred as Field of Global Tuning.

visual field, as well as information on the spatial correspondence between the positions of the hand and the eye on the target (see below). Secondly, for each individual cell, the preferred directions of eye and hand signals align with one another within a restricted part of space, referred to as the global tuning field (GTF) (Fig. 2.2) (Battaglia-Mayer *et al.* 2000, 2001). Within the GTF, different information is represented by different strengths. Therefore the GTF is an ideal combinatorial domain for eye–hand coordination during reaching, and a substrate for a spatial representation of reaching independent of eye and/or hand position. A third crucial feature of parieto-occipital neurons is the context dependency of neural activity. In fact, significant differences in cell activity can be observed (Battaglia-Mayer *et al.* 2000, 2001) when the same hand movement is made with or without prior information about its direction. Furthermore, neurons in areas 7m (Ferraina *et al.* 1997a), V6A (Battaglia-Mayer *et al.* 2000), and PEc (Battaglia-Mayer *et al.* 2001) discharge differently when hand movements are planned and performed in normal light conditions compared with total darkness, and when the hand, held immobile at different target locations, is visible or invisible. This modulation might reflect not only the visual monitoring of hand position and movement in the workspace, but also the structure of the visual space, which is known to exert a profound influence on the representation of endpoint position of reaches (Bridgeman *et al.* 1997). Finally, context dependency can also be found in the oculomotor domain (Battaglia-Mayer *et al.* 2000, 2001), since during saccades to a given spatial location, neurons in areas V6A, PEc and 7m fire differently depending on whether or not the target of the saccade is also the target for hand movement. This suggests that parietal activity that covaries with saccadic eye movements is often related not to the eye movement *per se*, but to the prediction of a future correspondence between eye and hand position on the target.

Functional architecture of the parietofrontal network for coordinated eye–hand movement

The functional architecture of the parietofrontal network can be established by comparing anatomical and physiological features across cortical areas. In this respect, the distribution of eye- and hand-related information in the tangential cortical domain is crucial to understanding early planning of reaching. Traditional topographic criteria are of little help in this analysis, as studies of receptive field properties indicate that there are no fine-grain maps of the somatosensory (Duffy and Burchfield 1971; Sakata *et al.* 1973; Mountcastle *et al.* 1975; Burbaud *et al.* 1991) or visual (Galletti *et al.* 1999; Battaglia-Mayer *et al.* 2000; Squatrito *et al.* 2001) peripheries in the superior parietal lobule or the dorsal premotor cortex (Wise *et al.* 1997; Fogassi *et al.* 1999). A recent microstimulation study of the dorsal premotor cortex (Raos *et al.* 2003) points to the same conclusion.

An interesting orderly arrangement emerges when the distribution of the dynamic (neural activity types) rather than the static (receptive field location) properties of cortical neurons is analysed in the tangential domain of the cortex. We have examined (Johnson *et al.* 1996; Battaglia-Mayer *et al.* 2001) the distribution of signals concerning the processes of target localization, hand and eye position, and movement direction in parietal areas V6A, PEc, PE, PEa and MIP, as well as in the dorsal premotor and primary motor cortices. It has been found that in the parietal cortex these activity types, which often coexist in individual neurons, are distributed in a trend-like fashion. While arm position signals have a rather uniform distribution, visually related information is represented mainly in the posterior part of the superior parietal lobule, and signals concerning planning and execution of eye and hand movement are represented at progressively more anterior locations. This trend is mirrored by a similar one in the frontal cortex, where visual, eye movement (see also Fujii *et al.* 2000) and eye position signals predominate in the rostral part of the dorsal premotor cortex (PMdr/F7), while information on plans for hand movement is more common in the caudal part of this area (PMdc/F2) and at its border with motor cortex. In M1, hand motor signals and hand-position-related activity dominate neural activity; however, the latter displays a rather uniform distribution across the frontal lobe. Furthermore, these studies (Johnson *et al.* 1996; Battaglia-Mayer *et al.* 2001) have shown that regions of similar activity types in the parietal and frontal cortex are linked by association connections.

This suggests that in the parietofrontal network eye- and hand-related information is probably shaped via recursive signaling operated by ipsilateral corticocortical connections. This interpretation is consistent with recent results (Chafee and Goldman-Rakic 2000) showing that association connections contribute to the shaping of common properties of prefrontal and inferior parietal neurons. Local parietal and frontal connections could be critical to this process. In fact, a network model (Mascaro *et al.* 2003) shows that the GTF of parietal neurons no longer emerges when inhibition is removed from a local recurrent network combining retinal, hand, and eye directional signals.

On the basis of these observations, one can speculate that, in the early planning of coordinated eye–hand movement, while the parietofrontal segment mainly performs coordinate transformation, the frontoparietal system, by providing information about the status of the motor system, is instrumental to predicting the sensory consequences of a motor plan, thus contributing to the composition of forward models of movement in the distributed network.

According to this view, reaching can no longer be regarded as the result of a top-down serial sequence of coordinate transformations, each performed by a given cortical area, but as the outcome of a recursive process where different signals are selected and combined in a context-dependent fashion throughout the network, and further developed locally via to intrinsic connections. This interpretation, derived from neuro-physiological studies, is in agreement with the results of psychophysical studies stressing the hybrid (Lacquaniti 1997), task-dependent (Carrozzo *et al.* 1999), and probabilistic (Vetter and Volpert 2000) nature of the reference frames for reaching, as well as the independent coexistence of multiple frames (Carrozzo *et al.* 2002). Taken together, these results do not support a recent proposal according to which different parietal areas encode reaching movements in a common eye-centered reference frame (reviewed by Cohen and Andersen 2002).

A parietofrontal network for oculomotor behavior

In the posterior parietal cortex of macaque monkeys (Figs. 2.1(b)–(d)), the intraparietal sulcus (Fig. 2.1(c)) separates the superior from the inferior parietal lobule. A number of studies (Brodmann 1909; Vogt and Vogt 1919; Von Bonin and Bailey 1947;

Pandya and Seltzer 1982) based on cytoarchitectonic criteria have provided conflicting parcellation schemes. Today, accepted subdivisions of parietal cortex are based on a combination of studies of cytoarchitecture, connectivity, and physiology. This is the case for the lateral intraparietal (LIP) and the medial intraparietal (MIP) areas, while the ventral intraparietal (VIP) area has been identified (Maunsell and Van Essen 1983) as the target of projections from the MT (middle temporal) area and V2. Other inferior parietal lobule areas, such as the anterior intraparietal (AIP) area, have been identified on the basis of physiological features (reviewed by Sakata *et al.* 1997).

Area LIP is one of the most intensely studied of the accepted subdivisions of the inferior parietal lobule. The functional role played by any area is largely dependent on its cortical connections. The input–output relationships of LIP (Petrides and Pandya 1984; Andersen *et al.* 1985; 1990; Ungerleider and Desimone 1986; Leichnetz and Goldberg 1988; Cavada and Goldman-Rakic 1989a,b; Blatt *et al.* 1990) suggest that this area is an important crossroads between extrastriate visual areas and the prefrontal cortex, and therefore is a crucial node of the neural network that processes visual information potentially related to the generation of eye movements.

Physiological approaches to cortical connectivity have recently benefited from the identification of the output neurons of LIP through antidromic stimulation from the target structures in behaving monkeys (Ferraina *et al.* 2002). The analysis of the dynamic properties of neurons with known axonal destination allows a detailed analysis of the nature of the efferent signals addressed, among the many represented in the input area, to different target regions. Since the frontal eye field (FEF) is a main target of the corticocortical output of LIP (Figs 2.1(b) and 2.3(a)), it was interesting to explore which aspects of the computations performed in LIP are addressed to FEF. In fact, saccadic signals could be computed *ex novo* in FEF, or be dependent on the association input from LIP (Schiller and Chou 1998), or even come from a different corticocortical source, such as that including temporal areas (Bullier *et al.* 1996). It has been found that LIP output neurons projecting to the FEF carry saccade-related signals (Ferraina *et al.* 2002; Figs. 2.3(b)–(c)). In LIP, neurons projecting to FEF are largely segregated from those antidromically activated from, and therefore projecting to, the superior colliculus (SC). This suggests that the efferent messages that LIP addresses to FEF and SC are, at least in part, different. A baffling result of this study was that the activity of two-thirds of LIP neurons projecting to FEF and of one-third of those projecting to the SC did not show any relationships with the oculomotor behavior tested. These projecting neurons could be active only while learning new tasks or be related to non-oculomotor functions. Both visual and visuomotor signals influenced cell activity in those neurons that displayed significant relations to oculomotor behavior. All information commonly observed in LIP seems to be conveyed to both the FEF and the SC (Fig. 2.3(c)). This includes a mixture of visual, delay, and saccade-related discharges, although with different proportions in the two output systems. Neurons projecting to FEF seem to be more concerned with visual events and less intimately related to saccade

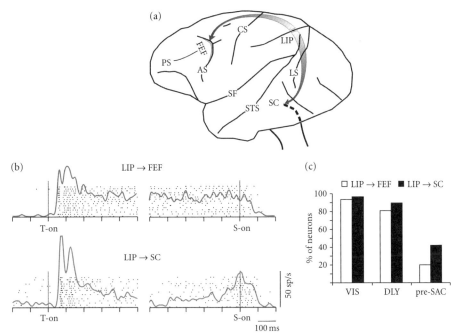

Fig. 2.3 In LIP, the output neurons projecting to the FEF and those projecting to the SC convey similar information, although presaccadic signals dominate in the corticocollicular pathway. (a) Brain diagram showing LIP projections to FEF and SC. Each neuron successfully isolated in LIP was tested for antidromic activation by stimulation in both FEF and SC. (b) Rasters and spike density functions illustrate neural activity aligned to the presentation of the visual-target stimulus (left) and to the onset of the saccade (right) of a delayed-saccade task. (c) Bar graph showing the percentage of neurons significantly modulated during different epochs of the delayed-saccade task. VIS, DLY and pre-SAC indicate the visual, delay and pre-saccadic activity modulation, respectively. White bars indicate LIP neurons antidromically activated from the FEF (LIP→FEF) and black bars show LIP neurons antidromically activated from the SC (LIP→SC).

generation, while those projecting to SC are more visuomotor in nature (Fig. 2.3(c)). The analysis of the delay and presaccadic period showed that their level of activity was lower in the memory trials than in the visual delay trials, and that this was true for both the neurons projecting to FEF and those projecting to the SC.

These results suggest that there is a gradual change of properties in the efferent messages addressed from LIP to different cortical and subcortical centers. Similar results have been obtained by all studies of LIP, FEF, and SC that have used comparable physiological procedures and the same behavioral tasks (Wurtz *et al.* 2001). The role of these structures is better illustrated by considering them as part of a distributed network rather than as separate nodes, each subserving a specific sensorimotor transformation.

Conceptual frameworks and models of parietofrontal operations

Neural networks can learn to perform sensorimotor transformations. Under these circumstances, network units can acquire tuning properties similar to those observed experimentally in the parietofrontal network (Zipser and Andersen 1988; Burnod *et al.* 1992; Bullock *et al.* 1993; Salinas and Abbot 1995; Pouget and Sejnowski 1997; Baraduc *et al.* 2001).

A major issue of modeling studies concerns the direct relationship between the distribution of local neuronal properties and the collective computation required to perform a sensorimotor task. Therefore, to provide general computational frameworks (Burnod *et al.* 1999), the properties of a cortical network must be related to its different sets of connections.

Three main computational principles emerge from the experimental results described above and from modeling studies on the parietofrontal system. First, each population of parietal neurons can learn an efficient sensorimotor transformation within a specific combinatorial domain, i.e. the space of all possible combinations of different signals from the sensory and motor modalities considered. Arm–hand movements in 3D space generate correlations between sensory signals that can be stored by neurons within a combinatorial domain. On experimental grounds, this learned computation is reflected by the positional and directional congruence between different sensory and motor signals observed at the neuronal level. Secondly, several bidirectional sensorimotor computations and different levels of sensorimotor predictions can coexist within the same cortical area, based on its pattern of corticocortical and subcortical relationships. Thirdly, neural computations for sensorimotor transformations are not segregated in different areas but are distributed over functional gradients across areas. Thus the parietofrontal system can be viewed as a network of neural populations (a network of networks) operating on the basis of its input–output relationships.

Sensorimotor transformation within specific combinatorial domains

A common property of parietal and frontal neurons is that they do not encode relevant parameters within pure sensory or motor 'reference frames' or in an abstract 'body-centered' representation, but rather combine them within 'hybrid' dimensions (Battaglia-Mayer *et al.* 2003). Each neuron is characterized by combinatorial tuning properties to different sensory and motor signals. These combinatorial properties are distributed over large gradients in both the parietal and frontal lobes. Neural net models have helped to understand how a population of cortical neurons with such hybrid properties can learn a visuomotor transformation in 3D space (Burnod *et al.* 1999; Baraduc *et al.* 2001; Pouget *et al.* 2002).

A second feature is that the tuning properties of neurons in different sensorimotor domains are not independent, but are closely related by congruent directional and positional properties in 3D space. For example, the sets of retinal, eye, and hand signals of parieto-occipital neurons are related to one another within the GTF (Battaglia-Mayer *et al.* 2000, 2001). These correlations may also arise naturally in the external world from signals generated by stereotypical forms of behavior.

The neural net approach suggests that the combinatorial properties of neurons emerge from network connectivity, while the congruency of directional and positional properties reflects the results of learning. Learning is due to coactivation on single neurons of different inputs, such as a motor command and its sensory consequences. Arm–hand movement produces powerful coactivation in sets of neurons that combine motor command signals with proprioceptive and visual (gaze and retinal) information. Computational studies show that, after learning, such neuronal populations can transform a visually derived input on target position into a motor command that aligns the hand on the target. Such a neuronal population becomes a 'matching unit' which implements specific visuomotor tranformations (Burnod *et al.* 1999). In general, signals come from peripheral sensory organs and muscles which are linked to different body segments, and their correlations can be learned only if neurons receive a third input concerning the postural relations between body segments; indeed, most parietal neurons are modulated by arm configuration and/or gaze position signals.

Neural network simulations show that such matching units can learn efficient transformations (Baraduc *et al.* 2001; Baraduc and Guigon 2002). This is not a trivial problem, since the control of movement in 3D space is shared by populations of broadly tuned neurons which code a distributed command of the muscles acting on several joints. Signaling hand position is based on a distributed information on muscle lengths and joint angles operated by monotonically tuned neurons; finally, representation of target location in 3D space is distributed over populations of neurons which code the stimulus position on the retina and the eye position in the orbit. It can be shown that an appropriate motor command is learned by a population of neurons in an unsupervised fashion through repeated action–perception cycles, simply by changing their synaptic weights on the arm-related proprioceptive information. After learning, this matching unit can transform distributed, visually derived information into a distributed motor command, with four remarkable features.

1 At both single unit and population level, the network properties resemble those of parietal and frontal areas.

2 The required transformation is performed accurately over a large part of the movement space, although few positions are actually learned;

3 The distribution of errors in the workspace is similar to that observed in psychophysical experiments.

4 When unexpected discrepancies occur among spatial modalities (such as an optical distortion), the same adaptive mechanism restores the correct perceptual-to-motor alignment.

Network models show that the distribution of preferred attributes within a population of neurons tuned to a given variable is crucial for generating the correct collective behavior of the population. For example, in the case of cosine tuning of cell activity related to movement direction, the distribution of preferred attributes has to be regular, and in the case of broad non-cosine tuning, it has to be uniform (Baraduc and Guigon 2001).

Several matching operations related to different sensorimotor situations (Burnod *et al.* 1999) can be learned in the same combinatorial domain. Examples refer to different situations, such as when the image of the hand is in the fovea, when the image of the hand moves toward the fovea, and when gaze tracks hand movement. Reaching to a foveated target can be computed by matching units storing congruent signals between actual hand and gaze positions. Reaching to non-foveated targets can be computed by the combination of two matching units: the first generates an internal signal which does not trigger an actual change in eye position, and the second computes hand movement direction by correlating this internal signal on predicted gaze position to actual hand position. Visual tracking of hand trajectory can result from the operations of matching units computing the position and direction of gaze that match the position and movement direction of the hand in space.

The coexistence of different matching operations in the same cortical area is largely supported by results from the parieto-occipital cortex where most neurons display a GTF when studied in a set of different visuomotor tasks requiring different forms of eye–hand coupling (Battaglia-Mayer *et al.* 1998, 2000, 2001). Similarly, several computations can coexist in relation to the different connections of a local population, as suggested by the different properties of LIP neurons projecting to the superior colliculus or the FEF (Ferraina *et al.* 2002).

Sensorimotor computations, predictions, and corticocortical connections

Each population of matching units can combine two distributed signals (e.g. arm position and visual direction) to compute a third one (motor command). Modeling studies suggest that the same matching unit can perform three parallel computations on each pair of input signals in order to compute a third one (Deneve *et al.* 2001; Pouget *et al.* 2002). Thus the same network can perform multidirectional computations, such as from one set of sensory coordinates to another (intersensory predictions), from any sensory to any motor coordinates (sensorimotor transformations or inverse models) and from any motor to any sensory coordinates (forward models). The network units combine three inputs and have bidirectional connections with them, shaping a recurrent network with attractor dynamics. For instance, the initial state of the network, characterized by two selective activations ('activation hills') in two of its inputs (e.g. retinal target position and eye position), evolves into three activations (retinal target position, eye position, head-centered target position) in the distributed input signals, thus computing appropriate transformations.

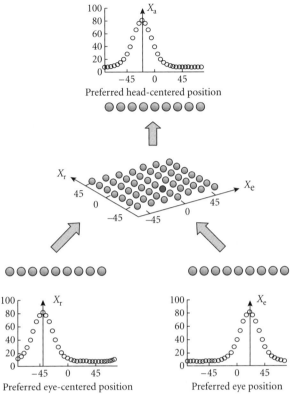

Fig. 2.4 Structure of a neural network using basis functions for coordinate transformations. In the two input layers, neurons code for eye-centered positions of a visual stimulus (left) and the proprioceptive eye position (right). The middle layer is composed of neurons that receive input from both input layers. Each neuron is modulated simultaneously by the two input signals, with preferred directions spanning the space of the Cartesian product of the two inputs. The output layer receives its input from the middle layer and is composed of neurons selective to the head-centered position of the stimulus. The desired coordinate transformation is performed by combining linearly the activities of the middle layer according to a synaptic matrix dependent on the specific transformation required. Modified from Pouget *et al.* (2002). *Nat Rev Neurosci*, **3**, 741–7.

Furthermore, such networks with combinatorial properties and attractor dynamics (recurrent connections) have a very interesting emergent property, resulting in partially shifting receptive fields of neurons, as observed experimentally in different parietal areas. If the parietal lobe is subdivided into several modules, each of which is associated with a particular frame of reference, each neuron is supposed to show multimodal response fields that are perfectly remapped in the frame of reference used by that module. In contrast, experimental results show partially shifting receptive fields, at least in VIP and LIP (Stricanne *et al.* 1996; Duhamel *et al.* 1997). This is exactly the prediction made by neural models (Fig. 2.4) with combinatorial properties (basis functions) and recurrent connections (Deneve *et al.* 2001; Pouget *et al.* 2002). Furthermore, it can be shown that such networks have optimal properties of (Bayesian) statistical inference and implement a close approximation of a maximum likelihood estimator. Different sensory modalities are not equally reliable but depend upon the context: the network dynamics weights each cue in proportion to its reliability, and modifies these weights when the context modified gain reliability (Deneve *et al.* 2001; Pouget *et al.* 2002). Attractor dynamics is also produced by recurrent excitatory and inhibitory connections within a population. It has been shown that these connections can play a major role in shaping the network activation in relation to both input activation and previous learning as a Bayesian collective decision process (Koechlin *et al.* 1999). Furthermore, a population of units with retinal, eye, and hand combinatorial properties, and recurrent excitatory and inhibitory connections, can generate a GTF (Mascaro *et al.* 2003), which no longer emerges when lateral inhibition is removed from the network.

Experimental results also show the coexistence of different temporal profiles of the rates of neurons sharing the same combinatorial tuning properties: neurons can be time-locked to a sensory stimulus or a motor command, or be active during a delay period between sensory stimuli and motor output. Neurons can be activated by a sensory event, and when a delay occurs or is imposed, their activity can selectively anticipate the upcoming motor output in relation to the task demands. Sustained activities during delay intervals are believed to predict the upcoming motor command. A computational interpretation of such sustained activation is that it reflects both the prediction of a future motor command computed by a matching unit, and a task-dependent control computed by a 'condition unit' which specifies when prediction is transformed into execution.

The dual relationship between condition and matching units sharing the same combinatorial domain can explain the two possible interpretations of the sustained activities that predict a motor command: sustained activities, including task-selective timing controls, can be viewed as subgoals in a plan to achieve reinforcement (condition units); otherwise they can be regarded as attentional controls (matching unit). Matching and condition units can be distributed in the same cortical area, but with a preferential distribution of the former in parietal areas and the latter in corticocortically related frontal areas.

A hypothesis concerning optic ataxia

Viewing the parietofrontal system as a network of networks allows a reinterpretation (Battaglia-Mayer and Caminiti 2002) of optic ataxia, a common higher-order motor disorder that follows superior parietal lesion. Optic ataxia is characterized by impaired visual control of arm reaching to a visual target (misreaching) and by defective hand orientation and grip formation. There are three the main features of this movement disorder (reviewed by Battaglia-Mayer and Caminiti 2002). The first is a defective control of the directional components of hand movement, which also includes failure to make smooth corrective adjustments after a target jump (Grea *et al.* 2002), and unawareness of the direction in which the movement occurred. Secondly, optic ataxia seems to affect mostly automatic on-line control, rather than planning *per se* (Pisella *et al.* 2000). Thirdly, optic ataxia only occurs when visual control of reaching is required and for real grasping, and not for pantomimic grasping to memorized objects (Milner *et al.* 2001). These last two features emphasize the task-dependent nature of the disorder in patients otherwise free of visual, somatosensory, or motor deficits.

A constant feature of patients suffering from optic ataxia is the site of the lesion, which mainly affects the superior parietal lobule at the parieto-occipital junction (reviewed by Battaglia-Mayer *et al.* 1998; Battaglia-Mayer and Caminiti 2002). Interestingly, a recent study (Nagaratnam *et al.* 1998) of five patients displaying optic ataxia has shown that three of them had posterior parietal lesions, while the remaining two suffered from frontal damage. Together with a case report of crossed optic ataxia involving the corpus callosum (Ferro *et al.* 1983), these observations support Bálint's (1909) original interpretation of this disorder as a corticocortical disconnection syndrome. The anatomical, physiological, and computational aspects of the parietofrontal system described above provide a frame for reinterpreting optic ataxia by taking into account the hypothesis of its subcortical origin (Classen *et al.* 1995).

Optic ataxia can be primarily seen as the result of a breakdown of the combinatorial mechanisms occurring within the GTFs of parietal neurons, where retinal, eye-related, and hand-related signals are combined on the basis of their directional congruence. As seen above, eye- and hand-related signals are arranged in a gradient-like fashion across the tangential domains of both the parietal and the frontal cortex, so that motor commands for reaching in the frontal lobe can only emerge as the result of a progressive match of information (Burnod *et al.* 1992, 1999), which mostly depends on reciprocal association connections. The 'collapse' of the gradient architecture of the network and the failure of re-entry might prevent the information match underlying the coordinate transformation necessary for motor commands. Thus it is not surprising that cases of optic ataxia have been reported in patients with frontal lesions (Nagaratnam *et al.* 1998), although this result awaits further confirmation. Finally, the task dependency of optic ataxia con only reside in the conditional nature of parietal cell activity, although the precise relationship between clinical signs and context dependency at the neural level remains to be determined.

Acknowledgements

This study was supported by the MIUR (FIRB- RBNE01SZB4, and COFIN) and the Ministry of Public Health of Italy, by the Commission of the European Communities (DG XII—contract number QLRT-1999–00448).

References

Andersen RA, Asanuma C, Cowan WM (1985). Callosal and prefrontal associational projecting cell populations in area 7A of the macaque monkey: a study using retrogradely transported fluorescent dyes. *J Comp Neurol*, **232**, 443–55.

Andersen RA, Asanuma C, Essik G, Siegel RM (1990). Cortico-cortical connections of anatomically and physiologically defined subdivisions within the inferior parietal lobule. *J Comp Neurol*, **296**, 65–113.

Bálint R (1909). Seelenlähmung des 'Schauens', optische Ataxie, räumliche Störung der Aufmerksamkeit. *Monatsschr Psychiatr Neurol*, **25**, 51–81.

Baraduc P, Guigon E (2002). Population computation of vectorial transformations. *Neural Comput*, **14**, 845–71.

Baraduc P, Guigon E, Burnod Y (2001). Recoding arm position to learn visuomotor transformations. *Cereb Cortex*, **11**, 906–17.

Battaglia-Mayer A, Caminiti R (2002). Optic ataxia as a result of the breakdown of the global tuning fields of parietal neurones. *Brain*, **125**, 225–37.

Battaglia-Mayer A, Ferraina S, Marconi B, Bullis JB, Lacquaniti F, Burnod Y, *et al.* (1998). Early motor influences on visuomotor transformations for reaching: a positive image of optic ataxia. *Exp Brain Res*, **123**, 172–89.

Battaglia-Mayer A, Ferraina S, Mitsuda T, Marconi B, Genovesio A, Onorati P, *et al.* (2000). Early coding of reaching in the parietooccipital cortex. *J Neurophysiol*, **83**, 2374–91.

Battaglia-Mayer A, Ferraina S, Genovesio A, Marconi B, Squatrito S, Molinari M, *et al.* (2001). Eye–hand coordination during reaching. II. An analysis of the relationships between visuomanual signals in parietal cortex and parieto-frontal association projections. *Cereb Cortex*, **11**, 528–44.

Battaglia-Mayer A, Caminiti R, Lacquaniti F, Zago M (2003). Multiple levels of representation of reaching in the parieto-frontal network. *Cereb Cortex*, **13**, 1009–22.

Blatt GJ, Andersen RA, Stoner GR (1990). Visual receptive field organization and cortico-cortical connections of the intraparietal area (area LIP) in the macaque. *J Comp Neurol*, **299**, 421–45.

Bridgeman B, Peery S, Anand S (1997). Interaction of cognitive and sensorimotor maps of visual space. *Percept Psychophys*, **59**, 456–69.

Brodmann K (1909). *Vergleichende Lokalisationslehre der Grosshirnrinde in ihren Prinzipien dargestellt auf Grund des Zellenbaues.* Leipzig: JA Barth.

Bullier J, Schall JD, Morel A (1996). Functional streams in occipito-frontal connections in the monkey. *Behav Brain Res*, **76**, 89–97.

Bullock D, Grossberg S, Guenther SH (1993). Self organizing neural model of motor equivalent reaching and tool use by multi-joint arm. *J Cogn Neurosci*, **4**, 408–435.

Burbaud P, Doegle C, Gross C, Bioulac B (1991). A quantitative study of neuronal discharge in area 5, 2, and 4 of the monkey during fast arm movements. *J Neurophysiol*, **66**, 429–43.

Burnod Y, Otto I, Grandguillaume P, Ferraina S, Johnson PB, Caminiti R (1992). Visuomotor transformations underlying arm movements toward visual targets: a neural network model of cerebral cortical operations. *J Neurosci*, **12**, 1435–53.

Burnod Y, Baraduc P, Battaglia-Mayer A, Guigon E, Koechlin E, Ferraina S, *et al.* (1999). Parieto-frontal coding of reaching: an integrated framework. *Exp Brain Res*, **129**, 325–46.

Caminiti R, Ferraina S, Johnson PB (1996). The sources of visual information to the primate frontal lobe: a novel role for the superior parietal lobule. *Cereb Cortex*, **6**, 319–328.

Carrozzo M, McIntyre J, Zago M, Lacquaniti F (1999). Viewer-centered and body-centered frames of reference in direct visuomotor transformations. *Exp Brain Res*, **129**, 201–10.

Carrozzo M, Stratta F, McIntyre J, Lacquaniti F (2002). Cognitive allocentric representations of visual space shape pointing errors. *Exp Brain Res*, **147**, 426–36.

Cavada C, Goldman-Rakic PS (1989a). Posterior parietal cortex in rhesus monkey: I. Parcellation of areas based on distinctive limbic and sensory corticocortical connections. *J Comp Neurol*, **287**, 393–421.

Cavada C, Goldman-Rakic PS (1989b). Posterior parietal cortex in rhesus monkey: evidence for segregated corticocortical networks linking sensory and limbic areas with the frontal lobe. *J Comp Neurol*, **287**, 422–45.

Chafee MV, Goldman-Rakic PS (2000). Inactivation of parietal and prefrontal cortex reveals interdependence of neural activity during memory-guided saccades. *J Neurophysiol*, **83**, 1550–66.

Classen J, Kunesch E, Binkofski F, Hilperath F, Schlaug G, Seitz RJ, *et al.* (1995). Subcortical origin of visuomotor apraxia. *Brain*, **118**, 1365–74.

Cohen YE, Andersen RA (2002). A common reference frame for movement plans in the posterior parietal cortex. *Nat Rev Neurosci*, **3**, 553–62.

Colby CL, Gattass R, Olson CR, Gross CG (1988). Topographical organization of cortical afferents to extrastriate visual area PO in the macaque: a dual tracer study. *J Comp Neurol*, **269**, 392–413

Deneve S, Latham PE, Pouget A (2001). Efficient computation and cue integration with noisy population codes. *Nat Neurosci*, **4**, 826–31.

Duffy FH, Burchfield JL (1971). Somatosensory system: organizational hierarchy from single units in monkey area 5. *Science*, **172**, 273–5.

Duhamel JR, Bremmer F, BenHamed S, Graf W (1997). Spatial invariance of visual receptive fields in parietal cortex neurons. *Nature*, **389**, 845–8.

Dum RP, Strick PL (1991a). The origin of the corticospinal projections from the premotor areas in the frontal lobe. *J Neurosci*, **11**, 667–689.

Dum RP, Strick PL (1991b). Premotor areas: nodal points for parallel efferente system involved in the central control of movement. In DR Humphrey, H-J Freund, (ed.) *Motor Control: Concepts and Issues*, pp. 383–97. New York: Wiley.

Fattori P, Gamberini M, Kutz DF, Galletti C (2001). 'Arm-reaching' neurons in the parietal area V6A of the macaque monkey. *Eur J Neurosci*, **13**, 2309–13.

Ferraina S, Garasto MR, Battaglia-Mayer A, Ferraresi P, Johnson PB, Lacquaniti F, *et al.* (1997a). Visual control of hand-reaching movement: activity in parietal area 7m. *Eur J Neurosci*, **9**, 1090–5.

Ferraina S, Johnson PB, Garasto MR, Battaglia-Mayer A, Ercolani L, Bianchi L, *et al.* (1997b). Combination of hand and gaze signals during reaching: activity in parietal area 7m of the monkey. *J Neurophysiol*, **77**, 1034–8.

Ferraina S, Battaglia-Mayer A, Genovesio A, Marconi B, Onorati P, Caminiti R (2001). Early coding of visuomanual coordination during reaching in parietal area PEc. *J Neurophysiol*, **85**, 462–7.

Ferraina S, Paré M, Wurtz RH (2002). Comparison of cortico-cortical and cortico-collicular signals for the generation of saccadic eye movements. *J Neurophysiol*, **87**, 845–858.

Ferro JM, Bravo-Marques JM, Castro-Caldas A, Antunes L (1983). Crossed optic ataxia: possible role of the dorsal splenium. *J Neurol Neurosurg Psychiatry*, **46**, 533–9.

Fogassi L, Raos V, Franchi G, Gallese V, Luppino G, Matelli M (1999). Visual responses in the dorsal premotor area F2 of the macaque monkey. *Exp Brain Res*, **128**, 194–9.

Fujii N, Mushiake H, Tanji J (2000). Rostrocaudal distinction of the dorsal premotor area based on oculomotor involvement. *J Neurophysiol*, **83**, 1764 -1769.

Galletti C, Battaglini PP, Fattori P (1991). Functional properties of neurons in the anterior bank of the parieto-occipital sulcus of the macaque monkey. *Eur J Neurosci*, **3**, 452–461.

Galletti C, Battaglini PP, Fattori P (1993). Parietal neurons encoding spatial locations in craniotopic coordinates. *Exp Brain Res*, **96**, 221–9.

Galletti C, Fattori P, Battaglini PP, Shipp S, Zeki S (1996). Functional demarcation of a border between areas V6 and V6A in the superior parietal gyrus of the macaque monkey. *Eur J Neurosci*, **8**, 30–52.

Galletti C, Fattori P, Kutz DF, Battaglini PP (1997). Arm movement-related neurons in the visual area V6A of the macaque superior parietal lobule. *Eur J Neurosci*, **9**, 410–3.

Galletti C, Fattori P, Kutz DF, Gamberini M (1999). Brain location and visual topography of cortical area V6A in the macaque monkey. *Eur J Neurosci*, **11**, 575–82.

Gattass R, Sousa APB, Covey E (1985). Cortical visual areas of the macaque: possible substrates for pattern recognition mechanisms. In R Chagas, R Gattass, CG Gross, (ed.) *Pattern Recognition Mechanisms*, pp. 1–20. Rome: Pontificiae Academia Scientia Scripta Varia.

Grea H, Pisella L, Rossetti Y, Desmurget M, Tilikete C, Grafton S, *et al.* (2002). A lesion of the posterior parietal cortex disrupts on-line adjustments during aiming movements. *Neuropsychologia*, **40**, 2471–80.

He S-Q, Dum RP, Strick PL (1995). Topographic organization of corticospinal projection from the frontal lobe: motor areas on the lateral surface of the hemisphere. *J Neurosci*, **13**, 952–980.

Johnson PB, Ferraina S, Caminiti R (1993). Cortical networks for visual reaching. *Exp Brain Res*, **97**, 361–5.

Johnson PB, Ferraina S, Bianchi L, Caminiti R (1996). Cortical networks for visual reaching. Physiological and anatomical organization of frontal and parietal lobe arm regions. *Cereb Cortex*, **6**, 102–19.

Johnson PB, Ferraina S, Garasto MR, *et al.*(1997). From vision to movement: cortico-cortical connections and combinatorial properties of reaching-related neurons in parietal areas V6 and V6A. Parietal lobe contributions to orientation in 3D space. *Exp Brain Res Suppl*, **25**, 221–36.

Koechlin E, Anton JL, Burnod Y (1999). Bayesian inference in populations of cortical neurons: a model of motion integration and segmentation in area MT. *Biol Cybern*, **80**, 25–34

Kutz DF, Fattori P, Gamberini M, Breveglieri R, Galletti C (2003). Early- and late-responding cells to saccadic eye movements in the cortical area V6A of macaque monkey. *Exp Brain Res*, **149**, 83–95.

Lacquaniti F (1997). Frames of reference in sensorimotor coordination. In Boller F, Grafman J, eds. *Handbook of Neuropsychology*, Vol 11.Amsterdam: Elsevier, 27–64.

Lacquaniti F, Caminiti R (1998). Visuo-motor transformations for arm reaching. *Eur J Neurosci*, **10**, 195–203.

Leichnetz GR, Goldberg ME (1988). Higher centers concerned with eye movement and visual attention: cerebral cortex and thalamus. *Rev Oculomot Res*, **2**, 365–429.

Marconi B, Genovesio A, Battaglia-Mayer A, Ferraina S, Squatrito S, Molinari M, *et al.* (2001). Eye–hand coordination during reaching. I. Anatomical relationships between parietal and frontal cortex. *Cereb Cortex*, **11**, 513–27.

Mascaro M, Battaglia-Mayer A, Nasi L, Amit DJ, Caminiti R (2003). The eye and the hand: neural mechanisms and network models for oculomanual coordination in parietal cortex. *Cereb Cortex*, **13**, 1276–86.

Matelli M, Govoni P, Galletti C, Kutz DF, Luppino G (1998). Superior area 6 afferents from the superior parietal lobule in the macaque monkey. *J Comp Neurol*, **402**, 327–52.

Maunsell JH, van Essen DC (1983). The connections of the middle temporal visual area (MT) and their relationship to a cortical hierarchy in the macaque monkey. *J Neurosci*, **3**, 2563–86.

Merchant H, Battaglia-Mayer A, Georgopoulos AP (2001). Effects of optic flow in motor cortex and area 7a. *J Neurophysiol*, **86**, 1937–54.

Milner AD, Dijkerman HC, Pisella L, McIntosh RD, Tilikete C, Vighetto A, *et al.* (2001). Grasping the past: delay can improve visuomotor performance. *Curr Biol*, **11**, 1896–901.

Mountcastle VB, Lynch JC, Georgopoulos A, Sakata H, Acuña C (1975). Posterior parietal association cortex of the monkey: command functions for operations within extrapersonal space. *J Neurophysiol*, **38**, 871–908.

Nagaratnam N, Grice D, Kalouche H (1998). Optic ataxia following unilateral stroke. *J Neurol Sci*, **155**, 204–7.

Nakamura K, Chung HH, Graziano MS, Gross CG (1999). Dynamic representation of eye position in the parieto-occipital sulcus. *J Neurophysiol*, **81**, 2374–85.

Pandya DN, Seltzer B (1982). Intrinsic connections and architectonics of posterior parietal cortex in the rhesus monkey. *J Comp Neurol*, **204**, 196–210.

Petrides M, Pandya DN (1984). Projections to the frontal cortex from the posterior parietal region in the rhesus monkey. *J Comp Neurol*, **228**, 105–16.

Picard N, Strick PL (1996). Motor areas of the medial wall: a review of their location and functional activation. *Cereb Cortex*, **6**, 342–53.

Pisella L, Gréa H, Tilikete C, Vighetto A, Desmurget M, Rode G, *et al.* (2000). An 'automatic pilot' for the hand in human posterior parietal cortex: toward reinterpreting optic ataxia. *Nat Neurosci*, **3**, 729–36.

Pouget A, Sejnowski T (1997). Spatial transformations in the parietal cortex using basis functions. *J Cogn Neurosci*, **9**, 222–37.

Pouget A., Deneve S, Duhamel JR (2002). A computational perspective on the neural basis of multisensory spatial representations. *Nat Rev Neurosci*, **3**, 741–7.

Raffi M, Squatrito S, Maioli MG (2002). Neuronal responses to optic flow in the monkey parietal area PEc. *Cereb Cortex*, **12**, 639–46.

Raos V, Franchi G, GalleseV, Fogassi L (2003). Somatotopic organization of the lateral part of area F2 (dorsal premotor cortex) of the macaque monkey. *J Neurophysiol*, **89**, 1503–18.

Sakata H, Takaoka Y, Kawarasaki A, Shibutani H (1973). Somatosensory properties of neurons in the superior parietal cortex (area 5) of the rhesus monkey. *Brain Res*, **64**, 85–102.

Sakata H, Taira M, Kusunoki M, Murata A, Tanaka Y (1997). The parietal association cortex in depth perception and visual control of hand action. *Trends Neurosci*, **20**, 350–7.

Salinas E, Abbott LF (1995). Transfer of coded information from sensory to motor networks. *J Neurosci*, **15**, 6461–74.

Schiller PH, Chou IH (1998). The effects of frontal eye field and dorsomedial frontal cortex lesions on visually guided eye movements. *Nat Neurosci*, **1**, 248–53.

Schlag J, Schlag-Rey M (1987). Evidence for a supplementary eye field. *J Neurophysiol*, **57**, 179–200.

Shipp S, Zeki S (1995). Direct visual inputs to premotor cortex from superior parietal cortex (areas V6 and V6A) in the macaque monkey. *Eur J Neurosci* **8** (Suppl), 75.

Shipp S, Blanton M, Zeki S (1998). A visuo-somatomotor pathway through superior parietal cortex in the macaque monkey: cortical connections of areas V6 and V6A. *Eur J Neurosci*, **10**, 3171–93.

Squatrito S, Raffi M, Maioli MG, Battaglia-Mayer A (2001). Visual motion responses of neurons in the caudal area PE of macaque monkeys. *J Neurosci*, **21**, RC130.

Stricanne B, Andersen RA, Mazzoni P (1996). Eye-centered, head-centered, and intermediate coding of remembered sound locations in area LIP. *J Neurophysiol*, **76**, 2071–6.

Tanné J, Boussaoud D, Boyer-Zeller N, Rouiller EM (1995). Direct visual pathways for reaching movements in the macaque monkey. *Neuroreport*, **7**, 267–72.

Tanné-Gariepy J, Rouiller EM, Boussaoud D (2002). Parietal inputs to dorsal versus ventral premotor areas in the macaque monkey: evidence for largely segregated visuomotor pathways. *Exp Brain Res*, **145**, 91–103.

Ungerleider LG, Desimone R (1986). Cortical connections of visual area MT in the macaque. *J Comp Neurol*, **248**, 190–222.

Vetter P, Wolpert D (2000). Context estimation for sensorimotor control. *J Neurophysiol*, **84**, 1026–34.

Vogt C, Vogt O (1919). Allgemeinere Ergebnisse unserer Hirnforschung. *J Psychol Neurol*, **25**, 279–461.

Von Bonin G, Bailey P (1947). *The Neocortex of Macaca mulatta*. Urbana, IL: University of Illinois Press.

Wise SP, Boussaoud D, Johnson PB, Caminiti R (1997). Premotor and parietal cortex: corticocortical connectivity and combinatorial computations. *Annu Rev Neurosci*, **20**, 25–42.

Wurtz RH, Sommer MA, Paré M, Ferraina S (2001). Signal transformations from cerebral cortex to superior colliculus for the generation of saccades. *Vision Res*, **41**, 3399–412.

Zipser D, Andersen RA (1988). A back-propagation programmed network that simulates response properties of a subset of posterior parietal neurons. *Nature*, **331**, 679–84.

Chapter 3

The planning and control of reaching and grasping movements

Michel Desmurget, Pierre Baraduc, and Emmanuel Guigon

Introduction

In our everyday life, we constantly interact with various objects. We reach for them, we manipulate them, and we grasp them with no apparent effort. Obviously, this simplicity has a cost in terms of the neural and functional organization of the nervous system. If our 'motor programs' are so powerful and easy to use, it is because their implementation is incredibly complex. A century of intense investigations have demonstrated that addressing this complexity is not a small challenge. In this chapter, we examine the most recent developments in this field of research. Because of space limitations, this presentation will focus on the most prominent models of motor control, often neglecting the details of some conceptual controversies. Four main questions will be addressed in succession. How is hand trajectory determined? How is the desired trajectory mapped into a set of motor commands? How is the ongoing trajectory monitored? How are grasping movements integrated into reaching behaviors?

Determining hand trajectory

It is generally agreed that spatiotemporal invariance can be used to identify the variables that are controlled by the motor system. As an illustration of this point, we consider the pioneering work of Morasso (1981). This author required naive subjects to point from a given initial position toward visual targets randomly distributed within the workspace. He observed that the morphology of the Cartesian hand path always remained roughly straight irrespective of the direction of movement, whereas the pattern of joint covariation exhibited systematic variations. Based on this extrinsic stability, he concluded that the hand trajectory in Cartesian space was the primary variable computed during movement planning, and that the pattern of joint covariation was defined in a second stage of the planning process to allow the hand to move along a predefined trajectory. This view has become dominant in the field of motor control, although it has been recently strongly disputed (Todorov and Jordan 2002). In a formal way, it suggests that reaching movements are planned in a hand-centered coordinate system, with direction and extent of the movement as the controlled parameters. Several arguments support this idea. Reaction times are reduced by prior information about either the direction or the distance of the target with respect to the hand (Bock and Arnold 1992). Changes of the visuomotor gain are learnt more easily than changes in movement direction and generalize to movements in all directions (Krakauer *et al.* 1999, 2000). The direction and extent variability or reaching movements are independent (Gordon *et al.* 1994). The direction of the hand-target vector is correlated with the neuronal activity in many cortical and cerebellar areas (Georgopoulos 1995). Pointings to targets symmetrically distributed around a starting position generate an average error that is strongly correlated with the errors observed when the subjects are required to localize their unseen hand on the movement starting position, as should be the case for a planning process based on the Cartesian hand-target vector (Vindras *et al.* 1998).

However, the hypothesis that reaching movements are planned to follow a straight-line path during visually directed movement was challenged in several studies showing that the Cartesian hand trajectory could be significantly curved and variable as a function of the movement direction (reviewed by Desmurget *et al.* 1998). According to several authors, this result can be attributed to incidental factors such as a distortion in the perception of straightness (Wolpert *et al.* 1994; but see Boessenkool *et al.* 1998) or the existence of biomechanical forces causing the real motion to deviate from the centrally programmed trajectory (Flash 1987). However, this explanation was questioned by converging observations suggesting that the morphological variations of the movement path reflected the nature of the planning process. For instance, Osu *et al.* (1997) investigated visually directed movements under two conditions: no path instruction (NI), and instruction to move the hand along a straight line (SI). Results showed that subjects generated much straighter movements in SI than in NI. As shown by electromyograms, this difference could not be related to an increase in arm stiffness. A similar conclusion was reached by our group in subsequent studies (Desmurget *et al.* 1997, 1999a). However, our data showed that the results reported by Osu and colleagues were only valid for unconstrained 3D movements. We failed to observe any kinematic differences between NI and SI for planar movements. This result suggests that planar and unconstrained movements might be planned in different frames of reference: while planar movements may be controlled in a Cartesian space, unrestrained movements may be defined in an intrinsic space.

With respect to this conclusion, several hypothesis have been proposed. A popular idea is that programmed trajectories must be optimal with respect to a cost measure. In the last 20 years, many different optimality criteria have been proposed such as minimum muscular energy (Alexander 1997), minimum effort (Cruse 1986), minimum jerk (Flash and Hogan 1985), minimum torque change (Uno *et al.* 1989), minimum work (Soechting *et al.* 1995) or minimum variance of the final position (Harris and Wolpert 1998). Because all these criteria were able to account for movement characteristics, none of them has achieved definitive success (although the idea that terminal movement conditions influence the shape of the whole trajectory has proved more attractive from a biological point of view). Another prominent theory suggest that hand trajectory is specified as a vector in the joint space. According to this view, the spatial characteristics of the target are initially converted into a set of arm and forearm orientations. The movement from the starting posture to the target posture is then implemented on the basis of an 'angular error vector' whose components represent the difference between the starting and target angles for each joint. During the movement, joint angle variations are not controlled independently but in a synergic way (temporal coupling). The curved hand path observed in the task space results directly from this temporal coupling. Computational (Rosenbaum *et al.* 1995), behavioral (Desmurget and Prablanc 1997), and electrophysiological evidence (Graziano *et al.* 2002a) supporting this model has been reported. For instance, Graziano *et al.* (2002b) showed that electrical stimulation of the motor cortex caused monkeys to produce coordinated complex movements toward a specific target posture. As shown in Figure 3.1, not only this posture was specified but also the entire coordinated trajectory aiming toward it.

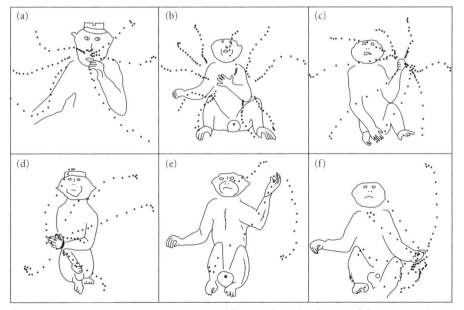

Fig. 3.1 Examples of complex postures evoked by electrical stimulations of the precentral gyrus. The dotted lines represent the trajectories from different starting point to the final posture. Reproduced from Graziano *et al.* (2002). *Neuron*, **34**, 841–51.

Mapping a desired trajectory into a set of motor commands

With respect to the present section, it should first be noted that the theoretical dissociation between inverse kinematics (specifying a desired trajectory) and inverse dynamics (specifying the actual motor command) could be an explanatory convenience referring to different levels of description rather than a neural reality (Uno *et al.* 1989). Such a dissociation is mainly supported by the demonstration that inverse kinematic and inverse dynamic models can be adapted independently (Krakauer *et al.* 1999). However, this result could not be replicated in a similar study (Tong *et al.* 2002). In addition, it was found that the transfer from learning new hand kinematics depended on the joint configurations used (Baraduc and Wolpert 2002) (Fig. 3.2) and the force environment (P. Baraduc and D. M. Wolpert, unpublished data), which is inconsistent with the independent specification of the desired hand or arm kinematics.

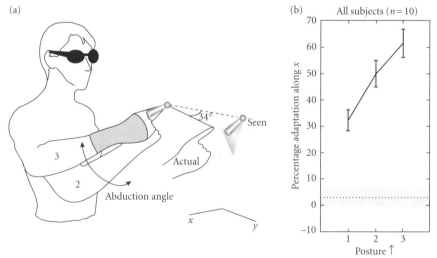

Fig. 3.2 (a) Subjects are immersed in a virtual reality environment where the tip of the finger is represented by a sphere and the forearm orientation by a cone section. The task is to point towards a target that constrains both fingertip position and forearm orientation (triangle). Visual feedback is progressively rotated when subjects repeatedly point using an adducted starting posture [training posture (3)]. After this training session, generalization of the visuomotor bias to other starting postures is tested. Specification of a final equilibrium posture would induce a complete generalization. (b) Percentage adaptation along the frontal axis. Although a specific final posture is required by the task, the final finger position depends strongly on the homology between the starting posture and the training posture (arrow). Reproduced from Baraduc and Wolpert (2002). *J Neurophysiol*, **88**, 973–81.

Bearing the previous comments in mind, one can classify the different models by explaining how the central nervous system (CNS) builds motor commands into two 'families'. On the one hand, the CNS could use internal models of the motor apparatus (Kawato 1999). In this case, an 'inverse' model calculates the necessary output required to reach a desired goal and, as will be discussed further below, a 'forward' model provides a fast internal feedback loop which can substitute for delayed sensory feedback (Desmurget and Grafton 2000). On the other hand, the CNS could avoid these complex computations by simply exploiting the viscoelastic properties of the neuro-muscular system. In this case, the movement is specified as a series of equilibrium postures (Bizzi et al. 1992; Feldman and Levin 1995). A large body of literature has been devoted to testing and discussing these conflicting theories.

The equilibrium point (EP) theory developed from early observations by A.G. Feldman and collaborators on invariant movement characteristics mediated by peripheral feedback (Feldman 1986). The idea developed by Feldman is that hand displacement may be generated by the mechanism responsible for static or quasi-static equilibrium. In this scenario, the brain defines a time-varying series of EPs and movement arises as a consequence of mechanical interactions between the moving limb and its environment. According to Feldman, the EP of a joint is fixed by setting the recruitment threshold (lambda command) of the muscles spanning the joint. In fact, assuming a simple model of joint agonist–antagonist organization, the lambda commands specify both the geometrical shape of the equilibrium (reciprocal command) and the apparent stiffness of the joint (coactivation command). This is known as the 'lambda model' of the EP theory.

Other proponents of the EP theory have suggested a different mechanism to specify the EP, which is sometimes referred to as the 'alpha model'. This model focuses on the viscoelastic properties of the muscles (as opposed to reflex). It suggests that muscles behave like springs whose stiffness can be controlled centrally. The desired EP is reached by setting the length–tension curves of all the muscles acting on the limb in such a way that the torques exerted by agonist and antagonist muscles nullify each other when the hand is at the desired position. Initial support of this view was provided by Polit and Bizzi (1979). These authors trained three monkeys to perform single-joint pointing toward visual targets presented in a dark room. Following the period of training, intrathecal deafferentation of the arm territory was performed. After recovery from surgery, deafferented monkeys were still able to reach to the targets with good accuracy. In a subsequent study using the same protocol, Bizzi et al. (1984) tested two additional conditions: arm held in its initial position, and arm displaced toward the target at movement onset. As predicted by the alpha model, the results showed, for both the intact and deafferented animals, that in the first condition the initial acceleration of the hand increased gradually with the duration of the holding period, and that in the second condition the forearm moved back in the direction of the starting point of the movement before reversing its displacement to return to the target. Evidence supporting a generalization of the 'continuous EP shift' hypothesis to multijoint movements was mainly provided by neurophysiological studies involving electrical stimulation of the spinal cord of the frog. Current injection at a given site was shown to induce forces at the extremity of the limb that pointed towards a fixed EP in space (reviewed by Bizzi *et al.* 1995). Moreover, the force fields produced by two simultaneous stimulations resembled the summation of the individual force fields (Mussa-Ivaldi *et al.* 1994). This is in accord with the suggestion that spinal networks could implement the building blocks (or 'primitives') of EP control. A simple (linear) combination of these primitives enables a broad repertoire of movements to be realized (Tresch *et al.* 1999). In this view, the EP is not determined by joint reciprocal commands but by a set of weights, one for each primitive.

A potential problem with the EP approach is that no fixed relationship exists between EP displacement and limb movement. Indeed, external forces can modify the geometry of the viscoelastic system. The CNS is routinely confronted with these external disturbances, for instance when carrying an object in the hand. The way external forces develop in reaction to arm motion is determined by the dynamic environment. It is now well documented that human subjects can quickly adapt to different dynamic environments, even those that they have never experienced before (Lackner and DiZio 1994; Shadmehr and Mussa-Ivaldi 1994; Burdet *et al.* 2001). The organization of descending commands in terms of EP control variables strongly constrains the interpretation of this plasticity. During adaptation to a novel dynamical environment, subjects progressively learn to cancel the effect of external perturbations and recover normal movement kinematics. In terms of EP, this involves modifying the equilibrium trajectory to compensate for the external force field. Muscular coactivation decreases as learning proceeds (Thoroughman and Shadmehr 1999), and this factor is probably not responsible for the adapted behavior. Thus the major attractive feature of the EP models, i.e. the fact that the equilibrium trajectory closely matches the desired trajectory, does not hold in these conditions. In a more general manner, it is unclear how any version of the EP theory can account for the adaptation to velocity-dependent force fields; a simple change in EP trajectory cannot explain how subjects generalize their learning to movement velocities (and hence forces) different from those encountered during adaptation (Goodbody and Wolpert 1998). These results are much easier to understand if a direct control of joint torque through inverse dynamic models is assumed (Kawato 1999).

The partial inability of the EP theory to account for some experimental results does not imply, as sometimes stated (e.g. Graziano *et al.* 2002a), that it should be considered obsolete. The original theory was based on the analysis of static and quasi-static equilibrium and it remains very attractive for the control of posture. As shown by Shadmehr and Arbib (1992), maintenance of a stable steady state against gravity for a single joint actuated by two muscles can be guaranteed by lambda control, but not by stiffness control (*a fortiori* torque control). As most motor behaviors start and finish at a stable equilibrium, efficient postural control is a desirable property. By its origin, the EP theory has nothing to do with voluntary muscular contractions. Extension to movement generation (in particular fast movements) is a challenging idea which has been widely criticized (reviewed by Desmurget *et al.* 1998) and which still needs to be elaborated. It should be noted that one of the most successful models of the formation of motor commands for single- and multijoint movements involves both stiffness control and EP control (Lan 1997).

Controlling the ongoing movement

Although now familiar, the idea that visually directed movements are controlled on line during their execution is quite recent. For a long time, researchers assumed that reaching movements were primarily under preprogrammed control and that feedback loops exerted a limited influence at the very end of the trajectory. This assumption was based on three main hypotheses (reviewed by Desmurget and Grafton 2003). First, feedback loops rely exclusively on sensory information. Secondly, accurate movements can be performed in the absence of sensory input. Thirdly, the minimum delay required to process sensory information is too long with respect to the duration of movement to allow efficient on-line control of the ongoing trajectory. To test these hypotheses, Prablanc and colleagues designed an experimental protocol known as the 'subliminal double-step paradigm' (Goodale *et al.* 1986; Prablanc and Martin 1992; Desmurget *et al.* 1999b). In this experiment, subjects are required to 'look and point' at peripheral visual targets that are displaced during the course of the initial saccade, when there is suppression of visual perception. Results gathered with this paradigm failed to confirm the feedforward concept of movement control. As shown by kinematic recordings, the initial motor command does not unfold in a ballistic manner, but is updated continuously by powerful feedback loops (Fig. 3.3). In order

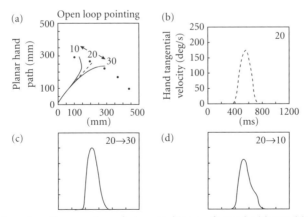

Fig. 3.3 Smooth early path corrections during reaching performed without vision of the limb. (a) Mean hand path performed by one subject to a stationary target (20°, broken line) and to displaced targets (20°→30°, 20°→10°; solid lines). (b–d) Corresponding velocity profiles. Reproduced from Prablanc and Martin (1992). *J Neurophysiol*, **67**, 455–69.

to account for this result it was proposed that feedback mechanisms might not rely exclusively on sensory information but on a forward model that integrates the sensory inflow and motor outflow to evaluate the consequences of the motor commands sent to the arm (reviewed by Miall and Wolpert 1996; Desmurget and Grafton 2000). The idea behind this concept is that the motor system can progressively learn to estimate its own behavior in response to a given command (efferent signal). During the movement, this prediction can be used to define the current state of the motor apparatus and to predict the final state. In parallel with this predictive activity, the system can also 'store' its successive predictions in a 'delayed buffer'. If the delay is equivalent to the time necessary to process sensory information, then the predicted and sensory estimated states can be compared directly. This comparison can be used to update the current estimation (Miall *et al.* 1993) and the learned forward model (Jordan and Rumelhart 1992). With such a model, the probable position and velocity of the effector can be estimated with negligible delays, and even predicted in advance, thus making feedback strategies possible for fast reaching movements.

A possible way in which forward modeling might allow on-line motor control has been proposed by Desmurget and Grafton (2000). The idea is that the subject first uses an inverse model to develop a motor plan. During the realization of the movement, a forward model of the arm's dynamics is generated. In its simplest version, this model receives as input a copy of the motor outflow. In a more general form, the model receives as input a copy of the motor outflow and an error signal defined by comparing a stored estimate of the motor state with the delayed sensory estimate (Kalman filtering) (Wolpert *et al.* 1995). The output of this forward model is a prediction of the movement endpoint. This prediction can be compared continuously with the target location. If there is a discrepancy an error signal is generated, triggering a modulation of the motor command.

In light of the previous results, one may wonder whether any movement needs to be planned in advance. Indeed, on-line feedback loops could theoretically underlie the development of the whole reaching movement, without a predefined motor plan (Feldman and Levin 1995). This would explain why movement variability is larger in the degrees of freedom that are irrelevant to the goal of the movement (Scholz *et al.* 2000). Although this possibility has never been formally rejected, it is challenged by three main results. First, fine predictive compensatory adjustments have been observed in single muscles (Flanagan and Wing 1997; Gribble and Ostry 1999). These adjustments can only be explained theoretically if the kinematic consequences of the upcoming motor command can be predicted precisely, i.e. if this motor command is, to some extent, known in advance. Secondly, when on-line feedback loops are inoperative due to a lesion (Pisella *et al.* 2000) or the application of a transcranial magnetic pulse over the posterior parietal cortex after onset of hand movement (Desmurget *et al.* 1999b), the subject can still reach the target with good accuracy (Fig. 3.4). Thirdly, recent computational studies suggest the existence of control models combining feedforward and feedback specification of the motor command (Wolpert *et al.* 1995; Bhushan and Shadmehr 1999).

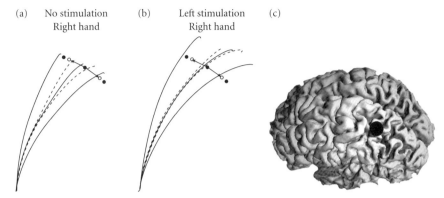

(a)   No stimulation   (b)   Left stimulation   (c)
        Right hand   Right hand

Fig. 3.4 Effect of disrupting on-line feedback loops on movement accuracy. Mean hand paths performed by one subject (right hand) (a) without and (b) with the application of a magnetic pulse over the left posterior parietal cortex. The solid curves represent the mean paths directed at stationary targets (20°, 30°, 40°). The broken curves represent the mean paths directed at jumping targets (30°→22.5°, 30°→37.5°). Solid circles indicate stationary target locations and open circles represent jumping target locations. (c) The transcranial magnetic stimulation (TMS) location site (solid circle) is determined by three-dimensional MRI. When TMS is applied, path corrections that normally occur in response to the target jump are disrupted. In addition, movements directed at stationary targets become less accurate although not erratic. Reproduced from Desmurget *et al*. (1999). *Nat Neurosci*, **2**, 563–7.

Integrating grasping movements to reaching behavior

As originally claimed by Descartes, it is possible reduce the complexity of any system by segmenting it into independent modules controlled in parallel. This analytic approach was successfully endorsed by Jeannerod (1981) who proposed partitioning prehension movements into two components ensuring, respectively, the transport of the arm to the vicinity of the target and the grasp itself. A third channel was added to account for the control of hand orientation (Arbib 1981). In addition, the existence of a coordinating meta-structure was assumed in order to explain the temporal coupling of each independently controlled module. This modular description of the reach-to-grasp action is supported by much behavioral, neurophysiological, imaging and clinical data (reviewed by Jeannerod *et al*. 1995; Paulignan and Jeannerod 1996). In particular, the corticospinal pathways responsible for the command of proximal and distal muscles are largely segregated. Neurons responding specifically to reaching or grasping behaviors are present in several cortical areas such as the premotor cortex and the posterior parietal cortex. The magnocellular red nucleus appears to be linked to the temporal coordination of reaching and grasping movements (van Kan and McCurdy 2002). Cortical lesions can selectively affect the transport of the arm or the preshaping of the hand. Variations of object location or size differentially influence the transport and grasping behaviors of normal subjects. When either the location or the size of the object to be grasped is modified after onset of hand movement, both components reorganize to reinstate their correct temporal coupling.

Despite the previous results, the modular conception of prehension movements is still widely debated. Alternative views have been proposed based on the claim that arm transport, hand orientation, and grip formation cannot be controlled and planned independently (Smeets and Brenner 1999). In particular, when the orientation of the object to be grasped changes, the transport of the arm is automatically affected (if you grasp an egg, the final location of the wrist will differ depending on which axis is orthogonal or parallel to your shoulder line). In addition, the muscular apparatus cannot be separated into independent proximal and distal entities. The biceps brachii controls not only the position of the hand but also its orientation through supination. Likewise, the flexor digitorum profundus controls not only the grip aperture by flexing the fingers, but also the hand orientation by flexing the wrist. To account for these observations a generalization of the 'joint space control hypothesis' was proposed, according to which the characteristics of the object to be grasped are transformed into a final posture specifying not only a set of arm and forearm orientations, but also a global posture involving the whole upper limb (Fig. 3.1) (Desmurget and Prablanc 1997; Graziano *et al.* 2002b). A promising alternative model has recently been developed based on the idea that prehension movements actually amount to a 'dual reaching task' in which the thumb and fingers are guided independently toward contact areas prespecified on the target object (Smeets and Brenner 1999). This idea is seductive inasmuch as it provides a unified framework within which prehension and reaching movements can be described and understood. However, it is mainly supported by computational evidence. Also, it is apparently challenged by the demonstration that the thumb and index finger cannot be flexed independently at the muscular level (Kilbreath and Gandevia 1994), despite the existence of indirect behavioral (Smeets and Brenner 2001) and computational evidence (Smeets *et al.* 2002).

Conclusion

As shown throughout this chapter, the literature offers several divergent models to account for the human ability to generate accurate hand movements. Strikingly, each of these models is supported and contradicted by sound experimental results. On the one hand, this might indicate that current theories of motor control might be partial or invalid. On the other hand, however, this might reflect the remarkable ability of the CNS to adapt to different experimental contexts. According to this view, different control strategies might coexist to form the large, diversified, and flexible motor repertory that characterizes primates.

References

Alexander RM (1997). A minimum energy cost hypothesis for human arm trajectories. *Biol Cybern*, **76**, 97–105.

Arbib MA (1981). Perceptual structures and distributed motor control. In WB Brooks, (ed.) *Handbook of Physiology. Section I: The Nervous System. Vol 2: Motor Control*, pp. 1449–80. Baltimore, MD: Williams & Wilkins.

Baraduc P, Wolpert DM (2002). Adaptation to a visuomotor shift depends on the starting posture. *J Neurophysiol*, **88**, 973–81.

Bhushan N, Shadmehr R (1999). Computational nature of human adaptive control during learning of reaching movements in force fields. *Biol Cybern*, **81**, 39–60.

Bizzi E, Accornero N, Chapple W, Hogan N (1984). Posture control and trajectory formation during arm movement. *J Neurosci*, **4**, 2738–44.

Bizzi E, Hogan N, Mussa-Ivaldi FA, Giszter S (1992). Does the nervous system use the equilibrium point control to guide single and multiple joint movements. *Behav Brain Sci*, **15**, 603–13.

Bizzi E, Giszter SF, Loeb E, Mussa-Ivaldi FA, Saltiel P (1995). Modular organization of motor behavior in the frog's spinal cord. *Trends Neurosci*, **18**, 442–6.

Bock O, Arnold K (1992). Motor control prior to movement onset: preparatory mechanisms for pointing at visual target. *Exp Brain Res*, **90**, 209–16.

Boessenkool JJ, Nijhof EJ, Erkelens CJ (1998). A comparison of curvatures of left and right hand movements in a simple pointing task. *Exp Brain Res*, **120**, 369–76.

Burdet E, Osu R, Franklin DW, Milner TE, Kawato M (2001). The central nervous system stabilizes unstable dynamics by learning optimal impedance. *Nature*, **414**, 446–9.

Cruse E (1986). Constraints for joint angle control of the human arm. *Biol Cybern*, **54**, 125–32.

Desmurget M, Grafton S (2000). Forward modeling allows feedback control for fast reaching movements. *Trends Cogn Sci*, **4**, 423–31.

Desmurget M, Grafton S (2003). Feedback or feedforward control, end of a dichotomy. In S Johnson, (ed.) *Taking Action: Cognitive Neuroscience Perspective on Intentional Acts*, pp. 289–338. Cambridge, MA: MIT Press.

Desmurget M, Prablanc C (1997). Postural control of three dimensional prehension movements. *J Neurophysiol*, **77**, 452–64.

Desmurget M, Jordan M, Prablanc C, Jeannerod M (1997). Constrained and Unconstrained movements involve different control strategies. *J Neurophysiol*, **77**, 1644–50.

Desmurget M, Pélisson D, Rossetti Y, Prablanc C (1998). From eye to hand: planning goal-directed movements. *Neurosci Biobehav Rev*, **22**, 761–88.

Desmurget M, Prablanc C, Jordan MI, Jeannerod M (1999a). Are reaching movements planned to be straight and invariant in the extrinsic space: kinematic comparison between compliant and unconstrained motions. *Q J Exp Psychol*, **52A**, 981–1020.

Desmurget M, Epstein CM, Turner RS, Prablanc C, Alexander GE, Grafton ST (1999b). Role of the posterior parietal cortex in updating reaching movements to a visual target. *Nat Neurosci*, **2**, 563–7.

Feldman AG (1986). Once more on the equilibrium-point hypothesis (L model) for motor control. *J Mot Behav*, **18**, 17–54.

Feldman AG, Levin MF (1995). The origin and use of positional frames of reference in motor control. *Behav Brain Sci*, **18**, 723–806.

Flanagan JR, Wing AM (1997). The role of internal models in motion planning and control: evidence from grip force adjustments during movements of hand- held loads. *J Neurosci*, **17**, 1519–28.

Flash T (1987). The control of hand equilibrium trajectories in multi-joint arm movements. *Biol Cybern*, **57**, 257–74.

Flash T, Hogan N (1985). The coordination of arm movements: an experimentally confirmed mathematical model. *J Neurosci*, **5**, 1688–1703.

Georgopoulos AP (1995). Current issues in directional motor control. *Trends Neurosci*, **18**, 506–10.

Goodale MA, Pélisson D, Prablanc C (1986). Large adjustments in visually guided reaching do not depend on vision of the hand and perception of target displacement. *Nature*, **320**, 748–50.

Goodbody SJ, Wolpert DM (1998). Temporal and amplitude generalization in motor learning. *J Neurophysiol*, **79**, 1825–38.

Gordon J, Ghilardi MF, Ghez C (1994). Accuracy of planar reaching movements: 1. Independence of direction and extent variability. *Exp Brain Res*, **99**, 97–111.

Graziano MS, Taylor CS, Moore T, Cooke DF (2002a). The cortical control of movement revisited. *Neuron*, **36**, 349–362.

Graziano MS, Taylor CS, Moore T (2002b). Complex movements evoked by microstimulation of precentral cortex. *Neuron*, **34**, 841–51.

Gribble PL, Ostry DJ (1999). Compensation for interaction torques during single- and multijoint limb movement. *J Neurophysiol*, **82**, 2310–26.

Harris CM, Wolpert DM (1998). Signal-dependent noise determines motor planning. *Nature*, **394**, 780–4.

Jeannerod M (1981). Intersegmental coordination during reaching at natural visual objects. In J Long, A Baddeley, (ed.) *Attention and Performance IX*, pp. 153–68. Hillsdale, NJ: Lawrence Erlbaum.

Jeannerod M, Arbib MA, Rizzolatti G, Sakata H (1995). Grasping objects: the cortical mechanisms of visuo-motor transformations. *Trends Neurosci*, **18**, 314–20.

Jordan M, Rumelhart D (1992). Forward models: supervised learning with a distal teacher. *Cogn Sci*, **16**, 307–54.

Kawato M (1999). Internal models for motor control and trajectory planning. *Curr Opin Neurobiol*, **9**, 718–27.

Kilbreath SL, Gandevia SC (1994). Limited independent flexion of the thumb and fingers in human subjects. *J Physiol (Lond)*, **479**, 487–97.

Krakauer JW, Ghilardi MF, Ghez C (1999). Independent learning of internal models for kinematic and dynamic control of reaching. *Nat Neurosci*, **2**, 1026–31.

Krakauer JW, Pine ZM, Ghilardi MF, Ghez C (2000). Learning of visuomotor transformations for vectorial planning of reaching trajectories. *J Neurosci*, **20**, 8916–24.

Lackner JR, Dizio P (1994). Rapid adaptation to coriolis force perturbations of arm trajectory. *J Neurophysiol*, **72**, 299–313.

Lan N (1997). Analysis of an optimal control model of multi-joint arm movements. *Biol Cybern*, **76**, 107–17.

Miall RC, Wolpert DM (1996). Forwards models for physiological motor control. *Neural Netw*, **9**, 1265–79.

Miall RC, Weir DJ, Wolpert DM, Stein JF (1993). Is the cerebellum a Smith predictor? *J Mot Behav*, **25**, 203–16.

Morasso P (1981). Spatial control of arm movements. *Exp Brain Res*, **42**, 223–7.

Mussa-Ivaldi FA, Giszter SF, Bizzi E (1994). Linear combinations of primitives in vertebrate motor control. *Proc Natl Acad Sci USA*, **91**, 7534–8.

Osu R, Uno Y, Koike Y, Kawato M (1997). Possible explanations for trajectory curvature in multijoint arm movements. *J Exp Psychol Hum Percept Perform*, **23**, 890–913.

Paulignan Y, Jeannerod M (1996). Prehension movements. The visuomotor channels hypothesis revisited. In P Haggard, R Flanagan, AM Wing, (ed.) *Hand and Brain: Neurophysiology and Psychology of Hand Movement*, pp. 265–82. Orlando, FL: Academic Press.

Pisella L, Grea H, Tilikete C, Vighetto A, Desmurget M, Rode G, *et al.* (2000). An 'automatic pilot' for the hand in human posterior parietal cortex: toward reinterpreting optic ataxia. *Nat Neurosci*, **3**, 729–36.

Polit A, Bizzi E (1979). Characteristics of motor programs underlying arm movements in monkeys. *J Neurophysiol*, **42**, 183–94.

Prablanc C, Martin O (1992). Automatic control during hand reaching at undetected two-dimensional target displacements. *J Neurophysiol*, **67**, 455–69.

Rosenbaum DA, Loukopoulos LD, Meulenbroek RGJ, Vaughan J, Engelbrecht SE (1995). Planning reaches by evaluating stored postures. *Psychol Rev*, **102**, 28–67.

Scholz JP, Schöner G, Latash ML (2000). Identifying the control structure of multijoint coordination during pistol shooting. *Exp Brain Res*, **135**, 382–404.

Sergio LE, Kalaska JF (1998). Changes in the temporal pattern of primary motor cortex activity in a directional isometric force versus limb movement task. *J Neurophysiol*, **80**, 1577–83.

Shadmehr R, Arbib MA (1992). A mathematical analysis of the force–stiffness characteristics of muscles in control of a single joint system. *Biol Cybern*, **66**, 463–77.

Shadmehr R, Mussa-Ivaldi FA (1994). Adaptive representation of dynamics during learning of a motor task. *J Neurosci*, **14**, 3208–24.

Smeets JB, Brenner E (1999). A new view on grasping. *Motor Control*, **3**, 237–71.

Smeets JB, Brenner E (2001). Independent movements of the digits in grasping. *Exp Brain Res*, **139**, 92–100.

Smeets JB, Brenner E, Biegstraaten M (2002). Independent control of the digits predicts an apparent hierarchy of visuomotor channels in grasping. *Behav Brain Res*, **136**, 427–32.

Soechting JF, Bueno CA, Herrmann U, Flanders M (1995). Moving effortlessly in three dimensions: does Donders law apply to arm movements? *J Neurosci*, **15**, 6271–80.

Thoroughman KA, Shadmehr R (1999). Electromyographic correlates of learning an internal model of reaching movements. *J Neurosci*, **19**, 8573–88.

Todorov E, Jordan MI (2002). Optimal feedback control as a theory of motor coordination. *Nat Neurosci*, **5**, 1226–35.

Tong C, Wolpert DM, Flanagan JR (2002). Kinematics and dynamics are not represented independently in motor working memory: evidence from an interference study. *J Neurosci*, **22**, 1108–13.

Tresch MC, Saltiel P, Bizzi E (1999). The construction of movement by the spinal cord. *Nat Neurosci*, **2**, 162–7.

Uno Y, Kawato M, Suzuki R (1989). Formation and control of optimal trajectory in human multijoint arm movement. Minimum torque-change model. *Biol Cybern*, **61**, 89–101.

Van Kan PL, McCurdy ML (2002). Contribution of primate magnocellular red nucleus to timing of hand preshaping during reaching to grasp. *J Neurophysiol*, **87**, 1473–87.

Vindras P, Desmurget M, Prablanc C, Viviani P (1998). Pointing errors reflect biases in the perception of the initial hand position. *J Neurophysiol*, **79**, 3290–4.

Wolpert DM, Ghahramani Z, Jordan MI (1994). Perceptual distorsion contributes to the curvature of human reaching movements. *Exp Brain Res*, **98**, 153–6.

Wolpert DM, Ghahramani Z, Jordan MI (1995). An internal model for sensorimotor integration. *Science*, **269**, 1880–1882.

Chapter 4

The premotor cortex: from attention to intention

Driss Boussaoud

Introduction

The capacity of the brain to process information about the external world and to plan and execute appropriate behavior has increased considerably throughout evolution, and has reached its highest level in mammals, especially the human and non-human primates. Our highly sophisticated sensory organs provide us with rich information about the external world, and our central nervous system has the capacity to extract relevant messages and process them in relation to context, previous experience, state of motivation, and other affective signals. Ultimately, the brain selects and executes one action from a diverse repertoire of actions which allow us to manipulate objects with tremendous skill. This sophistication in our sensorimotor systems requires selection mechanisms at both the input and output levels. At the sensory input level, the brain must select the pertinent information through selective attention. For example, the brain must select one object (e.g. a cup of tea) from a large number of images that fall on the retina. At the motor output level, neural activity must lead to the selection of one coordinated action (decision-making, motor preparation, intention) from many possible behaviors (grasp the cup of tea).

Selective attention and action are two intimately linked processes which overlap in time and space and are barely dissociable. This is particularly true for eye movements. A salient stimulus which attracts our attention automatically triggers a saccade toward it, indicating that attention and eye-movement commands might use the same brain networks. In line with this idea, it has been shown that brain circuits activated in relation to covert attention (without eye movements) and overt attention (with eye movements) overlap considerably (Corbetta *et al.* 1998). However, with the exception of eye movements, which are part of the orienting behavior, attention can be dissociated from actions involving other parts of our body, such as the hands. Attending to a target in space for identification purposes does not require moving the hand, or the intention to do so. In contrast, making a hand movement toward a target requires attention resources which vary with task difficulty and decrease with training. These observations raise the question of whether attention and intention rely on the same brain networks, or whether action uses an independent network which 'escapes' from the control of the attention system. In this chapter we review evidence suggesting that attention and intention activate two separate networks which converge at the level of the premotor cortex, a brain region which would play a key role in the interface between the two processes. We shall concentrate on the dorsal premotor cortex (PMd), where neurons can be selectively activated when a monkey prepares to move its arm in a particular direction, or when a human subject prepares to press a button with his or her finger. However, it should be stressed that this choice does not preclude the implication of other cortical areas (namely the medial premotor cortex) and subcortical structures (caudate nucleus) in bridging between attention and action.

The chapter is organized in three parts. In the first part, the current state of anatomical organization and connectivity of frontal cortex in the monkey is summarized. In the second part, the neural substrate of motor preparation (termed intention) is addressed by reviewing neurophysiological studies in the monkey and neuroimaging studies in humans. Finally, we review evidence from both monkey neurophysiology and neuroimaging in humans suggesting that the attention system is partially separated from the motor preparation system.

Anatomical and functional organization

Multiple subdivisions of premotor cortex

The frontal cortex, the cortex anterior to the central sulcus, involves two main architectonic regions: the agranular cortex comprises the primary motor cortex (M1) and the premotor cortex (PM, mainly Broadmann's areas 6 and 24), and the granular cortex involves the prefrontal cortex (Pf). Many areas have been identified within both the PM and Pf cortices, based on anatomical, physiological and neuropsychological evidence (Fig. 4.1). The prefrontal cortex is divided into three major regions along the lateral-to-medial axis: the orbitofrontal region (the inferior aspect), the lateral region (including the dorsolateral and dorsomedial aspects), and the medial region. The premotor cortex involves two main regions, one medial and one lateral. The medial premotor cortex involves the supplementary motor area (SMA) and the cingulate motor areas (CMA), whereas the lateral premotor cortex includes the dorsal (PMd) and ventral (PMv) premotor areas. Finer subdivisions have been identified within these premotor areas along the rostrocaudal axis, with pre-SMA, PMdr, and PMvr located rostrally, and SMA proper, PMdc, and PMvc located caudally (Matelli *et al.* 1985, 1991; Caminiti *et al.* 1996; Preuss *et al.* 1996; Tanné-Gariéppy *et al.* 2002). This chapter will concentrate on lateral premotor areas, especially the two divisions of PMd.

Connections with parietal cortex and prefrontal cortex

The posterior parietal cortex has long been considered as a bridge between vision and action (Critchley 1953), but early anatomical studies (Pandya and Kuypers 1969; Jones and Powell 1970) did not provide evidence for direct connections between the visual

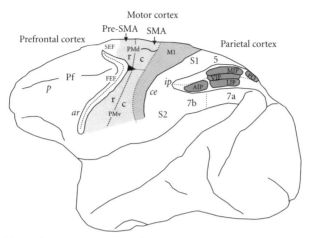

Fig. 4.1 Subdivisions of premotor cortex and parietal cortex shown on a lateral view of the macaque brain. Arcuate (ar) and intraparietal (ip) sulci are opened to expose hidden areas. Abbreviations: ce, central sulcus; p, principal sulcus; Pf, prefrontal cortex; PMd and PMv, dorsal and ventral premotor areas, with caudal (c) and rostral (r) subdivisions; M1, primary motor cortex; SMA, supplementary motor area; SEF, supplementary eye field; FEF, frontal eye field; AIP, LIP, MIP, and VIP, anterior, lateral, medial and ventral intraparietal areas, respectively; PO, parieto-occipital area; 7a, 7b, S1, S2, and 5, parietal subdivisions following Brodmann.

cortex and the motor cortex (Boussaoud *et al.* 1996; Wise *et al.* 1997). This has now been achieved due to progress made in the anatomy and physiology of the cortical networks. On the one hand, more sensitive anatomical tracing techniques have shown that some areas of the superior parietal lobule send direct projections to the premotor areas (Cavada and Goldman-Rakic 1989; Johnson *et al.* 1996; Tanné-Gariépy *et al.* 2002). On the other hand, understanding of the anatomical and functional organization of the posterior parietal cortex has improved substantially (Fig. 4.1). In particular, the superior parietal lobule (SPL), considered until the 1980s to be 'blind' in the sense of being devoid of visual inputs, is now known to contain areas with visual response properties and with direct connections with the visual cortex (Felleman and van Essen 1991). These parietal areas are the primary source of visual information to the premotor cortex (Pandya and Kuypers 1969; Petrides and Pandya 1984; Cavada and Goldman-Rakic 1989; Kurata 1994; Ghosh and Gattera 1995; Johnson *et al.* 1996; Matelli *et al.* 1998; Shipp *et al.* 1998; Tanné-Gariépy *et al.* 2002) as they are strongly connected to the extrastriate visual cortex, including areas V2, V3, MT, MST, and 7a (Colby *et al.* 1988; Cavada and Goldman-Rakic 1989; Boussaoud *et al.* 1990; Felleman and van Essen 1991; Shipp *et al.* 1998). The most direct pathway seems to originate from the parieto-occipital region (Johnson *et al.* 1996; Shipp *et al.* 1998; Tanné-Gariépy *et al.* 2002). These parieto-premotor pathways seem to be organized into parallel pathways which may serve different visuomotor functions (Fig. 4.2), see Chapter 2, this volume.

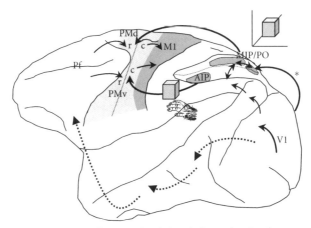

Fig. 4.2 Visual and visuomotor pathways. Visual signals from the visual cortex are directed to the posterior parietal cortex (dorsal stream) or the inferior temporal cortex (ventral stream). Both streams project to the prefrontal cortex (Pf), from which visual signals can reach the premotor cortex. In addition, the dorsal stream has direct inputs to the premotor cortex which are organized into at least two parallel pathways: one pathway rises from dorsomedial parietal areas (namely MIP and PO) and terminates in PMd, and the other originates from lateral parietal areas (namely area AIP) and terminates in PMv. The former mediates visuospatial information (represented by a cube in 3D space), and the latter processes object information for grasping and manipulation (represented by the cube and the hand). The asterisk indicates projections from the peripheral visual field representation of V1.

A parieto-premotor network for reaching and eye–hand coordination

Reaching movements are carried out by a parietofrontal network involving the superior parietal lobule (SPL) and the dorsal premotor cortex. Neurophysiological studies have shown that, within this network, areas share neuronal signals necessary for reaching movements and eye–hand coordination (Boussaoud *et al.* 1998; Caminiti *et al.* 1998; Shipp *et al.* 1998; Boussaoud and Bremmer 1999; Battaglia-Mayer *et al.* 2001; Marconi *et al.* 2001). In particular, in addition to visuospatial information, a variety of extra-retinal signals are present in both the parietal and premotor areas, including eye position signals and directional signals related to arm movements (Ferraina *et al.* 1997; Boussaoud *et al.* 1998; Jouffrais and Boussaoud 1999; Battaglia-Mayer *et al.* 2001; Fujii *et al.* 2000; Snyder *et al.* 2000; Buneo *et al.* 2002). Thus it appears that the superior parietal areas and PMd form a neuronal network that combines visual signals with other sensory and motor signals in order to build motor commands for reaching movements. These signals are also used to compute coordinate transformations. In this respect, it is worth stressing that several parietal areas use a common eye-centered frame of reference (reviewed by Andersen and Buneo 2002), and that neurons of the dorsal premotor cortex were also found to code limb movement direction in eye-centered coordinates (Boussaoud *et al.* 1998). Furthermore, modulation of eye-centered representation of eye and limb movement takes the form of gain fields when eye, head, or body position is changed systematically (Boussaoud and Bremmer 1999; Cohen and Andersen 2002). It was suggested that this common reference frame within the parietal cortex (Cohen and Andersen 2002) would facilitate communication between areas involved in coding movements of different effectors, such as LIP (for saccades) and parietal reach region (PRR, reaching). Such a facilitating role might also be important within the larger network formed by reciprocally connected areas of parietal and premotor cortex.

Another parieto-premotor network is specialized for grasping (Fig. 4.2). It involves mainly areas AIP (anterior intraparietal area) and 7b of the inferior parietal lobule, and the ventral premotor cortex (PMv). Area AIP, in particular, sends most of its frontal projections to PMv (Matelli *et al.* 1986, 1994; Ghosh and Gattera 1995; Sakata *et al.* 1997; Tanné-Gariéppy *et al.* 2002), and the two areas share neuronal properties pertinent to object manipulation and control of grasping movements (reviewed by Jeannerod *et al.* 1995; Sakata *et al.* 1997). Both areas contain neurons whose activity is related to hand manipulation of specific objects (Rizzolatti *et al.* 1988; Taira *et al.* 1990; Hepp-Reymond *et al.* 1994; Sakata *et al.* 1995, 1997; Murata *et al.* 1996; Shikata *et al.* 1996), and their lesion or reversible inactivation leads to grasping deficits (Gallese *et al.* 1994). A similar network seems to exist in the human brain, and its lesions cause deficits in grasping behavior (Jeannerod *et al.* 1994; Binkofski *et al.* 1999).

The problem of coordination

Sensorimotor transformations for reaching and grasping are clearly carried out by distinct parietofrontal systems, which are largely independent until the motor cortex. However, behavioral data suggest that these two components of prehension interact (Paulignan *et al.* 1991a,b; Roy *et al.* 2002). From the behavioral point of view, reaching to grasp an object can be described in terms of two parallel input–output visuomotor channels (Jeannerod and Biguer 1982), one for reaching and the other for grasping. The reaching channel requires information on the object's location in space and uses proximal arm muscles, whereas grasping needs information relative to the intrinsic attributes of the object (namely size and shape) and involves distal hand muscles. Behavioral studies have shown that changing one of the input variables (e.g. size or location) affects both reaching and grasping (Paulignan *et al.* 1991a,b; Roy *et al.* 2002), suggesting that the two visuomotor channels are coordinated. This coordination is partly due to biomechanical constraints, but central processes seem to be involved as well, allowing flexibility and adaptation to task demands, as suggested by Roy *et al.* (2002). One question is how this coordination is carried out in the brain, and more specifically in the parietofrontal anatomical circuits.

Anatomically, the dichotomy between reaching and grasping is an attractive and convincing model. If two distinct retrograde tracers are injected into the arm representation of PMd and the hand representation of PMv, respectively, the labeled neurons in the parietal cortex occupy largely separate regions (Fig. 4.3). This suggests that different sets of parietal signals are sent to the arm and hand representations and that coordination is not achieved by means of divergent/convergent parieto-premotor inputs, at least at first glance (but see Tanné-Gariépy *et al.* 2002). Physiologically, PMd contains the representation of proximal muscles, whereas PMv contains that of distal muscles of the hand (Sessle and Wiesendanger 1982; Weinrich and Wise 1982; Godschalk *et al.* 1995). However, other studies suggest that the body representation in PMd includes the hand and the eyes (Godschalk *et al.* 1995; Fogassi *et al.* 1999; Fujii *et al.* 2000;

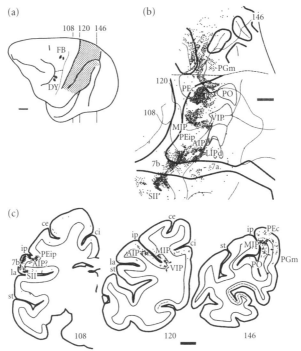

Fig. 4.3 Segregated parietal inputs to dorsal (PMd) and ventral (PMv) premotor areas. (a) Lateral view of the monkey left hemisphere showing the injection sites. (b) Two-dimensional map showing retrogradely labeled cells and the cortical areas concerned. Red dots represent labeled cells following DY injection; blue dots show the labeled cells following FB injection. Sulci and sulcal labels are shown in italics. Myeloarchitectonic borders are depicted by the thin green lines. (c) Representative coronal sections whose locations are indicated on the lateral view (a) and the 2D map (b). The small arrows indicate the myeloarchitectonic boundaries. Scale bar, 5 mm. Orientation is shown for (a), (b), and (c) (M, medial; R, rostral). Abbreviations: AIP, anterior intraparietal area; LIPd and LIPv, dorsal and ventral subdivisions of the lateral intraparietal area, respectively; MIP, medial intraparietal area; PEc, PEip and PGm, subdivisions used by Pandya and Seltzer (1982) and Matelli *et al.* (1998); PO, parieto-occipital area; VIP, ventral intraparietal area; SI and SII, first and second somatosensory areas. For other abbreviations see Figs 4.1 and 4.2.

Tanné-Gariépy *et al.* 2002). Also, PMv contains the representation of distal muscles of the hand and mouth in the anterior region (PMvr or F5), but has an arm representation caudally (F4) (Rizzolatti *et al.* 1988; Gentilucci *et al.* 1988; Hepp-Reymond *et al.* 1994; Preuss *et al.* 1996). In short, PMd and PMv contain representations of the forelimb, including proximal and distal muscles, which receive spatial and object information, respectively, from the parietal cortex. Thus the problem of coordination might have at least two solutions. The first is through shared parietal projections to PMd and PMv (Tanné-Gariépy *et al.* 2002). These projections are numerically weak, but they could play an important role. Another solution might be through interconnections between different body-part representations within the parietal cortex. Indeed, there are many interactions within the parietal cortex which may facilitate interactions between different representations in both parietal and premotor areas. For instance, local processing within PMv might allow coordination of arm, hand, and mouth representations during feeding behavior. On the other hand, interactions between eyes, hand, and proximal representations in PMd would allow eye–hand coordination during reaching to grasp an object in space or to point to a target.

Motor preparation, motor set, or intention

Neurophysiology

The involvement of the premotor cortex in motor preparation, or intention, has been studied since the early days of behavioral neurophysiology using tasks with an instructed delay period (Weinrich and Wise 1982). An instruction stimulus (IS), usually a visual cue, specifies the action to be made, but the subject has to wait until another visual or auditory stimulus (the GO signal) is given. The rationale in this design is to create a time window, the delay period, during which the animal knows what to do (and therefore forms an intention to do it) but has to wait for an instruction to do it. In other words, instructed delay paradigms allow the experimenter somehow to 'read' the intentions of the subject. Wise and coworkers have contributed considerably to the understanding of the fundamental neurophysiological correlates of motor intention (Wise 1984). Their early work showed that premotor cortex neurons are active during the preparatory delay, and that this delay activity appears to be correlated with movement direction (Weinrich *et al.* 1984; Wise and Mauritz 1982). Other studies have investigated the relation between the neuronal activity and other movement parameters, namely the amplitude (Riehle and Requin 1989; Kurata 1994; Fu *et al.* 1995). Neural activity during the instructed delay period was reported in a variety of cortical regions, including the prefrontal cortex, the parietal cortex and subcortical structures such as the basal ganglia. However, the functional interpretation of this apparently similar activity differs from one brain region to another. For example, delay activity has been interpreted in relation to working memory in the prefrontal cortex (Funahashi *et al.* 1990), intention in the premotor cortex (Boussaoud *et al.* 1996; Wise *et al.* 1997) and recently in the parietal cortex (Andersen and Buneo 2002). Further analysis shows that an important difference exists between the preparatory activity of the parietal cortex and that of the premotor cortex. Kalaska and Crammond (1995) have shown that the delay activity in the premotor cortex reflected the decision not to move, whereas in parietal area 5 neurons fire similarly in GO and NOGO trials. This finding suggests that the parietal cortex codes the direction of future actions even when they are not executed later, and their influence on the premotor cortex translates into activity only if those actions are executed. These neurophysiological findings might correspond to different hierarchical levels of intention.

Brain imaging

The role of premotor cortex in motor preparation has also been supported by brain imaging investigations in humans (Kawashima *et al.* 1994; Deiber *et al.* 1996, 1997; Richter *et al.* 1997; Lee *et al.* 1999; van Oostende *et al.* 1997; Grafton *et al.* 1998; Toni *et al.* 1999, 2001; Simon *et al.* 2002). In agreement with neurophysiological findings, these studies outlined, in addition to the dorsal premotor cortex, a frontal cortical network including the primary motor cortex and the medial premotor areas (pre-SMA, SMA, and cingulate motor areas) using positron emission tomography (Deiber *et al.* 1996; Krams *et al.* 1998; Rushworth *et al.* 2001) or event-related functional magnetic resonance imaging (fMRI) (Lee *et al.* 1999; Toni *et al.* 1999). Some of these studies also reported activation in the parietal cortex during movement preparation, but this is still an issue of debate (Simon *et al.* 2002).

Attention versus intention

There are several possible confounds in studies of motor preparation. For example, when activity changes with the direction of movement, it may of course reflect the intention to move in a specific direction, but it may also correlate partly or entirely with orientation of attention to a different part of space and/or directing gaze toward the region of interest. Experimental designs have been developed in order to dissociate these parameters one from another, in particular attention from intention. However, some theories argue that attention and intention are not dissociable. One of them is the 'premotor theory' of attention (Rizzolatti 1983), which postulates that attention results from the activity of premotor circuits signaling an intended action which then influences selective attention. This theory implies that attention and intention are mediated by the same brain network. However, others suggest that the attention system is separate from the systems involved in perception and action (Posner and Petersen 1990). The data accumulated in recent years tend to support an intermediate possibility where the two systems are distinct from each other, but partially overlap. Evidence from neurophysiology and from brain imaging work in favor of this alternative is presented in this section.

Neurophysiology

With the use of well-controlled experimental designs, it is possible to dissociate neuronal activity related to attention versus intention, as well as a variety of sensori-motor processes such as sensory processing from motor processing (Boussaoud and Wise 1993a,b; di Pellegrino and Wise 1993; Crammond and Kalaska 1994; Lebedev and Wise 2001). We will concentrate on the studies which have addressed the issue of how to dissociate attention from motor preparation (Boussaoud and Wise 1993a,b; di Pellegrino and Wise 1993; Lebedev and Wise 2001), and on the comparison of two frontal regions, the dorsolateral prefrontal cortex and the dorsal premotor cortex. We will review data showing that the premotor cortex codes the motor significance of visuospatial stimuli rather than merely the sensory attributes of instructional cues, or attention to such stimuli, whereas prefrontal cortex neurons are active with stimuli or attention to these stimuli, often independently of their instructional content.

The SAM–MIC task

Several studies have addressed the issue of dissociation between visual and visuomotor signals in the premotor cortex and elsewhere in the brain (Boussaoud *et al.* 1996; Wise *et al.* 1997), and have contributed significantly to the understanding of the sensorimotor transformations. However, few experimental designs have controlled for gaze, spatial attention, or the visuospatial attributes of the cues that guide an action (Boussaoud and Wise 1993a,b; di Pellegrino and Wise 1993). The general approach was to present identical visual stimuli that can either direct the focus of attention or instruct movement of the limb in a given direction. There were two assumptions. According to the first, cells related to intention would begin to discharge only after an instruction specifies the parameters of movement, here its direction; cells involved in selective attention would discharge in relation to cues that specify where relevant information is likely to appear (Fig. 4.4). The second assumption was that, during the instructed delay period, activity related to the intention to move in a given direction would remain insensitive to changes in stimulus attributes. Thus, if several different stimuli instruct a movement to the right, activity will remain constant. Conversely, if activity changes in this situation, then it reflects partly or entirely sensory input.

The experimental design has been described in detail elsewhere (Boussaoud and Wise 1993a,b; Boussaoud and Kemadi 1997). In summary, the design creates a situation where the same visual stimulus guided spatial attention and/or memory during the first part of the trial and instructed a limb movement during the second part of the same trial (Fig. 4.5). A neuron whose discharge rate is higher following the attentional cue than after the identical stimulus presented as an intentional stimulus is considered to be related to spatial attention and/or memory. In the opposite case, the neuron is considered to be related to intention. As expected, the activity of some neurons did not differ, possibly reflecting low-level sensory processing.

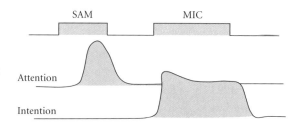

Fig. 4.4 Schematic representation of hypothetical neurons with attention versus intention activity: SAM, spatial attentional mnemonic cue; MIC, motor instructional cue.

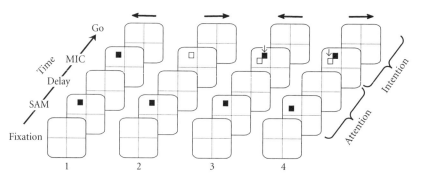

Fig. 4.5 Behavioral paradigm for attention–intention dissociation. Each diagonally oriented column represents one kind of trial among 56 types used. Time progresses from bottom left to upper right, as represented by the arrow on the left. In each screen (panel), the center represents the fixation point, the small squares indicate the location of the stimuli. A filled square indicates a red stimulus, and an open square represents a green stimulus. From bottom to top, the first panel shows the state of the video screen after the monkey has initiated the trial and put its gaze on the fixation point (fixation); the following panels represent the presentation of the spatial attentional mnemonic (SAM) cue, the post-SAM delay, the motor instructional cue (MIC) period including the instructed delay time, and finally the offset of MIC (the GO signal). The horizontal arrows indicate the direction of arm movement on each trial. The vertical arrows in trials 3 and 4 point to the square to select when there are two squares.

Previous neurophysiological studies led to the idea that the premotor cortex (PMd) codes intention. If so, they should be active when an intention to move is formed, not necessarily during attention. This is in fact the case for more than three-quarters of premotor cortex neurons. Figure 4.6 illustrates an example of cells with no activity during the first part of the trials (attention/memory), but with a high rate of activity during the intention phase. Additional indication that such activity reflects intention is further supported by the fact that it changes with direction of the intended movement when all other factors are controlled (gaze, attention). From these two observations, it can be concluded that most dorsal premotor cortex cells are not influenced by attention, at least not directly. In the prefrontal cortex, most cells are active during the first phase of the trials, i.e. in relation to spatial attention/memory (Figs 4.7 and 4.8(a)). Furthermore, during the intention phase, activity rate changes significantly when

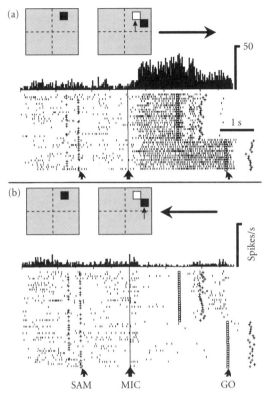

Fig. 4.6 Example of intention-related activity. Several trials are grouped by movement direction (indicated by the horizontal arrows), independently of the color or location of the SAM. In each raster, a vertical tick indicates the time of occurrence of an action potential. A line of vertical ticks represents the neuron's activity in one trial. The trials are aligned on the onset of the MIC cue (vertical line). Beneath each raster line, the plus signs mark the time of onset of the SAM cue, and the squares show the time of offset of MIC (the GO signal). Above each raster is a post-stimulus histogram (bin width, 20.4 ms). The MIC is composed of two adjacent squares, and the subject must select the square that matches the location of the SAM and respond following the rule (a) green = right or (b) red = left. Note that the neuron does not discharge after the SAM cue, and that the increase in activity after MIC onset and during the instructed delay period is observed only for movement to the right (a).

different stimuli instruct the same movement direction, suggesting the sensory nature of prefrontal activity.

This conclusion has been reached by other studies where attention and intention were dissociable (di Pellegrino and Wise 1993). di Pellegrino and Wise found many instances of PMd neurons with discharge modulations that could not be explained in terms of the attributes of the stimulus or of its role in directing spatial attention or memory. Instead, the activity of these cells reflects, at least in part, the instructional significance of those stimuli. Significantly fewer movement effects were observed in a relatively small

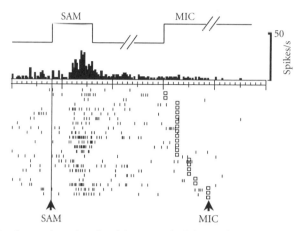

Fig. 4.7 Example of attention-related activity. Several trials are aligned on the onset of the SAM cue (vertical line). Same conventions as in Fig. 4.6.

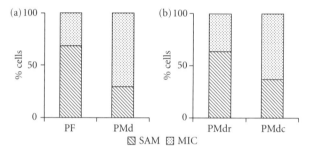

Fig. 4.8 (a) Comparison of the proportion of attention-related and intention-related cells in the dorsolateral prefrontal cortex (PF) and the dorsal premotor cortex (PMd). (b) Comparison of rostral versus caudal PMd.

population of cells in the prefrontal cortex, mainly ventral to the principal sulcus. Taken together, the comparison of cell activity in PMd and the prefrontal cortex indicates two main differences. One is that prefrontal cells are much more influenced by spatial attention/memory than by a specific intention to act. Secondly, during the intention phase of the trials, premotor activity is less prone to sensory influences than prefrontal activity. Thus activity of PMd neurons appears to represent the intentions created by stimuli, whereas activity of prefrontal cortex neurons codes factors other than instructional significance; one of them is spatial attention/memory.

Intrinsic organization of PMd

The dorsal premotor area is a large extent of cortex which can no longer be viewed as a homogeneous area. Several lines of evidence suggest that it contains at least two subregions, one rostral (PMdr) and one caudal (PMdc), which have different corticocortical connections and neuronal properties. Anatomically, the two PMd regions are part of two separate networks: a motor network and a cognitive network. Rostral PMd receives most of prefrontal inputs (Arikuni *et al.* 1980, 1988; Barbas and Pandya 1987; Boussaoud *et al.* 1996), but does not project to either the primary motor cortex (M1) or the spinal cord. On the contrary, PMdc receives weak inputs from the prefrontal cortex but projects strongly to both M1 and the spinal cord. The two subdivisions of PMd receive differential inputs from the parietal cortex (Johnson *et al.* 1996; Matelli *et al.* 1998; Shipp *et al.* 1998; Tanné-Gariépy *et al.* 2002). Visual signals from the parietal cortex are directed predominantly to PMdr, whereas parietal inputs to PMdc are likely to mediate motor and sensorimotor signals. There are two sources of physiological evidence that PMdr and PMdc could play differential roles. First, intracortical microstimulation elicits movements of the forelimb when applied to PMdc, whereas PMdr is not microexcitable (Sessle and Wiesendanger 1982; Weinrich and Wise 1982; Godschalk *et al.* 1995). This is compatible with the anatomical connections described above, especially regarding the projections to M1 and the spinal cord. Secondly, single-cell recordings in awake monkeys have reported differences in the neuronal properties of the two subdivisions (Johnson *et al.* 1996; Tanné-Gariépy *et al.* 2002). Cells in PMdr display activity in response to sensory cues, whereas cells in PMdc are less active in relation to the cues but discharge during the preparatory phase of movement as well as during movement execution.

Interestingly, it was found that the distribution of attention- and intention-related cells varies along the rostrocaudal axis in PMd (Boussaoud 2001; Lebedev and Wise 2001). Cells with spatial attention/memory properties tend to be found rostrally, whereas intention-related cells are mostly found caudally in PMd (Fig. 4.8(b)), in agreement with the anatomical and physiological data reviewed above. These data suggest that, in the monkey, PMdr and PMdc play different roles in movement planning. Given its links with the prefrontal cortex and posterior parietal areas, rostral PMd might play a role in high-order cognitive processes that precede action planning, such as selecting the goal of action and/or its temporal organization. In contrast, caudal PMd, which is connected to M1 and the spinal cord, would be more directly involved in movement preparation and execution. This hypothesis is supported by brain imaging studies in humans, which suggest that the distinction of the portions of PMd can be extended to the human brain, as reviewed below.

Brain imaging

The dorsal premotor cortex in humans has been implicated in a variety of functions, including overt and covert spatial attention, working memory (Petit *et al.* 1996, 1998; Corbetta *et al.* 1998; Coull and Nobre 1998; Courtney *et al.* 1998; D'Esposito *et al.* 1998; Kawashima *et al.* 1998; Stern *et al.* 2000), and motor preparation (Deiber *et al.* 1996; Krams *et al.* 1998; Lee *et al.* 1999; Toni *et al.* 1999; Rushworth *et al.* 2001). The question is whether the premotor cortex indeed plays a role in all these functions, and if so whether they are carried out by the same or different populations of premotor neurons. Neurophysiological studies in the monkey would predict the latter possibility for the distinction between attention/memory and intention.

In a recent fMRI study (Simon *et al.* 2002), the design used to dissociate attention/memory and intention was adapted and performed by normal volunteers while their brains were scanned using a 1.5 T machine. The subjects viewed visual stimuli and responded by pressing a key with their index or middle finger depending on a simple rule (red = index; green = middle). The experiment was run in four blocs of trials, two for attention and intention tasks and two for their respective controls. The general strategy was as follows.

1. The attention task emphasized shifting the locus of attention from one peripheral location to another, while fixating. The control for this task included the same stimuli and motor responses, except that subjects did not have to attend to the peripheral stimuli, but to the central cross.

2. The motor preparation task required subjects to prepare to respond with a button press for long and variable delays. Again, the control here was similar in all aspects, except that subjects did not have to wait for a GO signal; instead, they responded immediately after the instruction.

3. The two comparisons (attention–control; preparation–control) are made in the same group of subjects, which allows direct comparison of the spatial distribution of brain activation.

While fixating a central cross (Fig. 4.9), subjects shifted the locus of their attention to a peripheral stimulus (SAM) presented at various locations on a video screen. After the final presentation, two squares appeared, one at the exact location of the previous SAM, and one adjacent to it. Subjects were told to select the pre-cued square and respond by pressing a key with their index finger (if it was red) or middle finger (if it was green). The control bloc for this task was identical in terms of visual stimuli and motor response, but subjects were instructed to fixate the cross and respond when it changed color, based on the same color–response rule. Thus the design established two situations: one in which spatial attention and/or memory moved from one peripheral location to another, and the other where peripheral stimuli were irrelevant to the performance of the task (baseline task). Subtraction of baseline activation from the activation during the attention task should leave activity which is correlated with spatial attention/memory. In the intention paradigm, instructional cues lasted for a variable delay (up to 5.5 s) during which the subjects awaited for the GO signal (cue offset) to make the appropriate key press (Fig. 4.9). Again, the baseline bloc was identical in all visual and motor parameters, except that subjects were told to respond as soon as possible after MIC presentation and to keep fixating until the end of the trial. Subtraction of the baseline activation from the preparation activation should leave activation related to movement preparation.

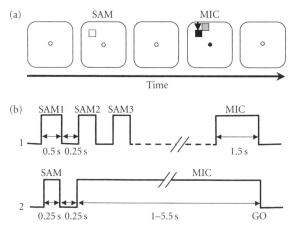

Fig. 4.9 Experimental design for the fMRI experiment. (a) Basic structure of the task. Each panel represents the stimulation screen at a particular point in time. First panel from left: a white cross at the screen center for fixation; Next panel: a white square (the SAM cue) is presented at one among several possible peripheral locations. After a delay (the last delay in the attention task), two squares are presented (MIC), one at the location of the previous SAM cue and the other at an adjacent location. They remain on for a fixed period of 1.5 s or a variable period of 1–5.5 s. After this period, MIC is extinguished and, simultaneously, the cross changes color from white to either red or green. (b) Sequence of events for (1) the attention and (2) the intention tasks. Note that in the attention task, SAM was presented 4, 8, or 12 times in each trial.

One limitation of this experimental was that spatial attention and memory were not dissociable, as subjects had to keep the location of the attentional cue in mind. Therefore activity associated with attention is probably at least partly due to working memory.

Premotor cortex is a site of convergence of attention and intention

Attention activates a large cortical network including the dorsal premotor cortex, parietal cortex, lateral prefrontal cortex, and medial premotor cortex (Fig. 4.10). Previous studies have already reported the involvement of this network in spatial attention and working memory (Corbetta *et al.* 1998; Coull and Nobre 1998; Kawashima *et al.* 1998; Smith and Jonides 1999; Haxby *et al.* 2000; Nobre *et al.* 2000; Beauchamp *et al.* 2001). One recurrent issue here, unlike in the monkey brain, is that the human premotor cortex is not easily distinguishable from the frontal eye field (FEF), which is activated by attention with and without eye movements (Corbetta *et al.* 1998; Gitelman *et al.* 1999; Beauchamp *et al.* 2001). Using a saccade task to locate FEF, Simon *et al.* (2002) have demonstrated that dorsal premotor activation during the attention task goes beyond the region activated by saccadic eye movements. This clearly demonstrates that the attentional network includes part of the dorsal premotor cortex.

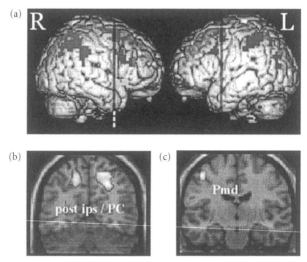

Fig. 4.10 Brain activation in relation to spatial attention/memory versus intention. Group analysis of the main effects of the two tasks relative to their baseline conditions. Red, attention minus baseline; yellow, intention minus baseline; green, overlap of the two activations. (a) Activation of surface view of left (L) and right (R) hemispheres. (b) Activity specifically associated with attention. (c) Activity specifically related to intention. Abbreviations as in previous figures.

Intention activates a frontal cortical network which includes the caudal portion of the dorsal premotor cortex bilaterally, the primary motor cortex contralateral to the moving finger, and the medial premotor cortex (both the pre-SMA and SMA regions and the underlying cingulate sulcus). This confirms the findings of other studies (Deiber *et al.* 1996; Krams *et al.* 1998; Lee *et al.* 1999; Toni *et al.* 1999; Rushworth *et al.* 2001). However, unlike previous studies, Simon *et al.* (2002) report no significant activation in the parietal cortex during the intention task.

Finally, attention and intention appear to activate different zones of dorsal premotor cortex, in line with the prediction made on the basis of monkey physiology. Spatial attention/memory preferentially activated a rostral region, in and anterior to the precentral sulcus, whereas intention engaged a more caudal portion of PMd located in the precentral gyrus (Simon *et al.* 2002).

Concluding remarks

Significant progress has been made in our understanding of the neuronal bases of attention and motor intention. With controlled experiments, it has been possible to dissociate the two processes and to identify their functional anatomy using modern techniques. Converging evidence from several sources supports the idea that the dorsal premotor cortex is organized functionally in the anterior to posterior axis. The anterior region receives direct, and perhaps very fast, visual pathways from the dorsal visual stream, and indirect ones from the prefrontal cortex (Fig. 4.11). Inputs mediated by these direct and indirect connections may trigger a wave of activity which propagates

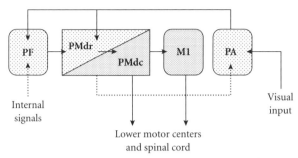

Fig. 4.11 A simplifying model of premotor function. Visual pathways from parietal cortex can reach PMd directly, or indirectly via the prefrontal cortex. Neural activity in rostral PMd is influenced by attention through these pathways. PMdr may in turn influence action selection in caudal PMd through intrinsic connections. The two subdivisions of PMd contain a gradient of neuronal properties (represented by the different shadings). Other signals may bias processing, such us internal inputs to PF (internally guided attention), or feedback signals from PMd to parietal cortex.

towards the caudal premotor cortex, and from there to the primary motor cortex and to lower motor centers. Attention and intention can be viewed as extremes of this complex chain of neural operations which meet at the level of premotor cortex, thereby allowing attention to influence intention and action selection.

Acknowledgement

This work was supported by the Centre National de la Recherche Scientifique.

References

Anderson RA, Buneo CA (2002). International maps in posterior prefrontal cortex. *Annu Rev Neurosci*, **25**, 189–220.

Arikuni T, Sakai M, Hamada I, Kubota K (1980). Topographical projections from the prefrontal cortex to the postarcuate area in the rhesus monkey, studied by retrograde axonal transport of horseradish peroxidase. *Neurosci Lett*, **19**, 155–60.

Arikuni T, Watanabe K, Kubota K (1988). Connections of area 8 with area 6 in the brain of the macaque monkey. *J Comp Neurol*, **277**, 21–40.

Barbas H, Pandya DN (1987). Architecture, and frontal cortical connections of the premotor cortex (area 6) in the rhesus monkey. *J Comp Neurol*, **256**, 211–28.

Battaglia-Mayer A, Ferraina S, Genovesio A, Marconi B, Squatrito S, Molinari M, *et al.* (2001). Eye–hand coordination during reaching. II. An analysis of the relationships between visuomanual signals in parietal cortex and parieto-frontal association projections. *Cereb Cortex*, **11**, 528–44.

Beauchamp MS, Petit L, Emmore TM, Ingeholm J, Haxby JV (2001). A parametric study of overt and covert shifts of visuospatial attention. *NeuroImage*, **14**, 310–21.

Binkofski F, Buccino G, Posse S, Seitz RJ, Rizzolatti G, Freund H (1999). A fronto-parietal circuit for object manipulation in man: evidence from an fMRI-study. *Eur J Neurosci*, **11**, 3276–86.

Boussaoud D (2001). Attention vs. intention in the primate premotor cortex. *NeuroImage*, **14**, S40–S45.

Boussaoud D, Bremmer F (1999). Gaze effects in the premotor cortex and parietal cortex: distributed processing and reference frames. *Exp Brain Res*, **128**, 170–80.

Boussaoud D, Kermadi I (1997). The primate striatum: effects of attention, stimulus and movement on the neuronal activity in the macaque monkey. *Eur J Neurosci*, **9**, 2152–68.

Boussaoud D, Wise SP (1993a). Primate frontal cortex: neuronal activity following attentional versus intentional cues. *Exp Brain Res*, **95**, 15–27.

Boussaoud D, Wise SP (1993b). Primate frontal cortex: effects of stimulus, and movement. *Exp Brain Res*, **95**, 28–40.

Boussaoud D, Ungerleider LG, Desimone R (1990). Pathways for motion analysis: cortical connections of the medial superior temporal, and fundus of the superior temporal visual areas in the macaque. *J Comp Neurol*, **296**, 462–95.

Boussaoud D, di Pellegrino G, Wise SP (1996). Frontal lobe mechanisms subserving vision-for-action versus vision-for-perception. *Behav Brain Res*, **72**, 1–15.

Boussaoud D, Jouffrais C, Bremmer F (1998). Eye position effects on the neuronal activity of dorsal premotor cortex in the macaque monkey. *J Neurophysiol*, **80**, 1132–50.

Buneo CA, Jarvis MR, Batista AP, Andersen RA (2002). Direct visuomotor transformations for reaching. *Nature*, **416**, 632–6.

Caminiti R, Ferraina S, Johnson PB (1996). The sources of visual information to the primate frontal lobe: a novel role for the superior parietal lobule. *Cereb Cortex*, **6**, 319–28.

Caminiti R, Ferraina S, Mayer AB (1998). Visuomotor transformations: early cortical mechanisms of reaching. *Curr Opin Neurobiol*, **8**, 753–61.

Cavada C, Goldman-Rakic PS (1989). Posterior parietal cortex in rhesus monkey: II. Evidence for segregated corticocortical networks linking sensory, and limbic areas with the frontal lobe. *J Comp Neurol*, **287**, 422–45.

Cohen YE, Andersen RA (2002). A common reference frame for movement plans in the posterior parietal cortex. *Nat Rev Neurosci*, **3**, 553–62.

Colby CL, Gattass R, Olson CR, Gross CG (1988). Topographical organization of cortical afferents to extrastriate area PO in the macaque, a dual tracer study. *J Comp Neurol*, **269**, 392–413.

Corbetta M, Akbudak E, Conturo TE, Snyder AZ, Ollinger JM, Drury MA, *et al.* (1998). A common network of functional areas for attention and eye movements. *Neuron*, **21**, 761–73.

Coull JT, Nobre AC (1998). Where and when to pay attention, the neural systems for directing attention to spatial locations and to time intervals as revealed by both PET and fMRI. *J Neurosci*, **18**, 7426–35.

Crammond DJ, Kalaska JF (1994). Modulation of preparatory neuronal activity in dorsal premotor cortex due to stimulus–response compatibility. *J Neurophysiol*, **71**, 1281–84.

Critchley M (1953). *The Parietal Lobes*. London: Edward Arnold.

D'Esposito M, Aguirre GK, Zarahn E, Ballard D, Shin RK, Lease J (1998). Functional MRI studies of spatial and nonspatial working memory. *Cogn Brain Res*, **7**, 1–13.

Deiber M-P, Ibanez V, Sadato N, Hallett M (1996). Cerebral structures participating in motor preparation in humans: a positron emission tomography study. *J Neurophysiol*, **75**, 233–47.

Deiber M-P, Wise SP, Honda M, Catalan MJ, Grafman J, Hallett M (1997). Frontal and parietal networks for conditional motor learning: a positron emission tomography study. *J Neurophysiol*, **78**, 977–91.

di Pellegrino G, Wise SP (1993). Visuospatial versus visuomotor activity in the premotor, and prefrontal cortex of a primate. *J Neurosci*, **13**, 1227–43.

Felleman DJ, van Essen DC (1991). Distributed hierarchical processing in the primate cerebral cortex. *Cereb Cortex*, **1**, 1–47.

Ferraina S, Johnson PB, Garasto MR, Battaglia-Mayer A, Ercolani L, Bianchi L, *et al.* (1997). Combination of hand and gaze signals during reaching : activity in parietal area 7m of the monkey. *J Neurophysiol*, **77**(2), 1034–8.

Fogassi L, Raos V, Franchi G, Gallese V, Luppino G, Matelli M, (1999). Visual responses in the dorsal premotor area F2 of the macaque monkey. *Exp Brain Res*, **128**, 194–9.

Fu QG, Flament D, Coltz JD, Ebner TJ (1995). Temporal encoding of movements kinematics in the discharge of primate primary motor and premotor neurons. *J Neurophysiol*, **73**, 836–54.

Fujii N, Mushiake H, Tanji J (2000). Rostrocaudal distinction of the dorsal premotor area based on oculomotor involvement. *J Neurophysiol*, **83**, 1764–69.

Funahashi S, Bruce CJ, Goldman-Rakic PS (1990). Visuospatial coding in primate prefrontal neurons revealed by oculomotor paradigms. *J Neurophysiol*, **63**, 814–31.

Gallese V, Murata A, Kaseda M, Niki N, Sakata H (1994). Deficit of hand preshaping after muscimol injection in monkey parietal cortex. *Neuroreport*, **5**, 1525–9.

Gentilucci M, Fogassi L, Luppino G, Matelli M, Camarda R, Rizzolatti G (1988). Functional organization of inferior area 6 in the macaque monkey: I. Somatotopy, and the control of proximal movements. *Exp Brain Res*, **71**, 475–90.

Ghosh S, Gattera R (1995). A comparison of the ipsilateral cortical projections to the dorsal and ventral subdivisions of the macaque premotor cortex. *Somatosens Mot Res*, **12**, 359–78.

Godschalk M, Mitz AR, van Duin B, van der Burg H (1995). Somatotopy of monkey premotor cortex examined with microstimulation. *Neurosci Res*, **23**, 269–79.

Grafton ST, Fagg AH, Arbib MA (1998). Dorsal premotor cortex and conditional movement selection: a PET functional mapping study. *J Neurophysiol*, **79**, 1092–7.

Haxby JV, Petit L, Ungerleider L, Courtney SM (2000). Distinguishing the functional roles of multiple regions in distributed neural systems for visual working memory. *NeuroImage*, **11**, 380–91.

Hepp-Reymond M-C, Huesler EJ, Maier MA, Qi H-X (1994). Force-related neuronal activity in two regions of the primate ventral premotor cortex. *Can J Physiol Pharmacol*, **72**, 571–9.

Jeannerod M, Biguer B (1982). Visuomotor mechanisms in reaching within extrapersonal space. In D Ingle, MA Goodale, R Mansfield, (ed). *Advances in the Analysis of Visual Behavior*, pp. 387–409. Cambridge, MA: MIT Press.

Jeannerod M, Decety J, Michel F (1994). Impairment of grasping movements following a bilateral posterior parietal lesion. *Neuropsychologia*, **32**, 369–80.

Jeannerod M, Arbib MA, Rizzolatti G, Sakata H (1995). Grasping objects : the cortical mechanism of visuomotor transformation. *Trends Neurosci*, **18**, 314–20.

Johnson PB, Ferraina S, Bianchi L, Caminiti R (1996). Cortical networks for visual reaching: physiological, and anatomical organization of frontal, and parietal lobe arm regions. *Cereb Cortex*, **6**, 102–19.

Jones EG, Powell TPS (1970). An anatomical study of converging sensory pathways within the cerebral cortex of the monkey. *Brain*, **93**, 793–820.

Jouffrais C, Boussaoud D (1999). Neuronal activity related to eye–hand coordination in the primate premotor cortex. *Exp Brain Res*, **128**, 205–9.

Kalaska JF, Crammond DJ (1995). Deciding not to go: neuronal correlates of response selection in GO/NOGO task in primate premotor, and parietal cortex. *Cereb Cortex*, **5**, 410–28.

Kawashima R, Roland PE, O'Sullivan RT (1994). Fields in human motor areas involved in preparation for reaching, actual reaching, and visuo-motor learning: a positron emission tomography study. *J Neurosci*, **14**, 3462–74.

Krams M, Rushworth M, Deiber M-P, Frackowiak RSJ, Passingham, RE (1998). The preparation, execution and suppression of copied movements in the human brain. *Exp Brain Res*, **120**, 386–98.

Kurata K (1994). Information processing for motor control in primate premotor cortex. *Behav Brain Res*, **61**, 135–42.

Lebedev MA, Wise SP (2001). Tuning for the orientation of spatial attention in dorsal premotor cortex. *Eur J Neurosci*, **13**, 1002–8.

Lee KM, Chang KH, Roh JK (1999). Subregions within the supplementary motor area activated at different stages of movement preparation and execution. *NeuroImage*, **9**, 117–23.

Marconi B, Genovesio A, Battaglia-Mayer A, Ferraina S, Squatrito S, Molinari M, *et al.* (2001). Eye–hand coordination during reaching. I. Anatomical relationships between parietal and frontal cortex. *Cereb Cortex*, **11**, 513–27.

Matelli M, Camarda R, Glickstein M, Rizzolatti G (1984). Interconnections within the postarcuate cortex (area 6) of the macaque monkey. *Brain Res* **310**, 388–92.

Matelli M, Luppino G, Rizzolatti G (1985). Patterns of cytochrome oxidase activity in the frontal agranular cortex of the macaque monkey. *Behav Brain Res*, **18**, 125–36.

Matelli M, Camarda R, Glichstein M, Rizzolatti G (1986). Afferent and efferent projections in the inferior areas in the macaque monkey. *J Comp Neurol*, **251**, 281–98.

Matelli M, Luppino G, Rizzolatti G (1991). Architecture of superior, and mesial area 6, and the adjacent cingulate cortex in the macaque monkey. *J Comp Neurol*, **311**, 445–62.

Matelli M, Luppino G, Murata A, Sakata H (1994). Independent, anatomical circuits for reaching, and grasping linking inferior parietal sulcus, and inferior area 6 in macaque monkey. *Soc Neurosci Abstr*, **20**, 984.

Matelli MP, Govoni C, Galletti P, Kutz F, Luppino G (1998). Superior area 6 afferents from the superior parietal lobule in the macaque monkey. *J Comp Neurol*, **402**, 327–52.

Murata A, Gallese V, Kaseda M, Sakata H (1996). Parietal neurons related to memoryguided hand manipulation. *J Neurophysiol*, **75**, 2180–86.

Nobre AC, Gitelman DR, Dias EC, Mesulam M-M (2000). Covert visual spatial orienting and saccades, overlapping neural systems. *NeuroImage*, **11**, 210–16.

Pandya DN, Kuypers HGJM (1969). Cortico-cortical connections in the rhesus monkey. *Brain Res*, **13**, 13–36.

Pandya DN, Seltzer B (1982). Intrinsic connections and archtectonics of the posterior parietal cortex in the rhesus monkey. *J. Comp Neurol*, **204**, 196–210.

Paulignan Y, MacKenzie C, Marteniuk R, Jeannerod M (1991a). Selective perturbation of visual input during prehension movements. 1. The effects of changing object position. *Exp Brain Res*, **83**, 502–12.

Paulignan Y, MacKenzie C, Marteniuk R, Jeannerod M (1991b). Selective perturbation of visual input during prehension movements. 2. The effects of changing object size. *Exp Brain Res*, **87**, 407–20.

Petit L, Orssaud C, Tzourio N, Crivello F, Berthoz A, Mazoyer B (1996). Functional anatomy of a prelearned sequence of horizontal saccades in humans. *J Neurosci*, **16**, 3714–26.

Petit L, Courtney SM, Ungerleider L, Haxby JV (1998). Sustained activity in the medial wall during working memory delays. *J Neurosci*, **18**, 9429–37.

Petrides M, Pandya DN (1984). Projections to the frontal cortex from the posterior parietal region in the rhesus monkey. *J Comp Neurol*, **228**, 105–16.

Posner MI, Peterson SE (1990). The attention system of the human brain. *Annu Rev Neurosci*, **13**, 25–42.

Preuss T.M, Stepniewska I, Kaas JH (1996). Movement representation in the dorsal, and ventral premotor areas of owl monkeys: a microstimulation study. *J Comp Neurol*, **371**, 649–75.

Richter W, Andersen PM, Georgopoulos AP, Kim S-G (1997). Sequential activity in human motor areas during a delayed cued finger movement task studied by time-resolved fMRI. *NeuroReport*, **8**, 1257–61.

Riehle A, Requin J (1989). Monkey primary motor, and premotor cortex, single-cell activity related to prior information about direction, and extent of an intended movement. *J Neurophysiol*, **61**, 534–49.

Rizzolatti G (1983). Mechanisms of selective attention in mammals. In JP Ewert, RR Capranica, DJ Ingle, (ed.) *Advances in Vertebrate Neuroethology*, pp. 261–297. London: Plenum Press.

Rizzolatti G, Camarda R, Fogassi L, Gentilucci M, Luppino G, Matelli M (1988). Functional organization of inferior area 6 in the macaque monkey: II. Area F5, and the control of distal movements. *Exp Brain Res*, **71**, 491–507.

Roy AC, Paulignan Y, Meunier M, Boussaoud D (2002). Prehension movements in the macaque monkey, effects of object location and size. *J Neurophysiol*, **88**, 1491–9.

Rushworth MF, Krams M, Passingham RE (2001). The attentional role of the left parietal cortex, the distinct lateralization and localization of motor attention in the human brain. *J Cogn Neurosci*, **13**, 698–710.

Sakata H, Taira M, Murata A, Mine S (1995). Neural mechanisms of visual guidance of hand action in the parietal cortex of the monkey. *Cereb Cortex*, **5**, 429–38.

Sakata H, Taira M, Kusunoki M, Murata A, Tanaka Y (1997). The TINS Lecture. The parietal association cortex in depth perception, and visual control of hand action. *Trends Neurosci*, **20**, 350–7.

Sessle BJ, Wiesendanger M (1982). Structural, and functional definition of the motor cortex in the monkey (*Macaca fascicularis*). *J Physiol*, **323**, 245–65.

Shikata E, Tanaka Y, Nakamura H, Taira M, Sakata H (1996). Selectivity of the parietal visual neurons in 3D orientation of surface of stereoscopic stimuli. *Neuroreport*, **7**, 2389–94.

Shipp S, Blanton M, Zeki S (1998). A visuo-somatomotor pathway through superior parietal cortex in the macaque monkey, cortical connections of areas V6, and V6A. *Eur J Neurosci*, **10**, 3171–93.

Simon S, Meunier M, Piettre L, Berardi A, Segebarth C, Boussaoud D (2002). Spatial attention and memory versus motor preparation, premotor cortex involvement as revealed by fMRI. *J Neurophysiol*, **88**, 2047–57.

Smith EE, Jonides J (1999). Storage and executive processes in the frontal lobes. *Science*, **283**, 1657–61.

Stern CE, Owen AM, Tracey I, Look RB, Rosen BR, Petrides M (2000). Activity in ventrolateral and mid-dorsolateral prefrontal cortex during nonspatial visual working memory processing, evidence fron functional magnetic resonance imaging. *NeuroImage*, **11**, 392–9.

Taira M, Mine S, Georgopoulos AP, Murata A, Sakata H (1990). Parietal cortex neurons of the monkey related to the visual guidance of hand movement. *Exp Brain Res*, **83**, 29–36.

Tanné-Gariéppy J, Rouiller EM, Boussaoud D (2002). Parietal inputs to the premotor cortex: evidence for segregated visuo-motor pathways. *Exp Brain Res*, **145**, 91–103.

Toni I, Schluter ND, Josephs O, Friston KJ, Passingham RE (1999). Signal-, set- and movement-related activity in the human brain, an event-related fMRI study. *Cereb Cortex*, **9**, 35–49.

Toni I, Thoenissen D, Zilles K (2001). Movement preparation and motor intention. *NeuroImage*, **14**, 110–17.

Ungerleider LG, Courtney SM, Haxby JV (1998). A neural system for human visual working memory. *Proc Natl Acad Sci USA*, **95**, 883–90.

van Oostende S, Hecke PV, Sunaert S, Nuttin B, Marchal G (1997). fMRI studies of the supplementary motor area and the premotor cortex. *NeuroImage*, **6**, 181–90.

Weinrich M, Wise SP (1982). The premotor cortex of the monkey. *J Neurosci*, **2**, 1329–45.

Weinrich M, Wise SP, Mauritz KH (1984). A neurophysiological study of the premotor cortex in the rhesus monkey. *Brain*, **107**, 385–414.

Wise SP (1984). Nonprimary motor cortex and its role in the cerebral control of movement. In G Edelman, WE Gall, WM Cowan, (ed). *Dynamic Aspects of Neocortical Function*, pp. 525–55. New York: Wiley.

Wise SP, Mauritz KH (1985). Set-related neuronal activity in the premotor cortex of rhesus monkey : effects of changes in motor set. *Proc Roy Soc Lond Biol Sci*, **223**, 331–54.

Wise SP, Weinrich M, Mauritz KH (1986). Movement-related activity in the premotor cortex of rhesus macaques. *Prog Brain Res*, **64**, 117–31.

Wise SP, Boussaoud D, Johnson PB, Caminiti R (1997). Premotor, and parietal cortex, corticocortical connectivity, and combinatorial computations. *Annu Rev Neurosci*, **20**, 25–42.

Chapter 5

Linking perception and action: an ideomotor approach

Günther Knoblich and Wolfgang Prinz

Theories addressing the links between perception and action normally take one of two clearly distinct perspectives. In sensorimotor approaches the focus is on the question of how certain patterns of stimulation evoke certain actions. Accordingly, actions are conceptualized as responses, i.e. as mere consequences of the preceding stimulation. A strict version of this view was defended in traditional behaviorism (Thorndike 1911, 1913; Hull 1930). Some recent versions of the sensorimotor account adopt the terminology of cognitive psychology and allow for additional factors, such as the influence of internal knowledge structures in encoding. However, essentially actions are still treated as being largely determined by perception.

The second perspective is the ideomotor perspective. It is fundamentally different from the sensorimotor perspective because it postulates that actions are not determined by the stimulation occurring in the outside world, but by volitional processes or intentions that cannot be directly observed. In other words, the causes for action are assumed to reside within the organism and not in the stimulation provided by the outside world. Although the fact that thinking is goal driven is a standard assumption in almost every cognitive science approach (Anderson and Lebiere 1998; Miller *et al.* 1960; Newell 1990), the claim of goal-directedness has not been fully acknowledged in research on action [see Jeannerod (1988, 1999) for an exception].

In the rest of this chapter, we will argue that one needs to adopt the ideomotor perspective in order to understand fully the links between perception and action. The chapter has three parts. In the first part, we will provide a short overview of the historical development and of the main ideas behind the ideomotor approach, and introduce a version of this approach that is compatible with the assumptions of modern cognitive science and the neurosciences. In the second part, we will report behavioral evidence that is easier explained when one adopts the ideomotor perspective, but is dfficult to explain when one adopts a sensorimotor perspective. In the third part, we will show how recent results obtained in neuroscience provide substantial support for the ideomotor approach.

Ideomotor theory

Historically, the ideomotor perspective is much younger than the sensorimotor perspective that dates back to Descartes (1664). The main ideas behind the ideomotor perspective were spelled out by the German philosopher Rudolf Hermann Lotze (1852) in his treatment of voluntary actions, i.e. those actions that cannot be explained by changes in the stimulation. According to Lotze, in order to carry out a voluntary action, two conditions must be fulfilled. First, there must be an idea or mental image of what is being willed (*Vorstellung des Gewollten*). Secondly, all conflicting ideas or mental images must be absent or removed (*Hinwegräumung aller Hemmungen*). When these two conditions are met, the mental image directly triggers the execution of the movements required to make the mental image a perceivable fact in the world without any additional volitional activity being required. In other words, Lotze assumed that mental images or ideas (cognitive representations in modern terminology) are by their very nature impulsive. Naturally, this should be particularly true for action representations.

Thirty years later, William James came to a very similar conclusion in his treatment of voluntary action and provided a classical definition of the ideomotor principle:

> Every representation of a movement awakens in some degree the actual movement which is its object; and awakens it in a maximum degree whenever it is not kept from doing so by an antagonistic representation present simultaneously in the mind. (James 1890, Vol. II, p. 526)

At first glance, there seems to be an obvious problem with this definition. It does not specify how the links between cognitive representations and actual movements arise in the first place. Both Lotze and James argue that these links arise during learning. Whenever a movement is performed it is accompanied by a number of perceivable consequences or action effects. Some are directly linked to carrying out the movement itself, such as the kinesthetic sensations that accompany each movement. Others are linked to the movement in a more indirect way because they occur at larger spatial and/or temporal distances from the actual movement. For example, when one's fingers operate a light switch, the light does not appear at the location of the switch but comes on at a distance. When one throws a basketball it will travel some time before it lands in the basket (if one is lucky). According to ideomotor theory, the regularities between actual movements and their more or less distant perceivable consequences are captured in associations. More exactly and in modern terms, representations coding the perceivable bodily and environmental consequences of a movement will become associated with motor representations coding the actual movement.

Such associations can then become functional in two different ways. First, they will allow one to expect certain perceivable consequences, given a certain movement or motor command, i.e. to predict the consequences of a movement. Secondly, they will allow one to select a certain movement or motor command, given an intention to achieve certain perceivable consequences, i.e. to derive the movement required to achieve a predefined goal. Note that these two different functional routes are also at the core of the distinction between forward models and inverse models in recent computational accounts of motor control (Wolpert and Kawato 1998). Forward models predict the sensory consequences of a given motor program, whereas inverse models specify the motor program required for achieving certain sensory consequences.

As mentioned above, the assumption that an intention to achieve certain perceivable consequences is sufficient to fully specify certain motor commands forms the functional basis of the ideomotor principle. Thus any representation of a perceivable event that is known to go along with, or follows from, a particular movement will exhibit the power to trigger the movement that will make this event appear in the perceptual input. This will apply not only to representations of body-related consequences of an action (e.g. thinking of how one's arms feel when intending to dance in the dark), but also to representations of more remote consequences in the environment (e.g. thinking of the light going on).

Extending the ideomotor perspective: ideomotor mapping and common coding

The principles of ideomotor theory, as outlined above, provide an attractive answer to the question of how voluntary actions are prompted and guided through internally generated anticipations of the consequences of an action. But how can these principles be applied to address the link between perception and action in general? If it is true that thinking of perceivable events prompts the corresponding movements to produce them, perceiving the same events happening in the environment (e.g. as the result of somebody else's action) should at least create a tendency to perform the movements required to produce the observed events. For instance, observing somebody throwing a dart at a dartboard should create a 'throwing tendency'. Hence representations of events that can either happen as a consequence of either one's own action or somebody else's actions might provide the required link.

Greenwald (1970, 1972) suggested an extension of the ideomotor theory along these lines and provided empirical evidence in its support. In his experiments, he varied the similarity between the stimuli participants needed to respond to and the feedback they received as a consequence of each response. According to the assumption that perceiving a certain action consequence creates a tendency to carry out the movement to produce that consequence, one would expect that a strong similarity between stimulus and feedback, such as when they share the same color, should speed up the response. This is exactly what Greenwald observed. For instance, participants were faster when a red stimulus light required a manual response which, in turn, triggered a red feedback flash than when it triggered a green feedback flash. According to Greenwald, the red stimulus speeded up the manual response because of its similarity with the perceivable consequences of the response (red feedback flash). Note that the sensorimotor account would predict that the similarity between stimulus and feedback does not matter, because only similarity in the stimulus–response relationship should affect the response times.

With this extension, the ideomotor approach provides a straightforward framework for conceptualizing the links between perception and action. The main principle underlying this framework is that the perception of an event that is similar to an event that has been learnt to accompany, or follow from, one's own action will tend to induce that action. If so, the strength of action induction should depend on the degree of similarity, or overlap, between stimulus events and the action-related events. In other words, perception should induce action when a perceived event has a strong similarity with an event that can result as a consequence of an action.

The extended ideomotor principle has two important functional implications: ideomotor mapping and common coding. The notion of ideomotor mapping addresses two learning requirements for a cognitive system that functions according to the similarity principle defined above. One is that the system is capable of inducing regularities between certain movements and their perceivable consequences. This type of induction can be achieved by, for instance, an associative network in which the link strength between a motor representation and an event representation increases when both representations are concurrently active (Hebb 1949; Hommel 1998). The second requirement is that the links between movements and their perceivable consequences, once established, can also function in a reversed temporal order. Specifically, the activation of a representation that codes the perceivable consequences of an action should automatically preactivate the respective motor command. In addition to Greenwald's original results, several recent behavioral studies (Elsner and Hommel 2001; Kunde 2001; Kunde *et al.* 2002; Stock and Hoffmann 2002) as well as a functional magnetic resonance imaging (fMRI) study (Elsner *et al.* 2002) provide evidence for the temporal reversibility claim.

The second functional implication of the extended ideomotor principle is captured in the notion of common coding. The common coding assumption defines a constraint on the architecture of systems that function according to this principle. Importantly, in such systems, the planning and control of action is not independent from the perceptual representation of environmental events. Instead, there is at least one representational level that is functionally involved in perception as well as action (Prinz 1984, 1990, 1997; MacKay 1987; Hommel *et al.* 2001; Prinz and Meltzoff 2002). The representations on such a level code events that can potentially follow from one's own actions. Perceiving events in the environment that match these representations will activate them. Because they are also associated with the motor commands that bring about the perceived event, the respective motor commands will also be activated. In addition, planning an action takes the form of internally activating a certain event representation that will automatically trigger the respective motor command if no conflicting event representations are concurrently active. The latter assumption incorporates the classical ideomotor principle into the extended version.

Common coding of perception and action: reciprocal modulations

The extended ideomotor principle, which from now on we will refer to as the common coding account of perception and action, provides an attractive alternative to, or at least an important extension of, sensorimotor accounts that address the link between perception and action. The latter have the problem that perception and action use separate and completely incommensurate representations. Perceptual representations code patterns of stimulation in the sense organs and certain properties that are derived from these patterns, whereas action representations represent patterns of excitations in muscles or certain regularities occurring in these patterns. Obviously, there is no way of determining different degrees of similarity between these two types of representations because they are incommensurate and thus not comparable. Accordingly, the only ways of linking perception and action are rule-based mappings between incommensurable representations.

The common coding account introduces another supposedly more powerful link between perception and action by defining principles that also allow for similarity-based matches. Such matches can only be conceived of when one assumes that perceptual and action representations are commensurate, at least at some representational level. Representations of events that are perceivable and 'produceable' are exactly that. The similarity principle implies that perception and action will modulate each other reciprocally whenever they are similar. This implication can be translated in two predictions that can be empirically tested.

The first prediction is that action planning and control can modulate perception. One possibile way of testing this prediction is to investigate situations in which a person perceives certain events or actions while she or he is concurrently planning an action. In these situations, the perception of events should be modulated by the similarity between the event that the action is anticipated to bring about and the perceived event. The second prediction is that perception can modulate action planning and control. One way of testing this prediction is to look at situations in which one person watches other people's actions and/or their consequences. In these situations, perceiving somebody else's actions and/or their consequences should be sufficient to activate event representations that are also functional in one's own planning and control of these actions, at least if one is able to carry out the observed action oneself. Thus the planning and control of an ongoing action should be modulated through concurrent perception of somebody else's actions. Obviously, this modulation should be content specific, i.e. it should depend on the similarity between the event representations involved in planning the one and perceiving the other action. We will review recent empirical evidence supporting both predictions in the next two sections.

Action modulates perception

In this section we will address three recent lines of research that provide evidence for the claim that action modulates perception: action effect blindness, apparent movement, and mental rotation.

Action effect blindness

Müsseler and coworkers conducted several studies in which they explicitly addressed the question of whether planning an action modulates the simultaneous perception of events in the environment in a specific way (Müsseler and Hommel 1997; Müsseler *et al.* 2000; Müsseler and Wühr 2002; Wühr and Müsseler 2002). In one study (Müsseler *et al.* 2000) they used a simple task in which the participants first planned to press either a left or a right key (Fig. 5.1). However, instead of immediately carrying out the left or right key press, they first initiated the presentation of a masked stimulus by simultaneously pressing both a left and a right key. Afterwards they carried out the left or right key press they had planned in advance as fast as possible. The stimulus that appeared with the double press was either a left- or a right-pointing arrow. The participants were instructed to identify the direction in which the arrow pointed (left or right) by providing an unspeeded judgment.

What is special about this task is that the participants needed to identify a spatial aspect (the pointing direction) of the stimulus while they were planning to carry out a response that was similar or dissimilar with regard to this spatial aspect. According to the common coding account, the spatial similarity between the planned action and the stimulus to be identified should affect the accuracy with which the stimulus direction can be correctly identified. To illustrate, when planning a left action and perceiving a stimulus pointing to the left, the event representations required for planning and identification are similar with respect to the spatial direction. When planning a right action

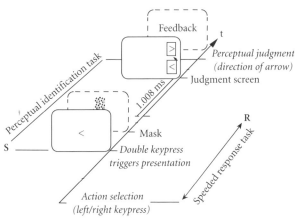

Fig. 5.1 Illustration of the action effect blindness paradigm (Müsseler *et al.* 2000). Participants chose to carry out either a left or a right key press. Afterwards they carried out a double key press to start the trial. The double press initiated the presentation of a left-pointing or a right-pointing arrow that was masked immediately afterwards. The participants' task was first to carry out the key press they had planned in advance, as fast as possible, and then to indicate the direction of the arrow as accurately as possible (without time pressure).

and perceiving a stimulus pointing to the left, the event representations required for planning and identification are dissimilar with respect to the spatial direction.

As predicted, there were differences between the similar and dissimilar conditions. Surprisingly, the identification rates for the pointing direction of the stimulus were lower when the planned action and the stimulus were similar than when they were dissimilar. For instance, arrows pointing to the right were less often correctly identified while planning a right action than while planning a left action. One conclusion that can be drawn from this result is that the planning of an action that produces a certain event in the environment clearly affects the perception of similar events in the environment. However, this influence could also have resulted in a better identification of events that are similar to the currently planned action. Müsseler and coworkers suggest that the disadvantage is due to the fact that event representations that are currently needed in order to plan an action are shielded from further perceptual input [see Hommel et al. (2001) for a specific explanation in terms of binding]. This 'blindness effect for response compatible stimuli' (Müsseler and Hommel 1997) has been demonstrated in a variety of different task contexts, including dual-task situations (reviewed by Müsseler and Wühr 2002).

Apparent movement

Wohlschläger (2000) conducted a further study that convincingly demonstrates that action modulates perception [see Ishimura and Shimojo (1994) for similar results]. In his experiments the participants observed an ambiguous motion display. The display consisted of a number of disks in a circular arrangement that were shifted by a constant angle about 6 times/s. When this display is observed under neutral conditions, one has roughly equally often the impression that the disks perform a clockwise or a counterclockwise circular movement. In other words, the movement direction experienced in the display is ambiguous. In the first experiment, Wohlschläger instructed participants to rotate a knob clockwise or counterclockwise in the same plane as the motion display. The motion display came on as soon as they started their movement. As predicted, the movement direction clearly affected the perceived direction of the ambiguous motion. For instance, when the participants rotated the knob in a clockwise direction, the ambiguous motion display was more often perceived as rotating clockwise.

A further experiment conducted by Wohlschläger demonstrates that it is not necessary actually to carry out a movement to obtain such effects. The participants were asked to either plan a clockwise or counterclockwise movement before the ambiguous motion display came on and to carry out the movement only after reporting the perceived direction of the ambiguous motion. The results were basically the same as for the experiment in which the participants concurrently carried out a movement. For instance, when they planned a clockwise movement they were more likely to perceive a clockwise movement in the ambiguous motion display. These results provide clear support for the predictions of the common coding account of perception action links.

Mental rotation

Another series of studies conducted by Wohlschläger and Wohlschläger (1998) demonstrates that action modulates not only perception but also mental imagery [see Wexler *et al.* 1998) for similar results]. The common coding account predicts such influences because the mental images generated in action planning are thought to be a sort of internally generated perceptual images just like the ones assumed to be generated during mental rotation (Shepard and Metzler 1971; Kosslyn and König 1992).

In one experiment, Wohlschläger and Wohlschläger asked the participants to rotate a knob continuously clockwise or counterclockwise while they simultaneously performed a mental rotation task. As in the standard task, the visual display showed two objects that were either identical or mirror versions of each other. In addition, the objects were rotated relative to each other by different angles. Participants were instructed to judge whether the objects were identical or not. It is well known that in order to solve this task one needs to rotate one object mentally to match the orientation of the other. Depending on the degree of rotation, the shortest way to rotate an object mentally is either clockwise or counterclockwise. According to the common coding account the direction of an action performed simultaneously should affect the time one needs to mentally rotate the object.

The results obtained by Wohlschläger and Wohlschläger support this assumption. When the direction of the movement matched the optimal rotation direction, it speeded up mental rotation. Conversely, when the direction of the movement ran counter to the optimal rotation direction, it slowed down mental rotation. To illustrate, when the optimal rotation direction to match two objects was clockwise, clockwise and counterclockwise movements performed simultaneously speeded up and slowed down, respectively, reaction times for the mental rotation task compared with a condition in which no movement was performed. As in the apparent motion studies, the same pattern of results was obtained when the participants were asked to plan a knob movement in a certain direction before working on the mental rotation and to carry it out after the mental rotation task had been finished. Again, planning an action was sufficient to modulate perception.

Perception modulates action

The second prediction of the common coding assumption is that the mere perception of an action should affect the way in which an observer plans or executes actions which resemble the observed action. In the following, we will provide an overview of recent behavioral evidence supporting this prediction. This support comes from a broad variety of research fields such as action initiation, action selection, action induction, goal-directed imitation, bimanual coordination, and action recognition.

Action initiation

In a recent study Brass *et al.* (2001) investigated whether initiating a simple finger action is affected by the concurrent perception of a related finger action (Fig. 5.2). In each experimental trial, their participants observed one of two stimulus sequences in random order. Both started with a static picture of an index finger. After a variable and therefore unpredictable amount of time the finger started moving upward in one sequence or downward in the other sequence. The participants were instructed to move their own index finger either upward or downward as soon as the observed finger started moving. Importantly, during a given block of trials the movement conducted by the participant remained the same. In other words, participants would see a randomized sequence of up and down movements of an index finger, but they always carried out the same action (e.g. moved their index finger downward). Accordingly, the action to be performed was prespecified throughout, and the identity of the triggering stimulus (moving up versus down) was completely irrelevant. The question was whether the irrelevant stimulus gesture would still affect the time needed to initiate the action.

The results of several experiments demonstrate that it took the participants longer to initiate a simple action when the observed action had a different direction than the one to be performed than when it had the same the direction. Upward movements were initiated faster when triggered by upward-moving stimulus gestures, and downward movements were initiated faster when triggered by downward-moving stimuli. This pattern of results implies a substantial stimulus–response compatibility effect. In previous studies (Hommel and Prinz 1997), such effects were only observed when

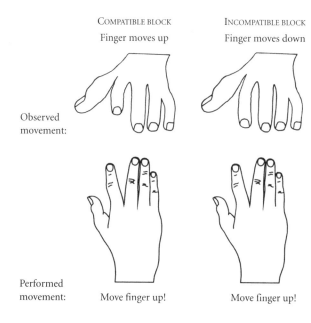

COMPATIBLE BLOCK
Finger moves up

INCOMPATIBLE BLOCK
Finger moves down

Observed
movement:

Performed
movement:

Move finger up!

Move finger up!

Fig. 5.2 Illustration of the finger lifting task (Brass *et al.* 2001). The up- and downward movement of the observed finger always started at a neutral position. The participants' task was to move their own finger as soon as they detected a movement in the observed finger. In a given experimental block, observed and performed movements were either compatible (left) or incompatible (right).

participants needed to select between two different actions. Hence the most surprising aspect of the study by Brass *et al.* (2001) is that a compatibility effect was observed for a simple and completely prespecified action. These results strongly suggest that the representations that are involved in initiating a certain action (e.g. move downward) are not separated from the representations involved in observing a similar action (a downward movement performed by somebody else). Otherwise, the time it takes to initiate a simple action should not be affected by the action observed. Thus these results provide evidence for the existence of common representations that contribute to perception and action, as postulated by the common coding assumption.

Action selection

In a further study, Stürmer *et al.* (2000) investigated whether similar compatibility effects are observed when the action to be performed is not prespecified and the stimulus dimension that defines this action is not related to the observed action. As mentioned above, there is ample empirical evidence demonstrating that a spatial overlap between stimuli and responses in choice reaction tasks results in compatibility effects (Simon 1990; Hommel and Prinz 1997). For example, when participants respond to a green object by pressing a left key and to a red object by pressing a right key, the responses are faster when the green object appears on the left and the red object appears on the right. Thus, although the spatial overlap between stimulus and response is completely task irrelevant, it affects the time required to select the appropriate response.

Stürmer *et al.* (2000) investigated whether such compatibility effects are also obtained when the irrelevant dimension consists in the similarity of a hand action to be performed and a hand action observed. If so, this would provide evidence that common codes are involved not only in initiating an action but also in selecting between different alternative actions. In the experiments performed by Stürmer and coworkers participants observed one of two hand movements after a neutral starting posture had been displayed (Fig. 5.3): either the fingers were extended to spread the hand apart or

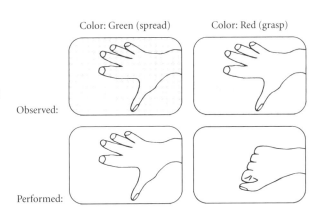

Fig. 5.3 Illustration of the task used by Stürmer *et al.* (2000). Participants observed a spreading movement, for example. Their task was to carry out a grasping or spreading movement depending on the color cue superimposed on the observed movement.

the fingers were flexed to form a grasping movement. With the onset of the movement a color cue was superimposed on the hand observed. Participants were instructed to perform a spreading action or a grasping action with their right dominant hand in response to the color cue. For instance, they performed the spreading action when the color cue was red and the grasping action when the color cue was blue. Thus the hand action observed was completely irrelevant for selecting the action to be performed. Nevertheless, Stürmer and coworkers observed substantial compatibility effects between the observed irrelevant hand action and the hand action to be performed. For example, when participants were instructed to perform a spreading action in response to a red color cue they selected the action faster when the observed hand also performed a spreading action.

Two additional findings are of interest. In some experiments the participants first observed how the irrelevant action unfolded for a given time (e.g. 400 ms) before the color cue was superimposed. Hence, there was additional time to process the irrelevant hand movement before the imperative signal indicated which action they needed to perform. One would expect that the additional time for processing the irrelevant movement should enhance the compatibility effect. However, this is not what happened. Instead, the compatibility effect was present to its full extent right from the outset. A similarly surprising result was obtained in a further experiment in which participants observed static hand postures instead of dynamic actions. The two postures represented the endstates of the spreading and grasping actions. In this situation, one would actually expect the compatibility effect to be smaller for observation of static postures than for dynamic action, because there is less overlap between a static gesture being observed and a dynamic action being performed. However, the compatibility effect was even somewhat larger for static postures.

Taken together, the results of these experiments suggest two conclusions. The first is that the similarity between an observed action and a performed action modulates action selection. The more similar the action to be performed is to the observed action, the faster it can be selected. Thus, not only action initiation but also action selection is affected by the concurrent perception of irrelevant actions. This finding lends further support to the claim that the same representations are involved in perceiving actions and performing actions. The second conclusion is that endstate postures of hand actions are particularly effective primes for the selection of the respective actions that would produce them as their result. This result is surprising because it suggests that endstates, or action goals, play a prominent role in the mechanisms underlying the compatibility effect in action selection and that the additional dynamic information provided by an actual movement does not contribute to this effect. In other words, it seems that the common representations do not code the actual movement by which an action goal is achieved, but the action goal itself. This implies that the codes are anticipatory in nature, just as postulated by the ideomotor approach.

Goal-directed imitation

Several recent studies on imitation in children in the age range of 3–5 years provide further support for the assumption that common representations might actually code action goals (Bekkering *et al.* 2000; Gleissner *et al.* 2000; Bekkering and Prinz 2002; Bekkering and Wohlschläger 2002). These studies used a task in which the same action goal could be achieved by performing different movements. The experimenter acted as a model and the child was asked to imitate the observed action. There were four possible actions (Fig. 5.4). The experimenter would (a) reach for her left ear with her left hand, (b) reach for her right ear with her right hand, (c) reach for her left ear with her right hand, or (d) reach for her right ear with her left hand. Note that there were only two possible action goals or end states for these actions, i.e. the left ear being touched [cases (a) and (c)] or the right ear being touched. Accordingly, there were two different movements by which the same action goal could be obtained: one that did not cross the body midline and one that crossed the body midline.

When adults imitate these actions they commit neither errors with regard to the action goal (touching the wrong ear) nor errors with regard to the movement (e.g. not crossing the body line). However, in the studies by Bekkering and coworkers the children showed a systematic pattern of errors. They never touched the wrong ear, i.e. they always correctly imitated the action goal. However, when the model performed an action in which the movement crossed the body midline [cases (c) and (d)], the children did not imitate it correctly. For instance, when the model touched her right ear with the left hand, the child touch her right ear with the right hand in

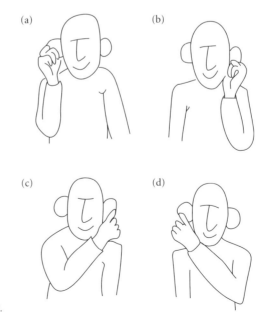

Fig. 5.4 Examples of the actions used in the goal-directed imitation task of Bekkering and coworkers.

approximately 50% of cases. The most likely explanation for these errors is that children focus on the action goal and not on the actual movement when imitating an action. Rather, they often choose the simplest movement to achieve the same action goal as the model that is imitated.

A study by Gleissner *et al.* (2000) provided further evidence for this explanation. This study used the same task as described above. In an additional condition the model carried out the four movements, but did not actually touch her ears. Hence, there was no obvious action goal connected to the endstate of the movement. Under these conditions, the children committed the same amount of errors with respect to the endstate of the movement, as with respect to the movement itself. For instance, children often moved a hand to the right side of their face when the model had moved a hand to the left side of her face.

Taken together, the studies on influences of perception on action reported so far demonstrate that perception and action use common representation in action initiation, action selection, and goal-directed imitation. These shared structures contain more information than just the kinematics of the perceived or to-be-performed movement patterns. Rather, they seem to represent several types of information about goal-directed actions, with action goals taking the functional lead over more specific movement-related information. This is, of course, in full accord with the central claim of ideomotor theory that actions are represented in terms of the consequences they should bring about.

Action induction

Further support for the assumption that action goals have a prominent role in linking perception and action comes from recent studies addressing action induction. Action induction refers to the phenomenon that the mere observation of others' actions and their outcomes can spontaneously induce or modulate actions on the part of the observer. The resulting spontaneous movements are often referred to in the literature as ideomotor movements (Prinz 1987). Consider the following situation. While watching an actor in a slapstick comedy film who walks along the edge of a plunging precipice, people are often unable to sit still and watch quietly. They will move their legs and their arms or displace their body weight from one side to the other.

Examples like above strongly suggest that action induction is a real phenomenon. However, they do not provide an indication of how the observed action and the induced action are related. The most straightforward assumption regarding this relationship would be that the action induced is similar to the action perceived. Thus, when the actor bends toward a precipice on the right, people in the audience should also bend toward the right. This classical perceptual induction assumption (Lotze 1852; Carpenter 1874; James 1890) invokes that people repeat through their induced movements what they see happening in the scene. Accordingly, one could say that action induction is considered to be a non-voluntary form of imitation. However, there is also a possible alternative assumption that has not been considered in classical approaches to action induction. This intentional induction assumption states that people realize through their induced movements what they would like to see happening in the scene (Knuf *et al.* 2001). In the film example this would imply that when the actor bends toward a precipice on the right, people in the audience should bend to the left (at least, if the actor is a likeable hero). Accordingly, the intentional induction assumption suggests that induced actions are a special class of goal-directed actions—futile instrumental activity, so to speak.

Two recent studies (Knuf *et al.* 2001; S. De Maeght and W. Prinz, unpublished data) addressed the question of whether action induction is perceptual and/or intentional in nature. The first study (Knuf *et al.* 2001) addressed action induction in a situation where participants watched the outcomes of their own preceding actions. The second study (De Maeght and Prinz, unpublished data) addressed action induction in a situation where participants watched the outcomes of somebody else's concurrent actions. We will address them in turn.

Knuf and coworkers developed a computerized version of a simple bowling game that allowed them to separate the influences of perceptual and intentional induction (Fig. 5.5). In each trial, the participants watched a ball moving toward a target object. At the beginning of the trial the ball was shown at its starting position at the bottom of

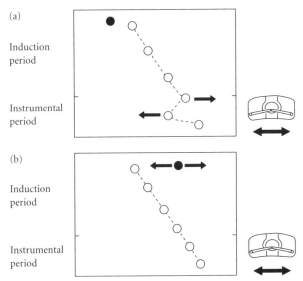

Fig. 5.5 Illustration of the ideomotor paradigm (Knuf *et al.* 2001). Participants watched a ball moving toward a target. (a) In the ball-manipulation condition they could change the horizontal position of the moving ball during the initial phase of the trial (instrumental period). (b) In the target-manipulation condition they could change the horizontal position of the target during the instrumental period. The main dependent variable was the direction of the 'futile' instrumental movements conducted during the induction phase.

the screen and the target object was shown at the top. The relative positions of the starting and target locations were chosen such that the ball needed to travel either leftward or rightward in order to hit the target. For instance, when the starting position was at the left bottom, the target position was at the right top. After 2 s the ball started moving toward the target with constant velocity, but always in a direction that would miss the target when no corrections were performed. There were two different conditions. In the ball-manipulation condition, participants moved a joystick to change the ball's horizontal position in order to change its trajectory to hit the target (Fig. 5.5(a)). In the target-manipulation condition, participants moved a joystick to change the horizontal position of the target in order to adjust the target to match the anticipated position of the ball at impact (Fig 5.5(b)). Importantly, the joystick only affected the ball or target position during the first part of the trial (a period of 1 s or roughly the first third of the distance covered). During the second part of the trial (a period of 2 s or roughly the remaining two-thirds of the distance covered) the joystick was not effective. It is likely that the movements performed during this induction phase are spontaneously induced by the observation of the events concurrently ongoing on the screen.

Knuf and coworkers were particularly interested in the joystick movements during the induction phase. The perceptual induction assumption predicts that these movements always reflect actions induced by the direction in which the ball moves, regardless of whether they previously affected the ball position or the target position. Moreover, perceptual induction should occur regardless of whether the ball will finally hit or miss the target. The intentional induction assumption makes different predictions. First, there should be no spontaneous joystick movements in trials with upcoming hits because participants should anticipate the target to be hit. Hence no further instrumental activity is required to achieve the goal and accordingly no intentional induction is expected. Secondly, on upcoming misses, participants should anticipate the target miss and this in turn should induce movements performed in an attempt to remedy the futile situation. The attempts at correction should depend on the object under previous instrumental control (ball versus target) and the side on which the ball is expected to miss the target (left versus right). In the ball-manipulation condition the joystick movements should act to push the ball toward the target. In the target-manipulation condition, joystick movements should act to push the target toward the ball.

The results obtained in several experiments fully support the predictions of the intentional induction assumption. First, the direction of the ball movement itself did not induce corresponding joystick movements. This rules out the perceptual induction assumption. Secondly, in trials with upcoming hits, induced movements were virtually absent, as predicted by the intentional induction assumption. Thirdly, in trials with upcoming misses, there were pronounced induced movements that depended on both the object under initial control (ball versus target) and the side of the upcoming target miss (left versus right), exactly in line with the pattern predicted by intentional induction.

In order to assess whether intentional induction is also present when another person's actions are observed, De Maeght and Prinz (2004) conducted a further study. Their participants observed the same displays as before, i.e. hits and misses in the bowling task. However, this time they did so on the understanding that they were watching the visible outcome of another individual's performance. While observing the game, participants controlled a marker that could be moved up and down on the right margin of the screen by moving a joystick. Their task was to move the marker to match as closely as possible the current vertical position of the ball on the screen. The main variable of interest was the direction of the movements on the irrelevant horizontal dimension. Because the tracker could only be moved vertically, horizontal movements were completely ineffective, and therefore could be used as a measure of spontaneously occurring movements induced by the observation of the bowling game. Action induction should exhibit itself in spontaneous unintentional drifts to the left or the right.

The experiment had two parts. In the first part participants played the bowling game themselves (player mode), just as in the earlier study (Knuf *et al.* 2001). In the second part, they tracked the visible outcome of another individual's performance on that game (observer mode). Hence the pattern of induced action for both the bowling and the tracking task could be assessed. The results for the player mode exactly replicated the earlier reported results. However, a different pattern of results emerged for the observer mode. In the tracking task perceptual induction was strong throughout, whereas intentional induction, although still present, was clearly weaker. A further experiment investigated action induction in participants who carried out the tracking task in the observer mode without having played the bowling game before. The results showed that action induction was generally much weaker than for observers who had acted as players before. Nevertheless, weak perceptual induction was obtained throughout which, in the ball condition, went along with weak intentional induction.

Together, the findings in the area of action induction provide further support for the notion of a common representational system for perception and action. The phenomenon of action induction is generally hard to explain without postulating such a system. The result that intentional induction prevails the more one is involved or the more familiar one is with a task, further underlines the claim that action goals play a major role in linking perception and action. The finding that perceptual induction prevails when others' actions are observed might indicate that the intentions behind others' actions are not derived by default.

Bimanual coordination

The common coding principle can also be applied to situations in which one person needs to coordinate two different actions, as in bimanual coordination. One standard assumption in theories of action coordination has been that the coordination of two actions is mainly achieved by the coupling of efferent motor signals (Kelso 1984). The common coding principle suggests a different assumption. Because action planning occurs on a level at which actions are represented in terms of the perceived outcomes, action coupling should occur on the level of perceivable action outcomes and not on the level of efferent motor commands. A recent series of studies provided substantial evidence for this assumption (Mechsner *et al.* 2001).

In the initial study Mechsner and co-workers addressed the symmetry tendency in a classical finger oscillation task. The participants were instructed to perform bimanual index-finger oscillations, either in symmetry or in parallel. In the standard task, both hands are held with the palm downward. To achieve symmetrical oscillations during the first part of the movement one concurrently moves the left index finger to the right and the right index finger to the left during the first part of the movement. During the second part of the movement, one moves the left index finger to the left and the right index finger to the right, and so on. To achieve parallel oscillations one concurrently moves both index fingers to the left, then to the right, and so on. The main result is that, as people move faster, parallel oscillations become harder to maintain and, at some point, the oscillations switch to the symmetrical mode. This result has been taken as evidence for the assumption that bimanual coupling occurs through concurrent activation of homologous muscles, as present in symmetrical oscillations.

A simple variation introduced by Mechnser and coworkers shows that this claim cannot be true. They introduced a further condition in which the participants were asked to carry out the finger oscillations with one hand held with the palm upward and one hand held with the palm downward. In this case, homologous muscle activation occurs during parallel oscillations. Therefore parallel oscillations should be more stable than symmetrical oscillations. However, this is not what happened. Rather, the results obtained under these conditions were exactly the same as in the standard task. The symmetrical oscillations were stable, and the parallel oscillations were harder to maintain and switched to symmetrical oscillations when the movements became faster. This result clearly supports the assumption that bimanual coupling occurs at a level of perceivable action outcomes and not at the level of efferent motor commands. The results obtained for a bimanual four-finger tapping task (Mechsner *et al.* 2001) support this conclusion and suggest that coupling generally occurs at the level of perceivable action outcomes and not only in specific tasks.

Even more surprising are the results obtained by Mechsner and coworkers in a study of the bimanual circling task. In this task participants carry out circular movements with both hands simultaneously. The standard finding is that there are only few stable patterns at high velocities (e.g. symmetrical movements). It is almost impossible for untrained persons to continuously produce circling patterns that are characterized by non-harmonic frequency ratios for the two hands. For instance, when asked to complete four circles with one hand and three circles with the other during a certain time interval, participants will invariably fail to produce a stable pattern at all, or will switch to a pattern with a harmonic frequency ratio (4:4 or 4:2).

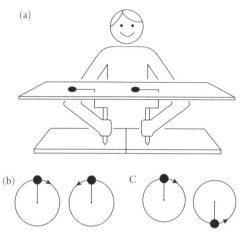

Fig. 5.6 Illustration of the circling task (Mechsner *et al.* 2001). (a) The apparatus used. The participants circled two visible flags by moving two cranks that were hidden under a table. The left flag circled directly above the left hand, whereas the right flag circled in a 4:3 frequency ratio to the right crank hand. Participants were instructed to move the two flags either (b) in symmetry (0° relative phase) or (C) in anti-phase (180° relative phase).

The standard interpretation for this finding is that efferent muscle commands can only be coupled when the frequency ratio is harmonic. However, according to the assumption that bimanual coupling occurs at the level of perceivable action outcomes, one would expect that movements with a non-harmonic frequency ratio are actually possible if salient action outcomes with a harmonic frequency ratio result from these movements. Mechsner *et al.* (2001) tested this assumption in an experiment in which they dissociated the actual movements and the perceivable action outcomes (Fig. 5.6). The participants circled two visible flags by moving two cranks that were hidden under a table. The left flag circled directly above the left crank (hand), whereas the right flag circled in a 4:3 frequency ratio to the right crank (hand) via a gear system. Thus a harmonic frequency in the visible action outcomes (4:4 in the flag movements) could be achieved by moving the two hands with a non-harmonic frequency (4:3).

The results confirmed the prediction that bimanual coupling is achieved on the level of perceivable action outcomes. All participants could produce stable flag movements, even at high velocities, by moving their hands in an otherwise impossible manner, i.e. by producing stable movements that had a non-harmonic frequency ratio of 4:3. This result is virtually impossible to explain if one assumes that bimanual coupling occurs between efferent motor commands. In this case, bimanual movements with non-harmonic frequencies should be impossible, regardless of the action outcomes observed.

Action recognition

A further line of research addressed recognition of one's own actions (Knoblich and Flach 2001; Knoblich and Prinz 2001, Knoblich *et al.* 2002; Flach *et al.*, 2003;

in press). An important implication of the common coding assumption is that the codes that govern action planning also contribute to the understanding of others' actions that are merely observed. The reason is that common codes provide a link between the observed action and one's own knowledge about how to carry out the observed action. This implies that the common coding system will not only match with the perceptual input but that it will also resonate with motor codes (Viviani and Stucchi 1992). One consequence of this assumption is that observing one's own earlier actions might lead to a higher resonance. The reason is that different people carry out the same actions in slightly different ways and these differences also show up in the perceivable outcomes of these actions. Because the producing and observing systems are only the same when one observes one's own actions, the perceptual input should be more similar to the common codes than when observing others' actions. As a consequence, the resonance with motor codes should be higher when one observes one's own actions. This in turn should allow one to recognize one's own earlier actions.

Knoblich and Prinz (2001) provided a first test of this hypothesis. They investigated whether persons can recognize the kinematics of their own drawing movements. The participants drew a large number of familiar and unfamiliar symbols on a writing pad and the movement trajectories were recorded. They could neither see their hands while drawing the symbols nor did they receive visual feedback about the emerging trace. About a week after the movement trajectories were recorded they participated in a second session. In each trial, they observed two of the movement trajectories produced earlier, one self-produced and one produced by another participant. A single moving point reproduced the movement kinematics without leaving a trace on the screen. Thus no static form information was provided. The two trajectories were presented in random order and the participants indicated whether they thought that they had produced the first or second movement trajectory themselves. They did not receive feedback about whether their judgment was correct.

The results showed that participants could recognize their own drawing actions based on the sparse kinematic information provided. Also, they could recognize the movement trajectories for familiar and unfamiliar symbols equally well. A further important result was that self-recognition was not possible when the movement trajectories were presented with constant velocity, i.e. when only the spatial and not the temporal characteristics of the production were retained. Accordingly, the self-recognition rates were always higher for movement trajectories of symbols whose production implied large discontinuities in velocity. All these results suggest that self-recognition is based on dynamic characteristics of the trajectory and not on static form information. This, in turn, suggests that self-recognition of actions is based on a higher resonance between perceptual and motor systems that is mediated by common codes. Recent results for the recognition of one's own clapping suggest a similar conclusion (Flach *et al.*, in press).

Two further studies investigated whether observing one's own earlier movements also facilitates the prediction of the future course of a movement or its underlying goal. In the first study (Knoblich *et al.* 2002), participants were asked to write either the whole symbol '2' or only the first stroke (to write the symbol '2' one needs to produce two strokes—a first bent one ending at the lower left corner and a second horizontal one). In a second session participants in each trial observed the movement trajectory of the first bent stroke. This stroke was either self- or other-produced, and had been produced either in isolation or as part of writing the complete symbol '2'. For each stroke, the participants indicated whether they thought it had been produced in isolation or as part of writing the complete symbol. Again, there was no feedback about the accuracy of the judgments. The results showed that participants' predictions were quite accurate when observing their own movement trajectories, but were no different from chance when observing others' movement trajectories.

The second study (Knoblich and Flach 2001) investigated whether one can also better predict the underlying action goal when one observes one's own movements. In the first session, the participants were videotaped while throwing darts at the upper, middle, or lower third of a target board. In a second session, they watched video clips that displayed either their own or somebody else's throwing movements (Fig. 5.7). Each video clip started with a person picking up the dart and immediately throwing it at the target board that was also visible. Each clip ended at exactly the moment when the dart left the person's hand. The task was to predict in which third of the target board the dart would land. Again, the participants were not told whether their predictions were correct throughout the whole session. During the initial trials the predictions were equally accurate for self- and other-generated throws. However, after some familiarity with the task had been acquired, the judgments became more accurate for self-generated than for other-generated throws.

The finding that people can not only recognize their own earlier actions but also derive more accurate predictions from them suggests that the common coding system might also play an important role in coupling currently observed perceptual input

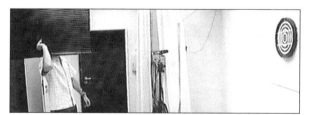

Fig. 5.7 Illustration of the prediction tak of Knoblich and Flach (2001). The participants watched video clips showing themselves or other persons throwing a dart at a target board. The clip stopped at the moment the dart left the person's hand. The task was to predict whether the dart would hit the upper, middle, or lower third of the target board displayed on the right.

with the motor system. Actually, it suggests a more specific interaction between perception and action than a mere resonance. It seems likely that the activation of a common code can initiate predictive mechanisms residing in the motor system, often referred to as action simulation mechanisms (Harris 1992; Gallese and Goldman 1998; Blakemore and Decety 2001; Chaminade *et al.* 2001; Knoblich *et al.* 2002, Proust 2002). Such mechanisms are normally used to predict the sensory consequences of motor programs during online action control. During observation of action, the output of such simulations might be fed back to the common coding level and thereby specify the future outcomes of currently observed actions.

Implementation of common coding in the brain

The common coding account provides a functional principle that does not necessarily imply that perception and action links are implemented by specific neuronal systems. For instance, binding or synchronization processes could link different neuronal systems in a way that could be functionally described as common coding (Müller *et al.* 2000; Hommel *et al.* 2001). However, there is a growing body of neurophysiological evidence suggesting that common coding of perception and action is also a principle that applies to the neuronal implementation of perception–action links. There are a number of areas in the brain that are active during planning and controlling an action as well as perceiving the actions of others, including specific frontal and parietal regions (Decety and Grèzes 1999; Blakemore and Decety 2001).

One frontal region seems to implement the common coding principle almost exactly. Using single-cell recordings Rizzolatti and coworkers discovered 'mirror neurons' in the premotor area of the macaque monkey (Di Pellegrino *et al.* 1992; Gallese *et al.* 1996; Rizzolatti *et al.* 2001). These neurons fire when the monkey carries out an object-directed action such as grasping a nut. They also fire when the monkey observes the experimenter carrying out the same specific action. Obviously, the existence of such neurons provides direct evidence for a common coding of perception and action on a neurophysiological level.

Recent positron emission tomography (PET) and fMRI studies suggest that humans possess a similar mirror system (Iacoboni *et al.* 1999; Buccino *et al.* 2001; Schubotz and von Cramon 2001; Decety *et al.* 2002; Koski *et al.* 2002). They show that the mere observation of actions and their consequences activates certain parts of the premotor cortex that might be homologous to the F5 area in the macaque monkey in which the mirror neurons are located (Rizzolatti and Arbib 1998). One problem of this homology is that large parts of the premotor cortex are traditionally considered as the center for speech production (Broca area). Thus the activation of premotor areas during action perception could be due to internal verbalization of the actions observed. However, recent studies (Buccino *et al.* 2001; Schubotz and Cramon 2001) suggest that the parts of the premotor area that are active during action perception are organized in a somatotopic manner. Such results seem to defy the inner verbalization hypothesis.

Further 'motor' areas that are often active while perceiving actions and their outcomes include the parietal cortex (Rizzolatti *et al.* 2001; Decety *et al.* 2002) and the supplementary area (Elsner *et al.* 2002).

Conclusion: added value of motor coding

The ideomotor approach we have outlined in this chapter suggests that the perception of action tends to induce related action tendencies and motor codings in the observer's mind and brain. As we have seen, this suggestion is widely supported by evidence from behavioral and brain studies. Theorists have summarized the evidence by stating that the proper function of those action tendencies and motor codings is to subserve action recognition or action understanding. For instance, Rizzolatti *et al.* (2001) claim 'that we understand actions when we map the visual representation of the observed action onto our motor representation of the same action (…) an action is understood when its observation causes the motor system of the observer to "resonate" '. Gallese and Goldman (1998) and Blakemore and Decety (2001) propose similar ideas.

At first glance, these seem to be plausible suggestions. However, if one takes a closer look at them, it is not obvious why the mechanisms for understanding actions should be so fundamentally different from those for understanding non-actions. For instance, when it comes to understanding mechanical events, such as a ball's trajectory when it rolls down a hill, theories would claim that we 'recognize', or 'understand', the movement pattern in exactly the same way as we understand everything else we perceive, i.e. by sensory analysis and semantic enrichment. Sensory analysis takes care of processing and identifying the physical surface structure of the event as far as it is contained in the stimulus pattern. Semantic enrichment takes care of linking the visual pattern to the perceiver's acquired knowledge in the pertinent domain. Hence recognizing or understanding an event is tantamount to performing these operations and making their results available to further processing.

If so, one may wonder what the added value of extra motor coding could be in the case of action perception. Like the perception of any other event, action perception will also rely on sensory analysis and semantic enrichment. What, then, can motor enrichment contribute above and beyond semantic enrichment?

There may be more than one answer to this question. The one that we find most convincing sees the added value of motor coding much more in its power of anticipating what is going to happen next, rather than recognizing what is happening now. Motor systems are anticipation engines: Their efficiency relies to a large extent on their power to generate forward models of the consequences arising from given actions. Hence, when perceived action is coded not only in terms of sensory and semantic codes, but also in terms of motor codes, these codes will deliver for free, as it were, anticipations of the future course of those actions. Accordingly, the trick that perceptual modules play when they engage the motor system to support them is to exploit that system's inbuilt power to predict the future course of events. With this view, the added value of motor coding does not so much arise from its contribution to the perception of the present (i.e. analyzing what is happening now) but rather to the anticipation of the future (i.e. forecasting what is going to happen next).

In fact the common-sense notion of action understanding may comprise both these aspects. To understand an action requires the build-up of a dynamical representation that will always extend, to some degree, over the past, the present, and the future. Sensory analysis and semantic enrichment take care of the past and the present. The future is taken care of by motor enrichment, supplied by a system whose proper function is to act as an anticipation engine. For social animals like humans, anticipating what the other is going to do next is often more important than recognizing what he or she is doing now. This may be a key to understanding why motor coding of action is so widespread among primates.

Acknowledgements

We thank Franz Mechsner and Jochen Müsseler for providing some of the figures and Max Schreder for drawing others.

References

Anderson JR, Lebiere C (1998). *The Atomic Components of Thought*. Mahwah, NJ: Lawrence Erlbaum.

Bekkering H, Prinz W (2002). Goal representations in imitative actions. In K Dautenhahn, CL Nehaniv, (ed.) *Imitation in Animals and Artifacts*, pp. 555–72. Cambridge, MA: MIT Press.

Bekkering H, Wohlschläger A (2002). Action perception and imitation. In W Prinz, B Hommel, (ed.) *Attention and Performance XIX: Common Mechanisms in Perception and Action*, pp. 294–314. Oxford, UK: Oxford University Press.

Bekkering H, Wohlschläger A, Gattis M (2000). Imitation of gestures in children is goal-directed. *Q J Exp Psychol*, **53A**, 153–64.

Blakemore S-J, Decety J (2001). From the perception of action to the understanding of intention. *Nat Rev Neurosc*, **2**, 561–7.

Brass M, Bekkering H, Prinz W (2001). Movement observation affects movement execution in a simple response task. *Acta Psychol*, **106**, 3–22.

Buccino G, Binkofski F, Fink GR, Fadiga L, Fogani L, Gallese V, *et al.* (2001). Action observation activates premotor and parietal areas in a somatotopic manner: an fMRI study. *Eur J Neurosci*, **13**, 400–4.

Carpenter WB (1874). *Principles of Mental Physiology*. London: John Churchill.

Chaminade T, Meary D, Orliaguet J-P, Decety J (2001). Is perceptual anticipation a motor simulation? A PET study. *Neuroreport*, **12**, 3669–74.

De Maeght, Prinz W (2004). Action induction through action observation. *Psychological Research*, **68**, 97–114.

Decety J, Grèzes J (1999). Neural mechanisms subserving the perception of human actions. *Trends Cogn Sci*, **3**, 172–8.

Decety J, Chaminade T, Grèzes J, Meltzoff AN (2002). A PET exploration of the neural mechanisms involved in reciprocal imitation. *Neuroimage*, **15**, 265–72.

Descartes R. (1664). *L'Homme*. Paris: Theodore Girard.

Di Pellegrino G, Fadiga L, Fogassi L, Gallese V, Rizzolatti G (1992). Understanding motor events: a neurophysiological study. *Exp Brain Res*, **91**, 176–80.

Elsner B, Hommel B (2001). Effect anticipation and action control. *J Exp Psychol Hum Percept Perform*, **27**, 229–40.

Elsner B, Hommel B, Mentschel C, Drzezga A, Prinz W, Conrad B, *et al.* (2002). Linking actions and their perceivable consequences in the human brain. *NeuroImage*, **17**, 364–72.

Flach R, Knoblich G, Prinz W. (2003). Synchronizing with self- and other-generated action effects. *Brain Cogn*, **153**, 503–13.

Flach R, Knoblich G, Prinz W. Temporal cues in self-recognition. *Psychological Research*, in press.

Gallese V, Goldman A (1998). Mirror neurons and the simulation theory of mind-reading. *Trends Cogn Sci*, **2**, 493–501.

Gallese V, Fadiga L, Fogassi L, Rizzolatti G. (1996). Action recognition in the premotor cortex. *Brain*, **119**, 593–609.

Gleissner B, Meltzoff AN, Bekkering H (2000). Children's coding of human action: cognitive factors influencing imitation in 3-year-olds. *Dev Sci*, **3**, 405–14.

Greenwald AG (1970). Sensory feedback mechanisms in performance control: with special reference to the ideo-motor mechanism. *Psychol Rev*, **77**, 73–99.

Greenwald AG (1972). On doing two things at once: time sharing as a function of ideomotor compatibility. *J Exp Psychol*, **94**, 52–7.

Harris P (1992). From simulation to folk psychology: the case for development. *Mind Lang*, **7**, 120–44.

Hebb DO (1949). *The Organization of Behavior*. New York: Wiley.

Hommel B (1998). Perceiving one's own action—and what it leads to. In Jordan JS, ed. *Systems Theory and A Priori Aspects of Perception*. Amsterdam: North-Holland, 143–79.

Hommel B, Prinz W (1997). *Theoretical Issues in Stimulus–Response Compatibility*. Amsterdam: North-Holland.

Hommel B, Müsseler J, Aschersleben G, Prinz W (2001). The theory of event coding (TEC): a framework for perception and action. *Behav Brain Sci*, **24**, 849–937.

Hull CL (1930). Knowledge and purpose as habit mechanisms. *Psychol Rev*, **37**, 511–25.

Iacoboni M, Woods R., Brass M, Bekkering H, Mazziotta JC, Rizzolatti G (1999). Cortical mechanisms of human imitation. *Science*, **286**, 2526–8.

Ishimura G, Shimojo S (1994). Voluntary action captures visual motion. *Invest Ophthalmol Vis Sci*, **36**, 1275.

James W (1890). *The Principles of Psychology*. New York: Holt.

Jeannerod M (1988). *The Neural and Behavioral Organization of Goal-Directed Movements*. New York: Oxford University Press.

Jeannerod M (1999). The 25th Bartlett Lecture. To act or not to act: perspectives on the representation of actions. *Qy J Exp Psychol*, **52A**, 1–29.

Kelso JAS (1984). Phase transitions and critical behavior in human bimanual coordination. *Am J Physiol*, **15**, R1000–4.

Knoblich G, Flach R (2001). Predicting action effects: interactions between perception and action. *Psychol Sci*, **12**, 467–72.

Knoblich G, Prinz W (2001). Recognition of self-generated actions from kinematic displays of drawing. *J Exp Psychol Hum Percept Perform*, **27**, 456–65.

Knoblich G, Seigerschmidt E, Flach R, Prinz W (2002). Authorship effects in the prediction of hand writing strokes: evidence for action simulation during action perception. *Q J Exp Psychol*, **55A**, 1027–46.

Knuf L, Aschersleben G, Prinz W (2001). An analysis of ideomotor action. *J Exp Psychol Gen*, **130**, 779–98.

Koski L, Wohlschläger A, Bekkering H, Woods RP, Dubeau MC, Mazziotta JC, *et al.* (2002). Modulation of motor and premotor activity during imitation of target-directed actions. *Cereb Cortex*, **12**, 847–55.

Kosslyn SM, König O (1992). *Wet Mind: The New Cognitive Neuroscience*. New York: Free Press.

Kunde W (2001). Response–effect compatibility in manual choice reaction tasks. *J Exp Psychol Hum Percept Perform*, **27**, 387–94.

Kunde W, Hoffmann J, Zellmann P (2002). The impact of anticipated action effects on action planning. *Acta Psychol*, **109**, 137–55.

Lotze RH (1852). *Medicinische Psychologie oder Physiologie der Seele*. Leipzig: Weidmann'sche Buchhandlung.

MacKay D (1987). *The Organization of Perception and Action: A Theory of Language and Other Cognitive Skills*. Berlin: Springer.

Mechsner F, Kerzel D, Knoblich G, Prinz W. (2001). What is coordinated in bimanual coordination. *Nature*, **414**, 69–72.

Miller GA, Galanter E, Pribram, H (1960). *Plans and the Structure of Behavior*. New York: Holt, Rinehart and Winston.

Müller K, Schmitz F, Schnitzler A, Freund M-J, Aschersleben G, Prinz W (2000). Neuromagnetic correlates of sensorimotor synchronization. *Journal of Cognitive Neuroscience*, **12**, 546–55.

Müsseler J, Hommel B (1997). Blindness to response-compatible stimuli. *J Exp Psychol Hum Percept Perform*, **23**, 861–72.

Müsseler J, Wühr P (2002). Response-evoked interference in visual encoding. In W Prinz, B Hommel, (ed.) *Attention and Performance XIX: Common Mechanisms in Perception and Action*, pp. 520–37. Oxford: Oxford University Press.

Müsseler J, Wühr P, Prinz W (2000). Varying the response code in the blindness to response-compatible stimuli. *Vis Cogn*, **7**, 743–67.

Newell A (1990). *Unified Theories of Cognition*. Cambridge, MA: Harvard University Press.

Prinz W (1984). Modes of linkage between perception and action. In W Prinz, AF Sanders, (ed.) *Cognition and Motor Processes*, pp. 185–93. Berlin: Springer-Verlag.

Prinz W (1987). Ideomotor action. In H Heuer, AF Sanders, (ed.) *Perspectives on Perception and Action*, pp. 47–76. Hillsdale, NJ: Lawrence Erlbaum.

Prinz W (1990). A common-coding approach to perception and action. In O Neumann, W Prinz, (ed.) *Relationships Between Perception and Action: Current Approaches*, pp. 167–201. Berlin: Springer-Verlag.

Prinz W (1997). Perception and action planning. *Eur J Cogn Psychol*, **9**, 129–54.

Prinz W, Meltzoff AN (2002). An introduction to the imitative mind and brain. In AN Meltzoff, W Prinz, (ed.) *The Imitative Mind: Development, Evolution, and Brain Bases*, pp. 1–15. Cambridge: Cambridge University Press.

Proust J (2002). Can 'radical' simulation theories explain psychological concept acquisition? In J Dokic, J Proust, (ed.) *Simulation and Understanding of Action*, pp. 201–28. Amsterdam: John Benjamins.

Rizzolatti G, Arbib MA (1998). Language within our grasp. *Trends Neurosci*, **21**, 188–94.

Rizzolatti G, Fogassi L, Gallese V (2001). Neurophysiological mechanisms underlying imitation and the understanding of action. *Nat Rev Neurosci*, **2**, 661–70.

Schubotz RI, von Cramon DY (2001). Functional organization of the lateral premotor cortex: fMRI reveals different regions activated by anticipation of object properties, location and speed. *Cogn Brain Res*, **11**, 97–112.

Shepard RN, Metzler J (1971). Mental rotation of three-dimensional objects. *Science*, **191**, 701–3.

Simon JR (1990). The effects of an irrelevant directional cue on human information processing. In RW Proctor, TG Reeve, (ed.) *Stimulus–Response Compatibility: An Integrated Perspective*, pp. 31–86. Amsterdam: Elsevier.

Stock A, Hoffmann J (2002). Intentional fixation of behavioural learning, or how R-O learning blocks S-R learning. *Eur J Cogn Psychol*, **14**, 127–53.

Stürmer B, Aschersleben G, Prinz W (2000). Correspondence effects with manual gestures and postures: a study on imitation. *J Exp Psychol Hum Percept Perform*, **26**, 1746–59.

Thorndike EL (1911). *Animal Intelligence*. New York: Macmillan.

Thorndike EL (1913). Ideo-motor action. *Psychol Rev*, **20**, 91–106.

Viviani P, Stucchi N (1992). Motor–perceptual interactions. In GE Stelmach, J Requin, (ed.) *Tutorials in Motor Behavior*, pp. 229–48. Amsterdam: North-Holland.

Wexler M, Kosslyn SM, Berthoz A (1998). Motor processes in mental rotation. *Cognition*, **68**, 77–94.

Wohlschläger A (2000). Visual motion priming by invisible actions. *Vision Res*, **40**, 925–30.

Wohlschläger A, Wohlschläger A (1998). Mental and manual rotation. *J Exp Psychol Hum Percept Perform*, **24**, 397–412.

Wolpert DM, Kawato M (1998). Multiple paired forward and inverse models for motor control. *Neural Netw*, **11**, 1317–29.

Wühr P, Müsseler J (2002). Blindness to response-compatible stimuli in the psychological refractory period paradigm. *Vis Cogn*, **9**, 421–57.

Chapter 6

Cerebellar motor and cognitive functions

Jeremy D. Schmahmann

Introduction

Cerebellar disorders typically manifest with deficits in motor control. It has become apparent that many cerebellar patients also experience changes in intellect and mood, and mounting evidence suggests that cerebellar pathology may be associated with alterations principally in mental function, rather than motor performance. There is a new realization that defining the role of the cerebellum in higher-order behavior is not only of academic interest to the fields of behavioral neurology and psychiatry, but has the potential to help explain the fundamental function of the cerebellum and to benefit patients with cerebellar diseases by devising optimal therapeutic and rehabilitation strategies.

The cerebellar motor syndrome

Impairment of gait (ataxia), extremity coordination (dysmetria), disordered eye movements, poor articulation (dysarthria), impaired swallowing (dysphagia), and tremor characterize the cerebellar motor syndrome. The basic deficit common to the motor incapacity is impairment of rate, rhythm, and force of contraction. In the early stages of cerebellar degenerative disorders, balance is poor and there is inability to stand on one leg or perform tandem gait. As the condition progresses, walking is characterized by widened base, turning is problematic and can result in falls, and there is high stepping, staggering, and lurching from side to side. When severe, ataxic individuals are no longer able to stand or walk without great assistance and effort. Dysmetria of the extremities is evident in dysdiadochokinesis (the impairment of alternating movements), dysrhythmic tapping of feet or hands, terminal dysmetria and swerving of the arm with finger to nose testing, side-to-side dysmetria and proximal overshoot with the heel to shin test, and decomposition of movement evident in the attempt to draw an imaginary circle in the air with the legs. The rebound phenomenon occurs (overcorrection of passive displacement of the limb) as well as overshoot of the affected extremity when following a stimulus rapidly, and sometimes tremor of extremities, head, and trunk (titubation). Tone is decreased, a sign formerly thought to be the pathophysiologic basis of the motor disability. Abnormal eye movements at rest include square-wave jerks, microsaccades, and chaotic movements termed opsoclonus and ocular flutter. The hallmark feature of nystagmus is present with horizontal gaze, and less often with vertical gaze; there are saccadic intrusions into the smooth pursuit reflex, hypometric or hypermetric saccades, slowing of saccades, impairment of the normal oculokinetic nystagmus, and loss of the ability to cancel the vestibulo-ocular reflex (as in focusing on a stationery object when the background is moving, performed with the patient rotating about an axis). Speech is characterized by 'scanning' dysarthria, with alteration in rate (slower), rhythm (irregular), and force (variable volume). There is slurring of speech, tremor of the voice, and ataxic respiration. When the cerebellar motor syndrome is fully manifest it is a striking and potentially severely disabling condition.

Unlike other disorders that affect the motor system, documenting disease severity and progression has been suboptimal for the ataxias. The development of the International Cooperative Ataxia Rating Scale (ICARS) (Trouillas *et al.* 1997) should be helpful in documenting response to the treatment options that will hopefully evolve in concert with the enhanced understanding of the neurobiology of disorders such as the spinocerebellar ataxias (SCAs)and multiple systems atrophy. More objective computerized tests of dysmetria are being developed and will hopefully complement and help validate the clinical scales.

The cerebellar motor syndrome does not necessarily occur in all cerebellar diseases. Indeed, in both monkeys and humans, lesions of the cerebellar dentate nucleus, the latter performed for the successful relief of parkinsonian tremor (Zervas *et al.* 1967), do not produce motor disability.

Non-motor aspects of cerebellar function

Around the time that Flourens (1824) concluded that the cerebellum is a motor control device, and long before the notion of cerebellum as a motor apparatus became entrenched by experimental work and clinical observations, investigators [perhaps starting with Combettes (1831)] described individuals with different forms of cerebellar damage, including failure of development (agenesis) and cerebellar atrophy, who demonstrated impairments of intellectual function and emotional or psychiatric disturbances (Schmahmann 1991). Later clinical studies identified a relationship between the cerebellum and personality, aggression and emotion (Heath *et al.* 1979), and they linked psychosis, and schizophrenia in particular, with enlargement of the fourth ventricle, smaller cerebellar vermis, and cerebellar atrophy (Moriguchi 1981; Lippmann *et al.* 1982). In the middle and later decades of the twentieth century, before the genetic basis of the ataxias was identified and multiple systems atrophy was classified with the synucleinopathies (Dickson *et al.* 1999), patients with cerebellar cortical atrophy and what was known as olivopontocerebellar atrophy (OPCA) were found to have cognitive problems. These included impairments in verbal intelligence, visuospatial abilities, learning and memory, and frontal system functions (Landis *et al.* 1974; Kish *et al.* 1988; Bracke-Tolkmitt *et al.* 1989; Botez-Marquard and Botez 1993). Tests showed deficits in strategy formation (Grafman *et al.* 1992) and procedural learning (Pascual-Leone *et al.* 1993).

Now that genetic diagnosis of many of the SCAs is available, new information suggests that there is some degree of cognitive change at different stages in most of them (Geschwind 1999). For example, impaired executive functions, deficits in verbal short-term memory, and mild generalized cognitive impairment (Burk *et al.* 2001) have been documented in SCA 1 (CAG repeat on chromosome 6). Patients with SCA 2 (triplet repeat on chromosome 12) may develop poor memory, concentration problems, impairments of conceptual reasoning, and frontal executive dysfunction on tests of verbal fluency and Luria's test of motor set switching, as well as emotional instability and impulsivity (Gambardella *et al.* 1998; Storey *et al.* 1999). Individuals with Machado–Joseph disease or SCA 3 (CAG expansion on chromosome 14) demonstrate deficits in visual and verbal attention, verbal fluency, and planning, and strategy tests such as the Wisconsin Card Sort Test (Zawacki *et al.* 2002). In SCA 13 (chromosome 19), moderate mental retardation (IQ 62–76) occurs in association with a progressive childhood-onset cerebellar 'motor' syndrome and developmental delay (Herman-Bert *et al.* 2000). Dementia is part of the diagnosis in SCA 17 [dementia, psychosis, extrapyramidal feature, and seizures, with a CAG repeat on chromosome 6 (Koide *et al.* 1999; Nakamura *et al.* 2001)] and in SCA 21 [ataxia with hyporeflexia, akinesia, rigidity, and cognitive impairment in a French kindred, with linkage to chromosome 7 (Devos *et al.* 2001)]. In Friedreich's ataxia the major pathology is located outside the cerebellum, and the extent of neuropsychological impairment has been studied with varying results. Some have noted impairments on tests of visual-perceptual and visual-constructive abilities, slowed information processing speed, decreased sustained attention, reduced verbal span, deficits in letter fluency, and impaired acquisition and consolidation of verbal information (Wollmann *et al.* 2002). In contrast, other studies have shown patients with Friedreich's ataxia to be relatively cognitively intact (White *et al.* 2000).

Pathological features are not confined to the cerebellum in most of these hereditary ataxias, and so the cognitive and emotional impairments are unlikely to be related exclusively to cerebellum.

In patients with focal cerebellar lesions, language problems include agrammatism (Silveri *et al.* 1994), decreased verbal fluency (Molinari *et al.* 1997), and inability to detect one's own errors in tasks such as the verb-for-noun generation paradigm (Fiez *et al.* 1992). Patients with ataxia have difficulties with attentional modulation (Courchesne *et al.* 1994), motor skill learning (Sanes *et al.* 1990; Thach *et al.* 1992; Doyon *et al.* 2002), and the ability to acquire conditional associative reflexes (Solomon *et al.* 1989). Experimental studies in animals reveal that electrical potentials are activated in the cerebellum by stimulation of somatosensory, visual, and auditory cortices (Snider 1950), stimulation of deep cerebellar nuclei evokes autonomic responses (Zanchetti and Zoccolini 1954; Martner 1975), grooming, predatory attack, and sham rage (Moruzzi 1947; Reis *et al.* 1973), and lesions of the cerebellar anterior interpositus nucleus prevent or abolish conditional associative learning tasks (Thompson *et al.* 1997).

This clinical and experimental background notwithstanding, a persistent set of clinical questions has limited the consideration of the cerebellum as an integral component of the circuits that subserve cognition and emotion. That is, are the reported cognitive impairments in cerebellar patients observed only with subtle neuropsychological tests, or are they indeed relevant for patients' lives? Do the deficits result from cerebellar damage itself, or from lesions in other brain regions affected by the neurodegenerative disorders?

The cerebellar cognitive affective syndrome: adults

In order to address the clinical uncertainties regarding the effect of focal cerebellar lesions on higher-order behaviors, Schmahmann and Sherman (1998) performed neurological examinations, bedside mental state tests, and neuropsychological testing in 20 patients with lesions confined to the cerebellum. Thirteen patients had stroke, three had post-infectious cerebellitis, three had cerebellar cortical atrophy, and one was studied following excision of a midline tumor. A pattern of clinically relevant behavioral changes was determined that could be diagnosed at the bedside and further quantified by neuropsychological tests. This constellation, termed the cerebellar cognitive affective syndrome (CCAS), was characterized by the following deficits:

(1) disturbances of executive function including deficient planning, set-shifting, abstract reasoning, working memory, and decreased verbal fluency;

(2) impaired spatial cognition, including visuospatial disorganization and impaired visuospatial memory;

(3) personality change manifesting as flattening or blunting of affect, and disinhibited or inappropriate behavior;

(4) linguistic difficulties, including dysprosodia, agrammatism, and mild anomia.

The net effect of these disturbances in cognitive functioning was a general lowering of overall intellectual function (Table 6.1).

These impairments were present on routine bedside mental state tests and were confirmed using standardized neuropsychological tests. They were clinically relevant, were noted by family members and the medical staff, and could not be explained by difficulties with motor control because in many cases the motor incoordination was mild. The neurobehavioral presentation was more pronounced and generalized in those with bilateral or large unilateral infarctions in the posterior lobes in the territory of the

Table 6.1 Principal clinical features of the cerebellar cognitive affective syndrome in adults

Executive function
Planning, set-shifting, verbal fluency, abstract reasoning, working memory
Spatial cognition
Visual spatial organization and memory
Personality change
Blunting of affect or disinhibited and inappropriate behavior
Language deficits
Agrammatism and aprosodia

Source: Schmahmann and Sherman 1998

posterior inferior cerebellar arteries, and in those with subacute onset of pancerebellar disorders such as occurs with post-infectious cerebellitis. It was less evident in patients with more slowly progressive cerebellar degenerations, in the recovery phase (3–4 months) after acute stroke, and in those with restricted cerebellar pathology (smaller strokes in the territory supplied by the superior cerebellar artery, i.e. in the anterior lobe of the cerebellum or the rostral part of the posterior lobe). The vermis was consistently involved in patients with pronounced affective presentations.

The clinical relevance of the CCAS has been replicated in subsequent reports of adults with cerebellar strokes. Malm *et al.* (1998) demonstrated deficits in attention, working memory, visuospatial skills, and cognitive flexibility, and stroke patients studied by Neau *et al.* (2000) had deficits in executive function, spatial cognition, attention, and some language tasks. Case reports have shown that patients with right cerebellar infarction develop impairments of linguistic processing, including agrammatism, decreased verbal fluency (Molinari *et al.* 1997), and deficits on antonym generation tasks (Gebhart *et al.* 2002).

The cerebellar cognitive affective syndrome: children

An under-recognized but important aspect of cerebellar function is its impact on cognition and emotion in children with cerebellar disorders. Levisohn *et al.* (2000) documented that the CCAS also occurs in children. Characteristic behavioral deficits in 19 children aged 3–14 years who had undergone resection of cerebellar tumors included difficulties with initiation of language, impaired verbal fluency and word-finding difficulties, decreased story retrieval, deficits in sequencing, planning, and maintaining sets, and visuospatial deficits. Impaired regulation of affect was seen in children with damage to the vermis, including irritability, impulsivity, disinhibition, and lability of affect with poor attentional and behavioral modulation. Riva and Giorgi (2000) observed similar phenomena in children following resection of cerebellar tumors, namely impairment in verbal intelligence and complex language tasks following right cerebellar hemisphere lesions, and deficient non-verbal tasks and prosody after left cerebellar hemisphere lesions. Children with vermal involvement developed irritability and autistic-like features. In the small series investigated by Scott *et al.* (2001), children with right cerebellar hemisphere tumors experienced a subsequent plateau in verbal and/or literacy skills, whereas those with left cerebellar damage were associated with delayed or impaired spatial skills.

The posterior fossa syndrome is observed in approximately 15% of children who undergo resection of midline cerebellar tumors (Wisoff and Epstein 1984; Kingma *et al.* 1994), although there was a higher incidence in our study (Levisohn *et al.* 2000). It is characterized by the development of mutism 1–4 days post-operatively, and in the recovery phase over a period of months it is accompanied by dysarthria, buccal and lingual apraxia, and a behavioral syndrome that includes regressive personality changes, apathy, withdrawal, and poverty of spontaneous movement. Emotional lability is marked, and there is rapid fluctuation of expression of emotion that gravitates between irritability, with inconsolable crying and agitation, to giggling and easy distractibility (Pollack *et al.* 1995).

Developmental anomalies

Cognitive and behavioral problems in children with cerebellar lesions have been observed in the setting of absence of the cerebellum (either complete or partial agenesis), as well as non-progressive cerebellar ataxia, previously called ataxic cerebral palsy. It used to be taught that cerebellar agenesis is asymptomatic, but this appears to be incorrect, from the perspective of motor symptoms (Glickstein 1994) as well as higher-order behavior. Gardner *et al.* (2001) reported delayed milestones, mild motor impairments, and intellectual handicap in three patients with near-total absence of the cerebellum. Chheda *et al.* (2002) found that near-complete or partial cerebellar agenesis in six children was accompanied by behavioral and motor deficits. The severity and range of the motor, cognitive, and psychiatric impairments were greater in those with more pronounced agenesis. The children presented with gross and fine motor delay, oral motor apraxia, impaired saccades and vestibulo-ocular reflex cancellation, clumsiness, and mild ataxia. Behavioral features included autistic-like stereotypical performance, obsessive rituals, and difficulty in understanding social cues. Tactile defensiveness (avoidance of, and adverse reaction to, touch) was a prominent feature in four children. Executive impairments included perseveration, disinhibition, and poor abstract reasoning, working memory, and verbal fluency. Spatial cognition was impaired for perceptual organization, visuospatial copying, and recall. Some children presented with expressive language delay as the principal manifestation; in two instances this was so severe as to require instruction in sign language. Impaired prosody was evident in all cases, and over-regularization of past-tense verbs was noted. In longitudinal follow-up, extensive rehabilitation enhanced motor, linguistic, and cognitive performance.

Several observations suggest a relationship between developmental anomalies of cerebellum and neurobehavioral syndromes. Quantitative morphometry of the cerebellum in attention-deficit hyperactivity disorder reveals smaller posterior lobes of the vermis in both males (Berquin *et al.* 1998; Mostofsky *et al.* 1998) and females (Castellanos *et al.* 2001), and the size of the vermis seems to be related to the severity of this disorder. Allin *et al.* (2001) found that the cerebellum is significantly smaller in children who were born very preterm (before 33 weeks of gestation), and this is correlated with impaired executive and visuospatial functions, as well as impaired language skills—the principal features of the CCAS. One of the theories of the pathophysiology of dyslexia is that cerebellar abnormalities prevent normal eye movements and interfere with the acquisition of lexical information (Nicolson *et al.* 2001). These investigators (Nicolson *et al.* 1999) found support for this hypothesis by showing that individuals with dyslexia have lower cerebellar activation than controls on positron emission tomography (PET) scans when learning novel sequences and when executing prelearned sequences of finger movements. Acquired dyslexia was also noted in patients with lesions of the vermis and paravermian region (Moretti *et al.* 2002).

Psychiatric disorders

Adults and children with CCAS may experience altered regulation of mood and personality, display obsessive–compulsive tendencies, and demonstrate psychotic thinking. As discussed above, early accounts of the behavioral consequences of cerebellar lesions focused on psychiatric manifestations, and the morphologic changes in the cerebellum in schizophrenia and other psychoses. The notion that there is a cerebellar component to the pathophysiology of schizophrenia is gaining momentum from current morphometric, metabolic, and functional imaging studies. Nopoulos *et al.* (1999) performed automated volumetric measures of subregions of the vermis in schizophrenics and found that the anterior lobe vermis was smaller than in controls, and was positively correlated with total cerebellar volume, reduced temporal lobe volume, and full-scale IQ. Further, lower cerebellar volume in schizophrenics was associated with the duration of negative and psychotic symptoms and with psychosocial impairment (Wassink *et al.* 1999). The vermis was decreased in size despite overall increased cerebellar blood volume in the schizophrenic patients studied by Loeber *et al.* (1999). These investigators (Loeber *et al.* 2001) also found that, compared with controls, schizophrenics have a significantly smaller inferior vermis and less cerebellar hemispheric asymmetry. Similarly, Ichimiya *et al.* (2001) found significantly reduced vermis volume in neuroleptic-naive schizophrenic patients wh correlated with the Depression and Paranoia subscores of the Brief Psychiatric Rating Scale, and Volz *et al.* (2000) found reduced volumes in the left cerebellar hemisphere and right cerebellar vermis, along with smaller volumes in the frontal lobe, temporal lobe, and thalamus. Not all studies demonstrate smaller cerebellar volumes (Staal *et al.* 2001). Levitt *et al.* (1999) observed that vermis volume was greater in their schizophrenia population, vermis white matter volume correlated with severity of positive symptoms, thought disorder, and impairment in verbal logical memory, and patients showed a trend for more cerebellar hemispheric volume asymmetry (left greater than right).

Metabolic abnormalities on magnetic resonance spectroscopy of chronically medicated male schizophrenics include decreased N-acetyl-aspartate, a putative neuronal/axonal marker, and creatine in the anterior cerebellar vermis, independent of duration of illness or neuroleptic dose (Deicken *et al.* 2001). PET in neuroleptic-naive patients with schizophrenia has revealed increased metabolic activity in the cerebellum, thalamus, and retrosplenial cortex, along with decreased metabolic activity in prefrontal, inferotemporal, and parietal cortices (Andreasen *et al.* 1997). Schizophrenic patients perform tests of word-list recall at similar levels to controls, but have decreased PET activation in the cerebellum, as well as in the frontal and temporal lobe areas and the thalamus (Crespo-Facorro *et al.* 1999).

Individuals with early infantile autism, once classified as juvenile schizophrenia, have enlarged fourth ventricles, loss of Purkinje cells in the lateral and inferior cerebellar cortex, and abnormal or reduced numbers of neurons in the deep cerebellar nuclei (Williams *et al.* 1980; Bauman and Kemper 1985; Ritvo *et al.* 1986; Kemper and Bauman 1998). Vermal atrophy (Courchesne *et al.* 1988) and hemispheric atrophy (Murakami *et al.* 1989) are evident on some magnetic resonance imaging (MRI) studies of autistic subjects, although these findings remain controversial (Rapin 1999). Pathological findings are present in other brain regions in autism, particularly in the limbic system, and thus it remains to be established which anatomic–pathologic features are most closely associated with the autistic features, and whether these pathologic findings cause the behavioral aberrations.

Depression has been shown to be a recurring problem in patients with SCA. Leroi *et al.* (2002) found that more than half their patients with cerebellar degeneration had psychopathology including depression, personality change, psychotic disorders, and impaired cognition. Affected individuals endorsed symptoms of depression that reached moderate to severe levels, as well as apathy. In another study (DelBello *et al.* 1999), cerebellar vermal lobules VIII–X were smaller in patients with bipolar disorder who experienced multiple episodes of depression. This suggested that cerebellar vermal atrophy may be a late neurodegenerative event in those who have multiple affective episodes. It is important that depression is recognized in cerebellar patients because it can be treated.

The mechanisms of the cerebellar modulation of complex behavior remain to be established. Case studies in patients with emotional dysregulation have begun to address this. Parvizi *et al.* (2001) explored the disequilibrium inherent in the emotional display of some patients with cerebellar lesions by considering the phenomenon of pathologic laughter and crying in a patient in whom the cerebellum was partially deafferented by multiple infarcts. The authors concluded that pathologic laughter and crying arose from disruption of the corticopontocerebellar pathways, preventing the cerebellum from automatically adjusting the execution of emotional display to cognitive and situational context, and resulting in inadequate or chaotic behavior. Annoni *et al.* (2003) studied a patient who underwent surgical excision of an infarcted left cerebellum (posterior and anterior inferior cerebellar artery territories). They noted prominent loss of emotional display and concern, and other aspects of the CCAS including impaired cognitive flexibility and decision-making ability, as well as increased risk taking on the gambling task of Bechara *et al.* (1997). Autonomic reactions, assessed by skin conductance to positively and negatively charged stimuli, were undifferentiated, suggesting that the healthy cerebellum is involved in the generation of emotionally congruent autonomic reactions.

Functional imaging

Functional brain imaging has revealed cerebellar activation by a number of cognitive tasks in the absence of overt movement. This large field cannot be summarized here, but it is worth noting that cerebellar activation occurs with tests of sensory processing and discrimination, mental imagery, motor learning, classical conditioning, non-motor learning and memory, linguistic processing, attentional modulation, timing estimation, emotion perception and experience, visuospatial memory, executive function (including verbal working memory, strategy, reasoning, and verbal fluency), and autonomic functions including the experience and anticipation of pain, thirst, hunger, and smell. There is evidence to suggest that these different functions are topographically arranged within the cerebellum. For reviews, see Desmond and Fiez (1998) and Schmahmann (1997, 2000a).

Dysmetria of thought and the universal cerebellar transform

The attempt to understand how the cerebellum may be involved in higher-order brain functions is facilitated by a consideration of its anatomy and its connections with the cerebral hemispheres and the brainstem. Whereas the microscopic anatomy of the cerebellum is quite uniform (Voogd and Glickstein 1998), the connections of the cerebellar cortex and nuclei are complex and diverse. Anatomic tract tracing studies indicate that there are pathways linking the cerebellum with autonomic areas (Haines and Dietrichs 1984; Andrezik *et al.* 1984) and limbic areas (Heath 1973) as well as with sensorimotor cortices (Brodal 1978). Leiner *et al.* (1986) postulated that the ventral part of the cerebellar dentate nucleus (the neodentate) expanded in concert with the prefrontal cortex, and the series of investigations by Schmahmann and Pandya (1997a,b) extended the work of earlier anatomists by demonstrating that the association areas in the prefrontal cortices, posterior parietal lobes, superior temporal regions, and parahippocampal areas send information in a precisely organized manner to the nuclei of the basilar pons, from where the information is conveyed to the cerebellum. Middleton and Strick (1994) demonstrated that the deep cerebellar nuclei, notably the dentate, send information back to those areas of the prefrontal cortex that send information into the cerebellum.

Further, just as there is a precise ordering in the way that information is sent from the cerebral cortex into the pons, and from there to the cerebellum, the feedback from the dentate nucleus of the cerebellum to the cerebral cortex is also precisely arranged. Thus there are circuits or anatomic loops that link the cerebellum in a bidirectional manner with brain areas concerned with instinctive behaviors, mood, and the highest levels of cognition and reasoning.

It has become necessary to develop a new way of thinking about the cerebellum which takes all the various cerebellar roles into consideration. If the cerebellum is not only a motor control device, then what does it do, and how does it do it? The early notion that the role of the cerebellum is to modulate neurologic function is compelling, and this has been adopted and amended as part of a conceptual approach to cerebellar function referred to as the 'dysmetria of thought hypothesis' (Schmahmann 1991, 1996, 2000b). In this view, because cerebellar anatomy is essentially uniform throughout the structure, the basic work that the cerebellum does in the nervous system should also be constant as well. This universal cerebellar transform (UCT) is characterized as the cerebellar modulation of behavior, serving as an oscillation dampener maintaining function automatically around a homeostatic baseline and smoothing out performance in all domains (Table 6.2).

The specificity of the anatomic subcircuits in the cerebrocerebellar system indicates that different areas in the cerebellum interact with precise and different areas of the cerebral cortex. These anatomic subcircuits are the structural basis for putative functional subunits and facilitate what appears to be topographic organization of motor and cognitive function in the cerebellum. In this proposed schema, the anterior lobe is mainly involved with motor control, whereas the posterior lobe is more concerned with higher-order behaviors. Further, whereas the lateral parts of the posterior lobe are hypothesized to be involved in cognitive operations, the vermis is considered to be the equivalent of the limbic cerebellum (Table 6.3).

According to the dysmetria of thought hypothesis, the UCT is the essential functional contribution that the cerebellum makes to the distributed neural system. Therefore, by analogy, there should be a universal cerebellar impairment (UCI). This UCI, the hypothesis holds, is dysmetria. When the dysmetria involves the motor domain the various manifestations of ataxia are evident in extremity movements, eye movements,

Table 6.2 Essential elements of the dysmetria of thought hypothesis

The universal cerebellar transform (UCT) is a fundamental function distributed throughout the cerebellum that modulates behavior automatically around a homeostatic baseline
Anatomic specificity within the cerebrocerebellar system permits the cerebellum to contribute to multiple domains of neurologic function
By corollary, there is a universal cerebellar impairment (UCI), namely dysmetria. This includes dysmetria of movement, **ataxia**, and dysmetria of thought and emotion, the **cerebellar cognitive affective syndrome**

Source: Schmahmann (1991, 1996, 2000b)

Table 6.3 Postulated topography of function in the human cerebellum

---

Anterior–posterior organization
Sensorimotor
    Anterior lobe (lobules I–V)
    'Secondary' representation (lobules VIII and IX)
Cognitive, affective
    Neocerebellum (lobules VI, VII—vermis and hemispheres)

Medial–lateral organization
Vermis and fastigial nucleus
    Autonomic regulation, affect, emotionally important memory
Cerebellar hemispheres and dentate nucleus
    Executive, visuospatial, linguistic, learning, and memory

---

Source: Schmahmann (1991, 1996, 2000b)

speech, and equilibrium. However, when the dysmetria involves non-motor functions subserved by cerebellum, this results in dysmetria of thought, or cognitive dysmetria, and manifests as the various components of the CCAS.

Other theories attempting to account for cerebellar involvement in sensorimotor, cognitive, and affective processing have been developed. These postulate that the cerebellum forms internal predictive models of behavior (Miall *et al.* 1993) related to generation of error signals (Ito 1997); it is involved in the anticipation and preparation for response (Courchesne and Allen 1997); it operates an internal timing system for precise representation of temporal information (Ivry 1997) and is primarily activated by timing irregularity (Dreher and Grafman 2002); it is a sensory processor, monitoring and adjusting the acquisition of most of the sensory data on which the rest of the nervous system depends (Bower 1997); it provides context linkage and the shaping of responses to trial and error learning (Thach 1997); it modulates cerebral cortical excitability in a discrete topographic manner, inducing coupling between sensory inputs and motor outputs, controlling plastic changes in the cerebral cortex (Molinari *et al.* 2002); it modulates activity in motor-related cerebral cortical regions and facilitates procedural motor learning (Doyon *et al.* 2002); and it is involved in the process by which motor tasks become automatic (Jenkins *et al.* 1994) and in motor sequence learning by virtue of a general operation that it performs in preparing responses to predictable sensory events (Nixon and Passingham 2001). The notion embodied in the dysmetria of thought hypothesis discussed above, namely that the cerebellum performs its unique computations in a topographically precise manner on diverse streams of information relating to almost all aspects of behavior, has brought to life the ideas and contributions of earlier investigators, such as Snider (1950), Dow (1974), and Heath (1977), and opened the way to a new era of cognitive neuroscience. This hypothesis has been specifically adapted, for example as 'cognitive dysmetria', to account for anatomic, clinical, and functional imaging observations implicating the cerebellum in the pathophysiology of schizophrenia (Andreasen *et al.* 1996).

Conclusions

The traditional view that the cerebellum is a motor control device arose out of experimental and clinical observations dating back to the early nineteenth century, but neglected to consider the lines of evidence initiated around the same time, indicating a role for the cerebellum in non-motor domains as well. The cerebellar cognitive affective syndrome follows acquired cerebellar lesions in adults and children, and also appears to be reflected in many degenerative and developmental cerebellar disorders. Further, disorders considered within the realm of psychiatry, including schizophrenia and autism, and behaviorally defined conditions ranging from dyslexia to attention deficit disorder, appear to have a link to cerebellar pathology. This realization has rekindled interest in earlier notions of the cerebellum as the great modulator of neurologic and psychiatric function. It has also required that models of cerebellar function be reconsidered to include not only the cerebellar control of movement, but also its contribution to cognition and affect. The dysmetria of thought hypothesis offers an overarching view of cerebellar function, harmonizing the essentially uniform architecture of the cerebellar corticonuclear microcomplex with the heterogeneity of the cerebrocerebellar anatomic subcircuits, and applicable to the postulated autonomic, sensorimotor, cognitive, and affective roles of the cerebellum.

These new ideas have practical relevance. Patients with cerebellar dysfunction may struggle with depression and other forms of psychological distress, limitations in cognitive ability and flexibility, slowed reaction times and impaired attentional modulation, and less ability to 'multitask' automatically. These deficits impact quality of life, employment, and personal relationships, and need to be recognized by the medical profession as well as by patients and their families. By working with available treatments and novel cognitive rehabilitation strategies, adults and children with inherited or acquired cerebellar disorders could benefit from the new recognition that the cerebellum is not only a motor control device, but it is also an essential component of the brain mechanisms for personality, mood, and intellect.

Acknowledgements

This chapter is based in part on a paper in *J Neuropsychiatry Clin Neurosci* 2004. The assistance of Jason MacMore is gratefully acknowledged. This work was supported in part by NIMH 1RO1MH067980–1 and the Birmingham Foundation.

References

Allin M, Matsumoto H, Santhouse AM, Nosarti C, Al Asady MH, Stewart AL, *et al.* (2001). Cognitive and motor function and the size of the cerebellum in adolescents born very pre-term. *Brain*, **124**, 60–6.

Andreasen NC, O'Leary DS, Cizadlo T, Arndt S, Rezai K, Ponto LL, *et al.* (1996). Schizophrenia and cognitive dysmetria: a positron-emission tomography study of dysfunctional prefrontal–thalamic–cerebellar circuitry. *Proc Natl Acad Sci USA*, **93**, 9985–90.

Andreasen NC, O'Leary DS, Flaum M, Nopoulos P, Watkins GL, Boles Ponto LL, *et al.* (1997). Hypofrontality in schizophrenia: distributed dysfunctional circuits in neuroleptic-naive patients. *Lancet*, **349**, 1730–4.

Andrezik JA, Dormer KJ, Foreman RD, Person RJ (1984). Fastigial nucleus projections to the brain stem in beagles: pathways for autonomic regulation. *Neuroscience*, **11**, 497–507.

Annoni JM, Ptak R, Caldara-Schnetzer AS, Khateb A, Pollermann BZ (2003). Decoupling of autonomic and cognitive emotional reactions after cerebellar stroke. *Ann Neurol*, **53**, 654–8.

Bauman M, Kemper TL (1985). Histoanatomic observations of the brain in early infantile autism. *Neurology*, **35**, 866–74.

Bechara A, Damasio H, Tranel D, Damasio AR (1997). Deciding advantageously before knowing the advantageous strategy. *Science*, **275**, 1293–5.

Berquin PC, Giedd JN, Jacobsen LK, Hamburger SD, Krain AL, Rapoport JL, *et al.* (1998). Cerebellum in attention-deficit hyperactivity disorder: a morphometric MRI study. *Neurology*, **50**, 1087–93.

Botez-Marquard T, Botez MI (1993). Cognitive behavior in heredodegenerative ataxias. *Eur Neurol*, **33**, 351–7.

Bower JM (1997). Control of sensory data acquisition. *Int Rev Neurobiol*, **41**, 489–513.

Bracke-Tolkmitt R, Linden A, Canavan AGM, *et al.* (1989). The cerebellum contributes to mental skills. *Behav Neurosci*, **103**, 442–6.

Brodal P (1978). The corticopontine projection in the rhesus monkey: origin and principles of organization. *Brain*, **101**, 251–83.

Burk K, Bosch S, Globas C, Zuhlke C, Daum I, Klockgether T, *et al.* (2001). Executive dysfunction in spinocerebellar ataxia type 1. *Eur Neurol*, **46**, 43–8.

Castellanos FX, Giedd JN, Berquin PC, Watter JM, Sharp W, Tran T, *et al.* (2001). Quantitative brain magnetic resonance imaging in girls with attention-deficit/hyperactivity disorder. *Arch Gen Psychiatry*, **58**, 289–95.

Chheda M, Sherman J, Schmahmann JD (2002). Neurologic, psychiatric and cognitive manifestations in cerebellar agenesis. *Neurology*, **58** (Suppl 3), 356.

Combettes (1831). Absence complete du cervelet, des pedoncles posterieurs et la protuberance cerebrale chez une jeune fille morte dans sa onzieme annee. *Bull Soc Anat Paris*, **5**, 148–57.

Courchesne E, Allen G (1997). Prediction and preparation, fundamental functions of the cerebellum. *Learn Mem*, **4**, 1–35.

Courchesne E, Yeung-Courchesne R, Press GA, Hesselink JR, Jernigan TL (1988). Hypoplasia of cerebellar vermal lobules VI and VII in autism. *N Engl J Med*, **318**, 1349–54.

Courchesne E, Townsend J, Akshoomoff NA, Saitoh O, Yeung-Courchesne R, Lincoln AJ, *et al.* (1994). Impairment in shifting attention in autistic and cerebellar patients. *Behav Neurosci*, **108**, 848–65.

Crespo-Facorro B, Paradiso S, Andreasen NC, O'Leary DS, Watkins GL, Boles Ponto LL, *et al.* (1999). Recalling word lists reveals 'cognitive dysmetria' in schizophrenia: a positron emission tomography study. *Am J Psychiatry*, **156**, 386–92.

Deicken RF, Feiwell R, Schuff N, Soher B (2001). Evidence for altered cerebellar vermis neuronal integrity in schizophrenia. *Psychiatry Res*, **107**, 125–34.

DelBello MP, Strakowski SM, Zimmerman ME, Hawkins JM, Sax KW (1999). MRI analysis of the cerebellum in bipolar disorder: a pilot study. *Neuropsychopharmacology*, **21**, 63–8.

Desmond JE, Fiez JA (1998). Neuroimaging studies of the cerebellum: language, learning and memory. *Trends Cogn Sci*, **2**, 355–62.

Devos D, Schraen-Maschke S, Vuillaume I, Dujardin K, Naze P, Willoteaux C, *et al.* (2001). Clinical features and genetic analysis of a new form of spinocerebellar ataxia. *Neurology*, **56**, 234–8.

Dickson DW, Lin W, Liu WK, Yen SH (1999). Multiple system atrophy: a sporadic synucleinopathy. *Brain Pathol.*, **9**, 721–32.

Dow RS (1974). Some novel concepts of cerebellar physiology. *Mt Sinai J Med*, **41**, 103–19.

Doyon J, Song AW, Karni A, Lalonde F, Adams MM, Ungerleider LG (2002). Experience-dependent changes in cerebellar contributions to motor sequence learning. *Proc Natl Acad Sci USA*, **99**, 1017–22.

Dreher JC, Grafman J (2002).The roles of the cerebellum and basal ganglia in timing and error prediction. *Eur J Neurosci*, **16**, 1609–19.

Fiez JA, Petersen SE, Cheney MK, Raichle ME (1992). Impaired non-motor learning and error detection associated with cerebellar damage. *Brain*, **115**, 155–78.

Flourens P (1824). *Recherches Expérimentales sur les Propriétés et les Fonctions du Système Nerveux dans les Animaux Vertébrés*. Paris: Crevot.

Gambardella A, Annesi G, Bono F, Spadafora P, Valentino P, Pasqua AA, *et al.* (1998). CAG repeat length and clinical features in three Italian families with spinocerebellar ataxia type 2 (SCA2): early impairment of Wisconsin Card Sorting Test and saccade velocity. *J Neurol*, **245**, 647–52.

Gardner RJ, Coleman LT, Mitchell LA, Smith LJ, Harvey AS, Scheffer IE, *et al.* (2001) Near-total absence of the cerebellum. *Neuropediatrics*, **32**, 62–8.

Gebhart AL, Petersen SE, Thach WT (2002). Role of the posterolateral cerebellum in language. *Ann NY Acad Sci*, **978**, 318–33.

Geschwind DH (1999). Focusing attention on cognitive impairment in spinocerebellar ataxia. *Arch Neurol*, **56**, 20–2.

Glickstein M (1994). Cerebellar agenesis. *Brain*, **117**, 1209–12.

Grafman J, Litvan I, Massaquoi S, Stewart M, Sirigu A, Hallett M. (1992). Cognitive planning deficit in patients with cerebellar atrophy. *Neurology*, **42**, 1493–6.

Haines DE, Dietrichs E (1984). An HRP study of hypothalamo-cerebellar and cerebello-hypothalamic connections in squirrel monkey (*Saimiri sciureus*). *J Comp Neurol*, **229**, 559–75.

Heath RG (1973). Fastigial nucleus connections to the septal region in monkey and cat: a demonstration with evoked potentials of a bilateral pathway. *Biol Psychiatry*, **6**, 193–96.

Heath RG (1977). Modulation of emotion with a brain pacemaker. Treatment for intractable psychiatric illness. *J Nerv Ment Dis*, **165**, 300–17.

Heath RG, Franklin DE, Shraberg D. (1979). Gross pathology of the cerebellum in patients diagnosed and treated as functional psychiatric disorders. *J Nerv Ment Dis*, **167**, 585–92.

Herman-Bert A, Stevanin G, Netter JC, Rascol O, Brassat D, Calvas P, *et al.* (2000). Mapping of spinocerebellar ataxia 13 to chromosome 19q13.3-q13.4 in a family with autosomal dominant cerebellar ataxia and mental retardation. *Am J Hum Genet*, **67**, 229–35.

Ichimiya T, Okubo Y, Suhara T, Sudo Y (2001). Reduced volume of the cerebellar vermis in neuroleptic-naive schizophrenia. *Biol Psychiatry*, **49**, 20–7.

Ito M (1997). Cerebellar microcomplexes. *Int Rev Neurobiol*, **41**, 475–89.

Ivry R (1997). Cerebellar timing systems. *Int Rev Neurobiol*, **41**, 556–71.

Jenkins IH, Brooks DJ, Nixon PD, Frackowiak RSJ, Passingham RE (1994). Motor sequence learning: a study with positron emission tomography. *J Neurosci*, **14**, 3775–90.

Kemper TL, Bauman M (1998). Neuropathology of infantile autism. *J Neuropathol Exp Neurol*, **57**, 645–52.

Kingma A, Mooij JJA, Metemaekers JDM, Leeuw JA (1994). Transient mutism and speech disorders after posterior fossa surgery in children with brain tumors. *Acta Neurochir*, **131**, 74–9.

Kish SJ, El-Awar M, Schut L, Leach L, Oscar-Berman M, Freedman M (1988). Cognitive deficits in olivopontocerebellar atrophy. Implications for the cholinergic hypothesis of Alzheimer's dementia. *Ann Neurol*, **24**, 200–6.

Koide R, Kobayashi S, Shimohata T, Ikeuchi T, Maruyama M, Saito M, *et al.* (1999). A neurological disease caused by an expanded CAG trinucleotide repeat in the TATA-binding protein gene: a new polyglutamine disease? *Hum Mol Genet*, **8**, 2047–53.

Landis DMD, Rosenberg RN, Landis SC, Schut L, Nyhan WL (1974). Olivopontocerebellar degeneration. *Arch Neurol*, **31**, 295–307.

Leiner HC, Leiner AL, Dow RS (1986). Does the cerebellum contribute to mental skills? *Behav Neurosci*, **100**, 443–54.

Leroi I, O'Hearn E, Marsh L, Lyketsos CG, Rosenblatt A, Ross CA, *et al.* (2002). Psychopathology in patients with degenerative cerebellar diseases: a comparison to Huntington's disease. *Am J Psychiatry*, **159**, 1306–14.

Levisohn L, Cronin-Golomb A, Schmahmann JD (2000). Neuropsychological consequences of cerebellar tumor resection in children: cerebellar cognitive affective syndrome in a paediatric population. *Brain*, **123**, 1041–50.

Levitt JJ, McCarley RW, Nestor PG, Petrescu C, Donnino R, Hirayasu Y, *et al.* (1999). Quantitative volumetric MRI study of the cerebellum and vermis in schizophrenia: clinical and cognitive correlates. *Am J Psychiatry*, **156**, 1105–7.

Lippmann S, Manshadi M, Baldwin H, Drasin G, Rice J, Alrajeh S (1982). Cerebellar vermis dimensions on computerized tomographic scans of schizophrenic and bipolar patients. *Am J Psychiatry*, **139**, 667–8.

Loeber RT, Sherwood AR, Renshaw PF, Cohen BM, Yurgelun-Todd DA (1999). Differences in cerebellar blood volume in schizophrenia and bipolar disorder. *Schizophr Res*, **37**, 81–9.

Loeber RT, Cintron CM, Yurgelun-Todd DA (2001). Morphometry of individual cerebellar lobules in schizophrenia. *Am J Psychiatry*, **158**, 952–4.

Malm J, Kristensen B, Karlsson T, Carlberg B, Fagerlund M, Olsson T (1998). Cognitive impairment in young adults with infratentorial infarcts. *Neurology*, **51**, 433–40.

Martner J (1975). Cerebellar influences on autonomic mechanisms. *Acta Physiol Scand (Suppl)*, **425**, 1–42.

Miall RC, Weir DJ, Wolpert DM, Stein JF (1993). Is the cerebellum a Smith predictor? *J Mot Behav*, **25**, 203–16.

Middleton FA, Strick PL (1994). Anatomical evidence for cerebellar and basal ganglia involvement in higher cognitive function. *Science*, **266**, 458–51.

Molinari M, Leggio MG, Silveri MC (1997). Verbal fluency and agrammatism. *Int Rev Neurobiol*, **41**, 325–39.

Molinari M, Filippini V, Leggio MG (2002). Neuronal plasticity of interrelated cerebellar and cortical networks. *Neuroscience*, **111**, 863–70.

Moretti R, Bava A, Torre P, Antonello RM, Cazzato G (2002). Reading errors in patients with cerebellar vermis lesions. *J Neurol*, **249**, 461–8.

Moriguchi I (1981). A study of schizophrenic brains by computerized tomography scans. *Folia Psychiatr Neurol Jpn*, **35**, 55–72.

Moruzzi G (1947). Sham rage and localized autonomic responses elicited by cerebellar stimulation in the acute thalamic cat. *Proc 17th Int Congr on Physiology*, Oxford, 114–15.

Mostofsky SH, Reiss AL, Lockhart P, Denckla MB (1998). Decreased cerebellar posterior vermis size in fragile X syndrome: correlation with neurocognitive performance. *Neurology*, **50**, 121–30.

Murakami JW, Courchesne E, Press GA, Yeung-Courchesne R, Hesselink JR (1989). Reduced cerebellar hemisphere size and its relationship to vermal hypoplasia in autism. *Arch Neurol*, **46**, 689–94.

Nakamura K, Jeong S-Y, Uchihara T, Anno M, Nagashima K, Ikeda S, *et al.* (2001) SCA17, a novel autosomal dominant cerebellar ataxia caused by an expanded polyglutamine in TATA-binding protein. *Hum Mol Genet*, **10**, 1441–8.

Neau JP, Arroyo-Anllo E, Bonnaud V, Ingrand P, Gil R (2000). Neuropsychological disturbances in cerebellar infarcts. *Acta Neurol Scand*, **102**, 363–70.

Nicolson RI, Fawcett AJ, Berry EL, Jenkins IH, Dean P, Brooks DJ (1999). Association of abnormal cerebellar activation with motor learning difficulties in dyslexic adults. *Lancet*, **353**, 1662–7.

Nicolson RI, Fawcett AJ, Dean P (2001). Developmental dyslexia: the cerebellar deficit hypothesis. *Trends Neurosci*, **24**, 508–11.

Nixon PD, Passingham RE (2001). Predicting sensory events. The role of the cerebellum in motor learning. *Exp Brain Res*, **138**, 251–7.

Nopoulos PC, Ceilley JW, Gailis EA, Andreasen NC (1999). An MRI study of cerebellar vermis morphology in patients with schizophrenia: evidence in support of the cognitive dysmetria concept. *Biol Psychiatry*, **46**, 703–11.

Parvizi J, Anderson SW, Martin CO, Damasio H, Damasio AR (2001). Pathological laughter and crying: a link to the cerebellum. *Brain*, **124**, 1708–19.

Pascual-Leone A, Grafman J, Clark K, Stewart M, Massaquoi S, Lou JS, *et al.* (1993). Procedural learning in Parkinson's disease and cerebellar degeneration. *Ann Neurol*, **34**, 594–602.

Pollack IF, Polinko P, Albright AL, Towbin R, Fitz C (1995). Mutism and pseudobulbar symptoms after resection of posterior fossa tumors in children: Incidence and pathophysiology. *Neurosurgery*, **37**, 885–93.

Rapin I (1999). Autism in search of a home in the brain. *Neurology*, **52**, 902–4.

Reis DJ, Doba N, Nathan MA (1973). Predatory attack, grooming and consummatory behaviors evoked by electrical stimulation of cat cerebellar nuclei. *Science*, **182**, 845–7.

Ritvo ER, Freeman BJ, Scheibel AB, Duong T, Robinson H, Guthrie D, *et al.* (1986). Lower Purkinje cell counts in the cerebella of four autistic subjects. Initial findings of the UCLA–NSAC autopsy research report. *Am J Psychiatry*, **143**, 8.

Riva D, Giorgi C (2000). The cerebellum contributes to higher function during development: evidence from a series of children surgically treated for posterior fossa tumors. *Brain*, **123**, 1051–61.

Sanes JN, Dimitrov B, Hallett M (1990). Motor learning in patients with cerebellar dysfunction. *Brain*, **113**, 103–20.

Schmahmann JD (1991). An emerging concept: the cerebellar contribution to higher function. *Archiv Neurol*, **48**, 1178–87.

Schmahmann JD (1996). From movement to thought: anatomic substrates of the cerebellar contribution to cognitive processing. *Hum Brain Mapping*, **4**, 174–98.

Schmahmann JD, (ed.) (1997). The Cerebellum and Cognition. *Int Rev Neurobiol*, **41**.

Schmahmann JD (2000a). Cerebellum and brainstem. In A Toga, J Mazziotta, (ed.) *Brain Mapping. The Systems*, pp. 207–59. San Diego, CA: Academic Press.

Schmahmann JD (2000b). The role of the cerebellum in affect and psychosis. *J Neurolinguistics*, **13**, 189–214.

Schmahmann JD (2004). Disorders of the cerebellum : ataxia, dysmetria of thought , and the cerebellar cognitive affective syndrome. *J Neuropsychiatry Clin Neurosci*, **16**, 367–78.

Schmahmann JD, Pandya DN (1997a). Anatomic organization of the basilar pontine projections from prefrontal cortices in rhesus monkey. *J Neurosci*, **17**, 438–58.

Schmahmann JD, Pandya DN (1997b). The cerebrocerebellar system. *Int Rev Neurobiol*, **41**, 31–60.

Schmahmann JD, Sherman JC (1998). The cerebellar cognitive affective syndrome. *Brain*, **121**, 561–79.

Scott RB, Stoodley CJ, Anslow P, Paul C, Stein JF, Sugden EM, *et al.* (2001). Lateralized cognitive deficits in children following cerebellar lesions. *Dev Med Child Neurol*, **43**, 685–91.

Silveri MC, Leggio MG, Molinari M (1994). The cerebellum contributes to linguistic production: a case of agrammatic speech following a right cerebellar lesion. *Neurology*, **44**, 2047–50.

Snider RS (1950). Recent contributions to the anatomy and physiology of the cerebellum. *Arch Neurol Psychiatry*, **64**, 196–219.

Solomon PR, Stowe GT, Pendlebury WW (1989). Disrupted eyelid conditioning in a patient with damage to cerebellar afferents. *Behav Neurosci*, **103**, 898–902.

Staal WG, Hulshoff Pol HE, Schnack HG, van Haren NE, Seifert N, Kahn RS (2001). Structural brain abnormalities in chronic schizophrenia at the extremes of the outcome spectrum. *Am J Psychiatry*, **158**, 1140–2.

Storey E, Forrest SM, Shaw JH, Mitchell P, Gardner RJ (1999). Spinocerebellar ataxia type 2: clinical features of a pedigree displaying prominent frontal-executive dysfunction. *Arch Neurol*, **56**, 43–50.

Thach WT (1997). Context–response linkage. *Int Rev Neurobiol*, **41**, 599–611.

Thach WT, Goodkin HP, Keating JG (1992). The cerebellum and the adaptive coordination of movement. *Annu Rev Neurosci*, **15**, 403–42.

Thompson RF, Bao S, Chen L, Cipriano BD, Grethe JS, Kim JJ, *et al.* (1997). Associative learning. *Int Rev Neurobiol*, **41**, 151–89.

Trouillas P, Takayanagi T, Hallett M, Currier RD, Subramony SH, Wessel K, *et al.* (1997). International Cooperative Ataxia Rating Scale for pharmacological assessment of the cerebellar syndrome. The Ataxia Neuropharmacology Committee of the World Federation of Neurology. *J Neurol Sci*, **145**, 205–11.

Volz H, Gaser C, Sauer H (2000). Supporting evidence for the model of cognitive dysmetria in schizophrenia—a structural magnetic resonance imaging study using deformation-based morphometry. *Schizophr Res*, **46**, 45–56.

Voogd J, Glickstein M (1998). The anatomy of the cerebellum. *Trends Neurosci*, **21**, 370–5.

Wassink TH, Andreasen NC, Nopoulos P, Flaum N (1999). Cerebellar morphology as a predictor of symptom and psychosocial outcome in schizophrenia. *Biol Psychiatry*, **45**, 41–8.

White M, Lalonde R, Botez-Marquard T (2000). Neuropsychologic and neuropsychiatric characteristics of patients with Friedreich's ataxia. *Acta Neurol Scand*, **102**, 222–6.

Williams RS, Hauser SL, Purpura DP, DeLong GR, Swisher CN (1980). Autism and mental retardation. *Arch Neurol*, **37**, 749–53.

Wisoff JH, Epstein FJ (1984). Pseudobulbar palsy after posterior fossa operation in children. *Neurosurgery*, **15**, 707–9.

Wollmann T, Barroso J, Monton F, Nieto A (2002). Neuropsychological test performance of patients with Friedreich's ataxia. *J Clin Exp Neuropsychol*, **24**, 677–86.

Zanchetti A, Zoccolini A (1954). Autonomic hypothalamic outbursts elicited by cerebellar stimulation. *J Neurophysiol*, **17**, 473–83.

Zawacki TM, Grace J, Friedman JH, Sudarsky L (2002). Executive and emotional dysfunction in Machado–Joseph disease. *Mov Disord*, **17**, 1004–10.

Zervas NT, Horner FG, Gordy PD (1967). Cerebellar dentatectomy in primates and humans. *Trans Am Neurol Assoc*, **92**, 27–30.

Chapter 7

Motor learning

Mark Hallett

Introduction

Very little of human motor performance is innate, and humans certainly need to modify performance constantly to meet environmental conditions. Therefore it is obvious that motor learning is a critical mechanism of integrative physiology. Motor learning is a complex phenomenon with a number of different components and has been defined in different ways. In this chapter, it will be defined as 'a change in motor performance with practice'. This will include a number of aspects such as increasing the repertoire of motor behavior and maintenance of a new behavior over a period of time. Motor learning is classified as a type of procedural learning, different from the more extensively studied declarative learning of facts and events (Squire 1986).

Even considering only the aspect of a change in motor performance, there are at least three different phenomena: classical conditioning, adaptation learning, and skill learning (Sanes *et al.* 1990; Hallett and Grafman 1997). Classical conditioning is a change in motor output in response to specific sensory stimuli. To distinguish adaptation and skill learning, it is probably easiest to refer to the concept of operating characteristic. An operating characteristic is a descriptor of a set of movements that relate different movement variables to each other. It describes the current state of capability of the system. Generally, a change in one variable will affect another. The best known operating characteristic of motor performance is Fitts' law which relates movement speed and accuracy (Fitts 1954). Movement from point A to point B can be made at various speeds, and each speed is associated with an accuracy. Slower speeds are more accurate, and faster speeds are less accurate. Mathematically, this is described as

$$MT = a + b \log_2(2A/W)$$

where MT is movement time, A is the required movement amplitude, W is the width (or size) of the target zone, and a and b are experimentally derived constants. Another operating characteristic would be the gain associated with a visuomotor tracking task. For a particular visual stimulus, there is an associated movement. With a change in gain, the appropriate movement might be smaller or larger.

Motor adaptation learning can be defined as a change in motor performance without a change in the operating characteristic. In a point-to-point movement, a faster movement with predictable increase in inaccuracy is a change in performance, but not a change in operating characteristic. This is not necessarily just a trivial change in performance. Learning the new speed may require considerable practice, but, if associated with an increase in inaccuracy, it does not indicate a new capability of the motor system. Likewise, a change in visuomotor gain by itself does not indicate anything more than a change in the point of working on the operating characteristic.

Motor skill learning can be defined as a change in motor performance with a change in the operating characteristic. It indicates a new capability of the motor system. If a point-to-point movement is made both faster and with greater accuracy, there is an apparent violation of Fitts' law. This means that there is a new operating characteristic. In many circumstances, this would be clearly recognized as a new skill. Skill learning can probably not stand alone, separate from adaptation learning. In satisfying a new motor requirement, it is not enough to achieve a new operating characteristic; it would probably also be necessary to find the correct place on the operating characteristic to work.

The next sections will discuss the physiology of these three types of motor learning.

Classical conditioning

In classical conditioning, a conditioned stimulus (CS) is paired with an unconditioned stimulus (UCS). The UCS ordinarily produces an unconditioned response (UCR). The CS ordinarily does not evoke any response, but after sufficient pairings it produces a response, called the conditioned response (CR), that is similar in appearance to the UCR. Hence there is a new motor response to a specific stimulus. Eyeblink conditioning is a form of classical conditioning that has been extensively studied. In nonhuman animal studies, eyeblink conditioning seems to require the cerebellum, at least for the expression and timing of the response (Thompson 1990). We have studied eyeblink conditioning in normal subjects and patients with cerebellar lesions to see if the intact cerebellum is required for eye-blink conditioning in humans (Topka *et al.* 1993). We employed a classical delay conditioning paradigm in five patients with pure cerebellar cortical atrophy and seven patients with olivopontocerebellar atrophy. The results were compared with those obtained in a group of neurologically healthy volunteers matched with the patients for age and sex. The two groups of patients had similar abnormalities in the acquisition of the conditioned response and produced fewer conditioned responses than in the control subjects in any given block of trials (Fig. 7.1). Many of the patients' conditioned responses were inappropriately timed with respect to the conditioned stimulus. Similar results have also been found by others (Daum *et al.* 1993). Gerwig *et al.* (2003) have studied a series of patients with lesions in the territory of the superior cerebellar artery and posterior inferior cerebellar artery. In accord with animal data that the critical cerebellar area, Larsell lobule H VI, is in the superior cerebellum, only patients with the superior cerebellar injury had a deficit.

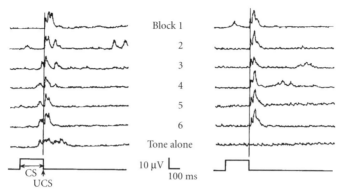

Fig. 7.1 Eyeblink conditioning of a normal subject on the left and a patient with cerebellar degeneration on the right. Records are rectified EMG from orbicularis oculi muscles. UCS is a shock to the supraorbital nerve and the CS is a tone. Records labeled blocks 1–6 are single trials from blocks with pairing of the CS and UCS. The records labeled 'tone alone' are with the CS without the UCS. In the normal subject, CRs are seen prior to the UCS in blocks 3–6 and with tone alone. No CRs are present in the cerebellar patient. Reproduced with permission from Topka *et al.* (1993). *Brain*, **116**, 961–69.

Neuroimaging studies have confirmed that the cerebellum is involved in eyeblink conditioning (Logan and Grafton 1995; Blaxton *et al.* 1996; Timmann *et al.* 1996; Schreurs *et al.* 1997; Dimitrova *et al.* 2002). The details of these studies differ and some other areas are sometimes involved, but these differences probably reflect differences in study design.

Eyeblink conditioning has been found to be normal in Parkinson's disease (Sommer *et al.* 1999) and Alzheimer's disease, indicating that basal ganglia circuitry does not seem necessary and that abnormalities of declarative learning have no influence.

The cerebellum also seems to be necessary for classical conditioning of lower-limb withdrawal reflexes (Timmann *et al.* 2000).

While it is appropriate to consider classical conditioning as a separate type of motor learning, it could be argued that it fits the definition proposed here for adaptation learning. Blinking of the eyelid to a conditioned stimulus may either occur or not. Whether it will or not, and how much, could be described by a single operating characteristic. At any one time, the amount of 'conditioning' could be the working point on the operating characteristic.

Adaptation learning

A standard example of adaptation learning is the change in gain of the vestibulo-ocular reflex (VOR). The gain of the VOR refers to the magnitude of eye movement resulting from head movement. The gain can change depending on environmental circumstances, such as a change in the magnification of eyeglasses. The amount of eye movement for a specific head movement depends on the working point on the operating characteristic defined by the gain. Selecting the appropriate gain is learning, but there is no apparent skill acquired when the gain changes. Adaptation of the VOR requires participation of the cerebellum and associated brainstem structures (Lisberger 1988).

Adaptation to lateral displacement of vision, such as that produced by prism glasses, is a method for assessing learning of a visuomotor task (Weiner *et al.* 1983). Pointing to a target is a clear example of the visual system directing the motor system. When prism glasses are used, there is at first a mismatch between where an object is seen and where the pointing is directed. With experience, normal human subjects adjust to this and begin to point correctly. This correct pointing can be a product of a true change in the visuomotor coordination or an intellectual decision to point in a different direction than where the object appears to be so that the correct movement is made. When the glasses are removed, typically the subject initially points in the opposite direction to that when the glasses were put on. In the naive subject, this is an excellent measure of true change in the visuomotor task since there is no reason for making any intellectual decision to point other than in the direction that the object appears to be. With additional experience, the subjects return to correct performance again. This type of motor learning fits well the definition of adaptation. With a stimulus, pointing could be anywhere. Choosing the correct visuomotor coordination to fit the current environmental situation is a type of adaptation learning. Patients with cerebellar damage show poor or no adaptation. On the first trial after the prisms are removed, cerebellar patients point almost exactly as they did before the experience with the prism glasses (Fig. 7.2).

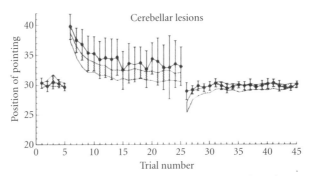

Fig. 7.2 Pointing performance before, during, and after wearing prism glasses. The shaded area is the performance of normal subjects, and the points with standard deviation bars show the performance of a group of patients with cerebellar dysfunction. The target was at 30. Prism glasses with shift to the right were worn for trials 6–25, and were taken off for trials 26–45. In trials 6–25, the cerebellar patients adapt less quickly than normal subjects. With the glasses off in trial 26, the cerebellar patients show no evidence of any adaptation learning. Reproduced with permission from Weiner *et al.* (1983). *Neurology*, **33**, 766–72.

Thus, no adaptation can be observed in this patient group. Patients with damage elsewhere in the brain, including basal ganglia and different regions of cortex, and including patients with verbal memory deficits, all show appropriate adaptation.

Prism adaptation has been further investigated by Thach and colleagues with several interesting results. Looking at the site of cerebellar lesions that impair prism adaptation, the important area seems to be the inferior cerebellum including the territory of the posterior inferior cerebellar artery (Martin *et al.* 1996a). Adaptation appears to be specific for the movements made in the training; when the movement was changed and if another body part (the other limb) was tested, there was no adaptation (Martin *et al.* 1996b). However, coordination of body parts in the training limb was variable so that there was not a highly specific pattern of interjoint coupling (Martin *et al.* 2002). This does suggest a 'dynamic and generalized' adaptation process, at least within the body part.

Another paradigm that can test adaptation learning is a task with a change in the visuomotor gain. An example is making movements of the elbow by matching targets on a computer screen. If the gain of the elbow with respect to the display on the computer screen is changed, then the amount of movement to match the targets will change. This simple gain change fits the definition of adaptation motor learning nicely. In the normal circumstance after a gain change, there would be an error which would gradually would be reduced with continued practice. We compared a group of 10 normal subjects with a group of 10 patients with cerebellar damage from degenerative diseases (Deuschl *et al.* 1996). We measured the rate of adaptation by fitting to a curve the amplitudes of successive movements during the learning. Patients showed much slower learning than did the normal controls (Fig. 7.3).

Neuroimaging studies have been done with adaptation learning. Clower *et al.* (1996) used positron emission tomography (PET) to investigate prism adaptation. When

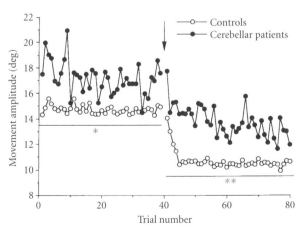

Fig. 7.3 Motor performance on an elbow flexion task with variable visuomotor gain. The gain was reduced at trial 40. The patients with cerebellar deficits show less rapid adaptation. Reproduced with permission from Deuschl *et al.* (1996). *J Neurol Neurosurg Psychiatry*, **60**, 515–19.

controlling for all other aspects of the performance, they found activation only in the posterior parietal cortex contralateral to the reaching limb. Inoue *et al.* (2000) studied movements distorted by optical rotation. Early in the process, they found regional cerebral blood flow (rCBF) increases in the rostral premotor cortex and superior parietal lobules bilaterally. In similar experiments, Ghilardi *et al.* (2000) found activation only in the posterior parietal cortex ipsilateral to the reaching limb. In other sensorimotor adaptation learning tasks, with attention to the cerebellum, it appears that cerebellar activity is prominent early in learning and then reduces (Flament *et al.* 1996; Imamizu *et al.* 2000). The decline in activity parallels the decline in errors, showing that the cerebellum plays some role in error reduction. Additionally, there is some area of the cerebellum that retains activity with the new state of adaptation, and this has been interpreted as the development of an internal model of the new state (Imamizu *et al.* 2000, 2003).

Like classical conditioning, adaptation learning does appear to depend significantly on the cerebellum; other parts of the brain play a role as well.

Skill learning

Complex multijoint arm movement tasks such a throwing a ball or playing the piano are typically considered skills. The ability to sequence all the component movements correctly, smoothly, and in an appropriate time is clearly difficult and appears to increase the behavioral repertoire. As such tasks are learned, they can be accomplished both more quickly and more accurately. This violates Fitts' law and establishes a new operating characteristic. Hence, by our definition, such learning would be skill learning.

We asked 18 patients with cerebellar degeneration and 15 normal controls to perform multijoint arm movements on a data tablet generating a trajectory connecting five via points in a given sequence (Topka *et al.* 1998). Subjects were asked to increase their accuracy but to maintain their movement time constant. If they become more accurate in the same time, this would indicate a new operating characteristic and the development of skill learning. The subjects performed 100 trials with a movement time of approximately 3500 ms (relatively slowly) and then did another 100 trials as fast as possible. In the slower task, both groups were successful in keeping time, and both improved relative accuracy at about the same rate. In the faster task, normal subjects performed more rapidly than the patients, yet they improved at a faster rate than the patients. A difference in learning rate with the faster task was confirmed by comparing a few normal subjects and patients doing the faster task first (before the slower task). These results made some facts clear. First, patients with cerebellar damage were able to learn new skills by our definition. Secondly, their ability to learn appeared to be speed related because it was worse when the required speed was fast. The coordination deficits of cerebellar patients is also speed dependent (Massaquoi and Hallett 1996). They do much better with slow movements than with fast. Thus their ability to refine movement variables needed for an adaptation component would probably be better with slow movements than with fast. We again come to the conclusion that the deficits of the cerebellar patients in this task could be related to an adaptation component. Deficits of cerebellar function do not impair skill learning as much as adaptation learning and classical conditioning.

In order to learn a skill, it is necessary to piece together numerous muscular contractions with precise timing. It would seem that cortical mechanisms are necessary for this degree of complexity. The cerebral motor cortex is clearly involved in movement, and investigations of it as well as other cortical regions do show their critical roles.

There is considerable evidence about the plasticity of the motor cortex as a function of use and motor learning. Using transcranial magnetic stimulation (TMS), it is possible to map the degree and extent of excitability of individual muscles on the scalp surface. Body parts that are used more have a larger representation (Pascual-Leone et al. 1993a), and this representation will shrink if the body part is not used (Liepert et al. 1995). We mapped the cortical motor areas, targeting the forearm finger flexor and extensor muscles in normal subjects learning a one-handed five-finger exercise on an electronic piano (Pascual-Leone et al. 1995a). The task was metronome paced so that improvement in accuracy should identify skill learning. The piano was connected by a MIDI interface to a personal computer for quantification of times of key presses. Subjects practised the task for 2 hrs daily. They improved in terms of ability to keep accurate time with the metronome and in reduction of errors. The size of the representation expanded over 5 days as the task was learned (Fig. 7.4). It is not unreasonable to consider the motor cortex as a relevant site for motor skill learning. It is clearly involved in movement, and cortical cells have complex patterns of connectivity, including variable influences on multiple muscles within a body part. Long-term potentiation (LTP) has been demonstrated in the motor cortex (Iriki et al. 1989).

Further evidence that cortical map plasticity is important in skill learning comes from primate experiments. Lesions of the basal forebrain cholinergeric pathways (which blocked cortical map plasticity) inhibited skill learning (Conner et al. 2003). However, this lesion did not block associative fear learning, again indicating the differences in different types of motor learning.

In motor learning tasks, a variety of brain regions have been demonstrated to be active with neuroimaging depending on the task (Friston et al. 1992; Grafton et al. 1992, 1994; Seitz and Roland 1992; Jenkins et al. 1994; Schlaug et al. 1994; Seitz et al. 1994; Karni et al. 1995). The primary motor cortex has almost always been activated to some extent, although because of resolution it has been often difficult to separate primary motor cortex from premotor cortex and/or primary sensory cortex. Moreover, the results have been somewhat confusing because techniques and experimental paradigms have differed, and because motor performance was not necessarily held constant over the course of learning.

One well known study used functional magnetic resonance imaging (fMRI) and focused attention on the contralateral primary motor cortex (Karni et al. 1995). Two finger-tapping sequences were compared, one that was in the process of being learned and a second that was already learned. Although the learned sequence could have been performed faster, both sequences were performed at the same rate paced by an auditory stimulus. As the motor task was learned, more area of the motor cortex was activated.

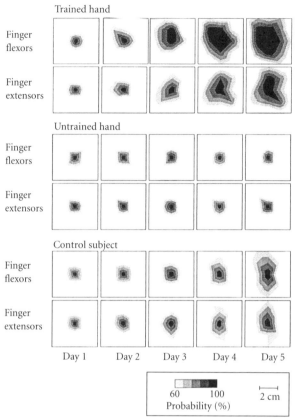

Fig. 7.4 Mapping of a 5 cm × 5 cm square region over the left motor cortex during learning of a five-finger exercise on a piano with the right hand. Maps show the probability of producing a motor evoked potential at each location. The trained hand worked 2 hrs/day; the untrained hand was the hand contralateral to the trained hand. The control subject shows the results from a subject who used his hand on the keys for 2 hrs/day, but did not learn a specific task. Reproduced with permission from Pascual-Leone *et al.* (1995). *J Neurophysiol*, **74**, 1037–45.

In most of these studies, cerebellar activation is evident in the learning phase and declines when the movement is learned. This certainly indicates a role in learning. The pattern is consistent with many possible roles, but certainly adaptation learning is one. That the cerebellar activation declines when the movement is learned is against the ideas that the cerebellum stores the movement and is in some way responsible for the automatic running of the motor program when it is well learned. On the other hand, the contralateral primary motor cortex and other cortical regions clearly play a major role in skill learning.

Late in motor skill learning, another relatively common neuroimaging result is that there is activation of parietal and premotor areas (Grafton *et al.* 1994; Jenkins *et al.* 1994;

Seitz *et al.* 1994). Sometimes the basal ganglia, particularly the putamen, are also activated (Grafton *et al.* 1994). We will see evidence for this network of structures as well with the serial reaction time task.

Sequence learning with the serial reaction time task

Many of the studies of motor learning are complicated, and it is difficult to separate out the different facets. One facet is learning the order of a number of components of a complex movement with sequential elements. The serial reaction time task (SRTT) appears to be a nice paradigm to study motor learning of sequences. The ability to carry out sequences of motor actions is clearly a critical part of most complex tasks, and the SRTT should be able to help in understanding this aspect of learning. The task is a choice reaction time with typically four possible responses. The responses can be carried out by key presses with four different fingers. A visual stimulus indicates which is the appropriate response. The completion of one response triggers the next stimulus. Each movement is simple and separate from the others, so that the movement aspect of this task is different (and easier) than other tasks considered previously such as finger tapping or piano playing. The trick in this task is that, unbeknown to the naive subject, the stimuli are a repeating sequence. With practice at this task, the responses become faster even though the subject has no conscious recognition that the sequence is repetitive. This is called implicit learning. With continuing practice and improvement, there is recognition that there is a sequence, but it may not be possible to specify what it is. Now knowledge is becoming explicit. With even more practice, the sequence can be specified and it has become declarative as well as procedural. Performance becomes even better at this stage, but the subject's strategy can change since the stimuli can be anticipated.

Thus, the SRTT appears to assess two processes relating to the sequencing of motor behavior while factoring out elements of motor coordination. As such, it might be considered a test of some components of motor skill learning.

We have looked at the intermanual transfer of implicit learning of the SRTT (Wachs *et al.* 1994). After a few blocks of training with one hand, subsequent blocks were performed with the other hand. Four groups of normal subjects were studied each under one of the following conditions: (1) random sequence, (2) a new sequence, (3) parallel image of the original sequence, and (4) mirror image of the original sequence. Only group 4 showed a carry-over effect from the original learning. This result suggests that what is stored as implicit learning is a specific sequence of motor outputs and not a spatial pattern.

Implicit learning in the SRTT is impaired in patients with cerebellar degenerations, Parkinson's disease, Huntington's disease, and progressive supranuclear palsy. (Pascual-Leone *et al.* 1993b). Patients with cerebellar degenerations were particularly severely affected. Not only was performance characterized by lack of improvement in reaction time, but there was also lack of development of explicit knowledge. Moreover, even giving the patients information about the sequence in advance (explicit knowledge) did not help with improvement in reaction time. On the other hand, implicit learning is preserved in patients with temporal lobe lesions and patients with short-term declarative memory disturbances such as most patients with Alzheimer's disease.

In relation to the question of the involvement of the primary motor cortex in implicit learning, we mapped the motor cortex with TMS contralateral to the hands of normal subjects performing the SRTT (Pascual-Leone *et al.* 1994). Mapping was done at intervals while the subjects were at rest between blocks of the SRTT. The map gradually enlarged during the implicit and explicit learning phases, but as soon as full explicit learning was achieved, the map size returned to baseline (Fig. 7.5). This suggests an important role for primary motor cortex in this task.

We examined the dynamic involvement of different brain regions in implicit and explicit motor sequence learning using PET (Honda *et al.* 1998). In an SRTT, subjects pressed each of four buttons with a different finger of the right hand in response to a visually presented number. Test sessions consisted of 10 cycles of the same 10-item sequence. The effects of explicit and implicit learning were assessed separately using a different behavioral parameter for each type of learning: correct recall of the test sequence for explicit learning, and improvement of reaction time before the successful recall of any component of the test sequence for implicit learning. During the implicit learning phase, when the subjects were not aware of the sequence, improvement of the reaction time was associated with increased activity in the contralateral primary sensorimotor cortex (Fig. 7.6). Explicit learning, shown as a positive correlation

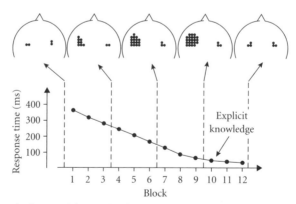

Fig. 7.5 Motor evoked potential mapping between blocks of an SRTT learned by the right hand. Bubbles show spots where motor evoked potentials were produced from both the right and left hemispheres to the contralateral hand muscles. Below are the response times in the blocks of the serial reaction time tasks; full explicit knowledge was developed by block 10. Excitability of the left motor cortex increases during the first part, but then declines after full explicit knowledge is achieved. Reproduced with permission from Pascual-Leone *et al.* (1995). In Grafman J, Boller F, Holyoak KJ, eds. *Structure and Function of the Human Prefrontal Cortex*. New York: New York Academy of Sciences, 61–70.

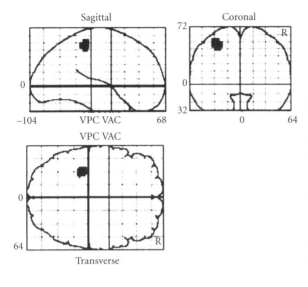

Fig. 7.6 Positron emission tomography (PET) study of an SRTT. Illustrated are sites of activation that correlate with reduction of response time in scans during blocks where there was no explicit knowledge of the sequence. Reproduced with permission from Honda *et al.* (1998). *Brain*, **121**, 2159–73.

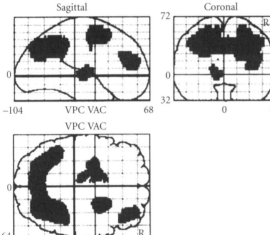

Fig. 7.7 Positron emission tomography (PET) study of an SRTT. Illustrated are sites of activation that correlate with length of the sequence that was explicitly known following the scan of that block. Reproduced with permission from Honda *et al.* (1998). *Brain*, **121**, 2159–73.

with the correct recall of the sequence, was associated with increased activity in the posterior parietal cortex, precuneus, and premotor cortex bilaterally, and also in the supplementary motor area (SMA) predominantly in the left anterior part, left thalamus, and right dorsolateral prefrontal cortex (DLPFC) (Fig. 7.7).

There have been a large number of other neuroimaging studies of the SRTT. Grafton *et al.* (1995) studied two situations. In one, a second distracting task was performed at the same time as the SRTT. Such distraction does not interfere with implicit learning, but makes explicit learning much less likely. Hence regions that were active are likely to reflect implicit learning. In a second experiment, there was no other task and subjects were scanned in the explicit learning phase. In the implicit learning situation, there was activation of the contralateral primary motor cortex, SMA and putamen. In the explicit learning situation, there was activation of the ipsilateral DLPFC and premotor cortex and of the parietal cortex bilaterally. Doyon *et al.* (2002, 2003) emphasized early cerebellar activation, a middle stage with premotor, anterior cingulate, and parietal activation, and a later stage with putamen, SMA, precuneus, and prefrontal activation. Penhune and Doyon (2002) investigated an SRTT with a different type of sequence; there was only one key, but the elements were of different duration. This begins to get at the issue of rhythm. Here again the cerebellum was active early, and later in learning the activation shifted to basal ganglia and medial frontal. Several days later, imaging during recall showed activation of primary motor cortex, premotor cortex, and parietal cortex, but not cerebellum or basal ganglia. Seidler *et al.* (2002), using an experimental paradigm similar to that of Grafton and coworkers, showed specifically that the cerebellum is not involved in early implicit learning in the SRTT. Using a distractor task during the SRTT, there was no cerebellar activation, but evaluation afterwards showed that implicit learning had indeed occurred. Cerebellar activation was present, however, upon first demonstration of the implicit learning after the distractor task was discontinued. The implication was that the cerebellar contribution related more to performance than learning itself.

Added evidence for the role of the motor cortex in SRTT learning comes from a study of transcranial direct current stimulation (TDC). Anodal TDC, which enhances cortical excitability, improves implicit learning in the SRTT, while similar stimulation of premotor and prefrontal stimulation does not (Nitsche *et al.* 2003).

Summarizing studies of the SRTT, it appears that multiple structures in the brain are involved, and that involvement comes at different stages. The primary motor cortex appears to play a definite role in implicit learning. Premotor and parietal cortical areas appear to play a role in explicit learning, perhaps in part by storage of the sequence. This concept is supported by the clinical finding that damage of premotor and parietal areas can lead to apraxia; this might be interpreted as a deficiency of motor memories for complex movements. The cerebellum also appears relevant in learning of movement sequences, given the results in the patients with cerebellar degeneration, but the nature of the role may relate more to the ability to manifest what is learned. The role of the basal ganglia is more obscure.

Consolidation

Consolidation is the process whereby learned skills become more permanent. Immediately after learning, the motor memory is fragile. In particular, it is vulnerable to disruption by learning something similar. However, if there is no disruption, with the passage of time, the memory becomes more robust. It is this process of becoming more robust with time that is designated consolidation. Consolidation was demonstrated clearly for the first time in the motor system in the study by Brashers-Krug *et al.* (1996). These investigators studied subjects making center-out movements on a two-dimensional surface under the

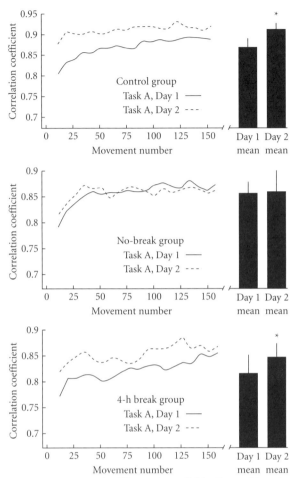

Fig. 7.8 Performance on movements in different force fields. Top: subjects learned task A, and then returned the next day and did task A again. Preservation of the learning was demonstrated at the beginning of day 2. Middle: subjects learned task A, then immediately learned task B, and then returned on day 2 and did task A again. There was no preservation of task A. Bottom: subjects learned task A, had a 4 hrs break, then learned task B, and then returned on day 2 to do task A. The learning of task A was consolidated during the 4 hrs period. Reproduced with permission from Brashers-Krug *et al.* (1996). *Nature*, **382**, 252–5.

influence of various force fields. Without the force field, the movements are made in straight paths. When first experiencing the field, the movements become distorted, but with practice the movements can become straight even in the force field. If a force field is learned, then the performance on the field is maintained the next day (Fig. 7.8). If a different force field is learned immediately after the first, the learning of the first field is completely lost. However, this disruption by a second force field does not occur if there is a delay of 4–6 hrs between learning the two fields. This demonstrates that consolidation of learning of the first field occurs during this several-hour period.

Imaging studies have been performed with force-field learning, and early in learning there was activation of motor cortex, putamen, and prefrontal cortex (Shadmehr and Holcomb 1997). In the recall of the force field, activation was now primarily in the parietal and premotor cortex and cerebellum. The pattern of early learning and late recall is similar to the pattern seen by Honda and coworkers with SRTT learning. A somewhat different pattern of activations was seen in another neuroimaging study of force-field learning (Krebs *et al.* 1998).

The learning of force fields can be reduced by lorazepam and dextromethorphan, suggesting that GABAergic and NMDA mechanisms are involved (Donchin *et al.* 2002). In the same study, there was evidence that scopolamine and lamotrigine did not inhibit the learning, implying that cholinergic mechanisms and membrane excitability do not play major roles.

Force-field learning is a nice model and has been used to advantage to illustrate certain principles. However, it is a complex task and, while often referred to as an example of adaptation learning, it is probably a combination of adaptation and skill. In general, there will be greater accuracy with similar timing implying a new operating characteristic.

We tested the possibility that the human M1 is essential to early motor consolidation (Muellbacher *et al.* 2002). We monitored changes in elementary motor behavior of pinching between the thumb and index finger while subjects practiced fast finger movements that rapidly improved in movement acceleration and muscle force generation. Low-frequency repetitive transcranial magnetic stimulation of M1, but not the frontal or occipital cortex, specifically disrupted the retention of the behavioral improvement, but did not affect basal motor behavior, task performance, or motor learning by subsequent practice (Fig. 7.9). However, if the repetitive TMS was given 6 hrs

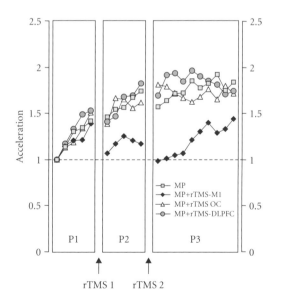

Fig. 7.9 Acceleration of pinching force with practice and various interventions. P1, P2, and P3 are practice periods. Repetitive TMS is given between the practice periods. Stimulation over M1, but not the occipital cortex (OC) or the dorsolateral prefrontal cortex (DLPFC), blocked the consolidation of learning. Reproduced with permission from Muellbacher *et al.* (2002). *Nature*, **415**, 640–4.

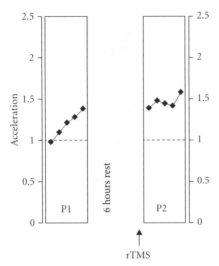

Fig. 7.10 Acceleration of pinching force in two practice periods, and with 6 hrs rest and then repetitive TMS of the primary motor cortex between the periods. P1 and P2 are practice periods. Stimulation over M1 in this circumstance does not block the consolidation of learning. Reproduced with permission from Muellbacher *et al.* (2002). *Nature*, **415**, 640–4.

after practice, it no longer disrupted the recall of the newly acquired motor skill (Fig. 7.10). These findings indicate that the human M1 is specifically engaged during the early stage of motor consolidation.

It appears that consolidation is stronger if a person sleeps after initial learning. For example, in learning a finger sequence task, a period of sleep will enhance performance if done during the day or night (Fischer *et al.* 2002). A similar situation was seen with learning a pursuit task, and in this circumstance neuroimaging was done as well (Maquet *et al.* 2003). Subjects either slept or were sleep deprived after learning. When tested 3 days later, those who slept performed better. Additionally, brain activation and functional connectivity were enhanced with sleep. More work is needed in this interesting area to explore physiology and to see if there are any therapeutic consequences.

Conclusion

Motor learning is a complex phenomenon with many components. Depending on the particular task, different anatomical structures are involved. It would be an oversimplification to say that only one part of the brain is involved with any task; it is more likely that a network is functional. On the other hand, it is possible to identify some aspects where particular structures play a major role. The cerebellum takes a principal role in classical conditioning and adaptation learning. On the other hand, skill learning seems more a cortical phenomenon. The development of new skills has many facets and probably engages large portions of the brain. The motor cortex is involved early, plays a role in consolidation, and, by map plasticity, may assign resources to different movements. A parietal and premotor network appears to play a major role in motor program storage. Subcortical structures appear to play more support roles. The cerebellum is clearly important for error correction and optimizing performance, including adaptation learning components. The basal ganglia may influence learning in several ways, including reward.

Acknowledgement

This chapter is revised and updated from Hallett and Grafman (1997).

References

Blaxton TA, Zeffiro TA, Gabrieli JD, Bookheimer SY, Carrillo MC, Theodore WH, *et al.* (1996). Functional mapping of human learning: a positron emission tomography activation study of eyeblink conditioning. *J Neurosci*, **16**, 4032–40.

Brashers-Krug T, Shadmehr R, Bizzi E (1996). Consolidation in human motor memory. *Nature*, **382**, 252–5.

Clower DM, Hoffman JM, Votaw JR, Faber TL, Woods RP, Alexander GE (1996). Role of posterior parietal cortex in the recalibration of visually guided reaching. *Nature*, **383**, 618–21.

Conner JM, Culberson A, Packowski C, Chiba AA, Tuszynski MH (2003). Lesions of the basal forebrain cholinergic system impair task acquisition and abolish cortical plasticity associated with motor skill learning. *Neuron*, **38**, 819–29.

Daum I, Schugens MM, Ackermann H, Lutzenberger W, Dichgans J, Birbaumer N (1993). Classical conditioning after cerebellar lesions in humans. *Behav Neurosci*, **107**, 748–56.

Deuschl G, Toro C, Zeffiro T, Massaquoi S, Hallett M (1996). Adaptation motor learning of arm movements in patients with cerebellar diseases. *J Neurol Neurosurg Psychiatry*, **60**, 515–19.

Dimitrova A, Weber J, Maschke M, Elles HG, Kolb FP, Forsting M, *et al.* (2002). Eyeblink-related areas in human cerebellum as shown by fMRI. *Hum Brain Mapping*, **17**, 100–15.

Donchin O, Sawaki L, Madupu G, Cohen LG, Shadmehr R (2002). Mechanisms influencing acquisition and recall of motor memories. *J Neurophysiol*, **88**, 2114–23.

Doyon J, Song AW, Karni A, Lalonde F, Adams MM, Ungerleider LG (2002). Experience-dependent changes in cerebellar contributions to motor sequence learning. *Proc Natl Acad Sci USA*, **99**, 1017–22.

Doyon J, Penhune V, Ungerleider LG (2003). Distinct contribution of the cortico-striatal and cortico-cerebellar systems to motor skill learning. *Neuropsychologia*, **41**, 252–62.

Fischer S, Hallschmid M, Elsner AL, Born J (2002). Sleep forms memory for finger skills. *Proc Natl Acad Sci USA*, **99**, 11987–91.

Fitts PM (1954). The information capacity of the human motor system controlling the amplitude of movement. *J Exp Psychol*, **47**, 381–91.

Flament D, Ellermann JM, Kim SG, Ugurbil K, Ebner TJ (1996). Functional magnetic resonance imaging of cerebellar activation during the learning of a visuomotor dissociation task. *Hum Brain Mapping*, **4**, 210–26.

Friston KJ, Frith CD, Passingham RE, Liddle PF, Frackowiak RSJ (1992). Motor practice and neurophysiological adaptation in the cerebellum: a positron tomography study. *Proc R Soc Lond B Biol Sci*, **248**, 223–8.

Gerwig M, Dimitrova A, Kolb FP, Maschke M, Brol B, Kunnel A, *et al.* (2003). Comparison of eyeblink conditioning in patients with superior and posterior inferior cerebellar lesions. *Brain*, **126**, 71–94.

Ghilardi M, Ghez C, Dhawan V, Moeller J, Mentis M, Nakamura T, *et al.* (2000). Patterns of regional brain activation associated with different forms of motor learning. *Brain Res*, **871**, 127–45.

Grafton ST, Mazziotta JC, Presty S, Friston KJ, Frackowiak RSJ, Phelps ME (1992). Functional anatomy of human procedural learning determined with regional cerebral blood flow and PET. *J Neurosci*, **12**, 2542–8.

Grafton ST, Woods RP, Tyszka M (1994). Functional imaging of procedural motor learning: Relating cerebral blood flow with individual subject performance. *Hum Brain Mapping*, **1**, 221–34.

Grafton ST, Hazeltine E, Ivry R (1995). Functional mapping of sequence learning in normal humans. *J Cogn Neurosci*, **7**, 497–510.

Hallett M, Grafman J (1997). Executive function and motor skill learning. *Int Rev Neurobiol*, **41**, 297–323.

Honda M, Deiber MP, Ibanez V, Pascual-Leone A, Zhuang P, Hallett M (1998). Dynamic cortical involvement in implicit and explicit motor sequence learning. A PET study. *Brain*, **121**, 2159–73.

Imamizu H, Miyauchi S, Tamada T, Sasaki Y, Takino R, Putz B, *et al.* (2000). Human cerebellar activity reflecting an acquired internal model of a new tool. *Nature*, **403**, 192–5.

Imamizu H, Kuroda T, Miyauchi S, Yoshioka T, Kawato M (2003). Modular organization of internal models of tools in the human cerebellum. *Proc Natl Acad Sci USA*, **100**, 5461–6.

Inoue K, Kawashima R, Satoh K, Kinomura S, Sugiura M, Goto R, *et al.* (2000). A PET study of visuomotor learning under optical rotation. *NeuroImage*, **11**, 505–16.

Iriki A, Pavlides C, Keller A, Asanuma H (1989). Long-term potentiation of motor cortex. *Science*, **245**, 1385–7.

Jenkins IH, Brooks DJ, Nixon PD, Frackowiak RSJ, Passingham RE (1994). Motor sequence learning: a study with positron emission tomography. *J Neurosci*, **14**, 3775–90.

Karni A, Meyer G, Jezzard P, Adams M, Turner R, Ungerleider LG (1995). Functional MRI evidence for adult motor cortex plasticity during motor skill learning. *Nature*, **377**, 155–8.

Krebs HI, Brashers-Krug T, Rauch SL, Savage CR, Hogan N, Rubin RH, *et al.* (1998). Robot-aided functional imaging: application to a motor learning study. *Hum Brain Mapping*, **6**, 59–72.

Liepert J, Tegenthoff M, Malin JP (1995). Changes of cortical motor area size during immobilization. *Electroencephalogr Clin Neurophysiol*, **97**, 382–6.

Lisberger SG (1988). The neural basis for learning of simple motor skills. *Science*, **242**, 728–35.

Logan CG, Grafton ST (1995). Functional anatomy of human eyeblink conditioning determined with regional cerebral glucose metabolism and positron-emission tomography. *Proc Natl Acad Sci USA*, **92**, 7500–4.

Maquet P, Schwartz S, Passingham R, Frith C (2003). Sleep-related consolidation of a visuomotor skill: brain mechanisms as assessed by functional magnetic resonance imaging. *J Neurosci*, **23**, 1432–40.

Martin TA, Keating JG, Goodkin HP, Bastian AJ, Thach WT (1996a). Throwing while looking through prisms. I. Focal olivocerebellar lesions impair adaptation. *Brain*, **119**, 1183–98.

Martin TA, Keating JG, Goodkin HP, Bastian AJ, Thach WT (1996b). Throwing while looking through prisms. II. Specificity and storage of multiple gaze-throw calibrations. *Brain*, **119**, 1199–1211.

Martin TA, Norris SA, Greger BE, Thach WT (2002). Dynamic coordination of body parts during prism adaptation. *J Neurophysiol*, **88**, 1685–94.

Massaquoi S, Hallett M (1996). Kinematics of initiating a two-joint arm movement in patients with cerebellar ataxia. *Can J Neurol Sci*, **23**, 3–14.

Muellbacher W, Ziemann U, Wissel J, Dang N, Kofler M, Facchini S, *et al.* (2002). Early consolidation in human primary motor cortex. *Nature*, **415**, 640–4.

Nitsche MA, Schauenburg A, Lang N, Liebetanz D, Exner C, Paulus W, *et al.* (2003). Facilitation of implicit motor learning by weak transcranial direct current stimulation of the primary motor cortex in the human. *J Cogn Neurosci*, **15**, 619–26.

Pascual-Leone A, Cammarota A, Wassermann EM, Brasil-Neto JP, Cohen LG, Hallett M (1993a). Modulation of motor cortical outputs to the reading hand of Braille readers. *Ann Neurol*, **34**, 33–7.

Pascual-Leone A, Grafman J, Clark K, Stewart M, Massaqoui S, Lou JS, *et al.* (1993b). Procedural learning in Parkinson's disease and cerebellar degeneration. *Ann Neurol*, **34**, 594–602.

Pascual-Leone A, Grafman J, Hallett M (1994). Modulation of cortical motor output maps during development of implicit and explicit knowledge. *Science*, **263**, 1287–9.

Pascual-Leone A, Dang N, Cohen LG, Brasil-Neto JP, Cammarota A, Hallett M (1995a). Modulation of muscle responses evoked by transcranial magnetic stimulation during the acquisition of new fine motor skills. *J Neurophysiol*, **74**, 1037–45.

Pascual-Leone A, Grafman J, Hallett M (1995b). Procedual learning and prefrontal cortex. In J Grafman, F Boller, KJ Holyoak, (ed.) *Structure and Function of the Human Prefrontal Cortex*, pp. 61–70. New York: New York Academy of Sciences.

Penhune VB, Doyon J (2002). Dynamic cortical and subcortical networks in learning and delayed recall of timed motor sequences. *J Neurosci*, **22**, 1397–1406.

Sanes JN, Dimitrov B, Hallett M (1990). Motor learning in patients with cerebellar dysfunction. *Brain*, **113**, 103–20.

Schlaug G, Knorr U, Seitz RJ (1994). Inter-subject variability of cerebral activations in acquiring a motor skill: a study with positron emission tomography. *Exp Brain Res*, **98**, 523–34.

Schreurs BG, McIntosh AR, Bahro M, Herscovitch P, Sunderland T, Molchan SE (1997). Lateralization and behavioral correlation of changes in regional cerebral blood flow with classical conditioning of the human eyeblink response. *J Neurophysiol*, **77**, 2153–63.

Seidler RD, Purushotham A, Kim SG, Ugurbil K, Willingham D, Ashe J (2002). Cerebellum activation associated with performance change but not motor learning. *Science*, **296**, 2043–6.

Seitz RJ, Roland PE (1992). Learning of sequential finger movements in man: a combined kinematic and positron emission tomography (PET) study. *Eur J Neurosci*, **4**, 154–65.

Seitz RJ, Canavan AG, Yaguez L, Herzog H, Tellmann L, Knorr U, *et al.* (1994). Successive roles of the cerebellum and premotor cortices in trajectorial learning. *NeuroReport*, **5**, 2541–4.

Shadmehr R, Holcomb HH (1997). Neural correlates of motor memory consolidation. *Science*, **277**, 821–5.

Sommer M, Grafman J, Clark K, Hallett M (1999). Learning in Parkinson's disease: eyeblink conditioning, declarative learning and procedural learning. *J Neurol Neurosurg Psychiatry*, **67**, 27–34.

Squire LR (1986). Mechanisms of memory. *Science*, **232**, 1612–19.

Thompson RF (1990). Neural mechanisms of classical conditioning in mammals. *Philos Trans R Soc Lond B Biol Sci*, **329**, 161–70.

Timmann D, Kolb FP, Baier C, Rijntjes M, Muller SP, Diener HC, *et al.* (1996). Cerebellar activation during classical conditioning of the human flexion reflex: a PET study. *NeuroReport*, **7**, 2056–60.

Timmann D, Baier PC, Diener HC, Kolb FP (2000). Classically conditioned withdrawal reflex in cerebellar patients. 1. Impaired conditioned responses. *Exp Brain Res*, **130**, 453–70.

Topka H, Valls-Solé J, Massaquoi S, Hallett M (1993). Deficit in classical conditioning in patients with cerebellar degeneration. *Brain*, **116**, 961–9.

Topka H, Massaquoi SG, Benda N, Hallett M (1998). Motor skill learning in patients with cerebellar degeneration. *J Neurol Sci*, **158**, 164–72.

Wachs J, Pascual-Leone A, Grafman J, Hallett M (1994). Intermanual transfer of implicit knowledge of sequential finger movements (abstract). *Neurology*, **44** (Suppl 2), A329.

Weiner MJ, Hallett M, Funkenstein HH (1983). Adaptation to lateral displacement of vision in patients with lesions of the central nervous system. *Neurology*, **33**, 766–72.

Chapter 8

The mirror neuron system and action recognition

Giacomo Rizzolatti and Luciano Fadiga

Introduction

Understanding actions made by others is a fundamental cognitive function on which social life and the survival of individuals depend. Despite its crucial role in social behavior, action understanding, unlike other cognitive capacities such as object or space perception, has never been a central topic in neuroscience. Only recently, with the discovery of mirror neurons (Gallese *et al.* 1996; Rizzolatti *et al.* 1996a), have action understanding and phenomena closely related to this function, such as imitation, become the object of intense investigation (reviewed by Rizzolatti *et al.* 2001).

How do we understand actions made by other individuals? What are the neurophysiological bases of this capacity? There are various accounts that might explain how action understanding may occur. The most intuitive one, which we will designate the 'visual hypothesis', is that action understanding is based on a visual analysis of the different elements forming an action and on their interrelations. Let us take as an example the observation of a girl biting an apple. The action is first decomposed into its elements: the hand, the apple, and the movement of the hand toward the apple. Then the combination of these elements, plus inferences from their semantics, allows the observer to understand the action witnessed. No motor or emotional involvement is required. This mechanism may be present in a living creature as well as in an artifact, for example in a robot that (obviously) has no idea whatsoever of what eating means.

If this view is correct, action understanding should be mediated by the activity of the extrastriate visual areas, the inferotemporal lobe, and the superior temporal sulcus (STS) areas. In both monkeys and humans these areas respond selectively to objects, body parts, biological motion, and, in the case of some neurons of STS, interactions between hands and objects (Gross *et al.* 1972; Perrett *et al.* 1989; Tanaka *et al.* 1991; Ungerleider and Haxby 1994; Carey *et al.* 1997; Allison *et al.* 2000; Kanwisher 2000).

A possible different hypothesis is that we understand actions when we map the visual representation of the observed action on the motor representations of the same action. We will designate this the 'direct matching hypothesis'. According to this hypothesis, an action is understood when its observation makes the motor system of the observer 'resonate'. Thus, when we observe the girl biting an apple, the same populations of neurons that control the execution of biting will resonate in the observer's motor areas. By means of such a mechanism, the 'motor knowledge' of the observer will be used to understand the observed action. The hypothesis that action understanding is based upon a direct matching mechanism does not exclude, of course, the possibility that other visual and cognitive processes based on object and movement descriptions may also play a role in action recognition. However, it stresses the primacy of direct action observation–execution matching.

The two accounts of action recognition presented above refer to 'cold' actions, i.e. to actions devoid of an emotional content. It is likely that different mechanisms are involved in the understanding of others' actions that induce emotions or have consequence on the welfare of the observer. In these cases there again appear to be two major possibilities. If the action of the others may produce harm, as in the case of attack or more generally in the case of aggressive behavior, the action is understood because its visual description is associated with its consequences. No involvement of the motor system of the observer is necessary. Note that here, unlike in the visual recognition of cold action, the correlation is between a visual event and what is going to occur and not between various visual events that is at the basis of action recognition.

Finally, also in the case of 'hot' actions (those with an emotional content), a resonance mechanism may play a fundamental role in action recognition ('direct matching hypothesis'). In this case, however, the resonating structures are not those coding the cold motor behavior, but those that mediate the visceromotor reactions expressing emotions. Preliminary evidence shows that structures such as insula are involved in this process (Carr *et al.* 2003; C. Keysers *et al.*, unpublished data).

The present chapter is structured as follows. First, we describe the mirror neuron system in the monkey. We then provide evidence that this system is also present in humans. Finally, we argue that the basic function of the mirror neuron system is action recognition and that, on the top of this older capacity, other faculties evolved in humans such as imitation and the faculty of language. Emotional behavior will be not dealt with.

The mirror neuron system in monkeys

Mirror neurons were first discovered in area F5 of the monkey premotor cortex (Di Pellegrino *et al.* 1992; Gallese *et al.* 1996; Rizzolatti *et al.* 1996a). F5 is basically a motor area that controls hand and mouth movements. A fundamental characteristic of this area is that many of its neurons discharge during specific goal-directed action such as grasping, holding, or tearing (Rizzolatti *et al.* 1988). Many of these neurons become active regardless of the effector (the right hand, the left hand, or the mouth) that is used to achieve the goal (e.g. grasping an object). Conversely, they do not fire when the monkey uses the same effectors but for another purpose (e.g. pushing away objects).

A second fundamental characteristic of area F5 is that many of its neurons specify how a goal can be achieved. For example, the majority of grasping neurons discharge only if grasping is made using a particular type of prehension, such as precision grip, finger prehension, or, more rarely, whole-hand prehension.

About 20% of F5 neurons respond to visual stimuli (Rizzolatti *et al.* 1988). One class of these visuomotor neurons, known as canonical neurons, discharge when the monkey sees an object that is congruent with the type of grip coded by the neuron (Murata *et al.* 1997). A second class of visuomotor neurons does not discharge in response to the presentation of 3D objects. The visual stimuli effective in triggering them are actions in which the experimenter (or a monkey) interacts with objects. Neurons with these properties are called mirror neurons (Gallese *et al.* 1996; Rizzolatti *et al.* 1996a).

Typically, F5 mirror neurons require an interaction between hand and object in order to be triggered. The sight of the object alone or of the agent mimicking an action is ineffective. The object significance for the animal has no influence on mirror neuron response. Grasping a piece of food or a geometric solid produces responses of the same intensity.

An important functional aspect of mirror neurons is the relation between their visual and motor properties. Virtually all mirror neurons show congruence between the visual actions they respond to and the motor response they code. According to the type of congruence they exhibit, mirror neurons have been subdivided into 'strictly congruent' and 'broadly congruent' neurons (Gallese *et al.* 1996).

Strictly congruent mirror neurons are defined as those mirror neurons in which the effective observed and effective executed actions correspond in terms of both goal (e.g. grasping) and means, i.e. how the action is executed (e.g. precision grip). They represent about 30% of F5 mirror neurons.

Broadly congruent mirror neurons are defined as those mirror neurons which, in order to be triggered, do not require the observation of exactly the same action that they code motorically. Some of them discharge during the execution of a particular type of action (e.g. grasping) when executed using a particular type of grip (e.g. precision grip). However, they respond to the observation of grasping made by another individual, regardless of the type of grip used. Other broadly congruent neurons discharge in association with a single motor action (e.g. holding), but respond to the observation of two actions (e.g. grasping and holding). Broadly congruent neurons are the class of mirror neurons usually represented (about 60%).

From this short review of basic properties of F5 neurons, it appears that this area stores potential actions or, as we previously described it, a 'vocabulary of actions' (Rizzolatti *et al.* 1988). The activation of F5 neurons does not necessarily determine an action. It evokes its representation. If other contingencies are met, this potential action becomes a real motor action (Rizzolatti and Luppino 2001). F5 potential actions can be activated endogenously or exogenously. Exogenous (visual) activation is caused by the observation of objects (canonical neurons) or by the observation of actions made by others (mirror neurons).

Another cortical area where there are mirror neurons is area PF (Fogassi *et al*. 1998; Gallese *et al*. 2002). This area forms the rostral part of the inferior parietal lobule. PF receives input from STS, where there are many neurons that become active during the observation of action (Perrett *et al*. 1989), and sends output to area F5.

Neurons in area PF are functionally heterogeneous. Most of them (about 90%) respond to sensory stimuli (Hyvarinen 1982; Leinonen and Nyman 1979; Fogassi *et al*. 1998; Gallese *et al*. 2002). About 50% of them also discharge in association with monkey active movements.

Neurons responding to sensory stimuli have been subdivided into three categories: 'somatosensory' neurons (33%), 'visual' neurons' (11%), and 'bimodal' somatosensory and visual stimuli (56%). Among the neurons with visual responses ('visual neurons' and 'bimodal neurons'), 41% respond to the observations of actions made by another individual. One-third of them, similarly to STS neurons, do not appear to have motor-related activity. The other two-thirds also discharge during the monkey's movement and, in most cases, showed the visuomotor congruence typical of mirror neurons—'PF mirror neurons' (Gallese *et al*. 2002).

New evidence for a role of F5 mirror neurons in action understanding

As soon as mirror neurons were discovered it was suggested that they play an important role in action understanding. The core of this proposal is the following. When an individual acts, he selects an action whose motor consequences are known to him. The mirror neurons allow this knowledge to be extended to actions performed by others. Each time an individual observes an action performed by another individual, neurons that represent that action are activated in his premotor cortex. Because the evoked motor representation corresponds to that generated internally during active action, the observer understands the witnessed action (Rizzolatti *et al*. 2001).

This action recognition hypothesis was recently tested by studying mirror neuron responses in conditions in which the monkey was able to understand the meaning of the occurring action, but without the visual stimuli that typically activate mirror neurons. The rationale of the experiments was the following. If mirror neurons are involved in action understanding, their activity should reflect the action meaning and not specific sensory contingencies.

In a series of experiments the hypothesis was tested by presenting the monkey with auditory stimuli able to evoke the idea of an action (Kohler *et al*. 2002). F5 mirror neuron activity was recorded while the monkey was observing a 'noisy' action (e.g. ripping a piece of paper), or was presented with the same noise without seeing it. The results (Fig. 8.1) showed that most mirror neurons that discharge to presentation of actions accompanied by sounds also discharge in response to the sound alone ('audiovisual' mirror neurons). The mere observation of the same 'noisy' action without sound was also effective. Further experiments showed that a large number of

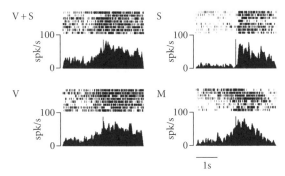

Fig. 8.1 Example of a mirror neuron selectively responding to action-related sounds. The neuron became active when the monkey observed a peanut breaking action: sound present (V + S). A similar response was present during the observation of the same action without sound (V) and during sound without vision (S). Panel M shows the motor discharge of the same neuron during active grasping. Vertical lines across the histograms indicate the time when the sound occurred (V + S, S). In the vision-only condition (V) the stimulus (peanuts) was modified and its breaking did not produce any sound. The vertical line indicates the time when the sound would have occurred under natural conditions. In the motor condition (M) the vertical lines indicates the moment when the monkey touched the object. Rasters above each histogram show the neuron's discharge during eight successive trials. Ordinates: spikes/s; Abscissae: time (s).

audiovisual mirror neurons respond selectively to specific action sounds. These results strongly support the notion that the discharge of F5 neurons correlates with action understanding and not with the stimuli that determine it. The effective stimuli may be visual or acoustic. Once they specify the action meaning, the neuron fires.

Another series of experiments aimed at testing the 'direct matching hypothesis' consisted in the study of mirror neuron responses in conditions in which monkey was prevented from seeing the occurring action (and listening to its sound), but was provided with clues as to what the action might be. If mirror neurons are involved in action understanding, they should also discharge in this condition.

This experiment was recently carried out by Umiltà *et al.* (2001). The experimental paradigm consisted of two basic conditions. In one, the monkey was shown a fully visible action directed toward an object ('full vision' condition). In the other, the monkey saw the same action but with its final critical part hidden ('hidden' condition). Before each trial the experimenter placed a piece of food behind the screen so that the monkey knew that there was an object behind it. The main result of the experiment was that more than half of the tested neurons discharged in the hidden condition. Some of them did not show any difference between hidden and full vision conditions, whereas others responded more strongly in the full vision condition.

In conclusion, both the experiments in which the stimulus conditions were altered showed that F5 mirror neuron activation correlates with action representation rather than with the stimulus properties leading to it. This finding strongly supports the notion that F5 activity plays a fundamental role in the understanding of action meaning.

The mirror neuron system in humans

Evidence that a mirror neuron system also exists in humans comes from three sources: transcranial magnetic stimulation (TMS) studies, electroencephalography (EEG) and magnetoencephalography (MEG) experiments, and brain imaging studies.

TMS studies

The first evidence in favor of the existence of a mirror system in humans came from a study by Fadiga *et al.* (1995) who stimulated the left motor cortex of normal volunteers. There were four experimental conditions: (i) observation of hand grasping movements; (ii) observation of meaningless intransitive arm movements; (iii) observation of three-dimensional objects; (iv) observation of the dimming of a small spot of light. Motor evoked potentials (MEPs) were recorded from hand muscles.

The rationale of the experiment was as follows. If the observation of the hand and arm movements made by another individual facilitates the observer's motor system, this facilitation should determine an increase in MEPs recorded from hand and arm muscles compared with the two control conditions (object observation and the dimming detection task). The results confirmed the hypothesis. A selective increase of MEPs was found in those muscles of the observer that she normally uses for producing them.

The facilitation of MEPs during movement observation can be explained in two ways. It may result from an enhancement of primary motor cortex excitability due to excitatory cortical connections reaching the primary motor cortex from the human cortical homologue of area F5 in the monkey. Alternatively, it may be to a facilitatory output to the spinal cord originating from the mirror human area homologue of F5. Data from an experiment by Strafella and Paus (2000) support the corticocortical hypothesis. By using a double-pulse TMS technique they demonstrated that the duration of intracortical recurrent inhibition occurring during action observation is similar to that occurring during action execution.

The same issue was also investigated by Baldissera *et al.* (2001). These authors examined the modulation of spinal cord excitability during observation of goal-directed hand actions by measuring the size of the H-reflex evoked in flexor and extensor muscles in normal human volunteers. They found that, in the absence of any detectable muscle activity, there was a modulation of the reflex amplitude during action observation, specifically related to the different phases of the observed movement. While the H-reflex recorded from flexors rapidly increased in size during hand opening, it was depressed during hand closing and quickly recovered during object lifting. The converse behavior was found in extensors. Thus, while modulation of cortical excitability varies in accordance with the observed movements, the spinal cord excitability changes in the opposite direction.

This result suggests that, at the spinal cord level, there is a mechanism that prevents execution of the observed actions, thus leaving the cortical motor system free to 're-enact' the observed actions without the risk of overt movement generation.

Changes in motor cortex excitability during the observation of actions made by others were also reported by Gangitano *et al.* (2001) and Maeda *et al.* (2002).

Gangitano *et al.* (2001) recorded MEPs from the hand muscles of normal volunteers while they were observing grasping movements made by another individual. The MEPs were recorded at different intervals following the onset of movement. The results showed that the motor cortical excitability faithfully followed the grasping movement phases of the observed action. This finding indicates that, in humans, the mirror neuron system codes for the temporal aspects of the observed movements and not only for the meaning of the observed action.

Maeda *et al.* (2002) also recorded MEPs from the hand muscles of normal volunteers. The recordings were made while the volunteers observed video clips of different finger movements such as thumb abduction/adduction. The finger movements were presented in two hand orientations: as if the actor was sitting next to the observer (hand 'away' position), and as if the actor was in front of the observer (hand 'toward' position). The results showed that the degree of cortical motor modulation depended on hand orientation. Modulation was greater when the observed movement was performed in the hand 'away' position (i.e. when the actor and the observer were in the same position) than in the hand 'toward' position.

In conclusion, the TMS studies reviewed above show that a mirror neuron system similar to that found in the monkey is also present in humans. In addition, they demonstrate two important properties of the human mirror neuron system that do not appear to exist in that of the monkey. First, intransitive meaningless movements produce mirror neuron activation in humans (Fadiga *et al.* 1995; Maeda *et al.* 2002), but not in monkeys. Secondly, the correlation between the time course of the observed movements and facilitation of the MEPs suggests that the human mirror neuron system codes for the movements forming an action, and not just for actions as in the monkey mirror neuron system. In a previous study (Rizzolatti *et al.* 1999) we referred to the mirror mechanism describing movements as the 'low-level resonance mechanism' contrasting it with the 'high-level resonance mechanism' of F5 where the coded element is the action. These properties of the human mirror neuron system may be an important factor in determining the human capacity for imitation.

EEG and MEG studies

Evidence in favor of a mirror neuron system in humans also comes from the study of the reactivity of cerebral rhythms during movement observation. It is a classical notion that, during motor activity, there is a desynchronization of a specific EEG rhythm (known as the 'mu' rhythm) present in the central cortical derivations. Pioneer experiments by Gastaut and Bert (1954) and Cohen-Seat *et al.* (1954) showed that action observation also may block the mu rhythm.

This finding was recently confirmed by Cochin *et al.* (1998) who showed desynchronization of central rhythms during the observation of leg movements. Control experiments in which non-biological motions (e.g. a waterfall) were presented to the subjects did not affect the rhythm activity. In a subsequent experiment the same authors compared the cortical electrical activity while participants observed and executed finger movements (Cochin *et al.* 1999). The results showed that the mu rhythm was blocked in correspondence to the central cortex in both conditions. Similar data were also obtained by Altschuler *et al.* (1997, 2000).

Further evidence for the existence of a mirror neuron system comes from MEG studies which showed that, among the various rhythms recorded from the central region, rhythmic oscillations around 20 Hz originate from the precentral cortex inside the central sulcus (Salmelin and Hari 1994; Hari and Salmelin 1997). The level of the 20 Hz activity enhances bilaterally within 500 ms after median nerve stimulation (Salmelin and Hari 1994; Salenius *et al.* 1997). This after-stimulation rebound is a highly reproducible and robust phenomenon that can be used as an indicator of the state of the precentral motor cortex. Most interestingly, it is abolished when the subject manipulates an object during the median nerve stimulation (Salenius *et al.* 1997) and is significantly diminished during motor imagery of manipulation movements (Schnitzler *et al.* 1997).

The post-stimulus rebound method was used to test whether action observation affects the 20 Hz rhythms (Hari *et al.* 1998). Participants were tested in three conditions: (i) rest, (ii) while they were manipulating a small object, and (iii) while they were observing another individual performing the same task. The left and right median nerves were stimulated alternately and the post-stimulus rebound (15–25 Hz activity) quantified. The results showed that the post-stimulus rebound was strongly suppressed bilaterally during object manipulation and, most interestingly, that it was significantly reduced during action observation. Because the recorded 15–25 Hz activity is known to originate mainly in the precentral motor cortex, these data indicate that the human motor cortex is activated during both execution of a motor task and action observation, a finding strongly supporting the existence of an action observation–execution system in humans.

Brain imaging studies

The neurophysiological experiments described above, while fundamental in showing that action observation elicits an activation of motor system, do not allow one to localize the areas where mirror neuron system is localized. Data on this issue have been obtained using brain imaging techniques.

Early brain imaging studies showed that the observation of hand actions activates (as well as various occipital visual areas) the STS region, the inferior parietal lobule, and the ventral premotor cortex plus Broca's area (Grafton *et al.* 1996; Rizzolatti *et al.* 1996b; Grèzes *et al.* 1998; Iacoboni *et al.* 1999). As previously mentioned, in the monkey neurons discharging during the observation of biological actions are present in the STS region and in the inferior parietal lobule. Furthermore, mirror neurons are present in the inferior parietal lobule and in the F5 sector of the ventral premotor cortex (PMv). Thus human and monkey cortical circuits that are active during action observation closely correspond.

A finding that raised some discussion was the activation of Broca's area during the observation of hand action. Although comparative cytoarchitectonic studies indicate that the pars opercularis of Broca's area (basically corresponding to area 44) is the human homologue of area F5 (Petrides and Pandya 1997), the traditional view is that area 44 is the speech motor area. In recent years, however, rich evidence has been accumulating that human area 44 contains, in addition to speech representation, a hand motor representation (as monkey area F5 does) (Krams *et al.* 1998; Binkofski *et al.* 1999; Iacoboni *et al.* 1999; Gerardin *et al.* 2000; Ehrsson *et al.* 2000; Schubotz and von Cramon 2001).

The deep-rooted idea that human area 44 is a speech area gave rise to speculation on the possibility that its activation in humans was due to verbal mediation, rather than to motor resonance due to mirror neurons (Grèzes and Decety 2001). New experiments on the general organization of the mirror neuron system showed that this interpretation of the findings is incorrect.

Buccino *et al.* (2001) extended the study of the organization of the mirror neuron system from hand actions to actions made with other effectors. Video clips showing transitive actions (actions directed toward an object) and intransitive actions made by mouth, hand, and foot were used. Action observation was contrasted with the observation of a static face, hand, and foot, respectively.

Observation of object-related mouth movements determined activation of the ventral premotor cortex and of the pars opercularis of the inferior frontal gyrus (IFG), bilaterally. In addition, two activation foci were found in the parietal lobe. One was located in the rostral part of the inferior parietal lobule (most likely area PF), while the other was located in the posterior part of the same lobule. The observation of intransitive actions determined activation of the same premotor areas, but there was no parietal lobe activation.

Observation of object-related hand–arm movements determined two areas of activation in the frontal lobe, one corresponding to the pars opercularis of IFG, and the other in the upper part of the precentral gyrus. The latter activation was more dorsally located than that found during the observation of mouth movements. Considering the motor organization of PMv, it is likely that the activation of pars opercularis was determined by observation of grasping hand movements, while that of dorsal PMv by observation of reaching. As for mouth movements, there were two activation foci in the parietal lobe. The rostral focus was, as in the case of mouth actions, in the rostral part of the inferior parietal lobule, but more posteriorly located, while the caudal focus was essentially in the same location as that for mouth actions. During the observation of intransitive movements the premotor activations were present, but the parietal activations were not.

Finally, the observation of object-related foot actions determined an activation of a dorsal sector of the precentral gyrus and an activation of the posterior parietal lobe, in part overlapping with those seen during mouth and hand actions, and in part extending more dorsally. Intransitive foot actions produced premotor, but not parietal, activation.

The results of this study are important for several reasons. First, they demonstrate that the mirror neuron system includes a large part of the premotor cortex and the rostral sector of the inferior parietal lobule. Secondly, they show that the activation map obtained during observation of actions made with different effectors is similar to the motor map obtained with electrical stimulation of the same region (Penfield and Rasmussen 1950; Woolsey 1958). Finally, they allow one to rule out the idea that the activation of area 44 is due to internal verbalization. Verbalization cannot be present during the observation of hand movements and disappear during the observation of foot movements.

Humans recognize not only actions performed by other human beings, but also actions performed by individuals belonging to other species. When we observe a monkey or a dog biting a piece of food, we have no difficulty in understanding what the observed animal is doing. How is this accomplished? Is the understanding of actions performed by animals based on the mirror neuron system? Or is there another mechanism that mediates action recognition in this case?

Recently, a functional magnetic resonance imaging (fMRI) experiment was carried out in order to answer these questions. Video clips showing mouth actions performed by humans, monkeys, and dogs were presented to normal individuals. Two types of actions were presented: biting and oral communication actions (speech reading, lip-smacking, barking). As a control, static images of the same actions were presented.

The results (Fig. 8.2) showed that the observation of biting, regardless of whether performed by a human, a monkey, or a dog, determined two activation foci in the inferior parietal lobule and activation in the pars opercularis of the IFG and the adjacent ventral premotor cortex. The left rostral parietal focus [located in the same position as in the experiments by Buccino *et al.* (2001) described above] and the left premotor focus were virtually identical for all three species, while the right-side foci were stronger during the observation of actions made by a human than by an individual of another species.

Observation of speech reading activated the left pars opercularis of IFG. Observation of lip-smacking, a monkey communicative gesture, activated a small focus in the right

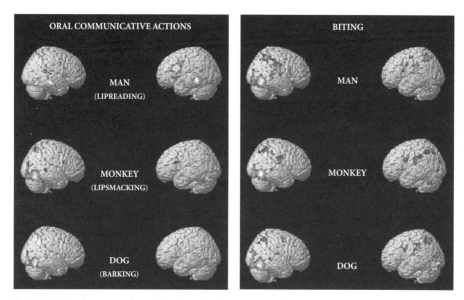

Fig. 8.2 Cortical areas activated during the observation of non-communicative and communicative actions performed by a human, a monkey, and a dog.

and left pars opercularis of the IFG. Finally, observation of barking did not produce any activation in the frontal lobe.

These results suggest that actions made by other individuals may be recognized through two different mechanisms. Actions belonging to the motor repertoire of the observer are mapped on his or her motor system. Actions that do not belong to this repertoire do not excite the motor system of the observer and appear to be recognized essentially on visual basis.

Mirror neuron system: action understanding and imitation

At first glance imitation seems to be a very simple concept: One sees something and one does it. However, as soon as the instances in which the term 'imitation' is used are examined, imitation looses its simplicity and appears to include different behaviors, some innate and others learned (Byrne 1995; Tomasello and Call 1997; Meltzoff and Prinz 2002).

Imitation, strictly defined, describes the capacity that individuals of some species (humans in particular) have so that they can learn to do an action from seeing it. This definition, which goes back to Thorndyke (1898), includes two fundamental concepts. Imitation implies learning. Imitation also implies a transformation of an action visually coded into an almost identical action done by the observer. Therefore imitation requires a 'translation' from the sensory to the motor domain.

In addition, there is another fundamental problem. Why does imitation occur? Why does an individual want to repeat an action made by another individual? It is obvious that this desire stems from the belief that doing the observed action will provide benefits.

Thus imitation of actions made by others requires (i) the comprehension of the goal of the observed action, (ii) a mechanism translating the observed action from the visual to the motor domain, and (iii) a learning mechanism that modifies internal motor programs matching them to the observed ones. The properties of mirror neuron meet these requirements.

As already discussed, there is convincing evidence that the mirror neuron system is involved in action understanding in both humans and monkeys. As far as imitation is concerned, the majority of ethologists agree that this faculty is absent in monkeys (Galef 1988; Byrne 1995; Whiten and Ham 1992). This indicates that monkeys, although endowed with a mechanism for generating internal copies of actions made by others, are unable to use them for replicating the observed actions. This capacity developed only later in evolution.

Do humans use the mirror neuron system for imitation? Evidence accumulating from fMRI and MEG experiments strongly suggests that is the case.

In an fMRI study Iacoboni *et al.* (1999) instructed normal human volunteers to observe and imitate a finger movement (imitation task) and, in other trials, to perform the same movement in response to a spatial or a symbolic cue (observation–execution tasks). In another series of trials, the same participants were asked to observe identical stimuli, but without responding to them (observation tasks). The results showed that activation was significantly stronger during imitation than in the two non-imitative observation–execution tasks in three cortical areas: the pars opercularis of the left inferior frontal cortex, the right anterior parietal region, and the right parietal operculum. The first two areas were also active during observation tasks, while the parietal operculum was active during observation–execution conditions only.

Remarkably similar results were obtained by Nishitani and Hari (2000) using the event-related neuromagnetic technique. In their experiment, Nishitani and Hari asked normal human volunteers to grasp a manipulandum, or to observe the same movement performed by an experimenter, or to observe and replicate the observed action on-line. The results showed that during the active grasping condition, there was an early activation in the pars opercularis of the inferior frontal cortex with a response peak appearing approximately 250 ms before the target was touched. This activation was followed within 100–200 ms by activation of the left precentral motor area and 150–250 ms later by activation of the right precentral motor area. During imitation,the pattern and sequence of frontal activations were similar to those found during execution, but area 44 activation was preceded by an occipital activation due to visual stimulation present in the imitation condition (see also Chapter 17, this volume).

It should be stressed that in the experiments described above, as well as in others on neural basis of imitation (Decety *et al.* 2002; Tanaka and Inui 2002; Koski *et al.* 2003), the 'imitation' studied was a special case of action execution in which action was elicited by the observation of an identical movement. However, according to its classical definition (see above), imitation includes learning. Imitation in this stricter sense has not yet been studied. Preliminary data from an event-related fMRI confirm the central role of the parietofrontal mirror circuits. However, they also show, contributions of prefrontal and anterior mesial cortical areas (G. Buccino *et al.*, unpublished data).

Mirror neuron system: the faculty of language

It has been proposed that the mirror neuron system represents the neurophysiological mechanism from which language evolved (Rizzolatti and Arbib 1998). This proposal is based on the consideration that the mirror neuron system creates a link between the sender of a message and its receiver. The action made by one individual determines the activation of a similar motor representation in the observer and allows him to understand the meaning of the observed action.

Although the primary function of the mirror neuron system, not only in monkeys but (most likely) in our ancestors as well, was that of action understanding, this system had the intrinsic potential to become the system for voluntary communication. An important step toward the voluntary use of the mirror neuron system was the development of a motor 'resonance' to intransitive (not object-directed) actions, including pointing to different directions and mimed actions (Fadiga *et al.* 1995; Buccino *et al.* 2001; Maeda *et al.* 2002). This type of resonance, which is present in humans but not in monkeys, most likely started to appear in primates belonging to the evolutionary line leading to *Homo sapiens*. Its appearance allowed the individuals to describe gesturally space positions, actions, and objects. It is worth noting that the semantics of these gestures is not arbitrarily imposed and does not result from an improbable agreement among different individuals, but is intrinsically present in the mirror system.

This evolutionary proposal stresses the importance of gestures in the evolution of language. However, the human language is typically based on the transmission of information via sounds. Recent experiments showed that, in the monkey, a set of mirror neurons, in addition to their visual response, also show a response to the sound of those actions that trigger a given neuron when they are observed or executed (Kohler *et al.* 2002). Although these audiovisual mirror neurons do not represent a step toward the development of spoken language, they show that, in the monkey, there is already auditory access to action representation. Furthermore, they indicate that, before the faculty of language appeared, primates were pre-adapted to associate sounds with actions and understand meaning from sound.

It is impossible at present to state how the sounds of words became attached to gestures and acquired meaning. However, we are inclined to think that during the initial phases of speech evolution the sounds accompanying actions were used as a common ground to evoke the meaning of a given action in the listener. Speculations in this sense were made in the 1930s in particular by Paget (1935), cited by Critchley (1939), who claimed that more than 70% of English words could be explained using this hypothesis.

Regardless of how words acquired meaning, a fundamental step toward the evolution of speech was the development of a mirror neuron system for sound imitation. The presence of this system was recently demonstrated in humans by a TMS study in which normal individuals were presented with words that require tongue movements in order to be generated (e.g. 'r'). Merely listening to these stimuli produced a strong increase in MEPs recorded from the listener's tongue muscles, in contrast with word stimuli that do not require tongue movements or non-linguistic sounds (Fadiga *et al.* 2002). This mirror phenomenon for linguistic material appears to be the equivalent of imitation of meaningless arm action in the gesture domain. This phenomenon is very similar to that originally proposed by Liberman (see Liberman and Whalen 2000). Note, however, that the existence of this auditory motor resonance does not necessary imply its involvement in speech perception.

In conclusion, the discovery of the mirror neuron system in primates and of its properties in humans allows one to propose some neurophysiological hypotheses on the evolution of the faculty of language in the broad sense (sensory–motor and conceptual–intentional systems). The issue of an evolutionary link between the language faculty in the narrow sense (computational mechanism for recursion) and the motor mechanism remains an open question (Hauser *et al.* 2002).

Acknowledgements

This work was supported by EC grants and by Italian Ministry of University grants to GR and LF.

References

Allison T, Puce A, McCarthy G (2000). Social perception from visual cues:role of the STS region. *Trends Cogn Sci*, **4**, 267–78.

Altschuler EL, Vankov A, Wang V, Ramachandran VS, Pineda JA (1997). Person see, person do: human cortical electrophysiological correlates of monkey see monkey do cell. *Soc Neurosci Abstr*, 719.17.

Altschuler EL, Vankov A, Hubbard EM, Roberts E, Ramachandran VS, Pineda JA (2000). Mu wave blocking by observation of movement and its possible use as a tool to study theory of other minds. *Soc Neurosci Abstr*, 68.1.

Baldissera F, Cavallari P, Craighero L, Fadiga L (2001). Modulation of spinal excitability during observation of hand actions in humans. *Eur J Neurosci*, **13**, 190–4.

Binkofski F, Buccino G, Posse S, Seitz RJ, Rizzolatti G, Freund H (1999). A fronto-parietal circuit for object manipulation in man: evidence from an fMRI-study. *Eur J Neurosci*, **11**, 3276–86.

Buccino G, Binkofski F, Fink GR, Fadiga L, Fogassi L, Gallese V, *et al.* (2001). Action observation activates premotor and parietal areas in a somatotopic manner: an fMRI study. *Eur J Neurosci*, **13**, 400–4.

Byrne RW (1995). *The Thinking Ape. Evolutionary Origins of Intelligence*. Oxford: Oxford University Press.

Carey DP, Perrett DI, Oram MW (1997). Recognizing, understanding and reproducing actions. In M Jeannerod, J Grafman, (ed.) *Handbook of Neuropsychology*. Vol 11 *Action and Cognition*, pp. 111–30. Amsterdam: Elsevier.

Carr L, Iacoboni M, Dubeau MC, Mazziotta JC, Lenzi GL (2003). Neural mechanisms of empathy in humans: a relay from neural systems for imitation to limbic areas. *Proc Natl Acad Sci USA*, **100**, 5497–502.

Cochin S, Barthelemy C, Lejeune B, Roux S, Martineau J (1998). Perception of motion and qEEG activity in human adults. *Electroencephalogr Clin Neurophysiol*, **107**, 287–95.

Cochin S, Barthelemy C, Roux S, Martineau J (1999). Observation and execution of movement: similarities demonstrated by quantified electroencephalograpy. *Eur J Neurosci*, **11**, 1839–42.

Cohen-Seat G, Gastaut H, Faure J, Heuyer G (1954). Etudes expérimentales de l'activité nerveuse pendant la projection cinématographique. *Rev Int Film*, **5**, 7–64.

Critchley M (1939). *The Language of Gestures*. London: Edward Arnold, 134.

Decety J, Chaminade T, Grezes J, Meltzoff AN (2002). A PET exploration of the neural mechanisms involved in reciprocal imitation. *Neuroimage*, **15**, 265–72.

Di Pellegrino G, Fadiga L, Fogassi L, Gallese V, Rizzolatti G (1992). Understanding motor events: a neurophysiological study. *Exp Brain Res*, **91**, 176–80.

Ehrsson HH, Fagergren A, Jonsson T, Westling G, Johansson RS, Forssberg H (2000). Cortical activity in precision- versus power-grip tasks: an fMRI study. *J Neurophysiol*, **83**, 528–36.

Fadiga L, Fogassi L, Pavesi G, Rizzolatti G (1995). Motor facilitation during action observation: a magnetic stimulation study. *J Neurophysiol*, **73**, 2608–11.

Fadiga L, Craighero L, Buccino G, Rizzolatti G (2002). Speech listening specifically modulates the excitability of tongue muscles: a TMS study. *Eur J Neurosci*, **15**, 399–402.

Fogassi L, Gallese V, Fadiga L, Rizzolatti G (1998). Neurons responding to the sight of goal directed hand/arm actions in the parietal area PF (7b) of the macaque monkey. *Soc Neurosci Abstr*, **24**, 257.5.

Galef BG (1988). Imitation in animals: history, definition and interpretation of data from psychological laboratory. In T Zental, BG Galef, (ed.) *Comparative Social Learning*, pp. 3–28. Hillsdale, NJ: Lawrence Erlbaum.

Gallese V, Fadiga L, Fogassi L, Rizzolatti G (1996). Action recognition in the premotor cortex. *Brain*, **119**, 593–609.

Gallese V, Fadiga L, Fogassi L, Rizzolatti G (2002). Action representation and the inferior parietal lobule. In W Prinz, B Hommel, (ed.) *Common Mechanisms in Perception and Action*. Vol 19 *Attention and Performance*, pp. 247–66. Oxford: Oxford University Press.

Gangitano M, Mottaghy FM, Pascual-Leone A (2001). Phase-specific modulation of cortical motor output during movement observation. *NeuroReport*, **12**, 1489–92.

Gastaut HJ, Bert J (1954). EEG changes during cinematographic presentation. *Electroencephalogr Clin Neurophysiol*, **6**, 433–44.

Gerardin E, Sirigu A, Lehericy S, Poline JB, Gaymard B, Marsault C, *et al*. (2000). Partially overlapping neural networks for real and imagined hand movements. *Cereb Cortex*, **10**, 1093–104.

Grafton ST, Arbib MA, Fadiga L, Rizzolatti G (1996). Localization of grasp representations in humans by PET: 2. Observation compared with imagination. *Exp Brain Res*, **112**, 103–11.

Grèzes J, Decety J (2001). Functional anatomy of execution, mental simulation, observation, and verb generation of actions: a meta-analysis. *Hum Brain Mapping*, **12**, 1–19.

Grèzes J, Costes N, Decety J (1998). Top-down effect of strategy on the perception of human biological motion: a PET investigation. *Cogn Neuropsychol*, **15**, 553–82.

Gross CG, Rocha-Miranda CE, Bender DB (1972). Visual properties of neurons in inferotemporal cortex of the macaque. *J Neurophysiol*, **35**, 96–111.

Hari R, Salmelin R (1997). Human cortical oscillations: a neuromagnetic view through the skull. *Trends Neurosci*, **20**, 44–9.

Hari R, Forss N, Avikainen S, Kirveskari E, Salenius S, Rizzolatti G (1998). Activation of human primary motor cortex during action observation: a neuromagnetic study. *Proc Natl Acad Sci USA*, **95**, 15061–5.

Hauser MD, Chomsky N, Fitch WT (2002). The faculty of language: what is it, who has it, and how did evolve? *Science*, **298**, 1569–79.

Hyvarinen J (1982). Posterior parietal lobe of the primate brain. *Physiol Rev*, **62**, 1060–129.

Iacoboni M, Woods RP, Brass M, Bekkering H, Mazziotta JC, Rizzolatti G (1999). Cortical mechanisms of human imitation. *Science*, **286**, 2526–8.

Kanwisher N (2000). Domain specificity in face perception. *Nat Neurosci,* **3**, 759–63.

Kohler E, Keysers C, Umilta MA, Fogassi L, Gallese V, Rizzolatti G (2002). Hearing sounds, understanding actions: action representation in mirror neurons. *Science*, **297**, 846–8.

Koski L, Iacoboni M, Dubeau MC, Woods RP, Mazziotta JC (2003). Modulation of cortical activity during different imitative behaviors. *J Neurophysiol*, **89**, 460–71.

Krams M, Rushworth MF, Deiber MP, Frackowiak RS, Passingham RE (1998). The preparation, execution and suppression of copied movements in the human brain. *Exp Brain Res*, **120**, 386–98.

Leinonen L, Nyman G (1979). Functional properties of cells in anterolateral part of area 7 associative face area of awake monkeys. *Exp Brain Res*, **34**, 321–33.

Liberman AM, Wahlen DH (2000). On the relation of speech to language. *Trends Cogn Neurosci*, **4**, 187–96.

Maeda F, Kleiner-Fisman G, Pascual-Leone A (2002). Motor facilitation while observing hand actions: specificity of the effect and role of observer's orientation. *J Neurophysiol*, **87**, 1329–35.

Meltzoff AN, Prinz W (ed.) (2002). *The Imitative Mind. Development, Evolution and Brain Bases.* Cambridge, UK: Cambridge University Press.

Murata A, Fadiga L, Fogassi L, Gallese V, Raos V, Rizzolatti G (1997). Object representation in the ventral premotor cortex (area F5) of the monkey. *J Neurophysiol*, **78**, 2226–30.

Nishitani N, Hari R (2000). Temporal dynamics of cortical representation for action. *Proc Natl Acad Sci USA*, **97**, 913–18.

Paget, R (1935). *This English*. London: Kegan Paul.

Penfield W, Rasmussen T (1950). *The Cerebral Cortex of Man. A Clinical Study of Localization of Function*. New York: Macmillan.

Perrett DI, Harries MH, Bevan R, Thomas S, Benson PJ, Mistlin AJ, *et al.* (1989). Frameworks of analysis for the neural representation of animate objects and actions. *J Exp Biol*, **146**, 87–113.

Petrides M, Pandya DN (1997). Comparative architectonic analysis of the human and the macaque frontal cortex. In F Boller, J Grafman, (ed.) *Handbook of Neuropsychology* Vol 9, pp. 17–58. New York: Elsevier.

Rizzolatti G, Arbib MA (1998). Language within our grasp. *Trends Neurosci*, **21**, 188–94.

Rizzolatti G, Luppino G (2001). The cortical motor system. *Neuron*, **31**, 889–901.

Rizzolatti G, Camarda R, Fogassi L, Gentilucci M, Luppino G, Matelli M (1988). Functional organization of inferior area 6 in the macaque monkey: II. Area F5 and the control of distal movements. *Exp Brain Res*, **71**, 491–507.

Rizzolatti G, Fadiga L, Gallese V, Fogassi L (1996a). Premotor cortex and the recognition of motor actions. *Cogn Brain Res*, **3**, 131–41.

Rizzolatti G, Fadiga L, Matelli M, Bettinardi V, Paulesu E, Perani D, *et al.* (1996b). Localization of grasp representation in humans by PET: 1. Observation versus execution. *Exp Brain Res*, **111**, 246–52.

Rizzolatti G, Fadiga L, Fogassi L, Gallese V (1999). Resonance behaviors and mirror neurons. *Arch Ital Biol*, **137**, 85–100.

Rizzolatti G, Fogassi L, Gallese V (2001). Neurophysiological mechanisms underlying the understanding and imitation of action. *Nat Rev Neurosci*, **2**, 661–70.

Salenius S, Schnitzler A, Salmelin R, Jousmaki V, Hari R (1997). Modulation of human cortical rolandic rhythms during natural sensorimotor tasks. *Neuroimage*, **5**, 221–8.

Salmelin R, Hari R (1994). Spatiotemporal characteristics of sensorimotor neuromagnetic rhythms related to thumb movement. *Neurosci*, **60**, 537–50.

Schnitzler A, Salenius S, Salmelin R, Jousmaki V, Hari R (1997). Involvement of primary motor cortex in motor imagery: a neuromagnetic study. *Neuroimage*, **6**, 201–8.

Schubotz RI, von Cramon DI (2001). Functional organization of the lateral premotor cortex: fMRI reveals different regions activated by anticipation of object properties, location, and speed. *Cogn Brain Res*, **11**, 97–112.

Strafella AP, Paus T (2000). Modulation of cortical excitability during action observation: a transcranial magnetic stimulation study. *NeuroReport*, **11**, 2289–92.

Tanaka K, Saito H, Fukada Y, Moriya M (1991). Coding visual images of objects in the inferotemporal cortex of the macaque monkey. *J Neurophysiol*, **66**, 170–89.

Tanaka S, Inui T (2002). Cortical involvement for action imitation of hand/arm postures versus finger configurations: an fMRI study. *NeuroReport*, **13**, 1599–1602.

Thorndyke EL (1898). Animal intelligence: an experimental study of the associative process in animals. *Psychol Rev Monogr*, **2**, 551–3.

Tomasello M, Call J (1997). *Primate Cognition*. Oxford: Oxford University Press.

Umiltà MA, Kohler E, Gallese V, Fogassi L, Fadiga L, Keysers C, *et al.* (2001). I know what you are doing. A neurophysiological study. *Neuron*, **31**, 155–65.

Ungerleider LG, Haxby JV (1994). 'What' and 'where' in the human brain. *Curr Opin Neurobiol*, **4**, 157–65.

Whiten A, Ham R (1992). On the nature and evolution of imitation in the animal kingdom: reappraisal of a century of research. *Adv Study Behav*, **21**, 239–83.

Woolsey CN (1958). Organization of somatic sensory and motor areas of the cerebral cortex. In HF Harlow, CN Woolsey, (ed.) *Biological and Biochemical Bases of Behavior*, pp. 63–81. Madison, WI: University of Wisconsin Press.

Chapter 9

Levels of representation of goal-directed actions

Marc Jeannerod

Introduction

This chapter deals with how an action can be neurally represented. The term 'action' includes a vast number of neural states, depending on whether the action is intended, planned, imagined, observed from another agent, or executed. Thus the definition of action that will be used here is broader than the behavioral motor aspect of the phenomenon that makes muscles contract and limbs move. Many of our actions remain unexecuted. It is essential to study the covert stages of action, the action representation, in order to understand the mechanisms that ultimately lead to overt behavior.

Neurophysiological concepts of action generation and representation

In the nineteenth century scientists developed concepts that tentatively accounted for the generation of goal-directed movements. The relatively simple input–output concept used for the generation of reflexes, which involved a strict contingency of the movement on the occurrence of an external stimulus, needed to be replaced. Indeed, it seems obvious that voluntary movements should remain independent of external events and should have greater autonomy with respect to biological needs (Jeannerod 1985).

Modern neurophysiologists encountered the same concept of an endogenous organization of action as the result of experiments demonstrating the ability of humans and animals to generate and execute actions without intervention of sensory afferences. The classical observations made by Lashley (1917, 1951) in a subject with a deafferented limb were quite influential in this respect. When blindfolded, this subject was able to place his anaesthetized limb in a predetermined position. A more recent experiment with a deafferented subject will be reported below. Deafferentation experiments in monkeys by section of the dorsal roots (Bizzi et al. 1971) showed that the complete structure of a monoarticular pointing movement could be predetermined centrally, including not only its initial ballistic phase, but also its the low-velocity phase and its endpoint. These results led to a minimalist formulation of the motor representation, the equilibrium point model, where the position of a joint was described as a single equilibrium point determined by the degree of stiffness (itself determined by a central command) of the muscles attached to that joint. A simple change in equilibrium point generated by a new motor command produced a rotation of the joint and a new position of the limb (Feldman 1966).

The contribution of cybernetics to neurophysiological concepts of action generation

Cyberneticians considered that a basic principle of the functioning of any machine was its ability to monitor its own functions. The desired output of the machine must be compared with its actual output in order to check for a possible mismatch between the two. The interaction between the effector and the external world may generate non-linearities in the response which cannot be entirely anticipated by the command generation mechanism; hence it is necessary for the command to be updated by signals arising from the execution. Nowadays, this idea is still the source of operational concepts for describing the functioning of biological motor systems.

In the 1930s Bernstein proposed that, in an action such as prehension of an object, the required position of the limb was established by the command apparatus and compared during execution with its factual position, as detected by the sensory receptors (Bernstein 1967). The discrepancy between the factual and the required values was used as a driving signal to the muscles until the system self-stabilized. A more complete model of this mechanism for regulating motor output was provided by von Holst and Mittelstaedt (1950). They assumed that each time the motor centers generate an outflow signal for producing a movement, a copy of this command (the 'efference copy') is retained. The reafferent inflow signals generated by the movement (e.g. visual, proprioceptive) are compared with the copy. If a mismatch between the efference copy and the reafferent signals is recorded, new commands are generated until the actual outcome of the movement corresponds to the desired movement. If the execution does not correspond to the expected outcome (or the movement is not executed because of some peripheral block, for example), a mismatch will arise between the sensory input and the copy. This mismatch signals that the actual movement departed from the desired movement.

von Helmholtz (1866) provided a pioneering and quite insightful description of this mechanism. Consider what happens when one moves one's eye to a target. If the actual movement corresponds to the desired command, the visual environment appears perfectly stable despite the displacement of the objects on the retina. von Helmholtz suggested that this is because the efforts of will (an antecedent of the efference copy) tell the visual system that the visual displacement is the result of an active movement, such that the visual effect of the movement is canceled. Conversely, if the eye is moved passively (by a gentle pressure on the ocular globe), no efforts of will are generated and

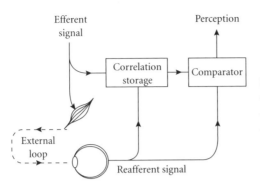

Fig. 9.1 The simple model of comparison between a desired movement and the actual output. Reproduced from Held (1961). *J Nerv Ment Dis*, **132**, 26–32.

the objects appear to be displaced as a result of the displacement of the retina. von Helmholtz predicted further that the same would happen if one attempted to move one's eye against a paralysis of an extraocular muscle. In that case, the expected outcome of the movement, the displacement of the objects on the retina, would not actually occur. Yet, the visual system would have received the signal to cancel this displacement and, paradoxically, the subject should see it.

A significant addition to the von Holst–Mittelstaedt model was made by Held (1961) (Fig. 9.1). Held was faced with the experimental fact that rearrangement of the relationships between a desired movement and its contingent reafferent consequences produces a progressive compensation for this atypical relationship. This effect can be observed after visual exposure of the subject's limb to a laterally displacing prism: the observed limb movement direction does not correspond to the expected one, and initially the subject systematically misreaches to a visual target in the direction of the prism displacement. A new visuomotor coordination then appears, which restores reaching accuracy (adaptation). Held proposed that a memory (the 'correlation storage' device) was used to match the efference copy to the new reafferent signal, and that this new correlation was stored. Indeed, the re-establishment of the normal relationship (e.g. by removing the prism) produces a transient misreaching in the direction opposite to that observed prior to adaptation. The existence of this after-effect is a demonstration of the fact that the new correlation had effectively been stored in the memory during the process of adaptation.

The above storage mechanisms for retaining the efference copy prior to and during execution of a movement, and for storing the optimal correlation between an efference copy and the corresponding reafferent signals, can be considered as one way of conceptualizing motor representations, a concept that will be amply developed later in this chapter. In the following sections, we will first examine the role of these representations in controlling goal-directed actions. Our questions will be as follows. How can a sensory effect produced by a self-generated action be distinguished from an externally produced event? How can the goal of an action be encoded in the command generation mechanism?

Compensation of the effects of self-produced motor activity on sensory perception

The main idea arising from these neurophysiological concepts was that a goal-directed action is signaled to the brain by neural events which are synchronous with its generation, i.e. which precede its execution. Indeed, this corresponds to the definition of what can be called a crude form of representation. These neural events can be thought of as anticipating the consequences (sensory or otherwise) of the action when it comes to execution. Following von Helmholtz's insight, one of the first functions to be proposed for such a mechanism anticipating the effects of a movement was the stability of visual perception during eye movements. Sperry (1950) had observed that a fish with inverted vision caused by surgical 180° eye rotation tended to turn continuously in circles when placed in a visual environment. He interpreted this circling behavior as the result of a disharmony between the retinal input generated by movement of the animal and a compensatory mechanism for maintaining the stability of the visual field. This mechanism proposed by Sperry was a centrally arising discharge that reached the visual centers as a corollary of any excitation generated by the motor centers and normally resulting in movement, hence the term 'corollary discharge' (CD) used by Sperry to designate this mechanism. In this way, the visual centers could distinguish the retinal displacement related to a movement of the animal from that produced by moving objects. Visual changes produced by a movement of the animal were normally 'canceled' by a CD of corresponding size and direction, and had no effect on behavior. However, if the CD did not correspond to the visual changes (e.g. after inversion of vision), these changes were not canceled and were read by the motor system as having their origin in the external world. The animal thus moved in the direction of this apparent visual displacement.

Experiments in animals have demonstrated the existence of eye-movement-related neural signals in the visual system, which would be consistent with a CD type of mechanism. For example, Jeannerod (1972) recorded changes in the discharge rate of visually responsive lateral geniculate neurons which correlated with the occurrence of eye movements. These changes were not due to visual displacement of the objects on the retina, as they were recorded in the dark. Further, they could not be due to the contraction of extra-ocular muscles either, as they persisted after the animal was paralyzed. The timing of these changes in discharge rate was compatible with an integration with retinal signals; they occurred some 100 ms after the onset of eye movement, which was congruent with the arrival of visual input corresponding to the next perceptual frame after the eye movement. Thus inflow (retinal) and outflow (extra-retinal) signals would combine to produce a perceived stability of the visual world. Note that the precise role of this mechanism in stabilizing vision is still a matter of debate. A mechanism based on extra-ocular proprioception could be equally likely.

Similar mechanisms have been proposed for explaining the effects of self-produced motor activity in other sensory domains. Following the idea of a dynamic cancellation observed in visuomotor interactions, the most consistent finding across different studies is that self-produced activity results in reducing the sensibility of the corresponding sensory recipient areas. For example, Müller-Preus and Ploog (1981) found that in monkeys the vocal utterance inhibits the activity of auditory cortical neurons. Similar observations have been reported in humans (Paus *et al.* 1995; Blakemore *et al.* 1999).

Internal models for anticipatory regulation of action

An essential aspect of this mechanism is its predictive nature. It predicts the interactions of the effector with the environment and the effects of these interactions in changing the state of the system itself. The metaphor of 'internal models', borrowed from computer science, has been used as a representation of the action generation system, which includes its current state and its desired, or predicted, state (see also Chapter 24, this volume). These internal models are constructed from stored knowledge and experience from previous interactions. Recent formulations of the internal model may even mimic the causal flow of the action generation process by predicting the next state in the sequence without waiting for sensory reafferences, or even without executing any movement. According to Wolpert *et al.* (1995), the predictive mechanism is a combination of two processes:

> The first process uses the current state estimate and motor command to predict the next state by simulating the movement dynamics with a forward model. The second process uses a model of the sensory output process to predict the sensory feedback from the current state estimate. The sensory error—the difference between actual and predicted sensory feedback—is used to correct the state estimate resulting from the forward model. (Wolpert *et al.* 1995, p. 1881)

This is exactly what one would expect from a mechanism accounting for planning and controlling execution of an action. Because reafferent signals during execution of a limb movement are necessarily delayed with respect to the command signal, the internal model must look ahead in time and produce an estimate of the movement parameters corresponding to the command. This estimate can be used for computing the current position of the limb with respect to the target. It is only because the current state of the action is monitored on-line (rather than after the movement terminates), that corrections can be applied without delay as soon as the deviation of the current trajectory from the desired trajectory is detected (Frith *et al.* 2000). The same mechanism can also be used at a lower level of control to produce a correspondence between the motor command and the amount of muscular contraction, even if the muscular plant is not linear. Non-linearities may also arise from interaction of the moving limb with external forces, specially if it is loaded (reviewed by Weiss and Jeannerod 1998).

Conscious action monitoring

So far, we have established the existence of mechanisms which represent a foregoing action before it reaches execution. These mechanisms have been shown to anticipate the execution of movements and to operate in relatively low-level aspects of visuomotor function, such as stabilization of the visual scene during eye movements or encoding of the position of a visual target. These functions are entirely automatic and do not reach conscious experience. In the present section, we are faced with a different set of problems: those that relate to the conscious monitoring of one's actions. How does an agent know that he is the author of his own movements? How does he distinguish a self-produced event from an external event? In simpler terms, to what extent are the neural signals involved in automatic regulation of action monitorable by the conscious self? Answering such questions obviously requires a methodology different from that used in the experiments reported in the above sections. It requires a direct participation of the subject from whom responses based on his introspection are requested. In the following, we review experimental data which address this problem of the conscious monitoring of intentions and actions.

In order to make a conscious judgment about one's own motor performance, several sources of information can be used. Visual cues, derived directly from vision of the moving segment or indirectly from the effects of the movement on external objects, provide a major contribution to monitoring one's actions. Another critical source is haptic perception, derived from movement-related mechanical deformations of the limb through receptors located in the skin, joints, and muscles. Position sense, the sense of the position of the limb at the end of a movement, is one of the conscious counterparts of these proprioceptive reafferences produced by the movement. Another classically considered source of information about one's own movements, which is highly relevant to the present discussion, relates not to sensory signals, but to the central discharges originating in the motor system during the production of a movement. As outlined earlier, the motor commands sent to the executive mechanisms are also sent to other areas of the nervous system, where a representation of the forthcoming movement (the same concept as that of the efference copy) is stored. This model of the control of action can be directly applied to the problem of self-recognition: self-recognition would be based on the degree of concordance between a desired (or intended) action (as reflected by the efference copy) and its sensory consequences. If the concordance is complete, such that the executed action corresponds to the desired action, the action is automatically attributed to the self. If, on the contrary, there is a discordance between the two and the automatic attribution fails, then the action is consciously monitored. As will be shown below, this view is supported by experimental data.

Limitations to the conscious monitoring of one's actions

In a classical debate, known as the 'the two Williams debate', William James defended the opinion that all that we know about our movements is based on a posteriori information from sensory organs, whereas Wilhelm Wundt, on the contrary, held that our knowledge is based on a priori efferent information of a central origin [for a detailed account of this debate, see Petit (1999)]. In this section, we examine some of the constraints involved in monitoring one's own actions. The first point is that there are limitations to the conscious monitoring of efferent activity. Several experimental results suggest that intentions for carrying out voluntary action are generated without explicit awareness. Libet *et al.* (1983) (see Libet 1985) instructed subjects to perform simple hand movements *ad libitum* and to report the instant W at which they became aware of wanting to move (by reporting the clock position of a revolving spot). In addition, readiness potentials were recorded from the subjects skull. Electromyographs were also recorded for measuring the precise onset of the movement. W was found to lag behind the onset of readiness potentials by about 345 ms. In Libet's terms:

> This leads to the conclusion that cerebral initiation . . . of a spontaneous voluntary act . . . can and usually does begin *unconsciously*'. . . . The brain 'decides' to initiate or, at least, to prepare to initiate the act before there is any reportable subjective awareness that such a decision has taken place. (Libet 1985, p. 536)

This interesting result is hardly compatible with the notion of monitorable sensations in relation to voluntary acts.

An experiment by Nielsen (1963) deals with the same question. Nielsen used a paradigm where subjects were unknowingly shown an alien hand in exact concordance with their own hand. Subjects were asked to follow with their (invisible) hand a straight line shown in a mirror; while they were doing so, the (visible) alien hand gently deviated to the right. Subjects were consistently found to deviate their own movement to the left, as if they tried to compensate for the visually perceived rightward deviation. In addition, most subjects experienced that the hand they saw was their own hand, and tried to interpret the rightward deviation as being due to inattention or fatigue, or to the action of external forces. In other words, the subjects preferred to rely on visual information rather than on their own motor outflow. These observations are consistent with the notion that conscious will is an illusion, as proposed by Wegner (2002). People tend to attribute to themselves actions that they have not performed but which present an appearance of mental causation. Indeed, simply looking at a moving limb superimposed on one's own limb creates a strong impression of having willed this movement and of being its author. Observations have been reported in amputated people who experience having a phantom limb. When their valid limb is visually transposed (by way of mirrors) to the amputated side, and when they produce movements with that limb, they experience a strong feeling of voluntary movement of the phantom limb. The same happens if the visually transposed limb is that of an experimenter (Ramachandran and Rogers-Ramachandran 1996). The same reasoning can be applied to Libet's experiments described above, where the subjects experience mental causation despite becoming aware of their intention to move after the movement started.

Although the sensation of will seems to be an illusion, it may become perceptible in some circumstances. One is the situation where a voluntary action is blocked or grossly impaired. This happens in abnormal situations like paralysis. The distinction made by Searle (1983) between 'intention in action' (the implicit step that precedes an overtly executed action) and 'prior intention' (a conscious desire to do something) is quite relevant here. This is because this distinction provides a phenomenological description of two different situations, however, and not because it corresponds to a radical difference between those situations. Consider, for example, the case where the movement of raising my arm is impossible because of paralysis. If I need to raise my arm to catch an object (an intention in action), the movement will not be performed. But I will shortly realize, in seeing my immobile arm, that in fact I intended to raise my arm (a prior intention). The obstacle on movement execution produces a shift from one type of action to another, i.e. from an automatic transfer of a representation into execution to a consciously performed action. It has been speculated, based on empirical observations, that consciousness of an action would arise as a consequence of lack of completion or failure of that action (Jeannerod 1994).

This hypothesis can be verified experimentally. Consider a situation where what a subject sees from his action does not correspond to what he is actually doing. Will this subject be able to monitor this discordance consciously? An experiment directed at this question was performed by Fourneret and Jeannerod (1998). In this experiment, inspired by that of Nielsen (1963), subjects were instructed to move a stylus with their unseen hand toward a visual target; only the trajectory of the stylus was visible as a line on a computer screen, superimposed on the hand movement (Fig. 9.2). In the perturbed condition, a directional bias was introduced electronically, such that the visible line no longer corresponded to that of the hand. In order to reach the target, the hand-held stylus had to be deviated in a direction opposite to the bias. In other words, although the line on the computer screen appeared to be directed to the target location, the hand movement was directed in a different direction. The novel aspect of the experiment is that, in addition to the data concerning subjects' accuracy in automatically correcting for the bias, other data were collected on subjects' judgments about their own performance. At the end of each trial, subjects were asked in which direction they thought their hand had moved (by indicating verbally a line in the corresponding direction on a chart).

This experiment revealed several important points. First, subjects accurately corrected for the bias in tracing a line which appeared visually to be directed to the target. This resulted from an automatic adjustment of the hand movement in a direction opposite to the bias and at the same angle. Secondly, subjects tended to ignore the veridical trajectory of their hand in making a conscious judgment about the direction of their hand. They tended to adhere to the direction seen on the screen and based their report on visual cues, thus ignoring non-visual (e.g. proprioceptive) cues. This result suggests that the visuomotor system may appropriately use information for producing accurate corrections, but that this same information cannot be accessed consciously.

In another experiment using the same apparatus, the bias was progressively increased from trial to trial (Slachewsky et al. 2001). Although in the previous experiment the bias was randomly presented and was limited to a maximum angle of 10° to the right

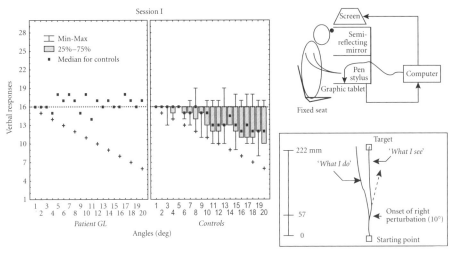

Fig. 9.2 Experiment of Fourneret and Jeannerod (1998). Upper right: the subject is facing a mirror hiding his hand and reflecting the trajectory of a hand held stylus on a digital tablet. Unknown to the subject, an electronically induced bias creates a discordance between the trajectory seen and the actual movement of the stylus. Although the subject compensates for the bias and correctly reaches the target, he remains unaware of the direction of his actual movement. Lower left: comparison of performance of the deafferented patient GL and normal controls in consciously monitoring their movements. The experimental design is the same as that of Fourneret and Jeannerod (1968). When the electronically induced bias increases above a mean value of 10°, normal subjects (right). become conscious of the discordance between the desired and the actual movement. This never happens with patient GL, who remains unaware of the discordance even for high bias values (20°). Reproduced from Fourneret *et al.* (2002). *NeuroReport*, **13**, 541–7.

or left, Slachewsky and colleagues used biases up to 42°, always presented in the same direction (e.g. to the right). When the bias amounted a mean value of about 14°, normal subjects changed strategy and began to use conscious monitoring of their hand movement to correct for the bias and to reach the target. In other words, the discrepancy between the seen trajectory and the felt trajectory became too large to be corrected automatically, and the failure of these corrections was compensated by conscious deviations of the hand movement in the appropriate direction. This was not true for a group of patients with frontal lesions, who apparently never became fully aware of this discrepancy, and continued to apply the automatic strategy with the consequence of larger and larger uncorrected errors in attempting to reach the target. The conclusion drawn from these results is twofold. First, failure of the automatic visuomotor system produces error signals which can be consciously monitored and which induce a shift to a different strategy. Secondly, prefrontal areas are likely to be involved in this strategic shift.

The respective roles of inflow and outflow information

The respective roles of the central discharges and of the sensory reafferences in determining conscious knowledge about actions has been the subject of a longstanding debate. At present, the question is more about whether a movement is recognized as one's own because it corresponds to the intention, or because the central discharges in themselves carry sufficient information. Answering this query would require manipulation of either the sensory signals or the central discharges, which raises difficult methodological problems, mainly because of the difficulty of suppressing haptic sensations in conscious humans. Several methods have been used. Ischemic block of one arm has been questioned because it affects not only sensory but also motor fibers (Philips 1986). Complete curarization of one limb, which excludes muscular contractions (and the correlative sensory input) from that limb, is another possibility; if subjects report sensations from their attempts to move their paralyzed limb, these sensations should arise from their motor commands and not from proprioceptive input. The available evidence shows that no perception of movement arises in this condition (McCloskey *et al.* 1983). Finally, experiments with partial curarization of the arm suggest a more balanced conclusion; subjects requested to estimate the heaviness of weights that they attempted to lift with their weakened arm report an increased perceived heaviness. This illusion was interpreted as reflecting the consecutive increase in motor outflow needed to lift the weights (Gandevia and McCloskey 1977). This result seems to provide indirect evidence as to the possibility that central signals influence conscious experience.

A more direct solution to this problem would be to examine patients with complete haptic deafferentation of pathological origin (e.g. by sensory neuropathy). However, the rare patients with such a pathology have mostly been tested for their ability to control their movements in the absence of proprioceptive input (in terms of accuracy, kinematics, or coordination, for example), and not for their ability to recognize movements they had performed (Ghez *et al.* 1990).

In the present study, we have taken advantage of the condition of GL, a well-documented haptically deafferented patient. GL presented a permanent and specific loss of the large sensory myelinated fibers (testified by a biopsy at the level of the sural nerve) from her whole body below the nose, following two episodes of sensory polyneuropathy. This illness resulted in absence of tendon reflexes in the four limbs as well as a total loss of the senses of touch, vibration, and pressure, and kinesthesia in neck, trunk, and limbs. Thus, despite normal motor nerve conduction velocities confirmed by electromyography, GL had no sensation or control of her head/neck and limb position or movement with her eyes closed. Confined to a wheelchair, she performs most of her daily manual activities under constant visual control [for a full clinical description, see Forget and Lamarre (1987)]. This clinical picture has been regarded as stable for the last 20 years.

Because GL has no haptic information about the movements she performs and visual feedback from the same movements can be either systematically distorted or suppressed, the only information on which she can rely to form a phenomenal experience about her own movements should be derived from the motor commands she generates for producing these movements. Thus, an experimental study of action recognition in this patient represents a unique opportunity to answer the open questions about the contribution of central signals to the conscious knowledge about one's behavior and one's own body. The device designed by Fourneret and Jeannerod (1998) was used (see above). In one session, an angular bias to the right, increasing from 1° to 20° over successive trials, was introduced (Fourneret *et al.* 2002). Patient GL performed the task without difficulty and was able to compensate for the bias. Her performance remained relatively stable and did not seem to be affected by the increasing discordance. Furthermore, she never explicitly reported a feeling of discordance between what she had seen and the movements she thought she had made with her hand. Conversely, control subjects recorded in the same situation became aware of the visuomotor conflict at an average angle of bias of about 6° (Fig. 9.2).

In another session, a mask placed on the screen occluded the first two-thirds of the trajectory. A constant bias of 15° to the right was introduced for all 20 trials. Thus in order to compensate for this bias, the subjects first had to discover the amplitude of the bias when they first saw the line coming out of the mask and then, in subsequent trials, to use a strategy of compensation beginning during the phase of the movement occluded by the mask. In this condition, GL's movements were fast, with no evidence for terminal braking, whereas control subjects moved more slowly. Secondly, the pattern of corrections made to orient the line toward the target was different in control subjects and in GL. Whereas in normal subjects corrections always appeared after the line became visible (i.e. they used the distance between the actual visual position of the line and the position of the target as a cue), GL's corrections were often generated while the line was still hidden by the mask. In fact, GL appeared to encode the required movement direction from the onset of the trajectory, and performed the movement in a completely open-loop fashion. This strategy was reflected in GL's everyday behavior. For grasping an object placed at a distance, GL tended to throw her hand in the direction of that object with great accuracy; in other words, her movements were based on computation of visual localization of the target and feedforward control of the movement. Vision was not used for on-line guidance, but only for calibrating motor output. The production of the corrections that she generated below the mask is more difficult to understand. As these corrections could not be due to a proprioceptive signal from the hand deviating from the target direction, they were likely to represent trajectory optimization or updating of an open-loop program rather than true corrections based on error feedback.

Despite expressing perplexity at the end of some trials, GL never became aware of the bias and, consequently, of any strategy of correction she had to apply to correct for it. However, despite the absence of any proprioceptive information resulting from her arm movement, GL explicitly mentioned the 'difficulty' of reaching the visual target and sometimes the 'effort' of concentration that this required from her. Conversely, all control subjects reported that they had to impose a leftward direction on their hand movements in order to achieve the task

Thus it is a striking finding that GL, despite achieving the visuomotor task correctly, was unaware of having to compensate for a bias introduced by the experimenter between the seen position of the target and the actual trajectory of her hand. This bias required the hand movement to be deviated by up to $20°$ away from the apparent position of the target in order to reach for it. Control subjects became aware of the existence of a bias when it exceeded $6°$ and realized that they had to shift from an automatic to a conscious strategy for achieving the task. In GL, the absence of proprioceptive cues from her movements and the strong reduction of the visual cues on which she could rely might account for the fact that she could not report how she reached the target. The vague feelings of effort and difficulty of the task that she reported were apparently the expression of non-sensory cues and possibly of central cues. Does this result mean that the role of central cues should be limited to such a secondary role and should not be the source of monitorable sensations? Before accepting this explanation, one should remember that, under normal conditions, central discharges do not work in isolation. During execution, the central discharges corollary to the motor commands are used as a reference for a desired action, against which reafferent sensory signals from the executed movement can be compared. It is likely that, in GL, the central discharges representing the desired movement were generated along with the motor commands but, because no reafference from the executed movement was present, the comparison process could not take place. The fact that GL could not report any sensation related to her movements implies that this conscious information would be derived, not from the central discharges themselves, but from the output of the comparison process.

This hypothesis is not incompatible with the fact that GL knew that she had attempted to perform the task at each trial, or with the fact that she was aware of her intention to move, if not of her actual movements. In other words, awareness of one's actions is only one aspect of the general problem of action consciousness. Our present results suggest that the cues for accessing awareness of mental states about action (like intending or imagining an action, for example) should be distinct from those that are generated at the time of execution (see below).

Brain mechanisms for consciousness of action

A further step in identifying the mechanism of consciousness of action is to examine brain activity during situations where the degree of congruence between the various signals produced by a self-generated movement can be modified. Consider, for example, the situation already described where a subject executes a given movement and receives a discordant visual feedback from this movement. This subject will experience a conflict between his intention and his senses, i.e. the anticipation of seeing a certain effect as the result of his intention (e.g. his hand moving in a certain direction) will be contradicted by the actual feedback he will observe. This situation should lead to attributing the action to a cause different from the self. An experiment using this paradigm was undertaken by Farrer *et al.* (2003). In this study, it was conjectured that the processes underlying the sense of agency (the recognition of self-generated actions) should not be all-or-none states, but rather should be based on continuous monitoring of the different action-related signals from sensory and central origin. To test this hypothesis, the degree of congruence of the visual feedback provided to the subjects about their own movements was varied. Visual feedback could be either fully congruent with the executed movements (i.e. the subject saw exactly what he did) or distorted up to the point where the seen movements were completely unrelated to the executed ones. Thus, in the congruent condition, the subjects were likely to feel in full control of their own movements, whereas in the maximally distorted condition, they were likely to feel that they were not in control, but rather were being overridden by the movements of another agent. To achieve this, subjects were instructed to move a joystick continuously with their right hand. The hand and the joystick were hidden from the subjects' view. Instead, the subjects saw the electronically reconstructed image of a hand holding a joystick appearing at the precise location of their own hand. When the subject moved, the electronic hand also moved by the same amount and in the same direction; subjects rapidly became acquainted with this situation and felt the movements of the electronic hand as their own (Franck *et al.* 2001). Distortions were introduced in this system, such that the direction of the movements seen by the subjects were rotated with respect to the direction of those that they actually performed. A graded rotation was produced by using a 25° rotation, a 50° rotation, and finally a situation where the movements appearing on the screen were unrelated to those of the subjects (they were actually produced by an experimenter). Subjects were instructed to concentrate on their own feelings of whether they felt in control of the movements that they saw.

The results of this and other experiments (e.g. Fink *et al.* 1999) demonstrate that a decreasing feeling of control was associated with changes in neural activity, measured using positron emission tomography (PET), in several specific brain areas. For the purpose of this chapter, we will concentrate on one of these areas, the inferior parietal lobule (Fig. 9.3). The reason for this choice is twofold: first, the inferior parietal lobule is an associative region where signals relevant to our present discussion (e.g. visuomotor and proprioceptive signals, signals related to motor commands) are likely to be processed; secondly, lesions of the inferior parietal lobule produce pathological effects which clearly indicate its involvement in action recognition. Patients suffering from lesions involving this brain area (usually in the right hemisphere) frequently deny ownership of the left side of their body. They may even report delusions about their left body half by contending that it belongs to another person despite contradictory evidence from touch or sight (Bisiach and Berti 1987; Daprati *et al.* 2000). Conversely, transient hyperactivity of a similar area of the parietal lobe (e.g. during epileptic fits)

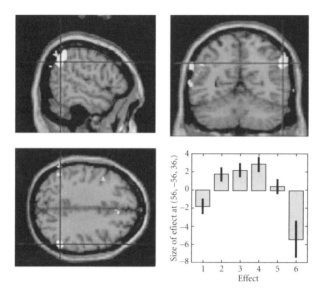

Fig. 9.3 Activity of the right posterior parietal cortex (at $x = 56$, $y = -56$, $z = 36$) during a discordance between an executed movement and its visual effect. The graph indicates the level of activity at these coordinates when the discordance increases. 1, No discordance; 2 and 3, 25° and 50° discordance, respectively; 4, complete discordance; 5 and 6, control conditions. Note the progressive increase in activity as the discordance increases. Reproduced from Farrer *et al.* (2003). *Neuroimage*, **18**, 324–33.

may produce impressions of an alien phantom limb (Spence *et al.* 1997). These observations stress the role of the parietal lobe in integrating signals for building representations essential for self-recognition (see also Chapter 24, this volume).

Thus, in the above neuroimaging experiment of Farrer *et al.* (2003), the degree of activation in the right inferior parietal lobule was modulated as a function of the feeling experienced by the subject of being in control of the action. Activation increased as a function of the degree of discordance between central signals arising from the motor intention and visual and kinesthetic signals arising from movement execution. A possible explanation for this effect is that the mismatch between normally congruent sets of movement-related signals should result in an increased level of processing of these signals and, consequently, in greater metabolic activity.

The problem raised by these results is to determine to what extent the modulation of neural activity for different degrees of discordance between an intended and an executed action, and the related feeling of being in control of an action, can be accounted for by the theory developed earlier in this chapter. This theory [the central monitoring theory (Frith *et al.* 2000)] capitalizes on neural signals produced by the subject's motor activity and postulates that they are used for comparing the end result with the internal model of the action. However, there are many situations where an action representation is formed but no movement is actually executed. In such situations, there are no output signals to the muscles, no reafferent (e.g. visual) signals from the outside world, no proprioceptive signals, and therefore no possibility for comparing execution with a desired output.

The simulation hypothesis: from motor imagery to action attribution

The notion that an action should be executed for self-recognition to operate, postulated by the central monitoring theory, is a problem in itself. The existence of overt behavior is not a prerequisite for self-attribution. It has often been argued that thinking, which normal subjects unambiguously attribute to themselves, is an equivalent of a weak form of behavior which does not activate muscles and therefore is invisible from the outside (Feinberg 1978; Hesslow 2002; Wegner 2002). A paradigmatic situation where this occurs is motor imagery. In this section, we will proceed in two steps. First, we will describe recent research on motor imagery in order to validate the notion of covert actions. We will try to access experimentally mental states characterized by absence of overt behavior by reintroducing introspection in the field of cognitive psychology, and by combining it with techniques for investigating brain activity. Secondly, we will propose another explanatory model of action recognition, attribution, and self-recognition based on central representations of actions.

Simulated actions

Our hypothesis postulates that covert actions are in fact actions in their own right, except for the fact that they are not executed. Covert and overt stages represent a continuum, such that every overtly executed action implies the existence of a covert stage, whereas a covert action does not necessarily become an overt action. As will be argued below, most of the neural events which lead to an overt action already seem to be present in the covert stages of that action. Being provocative, one might tentatively propose that a covert action includes everything that is involved in an overt action, except for the muscular contractions and the joint rotations. Even though this contention is factually incorrect, as we know that the musculo-articular events associated with a real movement generate a flow of (reafferent) signals which are not present as such in a covert action, it captures the functioning of the representation. Therefore the theory predicts a similarity, in neural terms, of the state where an action is simulated and the state which precedes execution of that action (Jeannerod 1994, 1997).

Motor imagery has become a major tool for the study of representational aspects of action. Among the most impressive behavioral findings revealed by motor imagery studies is the fact that motor images retain the same temporal characteristics as the corresponding real action when it comes to execution. For example, it takes the same time to walk mentally to a prespecified target as it takes actually to walk to the same place (Decety *et al.* 1989). Similarly, temporal regularities which are observed in executed actions, such as the classical speed–accuracy trade-off, are retained in their covert counterparts (Sirigu *et al.* 1996). Along the same lines, other situations have been described where the subject is requested to make a perceptually based 'motor' decision. These are situations where no conscious image is formed. Consider the situation where a subject is simply requested to make an estimate about the feasibility of an action, for example to determine the feasibility of grasping an object placed at different orientations. The time to give the response is a function of the object's orientation, suggesting that the arm has to be mentally moved to an appropriate position before the response can be given. Indeed, the time to make this estimate is closely similar to the time it takes to actually reach and grasp an object placed at the same orientation (Parsons 1994; Frak *et al.* 2001).

Motor imagery is only one of the forms an action representation can take. Another covert form of action is action observation. To observe an action with the purpose of understanding it or of understanding the intention behind it, is by no means a passive process. This idea was already present a century ago in the concept of empathy (Lipps 1903). Empathy expresses the possibility that one can understand other people's behavior (e.g. their actions, facial expressions, etc.) when one attempts to replicate and simulate their mental activity. In other words, the observed action would activate, in the observer's brain, the same mechanisms that would be activated if that action were intended or imagined by the observer (Gallese and Goldman 1998).

The concept of shared representations

A critical condition for assigning motor images and observed actions the status of covert and simulated actions is that they should activate brain areas known to be devoted to executing actions. Early work by Ingvar and Philipsson (1977), using measurement of local cerebral blood flow, had shown that 'pure motor ideation' (e.g. thinking of rhythmic clenching movements) produced a marked frontal activation and a more limited activation in the Rolandic area. More recent brain mapping experiments using PET or functional magnetic resonance (fMRI) have led to the conclusion that represented actions involve a subliminal activation of the motor system (Hari *et al.* 1998, Jeannerod 1999, 2001; Jeannerod and Frak 1999). They show the existence of a cortical and subcortical network activated during both motor imagery and action observation. This network involves structures directly concerned with motor execution, such as the motor cortex, dorsal and ventral premotor cortex, lateral cerebellum, and basal ganglia ; it also involves areas concerned with action planning, such as the dorsolateral prefrontal cortex and posterior parietal cortex. Concerning the primary motor cortex itself, fMRI studies unambiguously demonstrate that pixels activated during contraction of a muscle group are also activated during imagery of a movement involving the same muscles (Roth *et al.* 1996). During action observation, the involvement of primary motor pathways was demonstrated using a direct measurement of corticospinal excitability by transcranial magnetic stimulation (TMS) of the motor cortex (Fadiga *et al.* 1995).

In principle, a theory that postulates that both actions of the self and actions of the other can be distinguished solely on the basis of their central representations should predict separate representations for these two types of actions. At the neural level, one would expect the existence of different networks devoted to action recognition whether the action originates from the self or not. One network would be related to recognizing actions as belonging to the self. Another should correspond to attributing actions to another person. In the above sections, the idea was developed that brain areas activated during representing self-produced actions (executed or not) and observing actions of other people were partly overlapping. For example, the motor brain appeared to be activated in both cases. Thus, according to the concept of 'shared representations' introduced by Daprati *et al.* (1997) and Georgieff and Jeannerod (1998), different mental states concerning actions (e.g. intending an action and observing it from another person) should partly share the same neural representations.

To clarify this concept, let us briefly describe experimental results obtained from monkeys. A dramatic illustration of a shared representation is provided by the discovery of mirror neurons (di Pellegrino *et al.* 1992; Rizzolatti *et al.* 1995). Mirror neurons were identified in the monkey premotor cortex. They are activated in two conditions: first, they fire when the animal is involved in a specific motor action, like picking a piece of food with a precision grip; secondly, they also fire when the immobile animal watches the same action performed by an external agent (another monkey or an experimenter). In other words, mirror neurons represent one particular type of action, irrespective of the agent who performs it (see Chapter 8, this volume). At this point, it could be suspected that the signal produced by these neurons, and exploited by other elements downstream in the information-processing flow, would be the same for an action performed by the self and by another agent. Thus the two modalities of that action (executed and observed) would completely share the same neural representation. However, the problem of action identification is solved by the fact that other premotor neurons (the canonical neurons) and, presumably many other neuron populations as well, fire only when the monkey performs the action and not when it observes it from another agent. This is indeed another critical feature of the shared representations concept: they overlap only partially, and the non-overlapping part of a given representation can be the cue for attributing the action to the self or to the other. The same mechanism operates in humans. Brain activity during different conditions where subjects were simulating actions (e.g. intending actions and preparing for execution, imagining actions, or observing actions performed by other people) was compared (Decety *et al.* 1994; Grafton *et al.* 1996; Rizzolatti *et al.* 1996; Gérardin *et al.* 2000). The outcome of these studies is twofold: First, there exists a cortical network common to all conditions, to which the inferior parietal lobule (area 40), the ventral premotor area (ventral area 6), and part of SMA contribute; secondly, motor representations for each individual condition are clearly specified by the activation of cortical zones which do not overlap between conditions.

This view was confirmed in a recent investigation by Ruby and Decety (2001). They instructed subjects to imagine actions from different perspectives. In the first-person perspective, subjects received the instruction to imagine themselves doing the action; in the third-person perspective, subjects received the instruction to imagine that they were watching somebody else doing the action. This paradigm satisfies our requirement for demonstrating the validity of the simulation theory. The authors used two situations where the action representation was generated from within and therefore owed nothing to external stimuli. This experimental condition was not fulfilled in previous experiments where action observation and imagined actions were compared; in those experiments, the subjects built their representation of the observed action from perceptual cues which were absent from the imagination situation. The results obtained by Ruby and Decety (2001) demonstrate the existence of non-overlapping activation in the two situations. In the first-person perspective representation, a specific activation was observed in the inferior parietal lobule of the left hemisphere. In contrast, in the third-person perspective representation, activation was found in a symmetrical area of the right hemisphere. Other activated areas which were common to the two situations were also observed. Thus these data seem to provide a basis for an attribution mechanism, based on partially shared representations of different types of action simulation.

Conclusion: multiple levels of action representation

The results from the above experiments emphasize the existence of several levels of representation of action. First, at the lower level, automatic non-conscious mechanisms operate for visuomotor coordination. This is a highly automatized level which does not seem to participate directly in conscious monitoring of action.

Secondly, at a higher level, a mechanism of monitoring 'how to do' seems to operate. Its existence is demonstrated by the shift in strategy which occurs when the automatic system becomes insufficient for correcting the effects of a perturbation. A strategy based on the consciousness of the discrepancy is introduced; subjects become aware of the perturbation and can efficiently monitor the error correction. The involvement of prefrontal cortical areas in this mechanism is suggested by the experiment of Slachewsky *et al.* (2001); such patients do not notice the failure of their action when the degree of perturbation increases, and therefore do not shift to the explicit strategy of error correction. The fact that consciousness is called into operation when the normal course of action fails and when problems arise during execution is a good argument for attributing consciousness of action a dormant role in our everyday behavior. It wakes up when the normally automatic and implicit mode becomes inefficient in coping with the contingencies of the external world.

Finally, at a still higher level of representation, another conscious mechanism comes into play for assigning the action to its real origin. This function requires not only a simulation of the whole action and its consequences on the external world, but also the monitoring of intention-related signals. This is a key mechanism for correctly attributing intentions to their authors. Thus the attribution of intentional states to other people would rely on one's ability to monitor one's own mental states and to disentangle, between different representations of actions, those which pertain to oneself from those which pertain to other selves.

References

Bernstein N. (1967). *The Coordination and Regulation of Movements.* Oxford: Pergamon Press.

Bisiach E, Berti A (1987). Dyschiria. An attempt at its systemic explanation. In M Jeannerod, (ed.) *Neurophysiological and Neuropsychological Aspects of Spatial Neglect*, pp. 183–201. Amsterdam: North-Holland.

Bizzi E, Kalil RE, Tagliasco V (1971). Eye–head coordination in monkeys. Evidence for centrally patterned organization. *Science*, **173**, 452–4.

Blakemore SJ, Wolpert D, Frith CD (1998). Central cancellation of self-produced tickle sensation. *Nat Neurosci*, **1**, 635–40.

Blakemore SJ, Frith C, Wolpert, D (1999). Spatio-temporal prediction modulates the perception of self-produced stimuli. *J Cogn Neurosci*, **11**, 551–9.

Daprati E, Franck N, Georgieff N, Proust J, Pacherie E, Dalery J, *et al.* (1997). Looking for the agent: an investigation into consciousness of action and self-consciousness in schizophrenic patients. *Cognition*, **65**, 71–86.

Daprati E, Sirigu A, Pradat-Diehl P, Franck N, Jeannerod M (2000). Recognition of self produced movement in a case of severe neglect. *Neurocase*, **6**, 477–86.

Decety J, Jeannerod M, Prablanc C (1989). The timing of mentally represented actions. *Behav Brain Res*, **34**, 35–42.

Decety J, Perani D, Jeannerod M, Bettinardi V, Tadary B, Woods R, *et al.* (1994). Mapping motor representations with PET. *Nature*, **371**, 600–2.

Di Pellegrino G, Fadiga L, Fogassi L, Gallese V, Rizzolatti G (1992). Understanding motor events: a neurophysiological study. *Exp Brain Res*, **91**, 176–80.

Fadiga, L, Fogassi L, Pavesi G, Rizzolatti G (1995). Motor facilitation during action observation. A magnetic stimulation study. *J Neurophysiol*, **73**, 2608–11.

Farrer C, Franck N, Georgieff N, Frith CD, Decety J, Jeannerod M (2003). Modulating the experience of agency: a PET study. *Neuroimage*, **18**, 324–33.

Feinberg I (1978). Efference copy and corollary discharge. Implications for thinking and its disorders. *Schizophr Bull*, **4**, 636–40.

Feldman AG (1966). Functional tuning of the nervous system during control of movement or maintenance of a steady posture. II. Controllable parameters of the muscle. *Biophysics*, **11**, 565–78.

Fink GR, Marshall JC, Halligan PW, Frith CD, Driver J, Frackowiak RS, *et al.* (1999). The neural consequences of conflict between intention and the senses. *Brain*, **122**, 497–512.

Forget R, Lamarre Y (1987). Rapid elbow flexion in the absence of proprioceptive and cutaneous feedback. *Hum Neurobiol*, **6**, 27–37.

Fourneret P, Jeannerod M (1998). Limited conscious monitoring of motor performance in normal subjects. *Neuropsychologia*, **36**, 1133–40.

Fourneret P, Paillard J, Lamarre Y, Cole J, Jeannerod M (2002). Lack of conscious recognition of one's own actions in a haptically deafferented patient. *NeuroReport*, **13**, 541–7.

Frak VG, Paulignan Y, Jeannerod M (2001). Orientation of the opposition axis in mentally simulated grasping. *Exp Brain Res*, **136**, 120–7.

Franck N, Farrer C, Georgieff N, Marie-Cardine M, Dalery J, d'Amato T, *et al.* (2001). Defective recognition of one's own actions in schizophrenic patients. *Am J Psychiatry*, 158, 454–459.

Frith CD, Blakemore SJ, Wolpert DM. (2000). Abnormalities in the awareness and control of action. *Philos Trans R Soc Lond B Biol Sci*, **355**, 1771–88.

Gallese V, Goldman A (1998). Mirror neurons and the simulation theory of mind reading. *Trends Cogn Sci*, **2**, 493–501.

Gandevia SC, McCloskey DI (1977). Changes in motor commands, as shown by changes in perceived heaviness, during partial curarization and peripheral anaesthesia in man. *J Physiol*, **272**, 673–89.

Georgieff N, Jeannerod M (1998). Beyond consciousness of external reality. A 'Who' system for consciousness of action and self-consciousness. *Conscious Cogn*, **7**, 465–77.

Gérardin E, Sirigu A, Lehéricy S, Poline JB, Gaymard B, Marsault C, *et al.* (2000). Partially overlapping neural networks for real and imagined hand movements. *Cereb Cortex*, **10**, 1093–1104.

Ghez C, Gordon J, Ghilardi MF, Christakos CN, Cooper SE, (1990). Roles of proprioceptive input in the programming of arm trajectories. *Cold Spring Harb Symp Quant Biol*, **55**.

Grafton ST, Arbib MA, Fadiga L, Rizzolatti G (1996). Localization of grasp representations in humans by PET: 2. Observation compared with imagination. *Exp Brain Res*, **112**, 103–11.

Hari R, Forss N, Avikainen S, Kirveskari E, Salenius S, Rizzolatti G (1998). Activation of human primary motor cortex during action observation: a neuromagnetic study. *Proc Natl Acad Sci USA*, **95**, 15061–5.

Held R (1961). Exposure-history as a factor in maintaining stability of perception and coordination. *J Nerv Ment Dis*, **132**, 26–32.

Hesslow G (2002). Conscious thought as simulation of behavior and perception. *Trends Cogn Sci*, **6**, 242–7.

Ingvar D, Philipsson L (1977). Distribution of the cerebral blood flow in the dominant hemisphere during motor ideation and motor performance. *Ann Neurol*, **2**, 230–7.

Jeannerod, M (1972). Saccade-correlated events in the lateral geniculate body. *Bibl Ophthalmol*, **82**, 189–98.

Jeannerod M (1985). *The Brain-Machine. The History of Neurophysiological Thought*. Cambridge, MA: Harvard University Press.

Jeannerod M (1994). The representing brain. Neural correlates of motor intention and imagery. *Behav Brain Sci*, **17**, 187–245.

Jeannerod M (1997). *The Cognitive Neuroscience of Action*. Oxford: Blackwell.

Jeannerod M (1999). To act or not to act: perspectives on the representation of actions. *Q J Exp Psychol*, **52A**, 1–29.

Jeannerod, M. (2001). Neural simulation of action: a unifying mechanism for motor cognition. *Neuroimage*, **14**, S103–9.

Jeannerod M, Frak VG (1999). Mental simulation of action in human subjects. *Curr Opin Neurobiol*, **9**, 735–9.

Lashley KS (1917). The accuracy of movement in the absence of excitation from the moving organ. *Am J Physiol*, **43**, 169–94.

Lashley KS (1951). The problem of serial order in behavior. In LA Jeffress, (ed.) *Cerebral Mechanisms and Behavior*, pp. 112–36 New York: Wiley.

Libet B (1985). Unconscious cerebral initiative and the role of conscious will in voluntary action. *Behav Brain Sci*, **6**, 529–66.

Libet B, Gleason CA, Wright EW, Perl DK (1983). Time of conscious intention to act in relation to cerebral activities (readiness potential). The unconscious initiation of a freely voluntary act. *Brain*, **102,** 193–224.

Lipps T (1903). *Aesthetik: Psychologie des Schönen und der Kunst*. Hamburg: Voss.

McCloskey DI, Gandevia SC, Potter EK, Colebatch JG (1983). Muscle sense and effort. Motor commands and judgements about muscular contractions. In J Desmedt, (ed.) *Motor Control in Man*. New York: Raven Press.

Müller-Preuss P, Ploog D (1981). Inhibition of auditory cortical neurons during phonation. *Brain Res*, **215**, 61–76.

Nielsen TI (1963). Volition: a new experimental approach. *Scand J Psychol*, **4**, 225–30.

Parsons LM (1994). Temporal and kinematic properties of motor behavior reflected in mentally simulated action. *J Exp Psychol Hum Percept Perform*, **20**, 709–30.

Paus T, Marrett S, Worsley KJ, Evans AC (1995). Extraretinal modulation of cerebral blood-flow in the human visual cortex: implications for saccadic suppression. *J Neurophysiol*, **74**, 2179–83.

Petit JL (1999). In J Petitot, FJ Varela, B Pachoud, J-M Roy, (ed.) *Naturalizing Phenomenology*, pp. 220–44. Stanford, CA: Stanford University Press.

Philips CG (1986). *Movements of the Hand*. Liverpool: Liverpool University Press.

Ramachandran VS, Rogers-Ramachandran D (1996). Synaesthesia in phantom limbs induced with mirrors. *Proc R Soc Lond B Biol Sci*, **263**, 377–86.

Rizzolatti G, Fadiga L, Gallese V, Fogassi L (1995). Premotor cortex and the recognition of motor actions. *Cogn Brain Res*, **3**, 131–41.

Rizzolatti G, Fadiga L, Matelli M, Bettinardi V, Paulesu E, Perani D, *et al*. (1996). Localization of grasp representations in humans by PET: 1. Observation versus execution. *Exp Brain Res*, **111**, 246–52.

Roth M, Decety J, Raybaudi, Massarelli R, Delon-Martin C, Segebarth C, *et al*. (1996). Possible involvement of primary motor cortex in mentally simulated movement. A functional magnetic resonance imaging study. *Neuroreport*, **7**, 1280–84.

Ruby P, Decety J (2001). Effect of subjective perspective taking during simulation of action: a PET investigation of agency. *Nat Neurosci*, **4**, 546–50.

Searle J (1983). *Intentionality. An Essay in the Philosophy of Mind*. Cambridge, UK: Cambridge University Press.

Sirigu A, Duhamel J-R, Cohen L, Pillon B, Dubois B, Agid Y (1996). The mental representation of hand movements after parietal cortex damage. *Science*, **273**, 1564–8.

Slachewsky A, Pillon B, Fourneret P, Pradat-Diehl P, Jeannerod M, Dubois B (2001). Preserved adjustment but impaired awareness in a sensory-motor conflict following prefrontal lesions. *J Cogn Neurosci*, **13**, 332–40.

Spence SA, Brooks DJ, Hirsch SR, Liddle PF, Meehan J, Grasby PM (1997). A PET study of voluntary movement in schizophrenic patients experiencing passivity phenomena (delusions of alien control). *Brain*, **120**, 1997–2011.

Sperry RW (1950). Neural basis of the spontaneous optokinetic response produced by visual inversion. *J Comp Physiol Psycholo*, **43**, 482–9.

von Helmholtz H (1866). *Handbuch der physiologischen Optik*, Vol 3. Leipzig: Leopold Voss.

von Holst E, Mittelstaedt H (1950). Das Reafferenzprinzip. Wechselwirkungen zwischen Zentralnervensystem und Peripherie. *Naturwissenschaften*, **37**, 464–76.

Wegner D (2002). *The Illusion of Conscious Will*. Cambridge, MA: MIT Press.

Weiss P, Jeannerod M (1998). Getting a grasp on coordination. *News Physiol Sci*, **13**, 70–5.

Wolpert DM, Ghahramani Z, Jordan MI (1995). An internal model for sensorimotor integration. *Science*, **269**, 1880–2.

Part 2

Clinical studies of higher-order motor disorders

Chapter 10

Corticospinal deficits

Johannes Noth and Christoph Fromm

Introduction

Our knowledge about the consequences of corticospinal (CS) lesions in humans rests
on three lines of evidence: (i) behavioural studies on animals and, in particular, on
non-human primates which provide detailed anatomical and physiological information about the corticospinal system, (ii) conclusions drawn from experimental lesions
of the corticospinal tract in non-human primates, and (iii) case reports of neurological
syndromes following small well-defined cortical, peduncular, or pyramidal lesions of
the corticospinal tract. To avoid overlap with other contributions to this volume, only
those aspects that are essential for the understanding of corticospinal deficits will be
discussed here.

Organizational and functional aspects of the corticospinal tract

Sherrington's notion of the motor units forming 'the final common pathway of the
nervous system' can be transferred only in a cursory way to the CS tract as 'the final
common path of the motor cortex to the spinal cord'. There are other parapyramidal or
'indirect' systems arising from the motor cortex, such as the corticoreticulospinal
projections. The CS tract itself constitutes a distributed multicomponent system
(Kuypers 1981). It originates from many frontal and parietal areas of the peri-Rolandic
cortex which are distinguished by various motor, somatosensory, and limbic functions,
and by different connectivities, and its terminals are differentially distributed in
Rexed's laminae. In the monkey, the primary motor cortex (M1, area 4) contains the
largest proportion of CS neurons of any single area, giving rise to approximately
one-third to half of the CS fibres (Murray and Coulter 1981; Toyoshima and Sakai
1982). Other areas that directly project to the spinal cord are the supplementary motor
area (SMA proper), i.e. the medial part of area 6 together with the adjacent cingulate
motor areas (areas 23, 24) and a rostral portion of the precentral gyrus (the lateral part
of area 6), termed the arcuate premotor area in the monkey (Dum and Strick 1991).
The parietal lobe, i.e. the primary somatosensory cortex (from rostral area 3a to caudal
area 2), area 5 on the mesial surface and on the convexity of the posterior parietal
cortex, and the second somatosensory cortex, may contribute up to 40% of the CS

axons (Murray and Coulter 1981; Toyoshima and Sakai 1982). These distributions appear to be similar for the human peri-Rolandic cortex, yet realistic estimates of the exact proportions are not available.

Functional properties of identified corticospinal neurons

Relatively few investigations have directly compared the properties of CS neurons (identified antidromically by their responses to pyramidal stimulation) in the SMA (Tanji and Kurata 1982), arcuate premotor area (Werner *et al.* 1991), or parietal areas (Fromm and Evarts 1982) with their counterparts in M1. These studies indicate that CS neurons across these cortical subdivisions share 'muscle-like-activity' and preferential relations to small forces and precise joint positional changes. Furthermore, they receive fast feedback from proprioceptive and cutaneous receptors, while at the same time reflecting area-specific differences such as the different timing of activity in relation to voluntary movements. The fast somatosensory input and the crucial dependence of CS activity on the integrity of the dorsal columns are of paramount importance for our understanding of the function of the CS tract in active touch and accurate maintenance of steady force levels (Porter and Lemon 1993, pp. 247–271). Thus the activity of CS neurons in different cortical areas may contribute in a specific manner to the planning, initiation, execution, and somatosensory guidance of movements but with a gradient of operational activity of CS neurons working in functional groups and in parallel outputs across the fields of origin. When their functional similarities are stressed, it is because in studies on populations of M1 neurons *not* identified with respect to their efferent terminations quite different properties become apparent, i.e. extrinsic and more abstract parameter-encoding of movement (Georgopoulos *et al.* 1986; Kakei *et al.* 1999). These observations caution against equating the function of the CS tract with the function of any of its fields of origin, including M1.

Spinal terminations of corticospinal fibres and the cortico-motoneuronal connection

While the CS axons from M1 and the non-primary frontal motor fields mostly terminate within either the intermediate zone (laminae V–VIII) or the motoneuronal pools of the ventral horn (Kuypers 1981; Dum and Strick 1996), the CS fibres from post-central areas branch to specific sites within the dorsal horn (Coulter and Jones 1977) and the dorsal column nuclei (Catsman-Berrevoets and Kuypers 1976), but rarely to the ventral grey matter. These post-central areas, together with the caudal part of M1, are thus able to modulate afferent somatosensory transmission according to the requirements of a movement. In comparison with the monkey, there is a further ventral shift of CS terminals in humans with an increasing preponderance of monosynaptic linkages to the motoneurons in lamina IX, i.e. the cortico-motoneuronal (CM) connection; and these CS projections are almost entirely crossed. In humans, not only the dorsolaterally located motor nuclei (which innervate the distal muscles of the extremity) but also the ventromedially located motoneuronal pools (which innervate the proximal limb and girdle muscles) are densely contacted by CS fibres. The former are supplied by the lateral and the latter mainly by the anterior CS tract (Schoen 1964; Nathan *et al.* 1990). The CM component of the CS tract is a taxonomic feature of the primates, being virtually absent in other mammals, and has been regarded as crucial for the performance of relatively independent finger movements (Lawrence and Kuypers 1968).

Between half and three-quarters of identified CS tract neurons in the forelimb and digits representation of M1 in the macaque monkey have been shown to possess CM connections (Fetz and Cheney 1980; Lemon *et al.* 1986). These investigators have provided insight into the organization and physiology of 'CM cells' by applying a cross-correlation technique (spike-triggered averaging of the EMG) to define the extent of the 'muscle fields' of the CM cells, i.e. their monosynaptic excitatory or disynaptic inhibitory coupling with the spinal motoneurons. The proportions of CS neurons having CM synapses are vastly underestimated because of a methodical sampling bias towards large fast-conducting CS neurons which make up only 3% of the million pyramidal tract fibres in humans (Lassek 1954), and because small slowly conducting CS neurons have been demonstrated, at least in principle, to provide monosynaptic input to the motoneurons (Lemon *et al.* 1986). The transcranial magnetic stimulation technique (TMS) also selectively affects the fast CS output; thus we remain unaware of the role of the vast majority of slowly conducting elements. Regarding cortical areas outside M1, we know from a recent tracer study in the macaque that the SMA proper and the two cingulate motor areas definitively send efferents into the ventral horn, although the bulk of their terminations is within the intermediate zone (Dum and Strick 1996). In fact, CM connections with the hand and finger motoneurons originating from M1 are far more numerous and induce much stronger synaptic effects than those from the SMA (Lemon *et al.* 2002).

Organization and properties of cortico-motoneuronal cells

The work on CM neurons has shown that cells facilitating the same muscle form clusters, being separated by variable distances and extending over a considerable territory of M1, thus overlapping with multiple clusters for other muscles. Neighbouring CM cells in a cluster share the same target muscle but their muscle fields are not identical (Cheney *et al.* 1985). This convergent pattern is reciprocated by a substantial divergence of an individual CM axon to several motor nuclei and with graded degrees of synaptic influence which allow various combinations of functionally related agonist muscles— reciprocally inhibited antagonists as well as task-related synergies of the forearm and intrinsic hand muscles. Conversely, selective influence of a CM cell on a single muscle is the exception. The key function of CM neurons is their preferential relation to the small dynamic and static forces necessary for fine adjustments of muscular activity; most CM cells and identified CS neurons in M1 were found to be active with very small force changes, showing steep modulation of firing rate over the low force range and saturation at higher force levels (Cheney and Fetz 1980; Evarts *et al*. 1983). Maier *et al*. (1993) demonstrated this sigmoid relationship, especially for CM cells with restricted muscle fields, coding the force of index finger and thumb independently during the precision grip. Changes of regional cerebral blood flow (rCBF) in the human M1 with force gradation of the finger reflect this pattern (Dettmers *et al*. 1995). There is also a marked dissociation between the amount of a particular CM cell's discharge and the activity in its target muscle when precisely controlled slow movements are compared with forceful ballistic movements (Fromm and Evarts 1977, Cheney and Fetz 1980), or when a precision grip between thumb and index finger is changed to a power grip of the hand (Muir and Lemon 1983). Thus CM cells are not active during all movements in which their target muscles are involved.

As yet, no evidence for a non-monosynaptic excitation of spinal arm motoneurons by CS fibres has been obtained in the macaque (Olivier *et al*. 2001) or in humans (de Noordhout *et al*. 1999). The behavioural advantage of direct CM control over axial and proximal muscles is most likely the precise muscular control subserving reach and grasp. For example, piano playing and painting by '*Homo faber*' requires accurate positioning and stability around the shoulder and proximal arm muscles in close concert with the CM apparatus for the hand and fingers. Undoubtedly, however, there are important differences in CS influence over proximal and distal arm muscles at the cortical as well as spinal level with the well-known proximal-to-distal gradient of CM connections (Colebatch and Gandevia 1989; Turton and Lemon 1999).

Corticospinal deficits following experimental lesions in non-human primates

The adaptive processes following lesions of neurons or fibres within the CNS may completely conceal the initial deficits. In order to deduce from lesion studies which functional contribution is made by a neuronal network or a fibre tract to motor performance, it is essential to look not only at the chronic state of lesion-induced deficits but also at the initial symptoms. Therefore both the acute and chronic effects of CS lesions will be described here. Spasticity as a late response to lesions of descending fibres will not be discussed, because pure CS lesions are not considered to result in spasticity (reviewed by Denny-Brown 1980) and because an adequate discussion of this matter would go beyond the limits of this chapter (for references see Noth 1991; Dietz 1992; Young 1994).

David Ferrier (1873) was the first to demonstrate that after removal of the 'excitable' forelimb area of monkeys, the contralateral hand became plegic. This early observation was fully confirmed by later studies. When the arm or leg representation of M1 is excised, a flaccid paresis occurs in the respective contralateral muscles. During passive stretching of the plegic muscles, no stretch resistance can be felt and the tendon jerks are depressed on the affected side. Trunk muscles appear to be spared, and removal of

M1 never evokes a visible ipsilateral paresis. These findings demonstrate that before reorganization starts in primates, the descending projections from M1 to the spinal cord via direct or indirect pathways are so strong that without this synaptic drive no voluntary, proximal, or distal movements of the limbs are possible.

In order to achieve a more selective lesion of the CS system, pyramidotomy in monkeys was introduced by Tower (1940) and repeated later by many other groups. In this technique, CS fibres from all cortical fields of origin are disrupted at the level of the bulbar pyramid without a significant lesion of bulbospinal fibres. The consistent early effect of unilateral or bilateral lesions of the pyramid is a hypotonia of the contralateral limb muscles with slowing of movements and a severe impairment of digital dexterity (Tower 1940). Such lesioned monkeys are not able to retrieve small objects from the wells of a Klüver board by using the precision grip between thumb and index finger. Goal-directed arm movements are more affected than postural performance. The severe deficits of skilled finger movements last about a week, after which slow but never complete recovery of dexterity commences. Compared with the profound initial paresis of the contralateral extremities following M1 lesions, the muscular weakness after pyramidotomy is less pronounced, although in some of these experiments nearly all of the corticospinal fibres were severed. This difference demonstrates the important contribution of corticobulbospinal pathways to the control of arm and leg movements (Kuypers 1981).

The permanent behavioural deficits of the upper extremity mostly investigated after complete bilateral pyramidotomy are the inability to execute independent finger movements, and a persistent hypotonia and hyporeflexia in forelimb flexors (Woolsey *et al*. 1972). Another permanent deficit is a slowed development of isometric force between thumb and index (Hepp-Reymond and Wiesendanger 1972). The recovery of some discrete finger movements following unilateral pyramidotomy in some experiments has been attributed to a more vigorous effort to retrain the affected hand (Chapman and Wiesendanger 1982; Nudo *et al*. 1996), in contrast with experiments in which the animals recovered in a 'free situation'. However, in many of these preparations, and especially when histology revealed subtotal lesions of the pyramidal tract, spared CS fibres might have contributed to the recovery of discrete finger movements. This is supported by the observation that hand function of monkeys with a proven complete unilateral destruction of the pyramid recovers more slowly than in animals with an incomplete lesion, and that recovery is never complete in these cases (Schwartzman 1978). Persistent deficits include impairment of independent finger movements as well as inadequate use of somatosensory information, such as finely tuned movements to place the volar surface in contact with an offered object ('instinctive tactile grasp'). The loss of tactile exploration resembles the deficits seen after lesions of the dorsal columns at high spinal level, which underlines the close functional interaction between the CS tract and the dorsal column system in tactile guidance of individual finger movements (Davidoff 1989).

Even after complete unilateral pyramidotomy, the strategy to solve a manipulatory task is, in principle, unimpaired. Similar results were obtained in a study of conditioned step-tracking movements of the wrist of monkeys with resection of the contralateral arm area of M1 (Hoffman and Strick 1995). Despite intensive retraining, some specific deficits persisted in these animals, i.e. a profound slowing of wrist movements with deterioration of the precise spatiotemporal EMG pattern, lack of suppression of antagonistic muscle activity at movement onset, and a striking difficulty in accurately performing wrist movements, all of which can reasonably be attributed to CS neuronal dysfunction. However, the animals were able to perform movements in different directions, which indicates that the M1 cortex is not necessarily engaged in the basic programming of directional motor commands. Taken together, the substantial degree of recovery of skilled hand and finger movements following complete unilateral pyramidotomy does not argue against a prominent role of the CS system in the process of learning and executing these particular functions; rather, it emphasizes the high degree of plasticity within the CNS.

Corticospinal deficits in humans

Clinical descriptions of pure unilateral or bilateral lesions of the CS tract in humans are rare. Restoration of sensorimotor functions of the affected limbs following CS lesions involves a variety of plastic changes at different levels of the CNS. For a detailed commentary on plasticity and underlying mechanisms during recovery at the motorcortical level, we refer to Chapter 10 of this volume and the important work of Nudo *et al.* (1996). In the case of incomplete CS tract lesions, both terminal sprouting and an increase in gain of synaptic transmission of undamaged CS fibres at the spinal level are likely to play significant roles in functional recovery. Therefore convincing conclusions from permanent deficits of pure CS tract lesions can only be drawn if post-mortem histology reveals a complete unilateral destruction of the CS tract. Moreover, any permanent deficit (such as slowing of movements) may be influenced by pathological adaptive mechanisms inherent in the process of recovery (best illustrated by the occurrence of spasticity following lesions of the internal capsule).

By far the greatest number of case reports are based upon studies of patients with circumscribed lesions of the M1 cortex. Three major factors limit the interpretation of these clinical observations with regard to the function of the CS system.

1 M1 lesions affect not only other corticofugal fibres with a potential indirect spinal action but also its cortical output to other sensorimotor areas.

2 In the case of surgical excision of M1 for therapeutical reasons, the functional outcome cannot be compared with lesions of the intact cortex, as substantial reorganization may have taken place before surgical intervention.

3 Functional tests performed after recovery from the initial plegia may be 'contaminated' by post-lesional reorganization (see above).

There are many descriptions of 'pure motor plegia' in humans (reviewed by Fisher 1982), but they mostly refer to lesions of the internal capsule. Here, the relatively few CS fibres are intermingled with the bulk of axons directed to the pontine and bulbospinal nuclei. The contribution of these indirect pathways to the motor deficits remains difficult to assess. Nonetheless, it can be concluded from many clinical studies that, following any substantial damage of fibres in the course of the CS tract, weakness is much more pronounced in distal than proximal muscles of the contralateral limb (Twitchell 1951; Colebatch and Gandevia 1989). The much greater importance of the fast CM inputs for voluntary activation of hand rather than upper-arm muscles has been demonstrated by a number of TMS studies in normal subjects and patients (Turton and Lemon 1999). Yet again, it is an open question as to whether corticoreticulospinal projections and/or surviving slowly conducting CS inputs may compensate for the loss of the fast CM input to shoulder muscles.

A number of cases with histologically proven unilateral or even bilateral complete destruction of the medullary pyramid have been described in the literature (Bucy *et al.* 1964; reviewed by Kim *et al.* 1995). The acute clinical symptoms are a flaccid hemiplegia (or tetraplegia) sparing, to some degree, the axial and proximal limb muscles. The follow-up of these cases shows a persistent weakness of the contralateral arm and leg muscles with exaggerated tendon jerks. The ability to execute independent finger movements reappears to some extent, but in most of the published cases elaborate tests of hand functions were not performed. In one case, treatment of severe hemiballismus by surgical section of the right pyramid caused an initial contralateral flaccid hemiplegia which was followed, 24 hrs later, by a gradual recovery of voluntary hand movements (Bucy *et al.* 1964). Independent finger movements appeared after 4 weeks, but deficits in the execution of independent finger movements persisted until the patient died 30 months after the surgical procedure. Quantitative histology revealed that only 83% of the corticospinal fibres of the right pyramidal tract were damaged. The favourable outcome in this patient was likely to be due to the relatively high number of surviving CS fibres of the left pyramid.

The clinical symptoms of unilateral pyramidal lesions in humans resemble the functional deficits seen in monkeys following pyramidotomy and emphasize the powerful net excitatory action of the CS tract on the alpha-motoneurons (and possibly on fusimotoneurons) supplying the contralateral arm and leg muscles. Even after recovery from the initial plegia, dexterity of the contralateral hand never returns completely. Mild signs of spasticity, such as exaggerated tendon jerks, Babinski's sign, and spastic posture, were seen in most subjects, but spastic muscle tone in response to passive stretches was never observed. As far as M1 lesions are concerned, one of the best documented cases has been published by Foerster (1936). Following a complete surgical excision of the left arm and hand field of M1 in a young man, which resulted in a complete degeneration of the ipsilateral pyramid as proven at autopsy, a remarkable degree of functional recovery of hand and finger movements was observed. Initially, the right arm showed a complete flaccid plegia. Two years after the lesion, the patient was able to flex the fingers in synergy and to hold a pencil between thumb and index finger. However, individual finger movements never recovered. Another case with a circumscribed ischaemic lesion of the left-hand region of M1, as documented by CT scan, has been described by Freund (1987). The right-handed patient suffered a complete flaccid paresis of the right arm, sparing the proximal muscles. After 6–8 months of intensive rehabilitation, voluntary movements of the distal arm muscle reappeared, and the power grip of the right fist reached two-thirds of that of the left side. The precision grip between thumb and index finger also recovered. Tendon jerks of the right arm were slightly exaggerated. Permanent deficits included the inability to extend the fingers fully or to perform rapid alternating finger movements. These symptoms strikingly resemble the permanent deficits seen in monkeys after unilateral pyramidotomy.

There is accumulating evidence that the M1 cortex in humans is involved in motor learning and in particular in the early consolidation of newly acquired motor skills (see Chapter 9 of this volume). Therefore lesions of M1 should impede the acquisition and the execution of motor skills beyond the effects induced by lesion of the CS fibres. However, this is difficult to prove because of the inevitable paresis following M1 lesions. In recent years, progress in the understanding of the function of the human motor cortex, and in particular the dexterity of the human hand, has come from the application of the new non-invasive techniques such as TMS and functional magnetic resonance imaging in healthy subjects and in patients. Thus it can be expected that many of the open questions regarding the function of the CS system and the deficits following CS lesions will be solved in the near future.

References

Bucy PC, Keplinger JE, Sequeira EB (1964). Destruction of the 'pyramidal tract' in man. *J Neurosurg*, **21**, 385–98.

Catsman-Berrevoets CE, Kuypers HGJM (1976). Cells of origin of cortical projections to dorsal column nuclei, spinal cord and bulbar medial reticular formation in the rhesus monkey. *Neurosci Lett*, **3**, 245–52.

Chapman CE, Wiesendanger M (1982). Recovery of function following unilateral lesions of the bulbar pyramide in the monkey. *Electroencephalogr Clin Neurophysiol*, **53**, 374–87.

Cheney PD, Fetz EE (1980). Functional classes of primate corticomotoneuronal cells and their relation to active force. *J Neurophysiol*, **44,** 773–91.

Cheney PD, Fetz EE, Palmer SS (1985). Patterns of facilitation and suppression of antagonist forelimb muscles from motor cortex sites in the awake monkey. *J Neurophysiol*, **53**, 805–20.

Colebatch JG, Gandevia SC (1989). The distribution of muscular weakness in upper motor neuron lesions affecting the arm. *Brain*, **112**, 749–63.

Coulter JD, Jones EG (1977). Differential distribution of corticospinal projections from individual cytoarchitectonic fields in the monkey. *Brain Res*, **129**, 335–40.

Davidoff RA (1989). The dorsal columns. *Neurology*. **39**, 1377–85.

Denny-Brown D (1980). Preface: Historical aspects of the relation of spasticity to movement. In RG Feldmann, RR Young, WP Koella, (ed.) *Spasticity: Disordered Motor Control*, pp. 1–15. Chicago, IL: Year Book.

Dettmers C, Fink GR, Lemon RN, Stephan KM, Passingham RE, Silbersweig D, *et al.* (1995). The relation between cerebral activity and force in the motor areas of the human brain. *J Neurophysiol*, **74**, 802–15.

de Noordhout AM, Rapisarda G, Bogacz D, Gerard P, De Pasqua V, Pennisi G, *et al.* (1999). Corticomotoneuronal synaptic connections in normal man. An electrophysiological study. *Brain*, **122**, 1327–40.

Dietz V (1992). Human neuronal control of automatic functional movements: interaction between central programs and afferent input. *Physiol Rev*, **72**, 33–69.

Dum RP, Strick PL (1991). The origin of corticospinal projections from the premotor areas in the frontal lobe. *J Neurosci*, **11**, 667–89.

Dum RP, Strick PL (1996). Spinal cord terminations of the medial wall motor areas in macaque monkeys. *J Neurosci*, **16**, 6513–25.

Evarts EV, Fromm C, Kröller J, Jennings VA (1983). Motor cortex control of finely graded forces. *J Neurophysiol*, **49**, 1199–1215.

Ferrier D (1873). Experimental researches in cerebral physiology and pathology. *West Riding Lunatic Asylum Med Rep*, **3**, 1–50.

Fetz EE, Cheney PD (1980). Postspike facilitation of forelimb muscle activity by primate corticomotoneuronal cells. *J Neurophysiol*, **44**, 751–72.

Fisher CM (1982). Lacunar strokes and infarcts: a review. *Neurology*, **32**, 871–6.

Foerster O (1936). Motorische Felder und Bahnen. In H Bumke, O Foerster, (ed.) *Handbuch der Neurologie* Vol 6, pp. 1–357. Berlin: Springer-Verlag.

Freund HJ (1987). Abnormalities of motor behavior after cortical lesions in humans. In VB Brooks, (ed.) *Handbook of Physiology.* Vol 5. *The Nervous System.* Baltimore, MD: Williams & Wilkins, 763–810.

Fromm C, Evarts EV (1977). Relation of motor cortex neurons to precisely controlled and ballistic movements. *Neurosci Lett*, **5**, 259–65.

Fromm C, Evarts EV (1982). Pyramidal tract neurons in somatosensory cortex: central and peripheral inputs during voluntary movement. *Brain Res*, **238**, 186–91.

Georgopoulos AP, Schwartz AB, Kettner RE (1986). Neuronal population coding of movement direction. *Science*, **233**, 1416–19.

Hepp-Reymond M-C, Wiesendanger M (1972). Unilateral pyramidotomy in monkeys: effect on force and speed of a conditioned precision grip. *Brain Res*, **36**, 117–31.

Hoffman DS, Strick PL (1995). Effects of a primary motor cortex lesion on step-tracking movements of the wrist. *J Neurophysiol*, **73**, 891–5.

Kakei S, Hoffman DS, Strick PL (1999). Muscle and movement representations in the primary motor cortex. *Science*, **285**, 2136–9.

Kim JS, Chung CS, Kim HG (1995). Medial medullary syndrome: report of 18 new patients and a review of the literature. *Stroke*, **26**, 1548–52.

Kuypers HGJM (1981). Anatomy of the descending pathways. In VB Brooks, (ed.) *Handbook of Physiology*, Vol 2. pp. 597–666. Baltimore, MD: Williams & Wilkins.

Lassek AM (1954). *The Pyramidal Tract. Its Status in Medicine.* Springfield, IL: Charles C. Thomas.

Lawrence DG, Kuypers HGJM (1968). The functional organization of the motor system in the monkey. I. The effects of bilateral pyramidal lesions. *Brain*, **91**, 1–14.

Lemon RN, Mantel GWH, Muir RB (1986). Corticospinal facilitation of hand muscles during voluntary movement in the conscious monkey. *J Physiol*, **381**, 497–527.

Lemon RN, Maier MA, Armand J, Kirkwood PA, Yang HW (2002). Functional differences in the corticospinal projections from macaque primary motor cortex and supplementary motor area. *Adv Exp Med Biol*, **508**, 425–34.

Maier MA, Bennet KM, Hepp-Reymond MC, Lemon RN (1993). Contribution of the monkey cortico-motoneuronal system to the control of force in precision grip. *J Neurophysiol*, **69**, 772–85.

Muir RB, Lemon RN (1983). Corticospinal neurons with a special role in precision grip. *Brain Res*, **261**, 312–16.

Murray EA, Coulter JD (1981). Organization of corticospinal neurons in the monkey. *J Comp Neurol*, **195**, 339–65.

Nathan PW, Smith, MC, Deacon P (1990). The corticospinal tracts in man. *Brain*, **113**, 303–24.

Noth J (1991). Trends in the pathophysiology and pharmacotherapy of spasticity. *J Neurol*, **238**, 131–9.

Nudo RJ, Wise BM, SiFuentes F, Milken GW (1996). Neural substrates for the effects of rehabilitative training on motor recovery after ischemic infarct. *Science*, **271**, 1791–4.

Olivier E, Baker SN, Nakajima K, Brochier T, Lemon RN (2001). Investigation into non-monosynaptic corticospinal excitation of macaque upper limb single motor units. *J Neurophysiol*, **86**, 1573–86.

Porter R, Lemon RN (1993). *Corticospinal Function and Voluntary Movement*. Oxford: Clarendon Press.

Schoen JHR (1964). Comparative aspects of the descending fibre systems in the spinal cord. *Prog Brain Res*, **11**, 203–22.

Schwartzman RJ (1978). A behavioral analysis of complete unilateral section of the pyramidal tract at the medullary level in *Macaca mulatta*. *Ann Neurol*, **4**, 234–44.

Tanji J, Kurata K (1982). Comparison of movement-related activity in two cortical motor areas of primates. *J Neurophysiol*, **48**, 633–53.

Toyoshima K, Sakai H (1982). Exact cortical extent of the origin of the corticospinal tract (CST) and the quantitative contribution to the CST in different cytoarchitectonic areas. A study with horseradish peroxidase in the monkey. *J Hirnforsch*, **23**, 257–69.

Tower SS (1940). Pyramidal lesions in monkey. *Brain*, **63**, 36–90.

Turton A, Lemon RN (1999). The contribution of fast corticospinal input to the voluntary activation of proximal muscles in normal subjects and in stroke patients. *Exp Brain Res*, **129**, 559–72.

Twitchell TE (1951). The restoration of motor function following hemiplegia in man. *Brain*, **74**, 443–80.

Werner W, Bauswein E, Fromm C (1991). Static firing rates of premotor and primary motor cortical neurons associated with torque and joint position. *Exp Brain Res*, **86**, 293–302.

Woolsey CN, Gorska T, Wetzel A, Erickson TC, Earls FJ, Allman, JM (1972). Complete unilateral section of the pyramidal tract at the medullary level in Macaca mulatta. *Brain Res*, **40**, 119–24.

Young RR (1994). Spasticity: a review. *Neurology*, **44** (Suppl 9), S12–20.

Chapter 11

Bimanual coordination and its disorders

Mario Wiesendanger and Deborah J. Serrien

Overview

In human evolution, hand functions played a significant role in the emergence of toolmaking and tool use, as well as in expressing gestures. Tool use in everyday life, together with gestures and music performance, typically engage both hands in well-coordinated asymmetric synergies. A division of labor between hands is also an evolutionary trend, with the left engaging preferentially in posturing grasps, providing an egocentric reference frame for the right which manipulates the grasped object (MacNeilage 1987).

As techniques of functional brain imaging gradually improved, it became clear that coordinated manipulations engage widely distributed neural networks of cortical and subcortical structures, in varying combinations, depending on task constraints. Manipulative behavior strongly relies on cortical structures implicated in cognitive functions, such as action planning, attention, motivation, and reward, all of which are crucial ingredients of higher goal-directed motor behavior. In addition, coordination and adaptation to environmental constraints also require neural circuits at subcortical levels, notably cerebellar and basal ganglia circuits and also the brainstem and spinal cord with their motor and sensory pathways. Functional imaging and lesion studies have markedly advanced our knowledge about the implication of cerebral structures involved in bimanual tasks. They include the primary sensorimotor, premotor, mesial frontal, and posterior parietal cortical areas, the corpus callosum, and the cerebellum and basal ganglia. In order to understand neurological deficits in manipulative behavior, one needs to analyze and understand as far as possible the ingredients of the neural control of the highly complex hand dexterity.

The Russian neuropsychologist Luria (1969) was probably the first to point out the usefulness of in-phase versus anti-phase hand flexion/extension in neurological patients with brain lesions. This paradigm has been used frequently in normal subjects and patients with brain lesions, and almost exclusively to test bimanual coordination in functional imaging. Since the 1980s, a non-linear dynamic approach has been successfully introduced for interpreting coordination of bimanual rhythms (Kugler *et al.* 1980; Schöner and Kelso 1988). In this context, new terms are often used in the motor control literature. Thus the physical system of the motor apparatus follows dynamic self-organizing rules: the dynamic constraints. Moving in the physical world results in retroactions from the environment: the external constraints. Goal-oriented motor behavior needs to overcome and to compensate proactively for external constraints, and to adjust the neuronal control signals according to the goal representation. These are cognitive (internal) constraints, which include the intentional elements with all the attributes of motivation, goal, and stored movement plan with the necessary postural adjustment. Dynamic rules have now also been observed in the brain.

   Only a few attempts have been made to analyze 'natural' bimanual actions, although they dominate our daily motor repertoire. These actions are often complex and therefore are difficult to assess in detail. Characteristically, bimanual tasks in everyday life are goal directed, and achieving the goal may often be appropriate to overcoming the problem of task complexity. Coordinated goal invariance, such as goal synchronization, is a typical feature of bimanual behavior (Wiesendanger *et al.* 1996a).

Bilateral forelimb rhythms, coherence, and assimilation

Basic concepts

Rhythms, including breathing, chewing, and stepping, are fundamental semi-automatic components of motor behavior. In the 1930, von Holst (1973) pioneered studies in rhythmic movements, from fish to humans, by recording fin and limb movements. He came to the conclusion that these rhythms are not chains of reflexes (as previously thought), but rather are generated centrally by neuronal assemblies. Von Holst recognized the duality of interacting automatic patterns and command signals from higher levels of the neuraxis. Furthermore, he concluded that multiple rhythm generators compete to impose their frequency with a fixed phase relation to other rhythm generators, as if driven by attracting and repelling 'forces'. He termed this the 'magnet effect'. He referred to 'absolute coordination' when two effectors have the same frequency and phase relation. The tendency toward phase attraction, even when the component frequencies were originally not the same, was termed 'relative coordination' (see also Kelso 1994). Figure 11.1 is from an experiment of von Holst, recording movements of two pectoral fins in a fish (*Sargus*) displaying a sudden frequency and phase change (in this example from isodirectional to alternating movements). The same phenomenon (but more often from anti-phase to in-phase) can be observed in rhythmic movements of human limbs. Extensive treatment of the theoretical background to the application of non-linear dynamics in biomechanics, with many practical examples, can be found in Schöner *et al.* (1986); Swinnen *et al.* (1994); Turvey and Schmidt (1994); Kelso (1995); Swinnen (2002).

   Recent progress in neurobiology has been achieved in the areas of spinal interneurons, spinal circuitry, and pattern generators, and this work appears to be relevant to the problem of interlimb coupling. It includes the modification of activity in these circuits

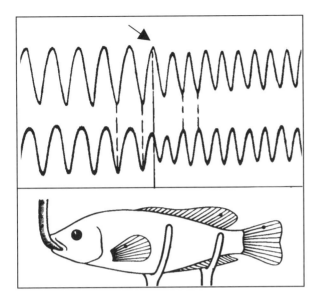

Fig. 11.1 Transition from in-phase to anti-phase rhythms of pectoral fins (arrow). In this case, the phase change is linked to a frequency change. Reproduced from von Holst (1973) The Behavioral Physiology of Animal and Man. Coral Gables, FL: Hillsdale (originally published in 1939).Reprinted with permission from Springer Verlag.

by modulators such as serotonin and norepinephrine (Hultborn 2001). Intracellular studies of the branching pattern of descending tract fibers with their rich collateralization in the spinal cord, provide important clues about bilateral control of the limbs (Shinoda *et al.* 1992). Interneurons that are likely to be responsible for interlimb coordination have been identified (Butt and Kiehn 2003). Natural locomotor rhythms exhibit in-phase as well as anti-phase bursts, for example in flexor–extensor muscle pairs. The neural mechanisms of the pattern generators can be studied in neonatal rat preparations and manipulated by transmitters or their agonists/antagonists (Cowley and Schmidt 1995). Unfortunately, there has been little communication between researchers working in the two fields of non-linear dynamics and neurobiology.

Rhythmic activity has also been observed at cortical levels. The dynamic waxing and waning of activation foci (dynamic 'maps') in human EEG and MEG-studies has established transient inter-areal coherences in the oscillation patterns. It has been suggested that coherent coupling of distributed synergistic foci reflects integration of large-scale neural networks, which in turn may be crucial for coordinating effectors for purposeful actions (Grossberg *et al.* 1997; Fuchs *et al.* 2000; Bressler and Kelso 2001; Engel *et al.* 2001; Varela *et al.* 2001; Gross *et al.* 2002). Manipulating the difficulty of the task was found to modify both motor output and coherence in the β-band of EEG oscillations. Note that the term coherence is used for interregional correlation of EEG oscillations, expressing functional interactions between distributed cortical areas. Furthermore, the β rhythm has been strongly associated with motor functions. For example, in cortical areas coherence was higher with anti-phase than with in-phase movements (**Serrien and Brown 2002**), which supports the idea that the more complex mode requires a relatively higher degree of neural communication. However, as stated by Varela *et al.* (2001), the mechanisms underlying 'binding' and its modulation are still largely unknown.

Temporal interactions in interlimb coupling

If pointing movements are executed to separate targets, one being more distant than the other, the timing for target reaching is about the same, i.e. the hand reaching to the nearer target moves more slowly than the hand reaching to the distant target (Kelso *et al.* 1979, 1983). However, later findings by Marteniuk *et al.* (1984) were not completely in line with the above results since, with additional loading of one arm, significant departures from synchronization were observed. Nonetheless, the tendency of temporal assimilation was observed in later experiments [but see exception in Hatzitaki and McKinley (2001)]. Dohle *et al.* (2000) reported that in bimanual prehension movements, temporal coupling during initial reaching was stronger than during the phase of grip aperture. The conclusion was that the process of grasping needed more independence of the hands, especially in asymmetrical manipulations, while the proximal limbs have to move together to initiate an action.

In-phase bimanual movements (e.g. two-handed finger tapping) are easily performed at frequencies of up to about 3 Hz, but need to be much higher in skilled pianists. With anti-phase tapping, the coordination relation tends to be less stable, with sudden transitions to the easier in-phase mode, particularly when rhythms get faster. Tapping at different frequencies between the hands (e.g. 2:3 polyrhythms) is difficult (Summers *et al.* 1993; Peper and Beek 1998). Learning to execute polyrhythms is essential for piano players. Thus, the coordination 'brain load' is rather higher for anti-phase than for in-phase rhythms, and is highest for polyrhythms. With an appropriate experimental design of a combination of rhythms, one should be able to gauge the amount of coordination load in bimanual tasks (Ullen *et al.* 2003). The 'in-phase–anti-phase paradigm' has been used extensively to assess central representations in brain imaging, or coordination deficits in patients. The rationale has been to capture the coordination 'load', assuming that any structure displaying a larger metabolic response in the anti-phase than in the in-phase mode reflects the extra work of coordination. As will be described later in this chapter, patients with neurological problems may indeed experience increased difficulty in maintaining an anti-phase rhythm.

Spatial and kinetic interactions in bimanual tasks and assimilation effects

In addition to temporal effects, spatial interactions have also been observed (Walter and Swinnen 1990; Franz *et al.* 1991; Semjen *et al.* 1995; Swinnen *et al.* 1997, 1998). For example, subjects have difficulties in drawing straight lines with the right hand while simultaneously drawing circles with the left hand. In our experiments (Serrien and Wiesendanger 2001b), subjects had to move hand-held objects rhythmically up and down in the in-phase and anti-phase modes. Loaded objects, one for each hand, were instrumented with force sensors to measure the normal grip force (GF) and the tangential load force (LF) exerted on the manipulanda (inset to Fig. 11.2). Each subject performed two series in changing order of left and right hands, and two bimanual series (Fig. 11.2). In this dynamic task, the two forces and their ratio oscillated with the movements. As one can easily verify, a load is felt to become lighter in an upward move and to become heavier in a downward move. This is shown in the GF and LF profiles on the right of Figure 11.2. However, the GF/LF ratio was minimal at the lower reversal and highest at the upper reversal. That means that GF diminishes less than LF as the object approaches the upper reversal point. The GF/LF ratio is considered as the controlling

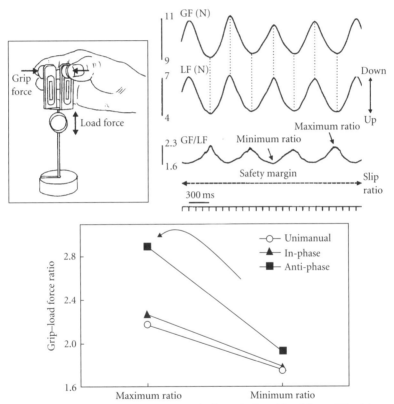

Fig. 11.2 Inset:manipulandum for measuring grip force (GF) and load force (LF) with exchangeable and variable weights. The task was to move the weights unimanually and bimanually, in-phase and anti-phase. Right: oscillations of the two forces and (below) of the GF/LF ratio considered to be the controlled variable. Arrowheads indicate the up and down direction changes. Maxima of the force ratio occur near peak vertical positions. The safety margin is between the dynamic GF/LF ratio and the slip ratio. When two objects were moved in the bimanual in-phase mode, the maximum force ratio was the same as in the unimanual series. However, in the bimanual anti-phase mode, the maximum force ratio of both hands increased significantly (graph below). Adapted from Serrien and Wiesendanger (2001b). Reprinted with permission from Elsevier.

variable determining the safety of object–hand coupling and the total load, including friction (Flanagan and Wing 1995; Serrien and Wiesendanger 2001c). The safety margin (Johansson and Westling 1988) is determined by asking the subject to release the grip slowly until the object slips out of the hand (equivalent to slip ratio); the safety margin represents the difference between the slip ratio, i.e. the minimum value determined by the friction between skin and object, and the grip-to-load force ratio employed by the subject. In the above dynamic situation, the observed ratio maxima at the upper reversal reflect an anticipatory safety strategy to secure coupling stability when LF is decreasing, becoming low at the reversal point. The new result of the bimanual experiment was that the ratio maxima were significantly larger during the anti-phase mode than during the in-phase mode (Fig. 11.2). Rescaling of the force ratio to higher values in the anti-phase paradigm suggests that the safety of hand–object coupling is automatically (and unconsciously) increased whenever the task is more difficult, probably because more monitoring and attention is required to maintain the phase relationship.

In a load-lifting experiment, Serrien and Wiesendanger (2001a) demonstrated that the object weight and also the moving distances (independent variables) affected the force ratio and movement time (the two dependent variables). Since the effects were similar for the two protocols, only the weight experiment will be discussed (Fig. 11.3). For the unimanual condition, a light weight produced a high force ratio (Fig. 3A, unimanual) and movement time was short (Fig. 3B, unimanual); the reverse was true for the heavy weight. This effect is explained by the parallel changes of load and velocity. Such manipulations had similar effects in the bimanual tasks. However, the main question is: Does a bimanual asymmetric condition (e.g. one hand light load, other hand heavy load) change the force ratio according to the unimanual specifications? As shown on the right of Figure 11.3, this was not the case; rather, the force ratios as well as the movement times of each hand are similar. Thus one can conclude that, in the asymmetric bimanual situation, the two commands to the individual hands are overruled and both force ratio and movement time are rescaled to a common control structure, with similar grasping forces and similar movement times.

In the above bimanual weight-lifting experiments, changes in external constraints were applied to an entire series and thus were predictable. In previous pioneering studies, Johansson and Westling (1988) investigated the mechanisms of grip force regulations when subjects had to lift single-handed a manipulandum with unexpected weight changes between lifts; the subjects regularly programmed their force according to the previous force. In a subsequent load-lifting experiment (Serrien and Wiesendanger 2001c), the effect of unpredictable load interference was examined in a bimanually coordinated task (Fig. 11.4; note that subject cannot see any load changes). The unpredictable weight constellations were (i) both hands heavy, (ii) both hands light, (iii) right hand heavy, left hand light, and (iv) left hand heavy, right hand light. As in the Johansson–Westling experiment, it was found that a preceding heavy weight had a transient influence on a subsequent lighter weight, with a prominent overshoot

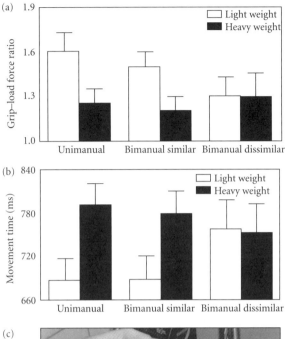

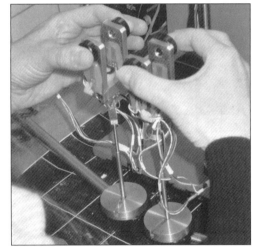

Fig. 11.3 Effects on (a) force ratio and (b) movement time in a bimanual load-lifting protocol with variable weights (c). When both hands carried the same weights (middle pair of white and black bars), the dependent variables were adjusted to the same values as in the unimanual protocol (left pair of bars). However, when the weights were dissimilar (right pair of bars), both force ratio and movement time assimilated. Reproduced from Serrien and Wiesendanger (2001a). Reprinted with permission from Elsevier.

in grip force in relation to the light weight. Figure 11.4(a) shows an example when a light weight lift was preceded by heavy weight lifts in the previous series. This resulted in a significant increase in force ratio for the first lift. However, the excessive force was rescaled to the expected level after only one trial. The reverse manipulation (light weight followed by heavy weight) had no or minimal effect. The new aspect of the study was the bimanual protocol; as illustrated in Fig. 11.4(c), the force ratio of the two hands, plotted for the first, second, and third trials showed, as expected,

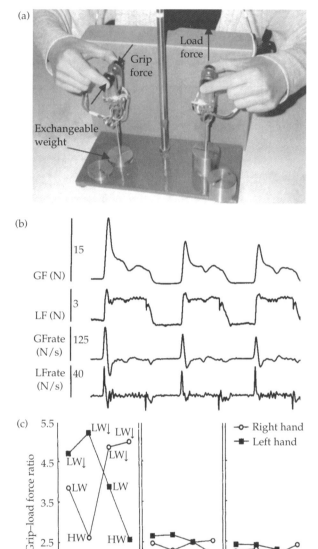

Fig. 11.4 (a) Bimanual lifting movements with unpredictable load distribution among hands. Note overshooting of GF (b) and irregular ratio (c), depending on the weight sequence in the first lifting trial when a light weight followed a heavy weight. From the second trial onward, GF is adjusted to appropriate values (b), with assimilation and stabilization of the force ratio (c). Reproduced from Serrien and Wiesendanger (2001c). Reprinted with permission from Blackwell.

a considerable initial variability for the four conditions, depending on the previous constellation. However, a remarkable bimanual similarity of the force ratio is already present in the second trial. Thus it appears that the bimanual assimilation of the grip forces takes place as soon as the physical properties become predictable, a further indication that the GF/LF ratio is the controlling variable for bimanual grasping behavior.

Neural networks for bimanual coordination

Rhythmic paradigms and brain imaging

The majority of functional magnetic resonance imaging (fMRI) studies compare the degree of activation obtained in the easier in-phase task with that of the more difficult anti-phase tasks. The rationale is that any surplus load in coordinating in the more difficult anti-phase mode would identify the critical region implicated in bimanual coordination. In a number of imaging studies, an increased metabolic response in the anti-phase paradigm is found in the mesial frontal cortex, including the supplementary motor area (SMA) and the anterior cingulate areas (Sadato *et al.* 1997; Goerres *et al.* 1998; Toyokura *et al.* 1999; Stephan *et al.* 1999b). An example from the work of Stephan *et al.* (1999a), illustrated in Figure 11.5, shows an 'extra-activation' in the cingulate area of the mesial frontal cortex. This was a particularly interesting case because the 'extra load' concerned a relatively small anatomical functional area of the mesial frontal

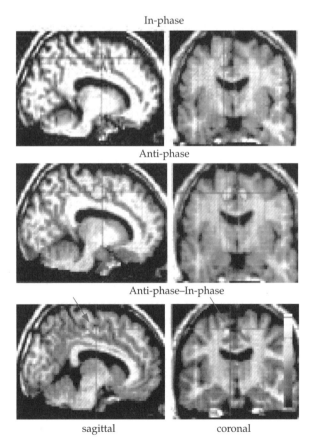

Fig. 11.5 Brain activation study (PET, saggital and coronal scans) in a healthy human subject performing the in-phase–anti-phase paradigm. It shows metabolic responses in the anterior ventral cingulate areas of the mesial cortex during both in-phase and anti-phase sequences. The lowest pair shows the surplus activation that results from the extra effort for coordination in the anti-phase mode (anti-phase–in-phase). Reproduced from Stephan *et al.* (1999a). *Brain*, **122**, 351–68. Reprinted with permission from Oxford University Press and from authors.

cortex. In a further fMRI study, bimanual tapping was executed at different beats between the hands (Jäncke *et al.* 2000). The result was an asymmetry in the activation pattern during bimanual movements, but only for the SMA and not for the primary sensorimotor cortex: 'During right fast versus left slow activity, the left SMA showed more activation than the right SMA, but during the left-fast versus right-slow movements, the right SMA was not significantly more activated than the left SMA' (Jäncke *et al.* 2000). Therefore it was concluded that the rate effect was restricted to the SMA of the dominant hemisphere.

Taken together, these results appear to be in agreement, but other studies on cyclic interlimb movements failed to confirm the notion of a crucial role of the SMA in bimanual coordination. Furthermore, the SMA has also been found to be implicated in rhythmic coordination of upper and lower limbs and thus seems to have a broader coordination function (Ehrsson *et al.* 2000). However, the imposed rhythm was very slow in that study (<1 Hz). Debaere *et al.* (2001), who also used the hand–foot paradigm, suggested ' . . . that interlimb coordination is mediated by motor representations shared by both limbs, rather than being mediated by specific additional neural populations'. Readiness potentials or sustained negativity during performance (EEG or MEG) were found to have highest amplitudes in mesial frontal recordings, and bimanual rhythms generated larger cortical sustained negativity than unimanual movements (Uhl *et al.* 1996). It should be remembered that this method has excellent temporal but relatively poor spatial resolution.

In two positron emission tomography (PET) studies (Fink *et al.* 1999; De Jong *et al.* 2002), the effect of anti-phase movements was not associated with a surplus metabolic response in the SMA, but rather in the posterior parietal, premotor, and prefrontal cortices. This is in line with another recent fMRI study revealing additional activation in the posterior parietal cortex during a bimanual finger opposition task (Nair *et al.* 2003). A further PET study showed that deliberate transitions from in-phase and anti-phase 'programs' were associated with metabolic responses in a more distributed pattern: posterior border of left angular gyrus, right precuneus, right premotor, and right medial–prefrontal cortices (De Jong *et al.* 1999). Finally, the responsibility of the dominant hemisphere for bimanual coordination has been emphasized by Jäncke *et al.* (1998, 2000) and by Serrien *et al.* (2003), and was also borne out in lesion studies (Haaland and Harrington 1994).

From functional imaging studies in humans it can be concluded that, overall, the evidence for one particular cortical area functioning as a 'center' for bimanual coordination is not convincing. Nevertheless, mesial frontal cortical networks appear to contribute to bimanual coordination in variable proportions and constellations, and probably together with the cerebellum and basal ganglia. As mentioned above, the posterior parietal cortex may also be an important structure for bimanual coordination.

The interpretation of whether differences between in-phase and anti-phase movements are due only to an additional coordination load is debatable and remains hypothetical. For example, one could argue that the increased metabolic demand in the anti-phase situation is due to attention (Jackson *et al.* 1999; Temprado *et al.* 2002). It should be remembered that, for most healthy people, both variants of the tasks are easily performed, at least at lower frequencies. Furthermore, performance tends to improve with practice and might also depend on the subject's daily activities, such as typing or playing music. However, discrepancies may be much more pronounced in neurological patients (see later in this chapter).

In search of 'bimanual neurons' in non-human primates

The question arises as to whether there are specific populations of neurons that engage in coordination processes of bimanual actions. Therefore we review briefly the evidence from single-neuron studies in non-human primates. A first report by Brinkman and Porter (1979) indicated that many neurons in the SMA have bilateral relationships with whole forelimb (and probably also trunk) movements. Tanji *et al.* (1987) identified neurons in M1 and SMA that were specifically related to discrete ipsilateral or bilateral hand–finger movements. In a subsequent single-unit study, we tested further the question of the bilaterality of SMA and M1 neurons and their potential involvement in a natural bimanual task. Monkeys were trained in a drawer-pulling task, which had been extensively used before by Kazennikov *et al.* (1994). In a series of single-unit recordings (Kazennikov *et al.* 1999), the monkeys had to perform three blocks of about 20–30 trials: (i) left-hand pulling movements and picking up food with the same hand (LEFT task), (ii) right-hand picking movement from an open drawer (RIGHT task), and (iii) a combined bimanual action in which the monkey picked up food with the right hand after fully opening the drawer with the left hand (BIM task). A total of about 100 neurons from each hemisphere was analyzed. The results for both hemispheres were straightforward: the majority of neurons had a strong association with the two contralateral unimanual tasks and a similar activation in the bimanual task, whereas the two ipsilateral tasks produced weak to moderate activation. This is illustrated in the population histograms in Fig. 11.6. When discharge patterns from individual neurons were examined, the majority reflected a prevailing contralateral association. A relatively small fraction of neurons of both M1 (14%) and SMA (16%) were also excited during execution of the ipsilateral task. Neurons with weak ipsilateral involvement were not assigned to the bimanual category. In addition, but rarely, neurons of M1 (2%) and of SMA (5%) had an exclusive association with the bimanual task. These neurons seem to belong to the same category of M1 and SMA neurons described by Tanji *et al.* (1987). Both motor areas may contribute to bimanual coordination, but we had no indication of a sizeable population of effector-independent neurons specifically involved in bimanual coordination.

Kermadi *et al.* (1998), using a similar bimanual drawer task, found a high proportion of neurons categorized as bimanual neurons: 87% in SMA and 53% in M1. However,

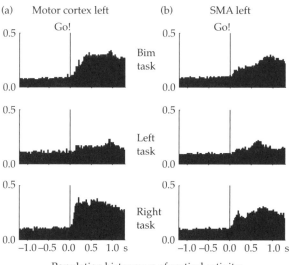

Population histograms of cortical activity
during drawer task performance (*n* = 100)

Fig. 11.6 Population histograms (*n* = 100 units) of neuronal activity recorded in M1 and SMA of the left hemisphere (*Macacca fascicularis*), for left hand reaching and opening drawer, for right hand reaching and picking food, and for the combined bimanual (Bim) task. Reproduced from Kazennikov *et al.* (1999). *Neuroscience*, **89**, 661–74. Reprinted with permission from Pergamon Press.

in a previous analysis, when we did not use stringent criteria for bimanuality, we also found a similarly high proportion of neurons modulated with the ipsilateral task, i.e. 63% in SMA and 35% in M1 for the right hemisphere, and 59% in SMA and 29% in M1 for the left hemisphere (Wiesendanger *et al.* 1996b). Whole-arm movements require considerable postural adjustments, which may well also activate muscles contralateral to the task arm, as we verified in EMG recordings (unpublished data). In line with our results, Cisek *et al.* (2003) found a strong contralateral bias for M1 neurons. These authors commented that the neurons recorded by Kermadi and coworkers were from a rostral zone of M1, i.e. at the border with PMC, which may favor M1 neurons with bilateral (and or proximal) projections. Kermadi and coworkers also changed the task protocol to pseudorandom occurrences of right, left, or bimanual trials, which was a progress in the paradigm but may also have contributed to a sustained preparedness for both arms. In a further experiment by the same group (Kermadi *et al.* 2000), the number of bimanual neurons was remarkably high in the dorsal premotor cortex (PMd), a finding that is in line with the results of Cisek *et al.* (2003). In addition, Kermadi and coworkers found also a high proportion of 'bimanual neurons' in the anterior cingulate motor cortex (CMA) and in the anterior intraparietal area of the posterior parietal cortex (AIP) related to grasping movements (Gallese *et al.* 1994; Wiesendanger *et al.* 1997).

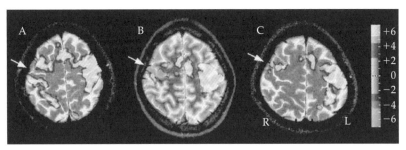

Fig. 11.7 Brain imaging (fMRI) showing representative activation patterns (metabolic responses) from three subjects (A, B, and C) performing self-paced finger opposition movements with the dominant right hand. To visualize the whole depth of the sulci, z scores of five slices were projected onto the center reference slice (slice orientation tilted 20–30° with respect to the bi-commissural line). The hand area of M1 is approximately in front of the omega-shaped 'hand notch' (lateral part of the central sulcus, indicated by arrows). Note lack of activation in the hand area of M1 in the hemisphere ipsilateral to finger movements in scans of subject B; the hand area was deactivated (blue color). Ipsilateral metabolic responses were seen outside M1, in the mesial frontal, premotor, and posterior parietal cortex, particularly in subject A. Reproduced from Nirkko *et al.* (2001). *Neuroimage*, **13**, 825–35. Reprinted with permission from Academic Press.

Donchin and coworkers (Donchin *et al.* 1998, 1999, 2001; Cardoso de Oliveira *et al.* 2002) made a strong case for the involvement of primary motor cortex in bimanual coordination. Again, the task involved whole-arm movements, which are likely to activate proximal and axial muscles on both sides. The involvement of the primary motor cortex in whole-limb movements is not surprising, considering the anatomical fact of ipsilateral motor cortex projections to motoneurons of proximal muscles (via corticospinal and, via brainstem, bilaterally descending pathways) (Brinkman and Kuypers 1973; Kuypers 1981). Together, these ipsilateral connections are rather strong. In humans subjected to functional imaging while performing unilateral proximal movements, ipsilateral activation of M1 was clearly present with proximal shoulder movements. However, when subjects performed fine distal finger and hand movements (Fig. 11.7), the activation of M1 was exclusively in the contralateral hand–finger representation (in front of the 'hand notch') and without activity in ipsilateral M1 (Nirkko *et al.* 2001). However, the bilateral metabolic activations in the secondary motor areas and the posterior parietal cortex should also be noted. In the human brain, the lateral PMC reaches well into the rostral portion of the precentral gyrus, and a relatively small strip of the gyrus is also strongly labeled with ipsilateral hand movements.

Fiber-tracing studies in monkeys revealed only a sparse callosal interconnection between left- and right-hand representations in M1 (Jenny 1979; Rouiller *et al.* 1994); in contrast, the distal forelimb representation in SMA (identified by intracortical stimulation) showed a strong projection to the opposite SMA. Recently, a comparison (from the same laboratory) of the callosal connectivity of the SMA and of the adjacent pre-SMA revealed an even stronger callosal interconnection in the latter (Liu *et al.* 2002).

Given the strong projections from the motor areas to the basal ganglia, including also a weaker projection from the contralateral cortex, one may also expect to find 'bimanual neurons' in these subcortical structures. A search of the caudate, putamen, and pallidum (Wannier *et al.* 2002) indeed confirmed the presence of 'bimanual' neurons (30% of task-related neurons) (see also Selezneva *et al.* 1999) . With respect to the cerebellum, the (relatively weak) contralateral projection of the sensorimotor cortex to the cerebellum, via pontine nuclei, suggests that bimanually related neurons also exist in the cerebellum; thus far no search has been performed.

On the basis of the above single-unit studies in non-human primates, together with imaging studies in humans, the evidence for a specific center for bimanual actions is tenuous. Some neurons which would satisfy the concept of an exclusive specificity for bimanual coordination (rather than for the unimanual movements *per se*) were observed in M1 and SMA. However, such neurons were rare. Rather, the results point to distributed networks of primary motor, dorsal premotor, anterior cingulate, and posterior parietal cortical areas, which may all participate in both uni- and bimanual movements depending on the task. The second somatosensory area SII, with its strong ipsilateral sensory representation (Simões and Hari 1999) and the presence of pyramidal tract neurons, may also be a candidate for bimanual controls. Finally, cortical activity from one hemisphere, engaged by bimanual actions, would also influence the opposite side of the neuraxis via the loops to the basal ganglia and the cerebellum.

Role of sensation in bimanual coordination

Cutaneous signals

The effect of sensation, or of sensory disturbances, on bimanual coordination has not been much explored, although it is well known that lack of sensation seriously hampers the execution of skillful motor behavior. Indirect evidence from bimanual tapping experiments has recently been reported (Drewing *et al.* 2002). It is known that temporal variability in bimanual tapping at a given pace is smaller in the bimanual than in the unimanual condition ('bimanual advantage') (Helmuth and Ivry 1996). The role of cutaneous afferents was inferred to play a role in this mechanism because, when one hand was tapping without hitting the surface with the fingers ('contact-free tapping'), the 'bimanual advantage' was reduced.

By means of the bimanual drawer pull-and-pick paradigm, extensively used in our laboratory, we tested whether a conduction block, transiently removing cutaneous sensation from the pulling thumb and index finger, affects bimanual coordination (Perrig *et al.* 1999). Without sensation, grasping and pulling were greatly affected, even with vision. Because of frequent slips of the pinch from the flat drawer handle, the pulling hand required much more time than normal to open the drawer. Interestingly, however, the unaffected hand immediately adapted to the situation; reaching slowed down at the same pace as the affected limb, resulting in synchronized goal achievement. The blindfolded subjects were not aware of any slowing of the picking hand. We interpret this 'adaptation' as an adaptive strategy to preserve bimanual goal coordination. Since the coordination was essentially preserved, also without vision, it was suggested that the intact proprioceptors in the pulling limb were sufficient to enable proper synchronization at the goal. It has also been suggested that tactile events function as triggering cues for adjusting the timing in an evolving action (Muller *et al.* 2000).

In bimanual symmetrical circle drawing at 1 Hz, the dominant arm typically showed a small phase advance of about 30 ms, which increased significantly when tendons of the dominant arm were vibrated whereas vibration of the non-dominant arm reduced the phase lag (Verschueren *et al.* 1999). Vibration has a disturbing effect on signaling of cutaneous and proprioceptive receptors; the authors therefore concluded that proper temporal coordination depends on intact proprioception.

Chronic deafferentation

Some of the above reports suggest that somatosensory signals, particularly proprioception, might be an important factor in bimanual coordination. The (rare) patients suffering from a chronic large-fiber neuropathy with a massive loss of cutaneous and proprioceptive information have severe problems in controlling their actions, as documented in a number of neurological and neurophysiological reports (Cole and Sedgwick 1992; Cole 1995; Forget and Lamarre 1995; Ghez *et al.* 1995; Voisin *et al.* 2002). Some relearning of important actions under visual control has been observed, including the generation of an adequate force level in a given task ('freezing'). In contrast with normal behavior, this relatively simple task requires constant (and tiring) mental concentration. Loss of proprioception leads to a lack of interjoint coordination (Sainburg *et al.* 1993). Therefore it is possible that bimanual dyscoordination would also occur in these patients. Except for a case with central deafferentation as a consequence of a lesion in the parietal cortex (Jackson *et al.* 2000b), only a few bimanual coordination tasks have been tested in a single deafferented patient, a Canadian woman with a chronic large-fiber neuropathy and subtotal deafferentation. Forget and Lamarre (1995) tested this patient using a bimanual load-lifting task introduced by Hugon *et al.* (1982). The task consists of an active unloading of a weight from the other load-bearing hand. Normally, EMG activity and force are rapidly reduced in a feedforward way, i.e. in anticipation to unloading, resulting in a relatively stable position of the load-bearing hand (passive unloading by another person results in a reflex silent period accompanied by a perturbing upward deflection of the forearm). It was found that the deafferented patient did the active unloading with normal anticipatory postural adjustments. This is in line with the hypothesis of a corollary discharge signaling the appropriate timing for force release in the load-bearing postural arm; this obviously occurs without need for proprioception. A similar result was obtained in the same deafferented patient when she moved an object in a 'passing task' toward the other grasping hand (Simoneau *et al.* 1999);

the hand opened proactively and performed an appropriate grasp without need of proprioception from the moving arm.

Cohen (1971) analyzed rhythmic mirror versus parallel bimanual movements and interpreted the higher variability in the latter mode to be caused by the asymmetric proprioceptive feedback from each moving arm. Asymmetric feedback would interfere with the other hand [termed 'cross-talk' by Marteniuk *et al.* (1984)] and therefore would increase interlimb variability by disturbing the central command. If this assumption holds, one would expect a reduced variability in a bimanual rhythmic task performed by a deafferented patient. This was investigated by Teasdale *et al.* (1994) in the same chronically deafferented patient. However, the results did not match Cohn's interpretation since the deafferent patient had an increased bimanual cross-talk compared with the control subjects. This was taken to indicate a positive regulatory smoothing function of sensory feedback on the bimanual cross-talk. This suggests that the role of proprioceptive feedback in bimanual coordination is task dependent.

The role of vision

To what extent is vision necessary for bimanual coordination in healthy human subjects? In a recent provocative study on interlimb rhythmic in-phase/anti-phase paradigms, Mechsner *et al.* (2001) argued that ' . . . coordination phenomena of this kind are purely perceptual in nature'. Furthermore, ' . . . that even highly complex . . . movements can easily be performed with only simple visual feedback', and that ' . . . a "motoric" representation of the performed perceptual oscillation patterns is not necessary'. Finally, the authors argue that there is no need for an internal feed-forward model as suggested by Wolpert and others (e.g. Wolpert and Ghahramani 2000). Note that updating by sensory feedback is a crucial attribute of the internal model theory. There is no doubt that vision is necessary for many actions (e.g. for catching a moving ball). Thus vision is one of a number of environmental constraints determining coordination. Recently, there have been a number of studies about the role of visual constraints in bimanual tasks (e.g. Bogaerts *et al.* 2003; Drewing and Aschersleben 2003). Coordinating rules depend, to a large extent, on environmental constraints and 'anchoring points' coded in sensory signals (Carson *et al.* 1994).

Different brain areas for visually guided versus internally generated bimanual rhythms

Bimanual coordination of cyclical hand movements was investigated with the aim of finding out whether an internally generated task engages different or the same brain structures when the same movements were performed under visual guidance. The task consisted of flexion–extension of the wrists at a phase offset of 90° (one limb leads the other by a quarter-cycle). This difficult task required extensive learning (Wenderoth and Bock 2001; Wenderoth *et al.* 2002). After stabilization of performance, subjects underwent fMRI investigations (Debaere *et al.* 2003). Comparison of the two tasks, one relying only on cognitive constraints and the other on vision as well, revealed different distributions of activated brain representations. The inferior temporal gyrus, the superior parietal cortex, the premotor cortex, the thalamus, and cerebellar lobule VI all had higher activation levels with visual feedback. On the other hand, the basal ganglia, SMA, cingulate motor cortex, inferior parietal cortex, frontal operculum, and cerebellar lobule IV–V/dentate nucleus had higher activation with internally guided movements (i.e. without visual feedback).

Goal-directed 'natural' bimanual synergies

As alluded to earlier, hands are most often used cooperatively and asymmetrically for skilful goal-oriented actions (Fagot and Vauclaire 1988). MacNeilage (1987) pointed to the typical ' . . . division between a holding hand and an operating hand'. This means that the left hand provides an egocentric spatial reference and stabilization ('frame'), whereas the right hand is used for skilful manipulations and acquiring knowledge of the object ('content element'). From the above frame-content model, it is possible to develop goal-directed 'routinized sequences of actions'. The concept of MacNeilage inspired us to develop the bimanual synergetic sequence that is near to goal-driven motor behavior with ecological significance. Jeannerod (1984) described an early attempt to quantify bimanual coordination in a natural sequence: grasping a small bottle with the left hand and removing the plug with the other hand. In this task, the velocity profiles of the two hands were almost superimposed.

As discussed above, it is difficult to draw straight lines with the left hand and circles with the right hand in continuous rhythmic movements. In contrast, in many goal-directed tasks, the two hands move independently without difficulty, i.e. in non-symmetrical trajectories and velocities. Therefore it appears that movement specifications are subordinate to goal coding (see also Weiss and Jeannerod 1998; Diedrichsen *et al.* 2001). Interlimb coupling is, of course, also task dependent. For example, when each hand attempted to reach and grasp an object simultaneously, coupling coefficients between reaching were higher than those between grasping (Dohle *et al.* 2000). During bimanual typing, wrist and finger movements occur with low correlation coefficients, i.e. largely independently (Flanders and Soechting 1992).

A drawer manipulandum for assessing goal-directed and 'natural' bimanual actions

The drawer task was first used in monkey experiments with the objective of testing the role of the SMA in bimanual synergy (Kazennikov *et al.* 1994). The animals quickly learned the task that was similar to the normal bimanual grasping behavior of monkeys. Most animals spontaneously used the left hand to pull the drawer while the right hand reached to the opening drawer to grasp a small food morsel from the completely open drawer (Fig. 11.8, bottom). Such sequences were repeated up to about 100 times per session and became 'routinized' (as are most of our daily actions). Series of about 20–30 trials were used to investigate different task conditions, such as vision–no vision, loading–no loading of drawer. The time structure was evaluated by means of discrete event markers and with occasional recordings of trajectories and time derivatives. In this way we could measure initiation of movements at the start positions, and the durations of the reach-and-pull phase and the reach–pick phase. Synchronization at onset and goal, as well as correlation of the movement phases, was computed from these data (Fig. 11.8). The goal was defined by the events 'drawer fully opened' (left-hand pinch) and 'pick-in' (reaching into the open drawer for the food morsel with the right precision grip). The left hand (performing a push–pull movement) led, while the right hand started later, moving at an appropriate speed in order to be in near-synchrony at the goal. Since the drawer was spring-loaded, the left hand had to maintain the pinch at the drawer handle as long as the right hand was picking up the food. The whole cycle was brief, usually less than 2 s. The major outcome was that, despite the asymmetric actions and the rather large variance of the individual limbs, goal synchronization was much less variable, with the mean centered a few milliseconds from zero (ideal synchronization). In addition, the two limb movements were highly correlated in time (histograms and regression plots in Fig. 11.8). Remarkably, this result was also present when the performance was in complete darkness, indicating an essentially feedforward performance, possibly aided by proprioceptive feedback. This paradigm was used successfully for investigating the role of the SMA in bimanual coordination, as briefly summarized in the section on bimanually tuned neurons. Although the drawer task appears to be rather complex, it has two major advantages: (i) it is an ecologically relevant task, which animals learn quickly, and (ii) it allows quantification of goal achievement.

Significance of the drawer task for goal coding and motor equivalence

The term 'motor equivalence', introduced by Lashley (1933), means 'variable means to invariant ends' (Abbs and Cole 1987). The principle provides ample flexibility in how to move individual components ('the means') while still preserving the goal (invariant means). Assessing goal achievement is the key for testing performance efficacy. Flexibility of the component movements comes in as an adaptive process, depending strongly on the actual external constraints. Furthermore, and of practical interest, motor equivalence also comes into play as an adaptive mechanism in pathological movement disorders, as will be shown later in this chapter.

The bimanual drawer task had to be introduced and evaluated in healthy human subjects (Perrig *et al.* 1999). The paradigm was similar to the above task in monkeys, but needed appropriate geometrical adjustments of the set-up. Subjects were instructed to reach for the flat drawer handle, pull it open to its mechanical stop, pick up a small

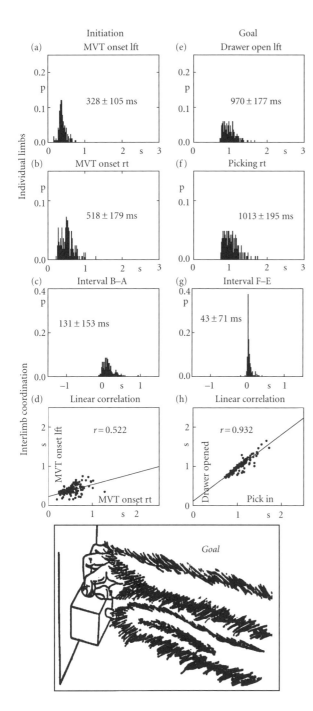

Fig. 11.8 Bimanual drawer task in *Macaca fascicularis*. Time markers are used to assess events at movement (MVT) initiation (left) and at goal reaching (right). Combined synchronization and regression at task onset (left) and goal (right) are plotted, together with means, standard deviations, and correlation coefficients. Reproduced from Kazennikov *et al.* (1994). Reprinted with permission from Blackwell Publisher.

peg inserted in the drawer recess, and reinsert it. Again, event markers provided the timing at onset of movement and at goal reaching, from which the synchronization and regression plots were calculated. Although the behavior seemed less automatized than in the monkeys and the data were more variable with a systematically longer synchronization interval at the goal of about 100 ms, a similar goal 'invariance' was obtained. Subjects were allowed to only a few preliminary trials to familiarize themselves with the procedure. All subjects performed in series with a full view on the

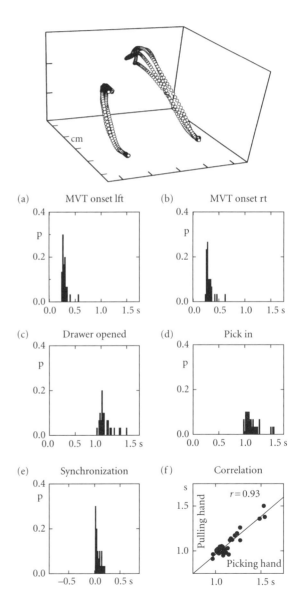

Fig. 11.9 Top: bimanual 3D trajectories of human subject performing drawer task. Below: time histograms of event markers. Bimanual coordination was expressed by goal synchronization intervals and the left–right correlation coefficients. Reproduced from Perrig *et al.* (1999). *Behav Brain Res*, **103**, 95–104. Reprinted with permission from Elsevier Publisher.

workspace and in other series without vision. The outcome with synchronization at the goal and high covariation of the two limb movements was similar to the more automated bimanual behavior in monkeys reported above (Kazennikov *et al.* 2002). Figure 11.9 shows that the trajectories of the pick-hand (top of figure) in the bimanual condition were more curved than the same limb movements in a unimanual control condition. It was suggested that a prolonged pathway serves as a time buffer to adjust timing of the more complex reach-and-pull movement of the leading limb. The kinematic analysis of the task furthermore suggested indirectly that discrete events in the leading hand ('anchor points') generated sensory signals for the companion limb to adjust its timing at the goal. Recently, this conclusion was reinforced by using interfering vibration, known to disturb sensory feedback. The result was a significant decay in goal synchronization, indicating that the vibration applied to the leading hand in motion perturbed the physiological–proprioceptive signaling to the non-leading hand (Kazennikov and Wiesendanger, unpublished data).

Breakdown of bimanual coordination in neurological patients

Lesions in the mesial frontal cortex, including the SMA (mesial area 6) and anterior cingulum

Since the earliest reports by Foerster (1936) and Penfield and Welch (1951), it was thought that the SMA (equivalent to Vogt's area 6ab on the mesial surface) is a bilaterally organized system. Essentially, this was based on stimulation effects from that area (also including the dorsal part on the lateral surface) consisting of 'contraversive' tonic head, trunk, and whole-arm contractions. Epileptic seizures with their origin in the SMA also suggested bilateral representations. This contrasted with the somatotopic organization in the precentral cortex. Later, neurosurgeons reported that the outcome following resections in the mesial frontal cortex in tumor and seizure cases was relatively benign, except for a short period of days or weeks when patients may have a poverty of talking and moving (Zentner *et al.* 1996). Laplane *et al.* (1977) observed that, as a remaining deficit, patients had some bimanual dyscoordination when asked to clench one hand and open the other simultaneously. However, these qualitative descriptions are of limited value. A deficit in bimanually coordinated complex movements was observed in a patient with a large mesial frontal lesion (Dick *et al.* 1986). Viallet *et al.* (1992) found that anticipatory postural reactions in the bimanual unloading task were abnormal in patients with mesial frontal lesions, including the SMA. Viallet *et al.* (1995), from the same laboratory, investigated the effect of unilateral SMA lesions of various causes, including cerebrovascular accidents within the territory of the anterior cerebral artery. Some of these lesions extended far beyond the SMA. Compared with the age-matched control subjects, the patient group had a significant increase in reaction time that was present with either right or left movements, but with a larger contralateral delay. However, reaction times in a group of patients who had undergone neurosurgical resection of the SMA did not differ from those in a control group (Bell and Traylor 1994).

One interesting patient was examined who had a lesion in the central part of the cingulate gyrus of the right hemisphere, just above and extending along the middle third of the corpus callosum, sparing the overlying SMA (Stephan *et al.* 1999a). Her complaint consisted of ' . . . a specific disturbance of everyday bimanual motor acts'. Neurologically, she also showed mild unimanual disturbances on the left side (dysdiadochokinesis, intermittent dystonia of the left hand and foot, and slightly impaired fractionated finger movements). However, the most subjective and objective impairments were bimanual actions, including bibrachial or bimanual rotations. Lacing shoes and buttoning were found to be much impaired. Formal testing of rhythmic index–thumb opposition movements revealed severe deficits, especially in the bimanual antiphase situation. A second patient with a tumor occupying anterior cingulate cortex, but with additional damage of the adjacent corpus callosum and SMA, also developed disturbances in bimanual coordination, as tested with the bimanual rhythmic paradigms. However, in contrast with the former case, this patient was not impaired in everyday bimanual tasks. Such cases might provide a more detailed functional 'specialization' in the vast domain of interlimb coordination. The interesting question raised by these two cases with similar but not identical lesions is: Why does the first patient have severe problems with over-learned familiar tasks of everyday life, and the other does not?

Dramatic interlimb disturbances were seen mainly in patients with mostly large cerebrovascular accidents in the territory of the anterior cerebral artery: neglect (Meador *et al.* 1986; Nakagawa *et al.* 1998), apraxia (Watson *et al.* 1986), inability to perform bimanual asymmetric movements (Schell *et al.* 1986), disturbance in producing non-mirror movements (Chan and Ross 1988), intermanual conflict (Graff-Radford *et al.* 1986; McNabb *et al.* 1988; Jason and Pajurkova 1992), and alien hand syndrome (Goldberg *et al.* 1981; McNabb *et al.* 1988; Goldberg and Bloom 1990; Leiguarda *et al.* 1994; Geschwind *et al.* 1995; Ventura *et al.* 1995; Baynes *et al.* 1997). The latter syndrome was first attributed to callosal damage alone (Brion and Jedynak 1972), but since, in most cases, cortical damage was large and not limited to the SMA, it sometimes also involved the corpus callosum or other structures supplied by the anterior cerebral artery. It can be concluded that lesions within the mesial frontal cortex and the anterior half of the corpus callosum can lead to bizarre interlimb dyscoordination (reviewed by Goldberg 1985; Wiesendanger 1993; Wiesendanger *et al.* 1994).

The newly available method of repetitive transcranial magnetic stimulation (rTMS) was found to produce transient dysfunctions in limited zones of the cerebral cortex. The technique was used to explore further the hypothesis about the role of the mesial frontal cortex in EEG coherence between the primary motor cortex of both hemispheres, as a marker for dynamic 'binding' of both motor-cortical areas

(Serrien *et al.* 2002c). rTMS of the mesial frontal cortex indeed resulted in a deterioration of bimanual coordination, and this was accompanied by a decrease in the functional coupling between left and right motor cortices (Serrien *et al.* 2002c). Therefore it is suggested that the mesial frontal cortex, including the SMA, contributes and modulates the coordination of the two limbs (Meyer-Lindenberg *et al.* 2002; Obhi *et al.* 2002; Steyvers *et al.* 2003).

In conclusion, the clinical descriptions of the above lesion effects are difficult to relate precisely to one 'responsible' structure, mainly because of the size differences and the exact topology of the damaged tissue. One could imagine that the most straightforward answers would come from the controlled neurosurgical excisions of the SMA in patients. However, interpretation on the basis of lost function(s) is particularly hampered in these cases since the pre-existing cortical tissue was already chronically abnormal (mostly due to epilepsy), probably also implying adaptive reorganizations. The initial post-surgery deficits included lack of spontaneous movements, poverty of speech, and a hemisyndrome, but these deficits usually disappeared within days or weeks and permanent symptoms were rare.

Lesions produced by ischemia or hemorrhage in the territory of the anterior cerebral artery are important because they demonstrate bizarre higher-order disorders of the normally skilful cooperation of the two hands. What seems clear, however, is that several cortical areas of the mesial frontal cortex, sometimes also including the corpus callosum, are involved in producing the behavioral deficits discussed above. Finally, one should also take into account the fact that, in addition to bimanual coordination, a number of other functions have been attributed to the SMA, including self-initiation of motor behavior, sequencing of movements, timing, and planning of movements, as reviewed elsewhere (Wiesendanger 1993). It is hoped that further case reports on lesions of the cingulate cortex may provide more indications about its special role in performing well-trained familiar bimanual actions, as recently reported for a patient within the cingulate gyrus (Stephan *et al.* 1999a).

Lesions in the lateral premotor cortex (lateral area 6)

Foerster (1936) described neurological deficits in 40 patients with lesions in area 6ab (i.e. the anterior part of area 6, probably also involving some mesial part of 6ab). No mention is made of bimanual disturbances, but the rather discrete symptoms concerned temporal uncoupling of movement elements, with loss of the fluency of the 'melody'. Freund and Hummelsheim (1985) carefully investigated the premotor deficit. In line with Foerster, the patients exhibited a lack of fluency and dyscoordination in bilateral forelimb movements, such as cyclic whole-arm movements. The most difficult exercise was the proper performance of windmill movements, forward and backward, with both arms moving in an anti-phase mode. The synergy was said to degrade and decompose from the beginning. Further support for the bimanual hypothesis of premotor cortex and SMA was provided by Halsband *et al.* (1993).

Effect of corpus callosum lesion on bimanual coordination

The corpus callosum is the largest interhemispheric commissure, which might suggest that its role in bimanual coordination is mandatory. The outcome in split-brain patients appears to speak against this. Apart from discrete, but clear-cut, signs in the immediate postoperative period (a few days or weeks postoperatively), patients can usually perform most of their familiar daily tasks requiring both hands (Sperry 1966). As mentioned before, recent studies in EEG coherence suggest that the corpus callosum is implicated in learning new and difficult bimanual finger movements, rather than in the execution of already learned bimanual habits (Andres *et al.* 1999; Serrien and Brown 2003). Franz *et al.* (2000) found that spatial planning and perceptual-motor learning indeed required an intact corpus callosum. Preilowski (1975, 1977, 1990) nicely demonstrated the immense difficulty that 'split-brain' patients encountered in using their hands in an unfamiliar and asymmetric cranking task when patients had to control the *x*-direction with one hand and the *y*-direction with the other in tracking either a straight oblique line or more complex trajectories. This was a persistent difficulty for split-brain patients, some of whom were repeatedly tested at intervals of years. As shown in Fig. 11.10, split-brain patients, even in the chronic stage, have greatest difficulties in coordinating their hands for copying a simple line drawing.

The concept of a 'disconnection syndrome', caused by callosal lesions, concerns mainly difficulties in 'sensory and high-level cognitive integration' (Seymour *et al.* 1994; Marangolo *et al.* 1998). On the motor side, the two hands become more independent than in normal subjects, such that split-brain patients are able to perform asymmetric spatial tasks without interactions (this begs the question of whether musicians who had a split-brain operation might improve their asymmetric fingering in piano playing!).

Kennerley *et al.* (2002) recently reported that callosotomy patients ' . . . exhibited a striking lack of temporal coupling during continuous movements, with the two hands oscillating at non-identical frequencies'. The task producing this effect was bimanual circling at different speeds and in symmetric versus asymmetric patterns. However, in a second paradigm, timing was not affected in those patients when index movements had discrete landmarks such as taps with contact. Therefore Kennerley and coworkers proposed that the deficit in split-brain patients is observed with the phasing in the continuous circling task, but not in tap-like movements without actual contact with the surface. The lack of a deficit in the tapping task was ascribed to movements that include discrete events. The temporal control would then come from another, possibly subcortical, source (see also Franz *et al.* 1996a; Ivry and Hazeltine 1999; Robertson *et al.* 1999). In split-brain patients performing with visual guidance, the task of bimanual and simultaneous button presses was only possible if the posterior callosal fibers had been spared (Eliassen *et al.* 2000). In a subject tested before and after an anterior callosal transection, the self-initiated movements of both hands were delayed

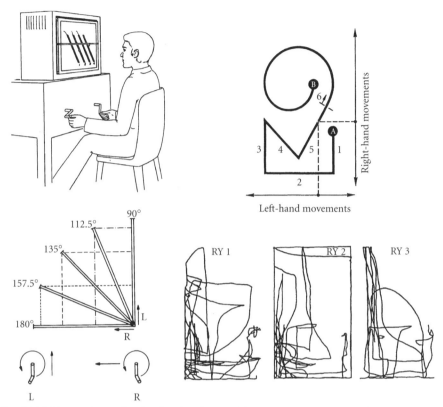

Fig. 11.10 Bimanual coordination for drawing straight trajectories or abstract figures, as used with chronic split-brain patients. Reproduced from Preilowski (1977). *J Mov Stud*, **3**, 169–81. Reprinted with permission from Author and Lippincott Williams and Wilkins.

postoperatively. Therefore it was concluded that the corpus callosum plays a role in bimanual synchronization at movement initiation.

We have compared two types of bimanual tasks, the drawer task and continuous rhythmic circle drawing, with the aim of assessing temporal coupling in three patients with callosal agenesis and three patients with acquired callosal lesions (Serrien *et al.* 2002b). The bimanual goal-directed drawer task, familiar from everyday life, was mastered by both healthy control subjects and congenital acallosal subjects. In subjects with chronic acquired callosal damage, synchronization at task initiation was increased in the no-vision condition or the task was performed sequentially: first pulling with one hand, and then grasping the object from the fully opened drawer. The results for the rhythmic task are shown in Fig. 11.11. Patients with an acquired lesion of the corpus callosum showed clear desynchronization at the peak positions of the displacement traces, whereas the congenital patients had almost normal timing, with the exception of one subject. It is likely that the congenital defect was accompanied by considerable

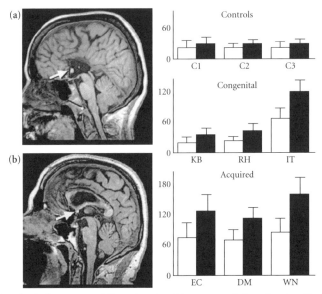

Fig. 11.11 MRI sagittal slices near midline showing (a) a congenital acallosal patient A and (b) a patient with acquired callosal pathology. Bar graphs (mean, standard deviation) of bimanual synchronization (ms) during cyclic in-phase (white) and anti-phase (black) vertical movements with the loaded objects (recorded with an optoelectrical system). Significant desynchronization occurs mainly in patients with acquired callosal lesions. The arrow in (A) points to the unusually large anterior commissure in the acallosal patient. Reproduced from **Serrien *et al.* (2002c)**. Reprinted with permission from Blackwell.

anatomical and functional adaptations (Jäncke *et al.* 1997). In MRI scans, a remarkable increase in the anterior commissure was noted in all our congenital acallosal subjects, as illustrated for one subject at the top of Fig. 11.11. This raises the question of whether the anterior commissure takes over some of the callosal function in the acallosal patients.

Involvement of the posterior parietal cortex in bimanual coordination

In an early report (Wyke 1971) on brain lesion effects from the frontal, temporal, and parietal lobes, it was found that all three sites could lead to deficits in bimanual coordination. The apparatus for testing was rather sophisticated and similar to the one used by Preilowski (see Fig. 11.10). Both hands controlled asymmetrically, via two handles, the trajectory of a pen for tracking a star figure. The task was also difficult for control subjects. Therefore both the learning phase and the end result were evaluated. The score consisted of the number of excursions outside the narrow path and of the required time to finish the task. The highest proportion of abnormal scores was in the left parietal lobe (nine out of 15 patients). The author concluded that ' . . . left-sided lesions show significant impairment of the ability to learn, as well as of the ultimate proficiency obtained in a bimanual coordination task'. Bilateral disturbances are typical for ideational and 'ideomotor' apraxia. A familiar test used to detect ideomotor apraxia is to pour water from a hand-held jug into a glass held by the other hand (Hécaen 1978), a typical asymmetric and goal-directed bimanual action. New advances in understanding the various motor-behavioral functions in apraxia, including manipulatory behavior, have been reported recently (Weiss *et al.* 2001) and will be treated elsewhere in this volume (Chapter 17). It has already been mentioned that evidence from functional imaging also points to a role of the posterior parietal cortex in bimanual actions (Fink *et al.* 1999). As pointed out later by Fink (2001), such goal-directed actions necessitate mechanisms that monitor sensory inputs to ensure that motor outputs are congruent with current intentions.

We have tested the capacity of three patients with lesions in the posterior parietal cortex of the dominant hemisphere, all confirmed with structural and functional MRI (Fig. 11.12, upper panel), to trace circles in the mirror or parallel mode simultaneously with the index fingers (**Serrien *et al.* 2001c**). A significant desynchronization was found for the patient group, mostly expressed in the parallel mode (Fig. 11.12).

Bimanual coordination in Parkinson's disease

One of the first quantitative reports about defective bimanual coordination in parkinsonian patients concerned the anticipatory postural adjustment produced by an active unloading of the upper limb, as described above. Normally, with self-unloading, the force and the underlying electromyogram augment in synchrony with the decay of these parameters in the unloaded limb. This anticipatory (not reactive) adjustment serves to stabilize the arm position (the 'waiter's test') and is likely to depend on an efference copy of the command signal (Diedrichsen *et al.* 2003). However, when unloading occurs passively (by another person), the load-bearing arm of the subject is not stabilized and moves upwards. This reactive response to an external load perturbation corresponds to the unloading reflex, which occurs at a latency of about 50 ms (Hugon *et al.* 1982; Kaluzny and Wiesendanger 1992). When parkinsonian patients were themselves unloading the other arm, no anticipatory postural mechanism was seen, but rather a slow decay of electromyographic activity and a prolonged upward move of the load-bearing arm. Viallet *et al.* (1992) found a similar disturbance in patients with lesions in the mesial frontal cortex, including the SMA.

Several reports have found that defective bimanual coordination was not due to a disorder of time sharing between the two limbs (Castiello and Bennett 1997), but to spatial incoordination (Caligiuri *et al.* 1992; Alberts *et al.* 1998; Jackson *et al.* 2000a) or decreased ability to shift attentional level (Horstink *et al.* 1990). In another study (Fattapposta *et al.* 2000), patients had to initiate the task with a left button press, followed by a second press on a right-hand button in a very rapid succession. The first press started an oscilloscope beam and the second press had to stop the beam

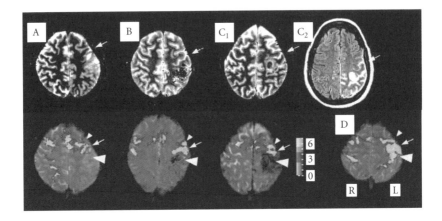

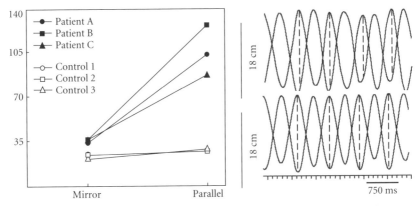

Fig. 11.12 (A), (B), (C₁), (C₂) MRI slices show posterior parietal lesions in three patients (upper row) and fMRI activation patterns of the same patients, demonstrating that the lesioned area was not functional. (D) normal activation pattern with the same task. Patients and control subjects performed in-phase and anti-phase circling movements (below right); on the left are the mean values of timing errors showing desynchronization in the three patients. Reproduced from Serrien *et al.* (2001c). Reprinted with permission from Lippincott Williams and Watkins.

within 20 ms in the middle of the screen. Since subjects were trained until they had a stable performance and since the target response time was set to an extremely short interval, the two-press sequence was considered to be preprogrammed. The outcome was twofold: (i) the patients' timing accuracy was lower than in controls; (ii) the patients did not improve the timing by learning, while controls did. This deficit cannot be interpreted as a deficit in bimanual coordination, but rather as a problem linked to self-initiation or, possibly, due to perception–action coupling. Similar conclusions were drawn by Stelmach and Worringham (1988).

Johnson *et al.* (1998) used Luria's classical in-phase–anti-phase paradigm in parkinsonian patients. However, rather than testing simple hand or finger tapping, the rhythmic metronome-paced movements were executed by right- or left-hand turns of manual cranks (two wheels in the vertical position) and the resulting circular trajectories were analyzed in terms of phase relations. With respect to bimanual criteria, the deficit was restricted to poor maintenance of an anti-phase rhythm. Because of the relative complexity of the rotating hand movements, it is possible that the deficit in the anti-phase mode was due to a higher attentional demand, especially because the patients improved their score with visual cues. Serrien *et al.* (2000) obtained concordant results with a coordination deficit in the anti-phase mode.

Bimanual coordination in Huntington's disease

Huntington's disease (HD) is a hereditary movement disorder, characterized by a progressive loss of neurons in the basal ganglia. Clinically, patients exhibit involuntary movements (chorea) and also show difficulties in the execution of complex movements. By means of a bimanual cranking task, as used before in parkinsonian patients, Johnson *et al.* (2000) investigated in-phase and anti-phase movements in HD patients. The results were similar to those obtained for parkinsonian patients, except that pacing with the metronome did not improve the performance. A comparative study in Parkinson's disease, HD, and cerebellar disease (Brown *et al.* 1993) showed that bimanual asymmetric tasks were particularly affected in all three diseases, including HD. Verbessem *et al.* (2002) confirmed that HD affects the quality of bimanual coordination negatively. In our own investigations of HD patients, we observed abnormalities in the appropriate regulation between grip force and load force when weighted objects were moved rhythmically (Serrien *et al.* 2001a). On the basis of these results, we made another study with specific attention to the force constraints in a bimanual task (Serrien *et al.* 2002a). This was explored in the rhythmic in-phase–anti-phase paradigm that also included the bimanual gripper task described and illustrated earlier in this chapter. In healthy subjects, it was shown that the amplitude of the grip–load force ratio oscillated in size with rhythmic up-and-down movements. In HD patients, the following abnormalities were observed: (i) significant increases of the force ratio compared with control subjects, by progressive amounts from unimanual to bimanual in-phase and bimanual anti-phase conditions; (ii) a temporal dissociation between grip and load force peaks, which resulted in pronounced irregularities of ratio profiles. Thus a disturbance of the grasp function was amplified in bimanual actions, whereby the grip–load force coupling deteriorated as a function of coordination complexity.

The role of the cerebellum in bimanual coordination

Holmes was probably first to comment on bimanual coordination in cerebellar patients [papers first published after the First World War and then reprinted as the Croonian Lectures in *Selected Papers of Sir Gordon Holmes* (Holmes 1956)]. He was an expert in cerebellar neurology and a pioneer in recording abnormal movements

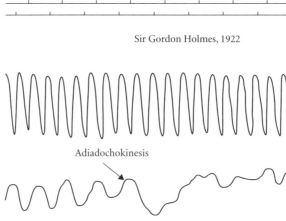

Sir Gordon Holmes, 1922

Adiadochokinesis

Fig. 11.13 Holmes' original tracing of rhythmic pronation-supination arm movements (diadochokinesis) in a patient with ipsilateral cerebellar lesion. Lower trace: highly abnormal trajectory, typical for adiadochkinesia; upper trace: arm contralateral to the lesion with regular sinusoidal movements. Time markers in seconds. Reproduced from Holmes (1956) *Selected Papers of Sir Gordon Holmes* (ed. FMR Walshe). London: Macmillan, 49–111. Reprinted with permission from Oxford University Press.

by means of a simple mechanical kymograph. In the third Croonian Lecture, Holmes discussed the phenomenon of adiadochokinesis in a patient with a unilateral cerebellar lesion. Figure 11.13 illustrates traces of the two hands moving rhythmically between pronation and supination. The affected arm moved at a distinct slow and irregular frequency, finally almost stopping altogether. Unfortunately, it is likely that the two illustrated traces were not recorded simultaneously (the two time markers in the figure do not coincide). Although we are not sure exactly how the hands interacted in a bimanual context, Holmes comments were that ' . . . the movements of the affected arm are almost invariably more inaccurate and less complete *when the patient attempts to perform them simultaneously with both limbs . . .* '. The reason, he commented, was 'insufficient attention' and 'confusion that naturally arises when, owing to lack of synchronicity, different acts are at the same time attempted by the two limbs'. Thus these comments indicate that the unilateral cerebellar lesion affected not only coordination of the ipsilesional limb, but also bimanual coordination.

Despite this early knowledge, there have been relatively few attempts to investigate the role of the cerebellum in bimanual coordination, even though it was recognized by neurologists that temporal decomposition of complex movement sequences is the hallmark of cerebellar lesions (Dichgans and Diener 1984; Inhoff *et al.* 1989). In contrast with Holmes' description of a bimanual disadvantage, Franz *et al.* (1996b), observed a bimanual advantage compared with unimanual actions in cerebellar patients with unilateral cerebellar lesions ('two hands are better than one . . . ') (Helmuth and Ivry 1996). The dependent variables in the finger-tapping task were the mean and standard deviation of the cycle duration in a trial. The underlying concept was that there are two sources of variability in movement production, one from planning ('central source', 'timekeeper') and the other from execution ('motor implementation process') (see also Wing 1982). It was assumed that lateral lesions (mainly the dentate nucleus, engaged in initiation of actions) would influence the central timer and medial lesions (medial nuclei related to execution) would affect execution. The result was that variability in the ipsilesional affected hand was augmented. However, it was reduced to near normal when the affected hand was used together with the intact hand. This was the case in subjects with lateral lesions, suggesting that central timing was impaired. The fact that variability was improved in the bimanual mode was taken to suggest that the remaining intact timer (on the uninjured side) is capable of achieving bimanual coupling (but note that Holmes' patient also had a unilateral lesion, but the performance deteriorated in the bimanual condition!). In a later study Cui et al. (2001) confirmed, by means of event-related fMRI, that preparation as well as execution of movement sequences is represented in each half of the cerebellum. In an elegant fMRI investigation (Tracy et al. 2001), normal adults executed series of rhythmic supination–pronation hand movements ('diadochokinesis'), either unimanually for each hand or bimanually in the anti-phase mode (parallel supination–pronation of both hands at about 1 Hz). Metabolic responses were observed, notably in the contralateral sensorimotor cortex and ipsilateral cerebellum for unimanual series, and a bilateral combination of these in the bimanual protocol. The special feature of this study was that subtraction of the sum of both unimanual tasks from the activation of the bimanual task revealed a specific BOLD response in the anterior and posterior medial stripes of the cerebellum that has been attributed to the extra load of bimanual coordination.

As mentioned before (Kennerley et al. 2002), the role of the corpus callosum in interlimb coupling was present only in rhythmic continuous movements, and not in event-driven tasks. Ivry et al. (2002) suggested that, in contrast, event-driven timing was likely to be the job of the cerebellum. Recently, a direct comparison in cerebellar patients appears to confirm this notion; the event-driven protocol disrupted the timing, whereas the continuous protocol did not (Spencer et al. 2003).

Goal representation (or goal coding) may be a special case of event-driven interlimb coupling. As mentioned before, in our bimanual drawer task, coordination at the goal was particularly prominent; the GO signal, grasping the drawer handle, the impact at full drawer-opening, onset of movement of the partner hand, and shaping of the grasp for picking up the object are all discrete events that may well contribute to temporal goal coordination (see also Kazennikov et al. 2002).

We assessed bimanual coordination in the drawer task in five cerebellar patients with bilateral lesions (Serrien and Wiesendanger 2000). The performance was grossly abnormal with a massive desynchronization at the start. In controls, the picking hand followed shortly after (~100 ms) initiation of the leading pull hand. In contrast, cerebellar patients were much more desynchronized at task initiation, the delay being

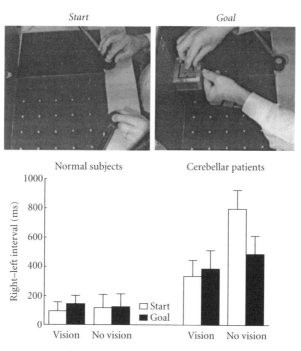

Fig. 11.14 Desynchronization of cerebellar patients in initiation of the bimanual drawer task, compared with control subjects, with and without vision. Patients were highly desynchronized at task initiation; particularly in the no-vision condition, movements were executed more sequentially. Goal synchronization remained the same (with vision) or even improved (no vision) with respect to initial synchronization, suggesting that mechanisms of goal synchronization were unaffected or only minimally affected by cerebellar lesions. Reproduced from Serrien and Wiesendanger (2000b). Reprinted with permission from Elsevier Publisher.

four times longer. It increased even more in the no-vision condition (Fig. 11.14). This means that the normal bimanual quasi-simultaneity at the start changed to an almost sequential strategy: one hand first reaching for pulling and then the other hand reaching for picking. Do cerebellar patients also have a deficit in goal coordination? Without any goal coordination, desynchronization at the start should further increase during reaching, but this was not the case in these patients. In the vision condition, the pronounced desynchronization was about the same at the goal, and in the no-vision condition, the initial desynchronization was reduced by about 40% at the goal. Therefore we concluded that at least some temporal goal coding was still functional. We propose that a higher-order goal-specification is engaging a different mechanism than the mechanism of task initiation, and that goal coordination was at least partly intact in cerebellar patients. The conjecture is that goal coordination is serving as an adaptive feedforward strategy to compensate for any temporal offset between hands at movement initiation (see also Kazennikov *et al.* 2002) . On the other hand, the massive desynchronization at the start of the bimanual synergy is compatible with the hypothesis of cerebellar event-driven timing (Ivry *et al.* 2002).

Final conclusions and outlook

Most studies of bimanual coordination used the rhythmic in-phase–anti-phase paradigm. More recently, movement dynamics has been related to that of neural populations. Theories of dynamics have brought new dimensions into neurosciences, particularly the discovery of coherences between cortical and peripheral oscillators which may improve understanding of coordination. An intensive search for one coordinating 'center' for bimanual coordination has not been successful. The SMA scored highest, but a picture of a number of widely distributed patches of activation in cortical and subcortical structures emerged, which are all likely to contribute to bimanual coordination. The distribution and intensity of participating neural networks also depend on task constraints. The larger region of the mesial frontal cortex, including the SMA, pre-SMA, anterior cingulate, prefrontal cortices, and corpus callosum, are all in the territory of the anterior cerebral artery. Larger lesions due to cerebrovascular accidents or large tumors within the mesial frontal cortex produced dramatic syndromes, such as the alien hand, mirror movements, and intermanual conflict, whereas smaller lesions may lead to discrete bimanual dysfunction, such as the cingulate case described by Stephan *et al.* (1999a). Several reports suggest that the posterior parietal association cortex of the dominant hemisphere plays a role in bimanual motor behavior.

At the spinal level, we are beginning to understand some of the sophisticated circuitry involving pattern generators, interneuronal circuits with their descending and segmental sensory influx, and neural modulators that finally drive motoneurons. Right–left coordination relies on commissural neurons and bilaterally descending neurons from the brainstem. At the cortical level, we are beginning to explore temporal 'binding' in terms of neuronal coherences. However, even in highly complex bimanual coordinated tasks, such as catching a ball, spinal 'binding' mechanisms for coupling more or less symmetrical motoneuron pools are likely to be involved as well. We have also discovered indirectly from lesion studies that the cerebellum is crucial in temporal coordination, including interlimb coordination, as first discussed by Holmes (1956) and Wing (1982).

As foreshadowed early by the eminent physiologist Bethe (1931), the dynamic principles of coordination are not in line with the doctrine of a coordinating center. Rather, his principle of *gleitende Koppelung* (gliding coupling) implied dynamically changing constellations of temporary coupling among effectors that in turn rely on temporary links of distributed neural networks, as we see today in functional imaging and electrophysiological coherence studies. The Russian psychologist Vygotsky (1965; originally published in 1934), viewed coordination 'as differentiated and hierarchically organized dynamic interrelation of separate zones'.

From the clinical point of view, including brain imaging, further studies of 'natural' bimanual tasks would be helpful because they potentially provide relevant information about progress in rehabilitation of everyday tasks and brain plasticity. For goal-oriented manipulations, post-lesion adaptive strategies often come into play, allowing goal achievement with changed component movements, i.e. Lashley's principle of motor equivalence (Lashley 1933; Hebb 1949; Abbs and Cole 1987). Ecologically relevant skills are goal related; most require both hands with different task assignments, the individual limbs being subordinate to goal coordination. In many higher skills, such as playing a musical instrument, hand movements often need to be uncoupled and steered individually. Therefore learning complex bimanual actions means allowing for separate non-simultaneous and/or non-symmetrical movements. It has been confirmed quantitatively that the two hands of an expert typist move independently (Flanders and Soechting 1992). The potential for independent actions of the two hands, required for music playing, emerges as a high-level perceptive goal. The hyper-complex skill of playing a musical instrument is based on years of practice and learning. Imagine the formidable complexity and speed in fingering of the left hand, up and down the fingerboard of the violin, the asymmetric right-hand bowing, with strokes and tilts for string changes. Exploration of the performance of complex 'natural' manipulations and artistic bimanual skills is quite an ambitious undertaking. However, more than 70 years ago Bernstein and Popowa (1929) published a remarkable and richly illustrated study of the dynamics and kinematics of keystrokes in professional concert pianists, using technical support far less sophisticated than that available today, although rather ingenious for the time.

References

Abbs JH, Cole KJ (1987). Neural mechanisms of motor equivalence and goal achievement. In Wise SP, ed. *Higher Brain Functions*. New York: Wiley, 15–43.

Alberts JL, Tresilian JR, Stelmach GE (1998). The co-ordination and phasing of a bilateral prehension task—the influence of Parkinson's disease. *Brain*, **121**, 725–42.

Andres FG, Mima T, Schulman AE, Dichgans J, Hallett M, Gerloff C (1999). Functional coupling of human cortical sensorimotor areas during bimanual skill acquisition. *Brain*, **122**, 855–70.

Baynes K, Tramo MJ, Reeves AG, Gazzaniga MS (1997). Isolation of a right hemisphere cognitive system in a patient with anarchic (alien) hand sign. *Neuropsychologia*, **35**, 1159–73.

Bell KR, Traylor GH, Anderson ME, Berger MS, Ojemann GA (1994). Features of targeted arm movement after unilateral excisions that included the supplementary motor area in humans. *Brain Res*, **655**, 202–12.

Bernstein N, Popowa T (1929). Untersuchung über die Biodynamik des Klavieranschlags. *Arbeitsphysiologie*, **1**, 396–432.

Bethe A (1931). Plastizität und Zentrenlehre. In A Bethe, G von Bergmann, (ed.) *Handbuch der Normalen und Pathologischen Physiologie. Arbeitsphysiologie II: Orientierung, Plastizität, Stimme und Sprach*, pp. 1175–221. Berlin: Springer.

Bogaerts H, Buekers MJ, Zaal FT, Swinnen SP (2003). When visuo-motor incongruence aids motor performance: the effect of perceiving motion structures during transformed visual feedback on bimanual coordination. *Behav Brain Res*, **138**, 45–57.

Bressler SL, Kelso JAS (2001). Cortical coordination dynamics and cognition. *Trends Cogn Sci*, **5**, 26–36.

Brinkman J, Kuypers HGJM (1973). Cerebral control of contralateral and ipsilateral arm, hand and finger movements in the split-brain rhesus monkey. *Brain*, **96**, 653–74.

Brinkman C, Porter R (1979). Supplementary motor area in the monkey: activity of neurons during performance of a learned motor task. *J Neurophysiol*, **42**, 681–709.

Brion S, Jedynak CP (1972). Troubles du transfert interhémisphérique (callosal disconnection) à propos de 3 observations de tumeurs du corps calleux. Le signe de la main étrangère. *Rev Neurol (Paris)*, **126**, 257–66.

Brown RG, Jahanshahi M, Marsden CD (1993). The execution of bimanual movements in patients with Parkinson's, Huntington's and cerebellar disease. *J Neurol Neurosurg Psychiatry*, **56**, 295–97.

Butt SJ, Kiehn O (2003). Functional identification of interneurons responsible for left-right coordination of hindlimbs in mammals. *Neuron*, **38**, 953–63.

Caligiuri MP, Heindel WC, Lohr JB (1992). Sensorimotor disinhibition in Parkinson's disease: effects of levadopa. *Ann Neurol*, **31**, 53–58.

Cardoso de Oliveira S, Gribova A, Donchin O, Bergman H, Vaadia E (2002). Neural interactions between motor cortical hemispheres during bimanual and unimanual arm movements. *Eur J Neurosci*, **14**, 1881–96.

Carson RG, Byblow WD, Goodman D (1994). The dynamical substructure of bimanual coordination. In S Swinnen, H Heuer, J Massion, *et al.*, (ed.) *Interlimb Coordination: Neural, Dynamical, and Cognitive Constraints*, pp. 319–37. San Diego, CA: Academic Press.

Castiello U, Bennett KMB (1997). The bilateral reach-to-grasp movement of Parkinson's disease subjects. *Brain*, **120**, 593–604.

Chan JL, Ross ED (1988). Left-handed mirror writing following right anterior cerebral artery infarction : evidence for nonmirror transformation of motor programs by supplementary motor area. *Neurology*, **38**, 59–63.

Cisek P, Crammond DJ, Kalaska JF (2003). Neural activity in primary motor and dorsal premotor cortex in reaching tasks with the contralateral versus ipsilateral arm. *J Neurophysiol*, **89**, 922.

Cohen L (1971). Synchronous bimanual movements performed by homologous and non-homologous muscles. *Percept Mot Skills*, **32**, 639–44.

Cole J (1995). *Pride and a Daily Marathon*. Cambridge, MA: MIT Press.

Cole JD, Sedgwick EM (1992). The perceptions of force and of movements in a man without large myelinated sensory afferents below the neck. *J Physiol*, **449**, 503–15.

Cowley KC, Schmidt BJ (1995). Effects of inhibitory amino acid antagonists on reciprocal inhibitory interactions during rhythmic motor activity in the in vitro neonatal rat spinal cord. *J Neurophysiol*, **74**, 1109–17.

Cui S-Z, Li E-Z, Zang Y-F, Weng X-C, Ivry, Wang J-J (2001). Both sides of human cerebellum involved in preparation and execution of sequential movements. *NeuroReport*, **11**, 3849–53.

De Jong BM, Willemsen AT, Paans AM (1999). Brain activation related to the change between bimanual motor programs. *Neuroimage*, **9**, 290–7.

De Jong BM, Leenders KL, Paans AM (2002). Right parieto-premotor activation related to limb-independent antiphase movement. *Cereb Cortex*, **12**, 1213–17.

Debaere F, Swinnen SP, Beatse E, Sunaert S, Van Hecke P, Duysens J (2001). Brain areas involved in interlimb coordination: a distributed network. *Neuroimage*, **14**, 947–58.

Debaere F, Wenderoth N, Sunaert S, Van Hecke P, Swinnen SP (2003). Internal versus external generation of movements: differential neural pathways involved in bimanual coordination performed in the presence or absence of augmented visual feedback. *Neuroimage*, **19**, 764–76.

Dichgans J, Diener HC (1984). Clinical evidence for functional compartmentalization of the cerebellum. In JR Bloedel, JD Dichgans, (ed.) *Cerebellar Functions*, pp. 126–47. Berlin: Springer.

Dick JPR, Benecke R, Rothwell JC, Day BL, Marsden CD (1986). Simple and complex movements in a patient with infarction of the right supplementary motor area. *Mov Disord*, **1**, 255–66.

Diedrichsen J, Hazeltine E, Kennerley S, Ivry RB (2001). Moving to directly cued locations abolishes spatial interference during bimanual actions. *Psychol Sci*, **12**, 493–8.

Diedrichsen J, Verstynen T, Hon A, Lehman SL, Ivry RB (2003). Anticipatory adjustments in the unloading task: Is an efference copy necessary for learning? *Exp Brain Res*, **148**, 272–6.

Dohle C, Ostermann G, Hefter H, Freund H-J (2000). Different coupling for the reach and grasp components in bimanual prehension movements. *NeuroReport*, **11**, 3787–91.

Donchin O, Gribova A, Steinberg O, Bergman H, Vaadia E (1998). Primary motor cortex is involved in bimanual coordination. *Nature*, **395**, 274–8.

Donchin O, De Oliveira SC, Vaadia E (1999). Who tells one hand what the other is doing: the neurophysiology of bimanual movements. *Neuron*, **23**, 15–18.

Donchin O, Gribova A, Steinberg O, Bergman H, Cardoso dO, Vaadia E (2001). Local field potentials related to bimanual movements in the primary and supplementary motor cortices. *Exp Brain Res*, **140**, 46–55.

Drewing K, Aschersleben G (2003). Reduced timing variability during bimanual coupling: a role for sensory information. *Q J Exp Psychol A*, **56**, 329–50.

Drewing K, Hennings M, Aschersleben G (2002). The contribution of tactile reafference to temporal regularity during bimanual finger tapping. *Psychol Res*, **66**, 60–70.

Ehrsson HH, Naito E, Geyer S, Amunts K, Zilles K, Forssberg H, *et al.* (2000). Simultaneous movements of upper and lower limbs are coordinated by motor representations that are shared by both limbs: a PET study. *Eur J Neurosci*, **12**, 3385–98.

Eliassen JC, Baynes K, Gazzaniga MS (2000). Anterior and posterior callosal contributions to simultaneous bimanual movements of the hands and fingers. *Brain*, **123**, 2501–11.

Engel AK, Fries P, Singer W (2001). Dynamic predictions: oscillations and synchrony in top-down processing. *Nat Rev Neurosci*, **2**, 705–16.

Fagot J, Vauclaire J (1988). Handedness and bimanual coordination in the lowland gorilla. *Brain Behav Evol*, **32**, 89–95.

Fattapposta F, Pierelli F, Traversa G, My F, Mostarda M, D'Alessio C, *et al.* (2000). Preprogramming and control activity of bimanual self-paced motor task in Parkinson's disease. *Clin Neurophysiol*, **111**, 873–83.

Fink GR (2001). What the brain needs for managing both hands at the same time. *NeuroReport*, **12**, A69.

Fink GR, Marshall JC, Halligan PW, Frith CD, Driver J, Frockowiak RS, *et al.* (1999). The neural consequences of conflict between intention and the senses. *Brain*, **122**, 497–512.

Flanagan JR, Wing AM (1995). The stability of precision grip forces during cyclic arm movements with a hand-held load. *Exp Brain Res*, **105**, 455–64.

Flanders M, Soechting JF (1992). Kinematics of typing: parallel control of the two hands. *J Neurophysiol*, **67**, 1264–74.

Foerster O (1936). Motorische Felder und Bahnen. In O Bumke, O Foerster, (ed.) *Handbuch der Neurologie VI*, pp. 1–357. Berlin: Springer.

Forget R, Lamarre Y (1995). Postural adjustments associated with different unloadings of the forearm: Effects of proprioceptive and cutaneous afferent deprivation. *Can J Physiol Pharmacol*, **73**, 285–94.

Franz EA, Zelaznik HN, McCabe G (1991). Spatial topological constraints in a bimanual task. *Acta Psychol*, **77**, 137–51.

Franz EA, Eliassen JC, Ivry RB, Gazzaniga MS (1996a). Dissociation of spatial and temporal coupling in the bimanual movements of callosotomy patients. *Psychol Sci*, **7**, 306–10.

Franz EA, Ivry RB, Helmuth LL (1996b). Reduced timing variability in patients with unilateral cerebellar lesions during bimanual movements. *J Cogn Neurosci*, **8**, 107–18.

Franz EA, Waldie KE, Smith MJ (2000). The effect of callosotomy on novel versus familiar bimanual actions: a neural dissociation between controlled and automatic processes? *Psychol Sci*, **11**, 82–85.

Freund H-J, Hummelsheim H (1985). Lesions of premotor cortex in man. *Brain*, **108**, 697–733.

Fuchs A, Jirsa VK, Kelso JAS (2000). Theory of the relation between human brain activity (MEG) and hand movements (comments and controversies). *Neuroimage*, **11**, 359–69.

Gallese V, Murata A, Kaseda M, Niki N, Sakata H (1994). Deficit of hand preshaping after muscimol injection in monkey parietal cortex. *NeuroReport*, **5**, 1525–9.

Geschwind DH, Iacoboni M, Mega MS, Zaidel DW, Cloughesy T, Zaidel E (1995). Alien hand syndrome: Interhemispheric motor disconnection due to a lesion in the midbody of the corpus callosum. *Neurology*, **45**, 802–8.

Ghez C, Gordon J, Ghilardi MF, Sainburg R (1995). Contributions of vision and proprioception to accuracy in limb movements. In MS Gazzaniga, (ed.) *The Cognitive Neurosciences*, pp. 549–64. Cambridge, MA: MIT Press.

Goerres GW, Samuel M, Jenkins IH, Brooks DJ (1998). Cerebral control of unimanual and bimanual movements: an H2(15)O PET study. *NeuroReport*, **9**, 3631–8.

Goldberg G (1985). Supplementary motor area structure and function: review and hypotheses. *Behav Brain Sci*, **8**, 567–616.

Goldberg G, Bloom KK (1990). The alien hand sign. Localization, lateralization and recovery. *Am J Phys Med Rehab*, **69**, 228–38.

Goldberg G, Mayer NH, Toglia JU (1981). Medial frontal cortex infarction and the alien hand sign. *Arch Neurol*, **38**, 683–6.

Graff-Radford NR, Welsh K, Godersky J (1986). Callosal apraxia and the supplementary motor area. *Neurology*, **36** (Suppl 1), 343–50.

Gross J, Timmermann L, Kujala J, Dirks M, Schmitz F, Salmelin R, *et al.* (2002). The neural basis of intermittent motor control in humans. *Proc Natl Acad Sci USA*, **99**, 2299–302.

Grossberg S, Pribe C, Cohen MA (1997). Neural control of interlimb oscillations.1. Human bimanual coordination. *Biol Cybern*, **77**, 131–40.

Haaland KY, Harrington DL (1994). Limb-sequencing deficits after left but not right hemisphere damage. *Brain Cogn*, **24**, 104–22.

Halsband U, Ito N, Tanji J, Freund H-J (1993). The role of premotor cortex and the supplementary motor area in the temporal control of movement in man. *Brain*, **116**, 243–66.

Hatzitaki V, McKinley P (2001). Effect of single-limb inertial loading on bilateral reaching: interlimb interactions. *Exp Brain Res*, **140**, 34–45.

Hebb DO (1949). *Organization of Behavior*. New York: Wiley, 112.

Hécaen H (1978). Les apraxies idéomotrices, essai de dissociation. In H Hécaen, M Jeannerod, (ed.) *Du contrôle moteur à l'organisation du geste*, pp. 343–58. Paris: Masson.

Helmuth LL, Ivry RB (1996). When two hands are better than one: reduced timing variability during bimanual movements. *J Exp Psychol Hum Percept Perform*, **22**, 278–93.

Holmes G (1956). The Croonian Lectures on the clinical symptoms of cerebellar disease and their interpretation. In FMR Walshe, (ed.)*Selected Papers of Sir Gordon Holmes*, pp. 49–111. London: Macmillan.

Horstink MWIM, Berger HJC, Van Spaendonek KPM, Van den Bercken JHL, Cools AR (1990). Bimanual simultaneous performance and impaired ability to shift attention in Parkinson's disease. *J Neurol Neurosurg Psychiatry*, **53**, 685–90.

Hugon M, Massion J, Wiesendanger M (1982). Anticipatory postural changes induced by active unloading and comparison with passive unloading in man. *Pflugers Archiv*, **392**, 292–6.

Hultborn H (2001). State-dependent modulation of sensory feedback (topical review). *J Physiol*, **533**, 5–13.

Inhoff AW, Diener HC, Rafal RD, Ivry R (1989). The role of cerebellar structures in the execution of serial movements. *Brain*, **112**, 565–81.

Ivry RB, Hazeltine E (1999). Subcortical locus of temporal coupling in the bimanual movements of a callosotomy patient. *Hum Mov Sci*, **18**, 345–75.

Ivry RB, Spencer RM, Zelaznik HN, Diedrichsen J (2002). The cerebellum and event timing. *Ann NY Acad Sci*, **978**, 302–17.

Jackson GM, Jackson SR, Kritikos A (1999). Attention for action: coordinating bimanual reach-to-grasp movements. *Br J Psychol*, **90**, 247–70.

Jackson GM, Jackson SR, Hindle JV (2000a). The control of bimanual reach-to-grasp movements in hemiparkinsonian patients. *Exp Brain Res*, **132**, 390–8.

Jackson GM, Jackson SR, Husain M, Harvey M, Kramer T, Dow L (2000b). The coordination of bimanual prehension movements in a centrally deafferented patient. *Brain*, **123**, 380–93.

Jäncke L, Wunderlich G, Schlaug G, Steinmetz H (1997). A case of callosal agenesis with strong anatomical and functional asymmetries. *Neuropsychologia*, **35**, 1389–94.

Jäncke J, Peters M, Schlaug G, Posse S, Steinmetz H, Müller-Gärtner HW (1998). Differential magnetic resonance signal change in human sensorimotor cortex to finger movements of different rate of the dominant and subdominant hand. *Cogn Brain Res*, **6**, 279–84.

Jäncke L, Peters M, Himmelbach M, Nösselt T, Shah J, Steinmetz H (2000). fMRI study of bimanual coordination. *Neuropsychologia*, **38**, 164–74.

Jason GW, Pajurkova EM (1992). Failure of metacontrol: breakdown in behavioural unity after lesion of the corpus callosum and inferomedial frontal lobes. *Cortex*, **28**, 241–60.

Jeannerod M (1984). The timing of natural prehension movements. *J Mot Behav*, **16**, 235–54.

Jenny AB (1979). Commissural projections of the cortical hand motor area in monkeys. *J Comp Neurol*, **188**, 137–46.

Johansson RS, Westling G (1988). Coordinated isometric muscle commands adequately and erroneously programmed for the weight during lifting task with precision grip. *Exp Brain Res*, **71**, 59–71.

Johnson KA, Cunnington R, Bradshaw JL, Phillips JG, Iansek R, Rogers MA (1998). Bimanual co-ordination in Parkinson's disease. *Brain*, **121**, 743–53.

Johnson KA, Bennett JE, Georgiou N, Bradshaw JL, Chiu E, Cunnington R, *et al.* (2000). Bimanual coordination in Huntington's disease. *Exp Brain Res*, **134**, 483–9.

Kaluzny P, Wiesendanger M (1992). Feedforward postural stabilization in a distal bimanual unloading task. *Exp Brain Res*, **92**, 173–82.

Kazennikov O, Wicki U, Corboz M, Hyland B, Palmeri A, Rouiller EM, *et al.* (1994). Temporal structure of a bimanual goal-directed movement sequence in monkeys. *Eur J Neurosci*, **6**, 203–10.

Kazennikov O, Hyland B, Corboz M, Babalian A, Rouiller EM, Wiesendanger M (1999). Neural activity of supplementary and primary motor areas in monkeys and its relation to bimanual and unimanual movement sequences. *Neuroscience*, **89**, 661–74.

Kazennikov O, Perrig S, Wiesendanger M (2002). Kinematics of a coordinated goal-directed bimanual task. *Behav Brain Res*, **134**, 83–91.

Kelso JAS (1994). Elementary coordination dynamics. In S Swinnen, H Heuer, J Massion, *et al.* (ed.) *Interlimb Coordination: Neural, Dynamical, and Cognitive Constraints*, pp. 301–18. San Diego, CA: Academic Press.

Kelso JAS (1995). *Dynamic Patterns: The Self-Organization of Brain and Behavior*. Cambridge, MA: MIT Press.

Kelso JAS, Southard DL, Goodman D (1979). On the nature of human interlimb coordination. *Science*, **203**, 1029–31.

Kelso JAS, Putnam CA, Goodman D (1983). On the space-time structure of human interlimb co-ordination. *Q J Exp Psychol*, **35A**, 347–75.

Kennerley SW, Diedrichsen J, Hazeltine E, Semjen A, Ivry RB (2002). Callosotomy patients exhibit temporal uncoupling during continuous bimanual movements. *Nat Neurosci*, **5**, 376–81.

Kermadi I, Liu Y, Tempini A, Calciati E, Rouiller EM (1998). Neuronal activity in the primate supplementary motor area and the primary motor cortex in the relation to spatio-temporal bimanual coordination. *Somatosens Mot Res*, **15**, 287–308.

Kermadi I, Liu Y, Rouiller EM (2000). Do bimanual motor actions involve the dorsal premotor (PMd), cingulate (CMA) and posterior parietal (PPC) cortices? Comparison with primary and supplementary motor cortical areas. *Somatosens Mot Res*, **17**, 255–71.

Kugler PN, Kelso JAS, Turvey MT (1980). On the concept of coordinative structures as dissipative structures: I. Theoretical lines of convergence. In GE Stelmach, J Requin, (ed.) *Tutorials in Motor Behavior*, pp. 3–47. Amsterdam: North-Holland.

Kuypers HGJM (1981). Anatomy of descending pathways. In VB Brooks, (ed.) *Handbook of Physiology (The Nervous System)*, Vol 2, Part 1, pp. 597–666. Bethesda, MD: American Physiological Society.

Laplane D, Talairach J, Meininger V, Bancaud J, Orgogozo JM (1977). Clinical consequences of corticectomies involving the supplementary motor area in man. *J Neurol Sci*, **34**, 301–14.

Lashley KS (1933). Integrative functions of the cerebral cortex. *Physiol Rev*, **13**, 1–42.

Leiguarda R, Lees AJ, Merello M, Starkstein S, Marsden CD (1994). The nature of apraxia in corticobasal degeneration. *J Neurol Neurosurg Psychiatry*, **57**, 455–9.

Liu J, Morel A, Wannier T, Rouiller EM (2002). Origins of callosal projections to the supplementary motor area (SMA): a direct comparison between pre-SMA and SMA-proper in macaque monkeys. *J Comp Neurol*, **443**, 71–85.

Luria AR (1969). Frontal lobe syndromes. In PJBGW, Vinken, (ed.) *Handbook of Clinical Neurology*, Vol 2. pp. 725–57, Amsterdam: Elsevier.

McNabb AW, Carroll WM, Mastaglia FL (1988). 'Alien hand' and loss of bimanual coordination after dominant anterior cerebral artery territory infarction. *J Neurol Neurosurg Psychiatry*, **51**, 218–22.

MacNeilage PF (1987). The evolution of hemispheric specialization for manual function and language. In SP Wise, (ed.) *Higher Brain Functions*, pp. 285–309, New York: Wiley.

Marangolo P, De Renzi E, Di Pace E, Castriota-Scanderbeg A (1998). Let not thy left hand know what thy right hand knoweth—the case of a patient with an infarct involving the callosal pathways. *Brain*, **121**, 1459–67.

Marteniuk RG, MacKenzie CL, Baba DM (1984). Bimanual movement control: information processing and interaction effects. *Q J Exp Psychol*, **36A**, 335–65.

Meador KJ, Watson RT, Bowers D, Heilman KM (1986). Hypometria with hemispatial and limb motor neglect. *Brain*, **109**, 293–305.

Mechsner F, Kerzel D, Knoblich G, Prinz W (2001). Perceptual basis of bimanual coordination. *Nature*, **414**, 69–73.

Meyer-Lindenberg A, Ziemann U, Hajak G, Cohen L, Berman KF (2002). Transitions between dynamical states of differing stability in the human brain. *Proc Natl Acad Sci USA*, **99**, 10948–53.

Muller K, Schmitz F, Schnitzler A, Freund HJ, Aschersleben G, Prinz W (2000). Neuromagnetic correlates of sensorimotor synchronization. *J Cogn Neurosci*, **12**, 546–55.

Nair DG, Purcott KL, Fuchs A, Steinberg F, Kelso JA (2003). Cortical and cerebellar activity of the human brain during imagined and executed unimanual and bimanual action sequences: a functional MRI study. *Brain Res Cogn Brain Res*, **15**, 250–60.

Nakagawa Y, Tanabe H, Kazui H, Kato A, Yoshimine T (1998). Motor neglect following damage to the supplementary motor area. *Neurocase*, **4**, 55–63.

Nirkko AC, Ozdoba C, Redmond SM, Bürki M, Hess CW, Wiesendanger M (2001). Different ipsilateral representations for distal and proximal movements in the sensorimotor cortex: activation and deactivation patterns. *Neuroimage*, **13**, 825–35.

Obhi SS, Haggard P, Taylor J, Pascual-Leone A (2002). rTMS to the supplementary motor area disrupts bimanual coordination. *Mot Control*, **6**, 319–32.

Penfield W, Welch K (1951). The supplementary motor area of the cerebral cortex. *Arch Neurol Psychiatry (Chic)*, **66**, 289–317.

Peper CE, Beek PJ (1998). Distinguishing between the effects of frequency and amplitude on interlimb coupling in tapping a 2 : 3 polyrhythm. *Exp Brain Res*, **118**, 78–92.

Perrig S, Kazennikov O, Wiesendanger M (1999). Time structure of a goal-directed bimanual skill and its dependence on task constraints. *Behav Brain Res*, **103**, 95–104.

Preilowski B (1975). Bilateral motor interaction : perceptual-motor performance of partial and complete 'split-brain' patients. In KS Zülch, O Creutzfeldt, (ed.) *Cerebral Localization*, pp. 115–32. Berlin: Springer.

Preilowski B (1977). Phases of motor-skills acquisition : a neuropsychological approach. *J Mov Stud*, **3**, 169–81.

Preilowski B (1990). Intermanual transfer, interhemispheric interaction and handedness in man and monkeys. In C Trevarthen, (ed.) *Brain Circuits and Functions of the Mind*, pp. 168–80. Cambridge: Cambridge University Press.

Robertson SD, Zelaznik HN, Lantero DA, Bojczyk KG, Spencer RM, Doffin JG, *et al.* (1999). Correlations for timing consistency among tapping and drawing tasks: evidence against a single timing process for motor control. *J Exp Psychol Hum Percept Perform*, **25**, 1316–30.

Rouiller EM, Babalian A, Kazennikov O, Moret V, Yu X-H, Wiesendanger M (1994). Transcallosal connections of the distal forelimb representations of the primary and supplementary motor cortical areas in macaque monkeys. *Exp Brain Res*, **102**, 227–43.

Sadato N, Yonekura Y, Waki A, Yamada H, Ishii Y (1997). Role of the supplementary motor area and the right premotor cortex in the coordination of bimanual finger movements. *J Neurosci*, **17**, 9667–74.

Sainburg RL, Poizner H, Ghez C (1993). Loss of proprioception produces deficits in interjoint coordination. *J Neurophysiol*, **70**, 2136–47.

Schell GL, Hodge CJ, Cacayosin E (1986). Transient neurological deficits after therapeutic embolization of the arteries supplying the medial wall of the hemisphere including the supplementary motor area. *Neurosurgery*, **18**, 353–6.

Schöner G, Kelso JAS (1988). Dynamic pattern generation in behavioral and neural systems. *Science*, **239**, 1513–20.

Schöner G, Haken H, Kelso JAS (1986). A stochastic theory of phase transitions in human hand movemnet. *Biol Cybern*, **53**, 247–57.

Selezneva OAA, Afanas'ev E, Tolkunov B (1999). Correlates of sequential elements of bimanual behavior in the neuronal activity of the neostriatum in monkeys. *Neurosci Behav Physiol*, **29**, 53–9.

Semjen A, Summers JJ, Cattaert D (1995). Hand coordination in bimanual circle drawing. *J Exp Psychol*, **21**, 1139–57.

Serrien DJ, Brown P (2002). The functional role of interhemispheric synchronization in the control of bimanual timing tasks. *Exp Brain Res*, **147**, 268–72.

Serrien DJ, Brown P (2003). The integration of cortical and behavioural dynamics during initial learning of a motor task. *Eur J Neurosci*, **17**, 1098–104.

Serrien DJ, Wiesendanger M (2000). Temporal control of a bimanual task in patients with cerebellar dysfunction. *Neuropsychologia*, **38**, 558–65.

Serrien DJ, Wiesendanger M (2001a). A higher-order mechanism overrules the automatic grip-load force constraint during bimanual asymmetrical movements. *Behav Brain Res*, **118**, 153–60.

Serrien DJ, Wiesendanger M (2001b). Regulation of grasping forces during bimanual in-phase and anti-phase coordination. *Neuropsychologia*, **39**, 1379–84.

Serrien DJ, Wiesendanger M (2001c). Bimanual organization of manipulative forces: evidence from erroneous feedforward programming of precision grip. *Eur J Neurosci*, **13**, 1825–32.

Serrien DJ, Steyvers M, Debaere F, Stelmach GE, Swinnen SP (2000). Bimanual coordination and limb-specific parameterization in patients with Parkinson's disease. *Neuropsychologia*, **38**, 1714–22.

Serrien DJ, Burgunder J-M, Wiesendanger M (2001a). Grip force scaling and sequencing of events during a manipulative task in Huntington's disease. *Neuropsychologia*, **39**, 734–41.

Serrien DJ, Nirkko AC, Wiesendanger M (2001b). Damage to the parietal lobe impairs bimanual coordination. *NeuroReport*, **12**, 2721–4.

Serrien DJ, Burgunder JM, Wiesendanger M (2002a). Control of manipulative forces during unimanual and bimanual tasks in patients with Huntington's disease. *Exp Brain Res*, **143**, 328–34.

Serrien DJ, Nirkko AC, Wiesendanger M (2002b). Role of the corpus callosum in bimanual coordination: a comparison of patients with congenital and acquirewd callosal damage. *Eur J Neurosci*, **14**, 1897–905.

Serrien DJ, Strens LH, Oliviero A, Brown P (2002c). Repetitive transcranial magnetic stimulation of the supplementary motor area (SMA) degrades bimanual movement control in humans. *Neurosci Lett*, **328**, 89–92.

Serrien DJ, Cassidy MJ, Brown P (2003). The importance of the dominant hemisphere in the organization of bimanual movements. *Hum Brain Mapping*, **18**, 296–305.

Seymour SE, Reuter-Lorenz PA, Gazzaniga MS (1994). The disconnection syndrome—basic findings reaffirmed. *Brain*, **117**, 105–15.

Shinoda Y, Ohgaki T, Sugiuchi Y, Futami T (1992). Morphology of single medial vestibulospinal tract axons in the upper cervical spinal cord of the cat. *J Comp Neurol*, **316**, 151–72.

Simóes C, Hari R (1999). Relationship between responses to contra- and ipsilateral stimuli in the human second somatosensory cortex SII. *Neuroimage*, **10**, 408–16.

Simoneau M, Paillard J, Bard C, Teasdale N, Martin O, Fleury M, *et al.* (1999). Role of the feedforward command and reafferent information in the coordination of a passing prehension task. *Exp Brain Res*, **128**, 236–42.

Spencer RM, Zelaznik HN, Diedrichsen J, Ivry RB (2003). Disrupted timing of discontinuous but not continuous movements by cerebellar lesions. *Science*, **300**, 1437–9.

Sperry RW (1966). Brain bisection and mechanisms of consciousness. In JC Eccles, (ed.) *Brain and Conscious Experience*, pp. 298–313. Berlin: Springer.

Stelmach GE, Worringham CJ (1988). The control of bimanual aiming movements in Parkinson's disease. *J Neurol Neurosurg Psychiatry*, **51**, 223–31.

Stephan KM, Binkofski F, Halsband U, Dohle C, Wunderlich G, Schnitzler A, *et al.* (1999a). The role of ventral medial wall motor areas in bimanual co-ordination—a combined lesion and activation study. *Brain*, **122**, 351–68.

Stephan KM, Binkofski F, Posse S, Seitz RJ, Freund H (1999b). Cerebral midline structures in bimanual coordination. *Exp Brain Res*, **128**, 243–9.

Steyvers M, Etoh S, Sauner D, Levin O, Siebner HR, Swinnen SP, *et al.* (2003). High-frequency transcranial magnetic stimulation of the supplementary motor area reduces bimanual coupling during anti-phase but not in-phase movements. *Exp Brain Res*, **151**, 309–17.

Summers JJ, Rosenbaum DA, Burns BD, Ford SK (1993). Production of polyrhythms. *J Exp Psychol Hum Percept Perform*, **19**, 416–28.

Swinnen SP (2002). Intermanual coordination: from behavioural principles to neural-network interactions. *Nat Rev Neurosci*, **3**, 348–59.

Swinnen S, Heuer H, Massion J, Casaer P (ed.) (1994). *Interlimb Coordination: Neural, Dynamical, and Cognitive Constraints.* San Diego, CA: Academic Press.

Swinnen SP, Jardin K, Meulenbroek R, Dounskaia N, Hofkens-Van den Brandt M (1997). Egocentric and allocentric constraints in the expression of patterns of interlimb coordination. *J Cogn Neurosci*, **9**, 348–77.

Swinnen SP, Jardin K, Verschueren S, Meulenbroek R, Franz L, Dounskaia N, *et al.* (1998). Exploring interlimb constraints during bimanual graphic performance: effects of muscle grouping and direction. *Behav Brain Res*, **90**, 79–87.

Tanji J, Okano K, Sato KC (1987). Relation of neurons in the nonprimary motor cortex to bilateral hand movement. *Nature*, **327**, 618–20.

Teasdale N, Bard C, Fleury M (1994). Bimanual interference in a deafferented patient and control subjects. In S Swinnen, H Heuer, J Massion, P Casaer *et al.*, (ed.) *Interlimb Coordination: Neural, Dynamical, and Cognitive Constraints*, pp. 243–58. San Diego, CA: Academic Press.

Temprado JJ, Monno A, Zanone PG, Kelso JA (2002). Attentional demands reflect learning-induced alterations of bimanual coordination dynamics. *Eur J Neurosci*, **16**, 1390–4.

Toyokura M, Muro I, Komiya T, Obara M (1999). Relation of bimanual coordination to activation in the sensorimotor cortex and supplementary motor area: analysis using functional magnetic resonance imaging. *Brain Res Bull*, **48**, 211–17.

Tracy JI, Faro SS, Mohammed FB, Pinus AB, Madi SM, Laskas JW (2001). Cerebellar mediation of the complexity of bimanual compared to unimanual movements. *Neurology*, **57**, 1862–9.

Turvey MT, Schmidt RC (1994). A low-dimensional nonlinear dynamic governing interlimb rhythmic coordination. In S Swinnen, H Heuer, J Massion, P Casaer, ed. *Interlimb Coordination: Neural, Dynamical, and Cognitive Constraints.* San Diego, CA: Academic Press, 277–318.

Uhl F, Kornhuber AW, Wartberger P, Lindinger G, Lang W, Deecke L (1996). Supplementary motor area in spatial coordination of bilateral movements: A new aspect to 'the SMA debate'? *Electroencephalogr Clin Neurophysiol*, **101**, 469–77.

Ullen F, Forssberg H, Ehrsson HH (2003). Neural networks for the coordination of the hands in time. *J Neurophysiol*, **89**, 1126.

Varela F, Lachaux JP, Rodriguez E, Martinerie J (2001). The brainweb: phase synchronization and large-scale integration. *Nat Rev Neurosci*, **2**, 229–39.

Ventura MG, Goldman S, Hildebrand J (1995). Alien hand syndrome without a corpus callosum lesion. *J Neurol Neurosurg Psychiatry*, **58**, 735–7.

Verbessem P, Op't EB, Swinnen SP, Vangheluwe S, Hespel P, Dom R (2002). Unimanual and bimanual voluntary movement in Huntington's disease. *Exp Brain Res*, **147**, 529–37.

Verschueren SMP, Swinnen SP, Cordo PJ, Dounskaia NV (1999). Proprioceptive control of multijoint movement: bimanual circle drawing. *Exp Brain Res*, **127**, 182–92.

Viallet F, Massion J, Massarino R, Khalil R (1992). Coordination between posture and movement in a bimanual load lifting task: Putative role of a medial frontal region including the supplementary motor area. *Exp Brain Res*, **88**, 674–84.

Viallet F, Vuillon-Cacciuttolo G, Legallet E, Bonnefoi-Kyriacou B, Trouche E (1995). Bilateral and side-related reaction time impairments in patients with unilateral cerebral lesions of a medial frontal region involving the supplementary motor area. *Neuropsychologia*, **33**, 215–23.

Voisin J, Lamarre Y, Chapman CE (2002). Haptic discrimination of object shape in humans: contribution of cutaneous and proprioceptive inputs. *Exp Brain Res*, **145**, 251–60.

von Holst E (1973). *The Behavioral Physiology of Animal and Man*. Coral Gables, FL: Hillsdale. (Originally published in German in 1937 and 1939.)

Vygotsky LS (1965). Psychology and localization of functions *Neuropsychologia*, **3**, 381–6. (Originally published in Russian in 1934.)

Walter CB, Swinnen SP (1990). Asymmetric interlimb interference during the performance of a dynamic bimanual task. *Brain Cogn*, **14**, 185–200.

Wannier T, Liu J, Morel A, Jouffrais C, Rouiller EM (2002). Neuronal activity in primate striatum and pallidum related to bimanual motor actions. *NeuroReport*, **13**, 1–5.

Watson RT, Fleet WS, Gonzales-Rothi L, Heilman KM (1986). Apraxia and the supplementary motor area. *Arch Neurol*, **43**, 787–92.

Weiss P, Jeannerod M (1998). Getting a grasp on coordination. *News Physiol Sci*, **13**, 70–5.

Weiss PH, Dohle C, Binkofski F, Schnitzler A, Freund H-J, Hefter H (2001). Motor impairment in patients with parietal lesions: disturbances of meaningless arm movement sequences. *Neuropsychologia*, **39**, 397–405.

Wenderoth N, Bock O (2001). Learning of a new bimanual coordination pattern is governed by three distinct processes. *Mot Control*, **5**, 23–35.

Wenderoth N, Bock O, Krohn R (2002). Learning a new bimanual coordination pattern is influenced by existing attractors. *Mot Control*, **6**, 166–82.

Wiesendanger M (1993). The riddle of supplementary motor area function. In N Mano, I Hamada, (ed.) *Role of the Cerebellum and Basal Ganglia in Voluntary Movement*, pp. 253–66. Amsterdam: Elsevier.

Wiesendanger M, Wicki U, Rouiller EM (1994). Are there unifying structures in the brain responsible for interlimb coordination? In S Swinnen, H Heuer, J Massion, P Casaer, (ed.) *Interlimb Coordination: Neural, Dynamical, and Cognitive Constraints*, pp. 179–207. San Diego, CA: Academic Press.

Wiesendanger M, Kazennikov O, Perrig S, Kaluzny P (1996a). Two hands—one action. In AM Wing, P Haggard, (ed.), *Hand and Brain*, pp. 283–300. Oxford: Oxford University Press.

Wiesendanger M, Rouiller EM, Kazennikov O, Perrig S (1996b). Is the supplementary motor area a bilaterally organized system? In HO Lüders, (ed.) *Supplementary Sensorimotor Area*, pp. 85–93. New York: Raven Press.

Wiesendanger M, Kazennikov O, Perrig S, Rouiller EM, Kermadi I (1997). Reaching, grasping, and bimanual coordination with special reference to the parietal cortex. In P Thier, HO Karnath, (ed.) *Parietal Lobe Contributions to Orientation in 3D Space*, pp. 271–88. Berlin: Springer.

Wing AM (1982). Timing and coordination of repetitive bimanual movements. *Q J Exp Physiol*, **34A**, 339–48.

Wolpert DM, Ghahramani Z (2000). Computational principles of movement neuroscience. *Nat Neurosci*, **3**, 1212–17.

Wyke M (1971). The effects of brain lesions on the learning performance of a bimanual co-ordination task. *Cortex*, **7**, 59–72.

Zentner J, Hufnagel A, Pechstein U, Wolf HK, Schramm J (1996). Functional results after resective procedures involving the supplementary motor area. *J Neurosurg*, **85**, 542–9.

Chapter 12

Higher-order disorders of gait

John G. Nutt

Introduction

The term 'highest-level (or higher-order) gait disorders' is derived from Hughlings Jackson's concept of lowest, middle and highest levels of function in the nervous system (Jackson 1932). The highest levels of neurological function were those requiring the most complex sensory–motor integration. As an example of the anatomical distribution of these functions, Jackson assigned the anterior horn motor neurons to the lowest level, the primary motor strip to the middle-level, and the prefrontal cortex to highest level. He considered spinal muscular atrophy as a lowest-level disorder, paralysis agitans as a middle-level disorder, and general paresis as a highest-level disorder. In terms of gait and balance disorders, Jackson's highest-level disorders refer to gait abnormalities that arise from impaired integration of sensory and contextual information to produce appropriate and purposeful gait and balance synergies. Although Jackson used lowest and highest levels, lower and higher levels or orders will be used in this chapter, partially because there may be gradations within lower and higher functions.

It is helpful to first consider lower- and middle-level gait and balance disorders to help define higher-order disorders by exclusion (Tables 12.1 and 12.2). At the lower level, disturbances of force production, such as arise from muscle diseases, motor neuropathies, and motor neuron diseases, produce foot drop and waddling gait patterns. Also at the lower level, end-organ vestibular, somatosensory, and visual disturbances cause weaving, ataxic, and cautious gait patterns. The origins of these lower-level gait and balance disorders are generally obvious from clinical history and examination. At the middle level are disturbances of gait arising from impaired modulation of lower-level functions. These patterns include dysmetric locomotor and balance synergies with cerebellar disorders, spasticity with corticospinal dysfunction, and bradykinetic, dystonic, and choreic gaits with basal ganglia disorders. Middle-level sensory dysfunction is less clear, although interruption of vestibular pathways in the brainstem and subcortical regions might be examples (Dieterich and Brandt 1992). Middle-level motor patterns of gait and balance are also readily recognized by clinicians. Gait problems that cannot be explained by lower- and middle-level nervous system dysfunction are, by exclusion, considered as higher-level nervous system dysfunction.

Table 12.1 Lower-level gait disorders

	Disorder	Gait pattern
Sensory		
Proprioception	Peripheral neuropathy	Ataxic
	Posterior column lesions	Ataxic
Vestibular	Vestibular labyrinth lesions	Weaving
Visual	Cataracts, macular degeneration	Cautious
Motor		
Muscle	Muscular dystrophy	Waddling
Peripheral nerve	Motor neuropathy	Food drop
Motor neuron	Spinal muscular atrophy	Mixed

Table 12.2 Middle-level gait disorders

	Disorder	Gait pattern
Sensory		
Central vestibular	Wallenberg's syndrome	Lateropulsion
Motor		
Corticospinal	Spastic paraparesis	Spastic
Cerebellar	Spinocerebellar	Ataxic
Basal ganglia	Huntington's chorea	Dancing
	Parkinson's disease[a]	Shuffling

[a] Mild and moderate disease

The preceding paragraph suggests that if no lower- or middle-level dysfunction is identified, the problem is a higher-level dysfunction. There are other possibilities that must be kept in mind. One possibility is that gait disorders not explained by lower- and middle-level dysfunction are multifactorial in origin, with no single factor in isolation being sufficient to disturb gait or balance. With this scenario, multiple deficits might give rise to a clinical history and examination that contain no indications of significant dysfunction in any motor, sensory, or higher function to account for the difficulties in gait and balance. A second possibility is that abnormalities in what are considered lower- or middle-level functions are not detected clinically; disturbances of central vestibular pathways or midline cerebellar and brainstem structures important to balance might cause balance disorders without the usual clinical findings that point to lesions in these structures.

At a clinical level, higher-level gait and balance disorders are defined as impaired execution of learned locomotor and equilibrium responses that are not explicable by weakness, altered muscle tone, primary sensory loss, incoordination, involuntary movements, inattention, or incomprehension. This definition is, of course, that commonly used for apraxia (Geschwind 1975). Thus, higher-level gait disorders could be considered apraxia. However, the term apraxia generally implies abnormalities in motor programs. But the definition of apraxia by exclusion of other motor, sensory, or comprehension disturbances allows inclusion of gait dysfunction that could be attributed to abnormal sensory integration, sensory or motor neglect, loss of access to automatic ('lower-level') brainstem and spinal motor programs, lack of attention, and impaired insight/cognitive functioning.

The higher-level gait and balance disorders need not arise from cortical pathology. Subcortical lesions, particularly those in thalamus, basal ganglia, and tracts connecting these subcortical nuclei with the cortex, may disturb cortical function indirectly and also account for cortical dysfunction. This formulation parallels that for limb apraxia and spatial neglect which may arise from subcortical as well as cortical lesions (de Renzi *et al.* 1986; Hanna-Pladdy *et al.* 2001; Karnath *et al.* 2002). The subcortical nuclei may have direct influences on gait and balance that are envisioned as middle-level function as well as indirect influences through interaction with frontal cortical areas that are critical to higher-level functions. For example, some deficits in parkinsonism may be explained by ineffective recruitment of motor units producing slowed gait and postural responses, features that are generally responsive to levodopa, and in this scheme are considered middle-level functions. Postural and gait abnormalities of advanced parkinsonism that are not corrected by levodopa may be due to basal ganglia influences on 'higher-level' frontal and prefrontal regions. It should also be noted that frontal cortex lesions and their connections to subcortical areas are often considered as the exclusive origin of higher-level gait and balance disorders. However, other cortical dysfunction, particularly parietal, may produce higher-level balance problems as well.

Gait patterns of higher-level disorders

The sections below describe locomotor and balance patterns or syndromes that appear to result from higher-level dysfunction. Some of the disorders are well- recognized clinical patterns, others are more obscure, and two are based on personal observation. This classification is a work in progress and does not pretend to account for all gait patterns that may be encountered in the clinic.

The terminology for higher-level locomotor and balance disorders is confusing, with many synonyms for similar or identical disorders. The approach in this chapter is to name locomotor and balance patterns by characteristic clinical features. Anatomical names, such as 'frontal gait', are not used because the dysfunction does not necessarily arise from the area implied by the name. Neurological function or dysfunction, such as agnosia or apraxia, is also avoided because the nature of the disorders is often speculative. Finally, gaits are not named by the disease process, such as gait of normal pressure hydrocephalus, because there are few, if any, gait and balance patterns that are pathognomonic for any disease or disorder.

Gait, in the clinical sense, encompasses two functions: locomotion and balance. Locomotion, the rhythmical limb movements that produce progression of the body through space, is hard-wired at the spinal level, and is turned on and off and adapted to a person's goals by descending influences from the brainstem and hemispheres. Balance, postural responses that support the body in the upright or desired position for locomotion and preserve balance during changes in body position and purposeful locomotion, arise from brainstem structures and are influenced by higher centers. Although both locomotion and postural responses are physiologically linked (Mori and Takakusaki 1988) in some human disorders, they may be relatively dissociated so that disequilibrium may dominate the clinical picture in some situations and locomotor abnormalities in others. For this reason, gait disorders are divided into those in which locomotion is the predominant difficulty (Table 12.3) and those in which balance is the major difficulty (Table 12.4).

Table 12.3 Higher-level gait (locomotor) disorders

Gait pattern	Lesions	Gait features
Freezing		
Narrow-based	Basal ganglia and subcortical white matter	Start and turn hesitation
Wide-based	Subcortical white matter	Start and turn hesitation
Marche à petits pas	Subcortical white matter	Wide-based, very short steps without freezing
Cautious gait	Non-specific, multifactional and environmental	Minimal widening, shortened stride and en bloc turns
Careless gait	Dementia or delirium	Falls from carelessness
Psychogenic gait	—	May resemble lower- and middle-level disorders or be bizarre

Table 12.4 Higher-level gait (balance) disorders

Gait pattern	Lesions	Gait features
Lateral pusher syndrome	Thalamus-parietal	Actively pushing contralateral to the lesion
Posterior pusher syndrome	Widespread cortical and subcortical lesions	Actively pushing backwards
Drifting astasia	Thalamus and basal ganglia	Drifting backwards and laterally into falls
Balance disorganization	Medial frontal	Bizarre postural synergies

Higher-level gait (locomotor) disorders

Freezing gaits

Freezing gaits are characterized by difficulty in initiating stepping and interruption of gait by distraction, visual obstacles, and turning (Giladi *et al*. 1992, 1997). This pattern has also been called gait ignition failure (Atchison *et al*. 1993; Nutt *et al*. 1993). The difficulty in initiating locomotion can take several forms. The first is a complete immobility on attempting to walk, with no movement apparent to an observer; the person appears 'frozen' or 'fixed to the spot'. Surface EMGs of leg and truncal muscles show no activation in this situation. In another form, patients are immobile but develop an alternating tremor in the legs, generally an alternating flexion of one knee with extension of the other knee. The tremor may be brief, may involve several alterations, or may persist for 5–10 s. The base is normal or even narrowed. These forms of gait initiation failure are generally seen in parkinsonism. A third pattern of gait initiation difficulty is the initiation of gait with small steps that progressively increase in length, the so-called 'slipping clutch' gait. The slipping clutch form may be associated with exaggerated lateral truncal sway and arm swing as though the person is attempting to free a foot that is stuck to the floor. Examination of these people during initiation of gait shows that they have multiple small weight shifts but with aborted steps as they start to walk (Elble *et al*. 1996). The base may be normal but is more commonly widened. This pattern of initiation difficulty is particularly characteristic of multi-infarct states or subcortical white matter lesions. In general, the base is an important clue to the cause of freezing. Narrow base implies that parkinsonism is most likely; a wide base suggests a parkinsonism plus syndrome or multi-infarct etiology. Exaggerated truncal sway and arm swing is very suggestive of multi-infarct etiology.

Interruption of gait by distraction (such as asking the person a question), obstacles in the path of progression (such as a telephone cord on the floor and narrow openings like doorways), or approaching the destination will interrupt locomotion. Of interest, very similar stimuli can aid gait. For example, another person counting cadence, having the person try to step on marks on the floor, or stepping over an inverted cane may help a person start or maintain locomotion. These various stimuli that aid or hinder gait may have in common the fact that they either help the person to concentrate on walking or they distract the person from the task of walking. This interpretation suggests that gait is under conscious cortical control in these people, unlike normal people in whom gait requires little direct attention. People with freezing are like normal people learning a new dance step. The instructor's counting cadence aloud, the music, and the dance partner's ability all aid the novice dancer. If these clues are withdrawn or the dance partner makes a sarcastic comment, the novice dancer is likely to lose the dance rhythm or even to freeze.

The question is why in people with freezing has walking come under direct conscious control or, in common parlance, why can they no longer 'walk and chew gum'? It seems that subconscious access to locomotor programs is impaired and direct cortical control, as in learning a new motor task, is required. As freezing is associated with parkinsonism, in which there is impaired activation of frontal motor areas, and with ischemic subcortical lesions, in which damage to connections between frontal motor areas and diencephalon and brainstem locomotor areas is likely, a 'disconnection' syndrome is an appealing explanation.

Marche à petits pas

This is a stereotyped gait pattern characterized by short steps (often only an inch or so), generally a widened base, en bloc turns, minimal freezing and mild to moderate impairment of balance. It is frequently associated with subcortical ischemic lesions and hydrocephalus. This gait pattern has been described as a frontal gait (Nutt *et al.* 1993). Frontal gait may not be an appropriate name because the pattern is not necessarily associated with frontal lesions. Marche à petits pas pattern is also commonly referred to as gait apraxia. Because the pattern is so stereotyped, it seems that gait apraxia or disordered locomotor programs is not a likely explanation for this gait pattern. In apraxia of the limbs, the incorrect response is not stereotyped. Marche à petits pas is chosen here because it is a description of the most salient feature of the gait.

Is there such a thing as apraxia of gait? The term is commonly used in the United States for the gait pattern described above for Marche à petits pas, a rather stereotyped gait pattern. There are gait patterns that are bizarre, not stereotyped, and appear to be a true disruption of locomotor programs. However, the few patients with this bizarre gait pattern that are described in the medical literature also had profound abnormalities of balance that often precluded standing or ambulating without assistance. For this reason, these cases may be better considered as apraxia of balance rather than of gait, and they are classified as disorganized balance strategies and described below.

Cautious gait

This gait pattern is characterized by slowing of gait velocity, shortened steps, no or minimal widening of base, en bloc turns but no freezing, and minimal imbalance (Nutt *et al.* 1993). It is a non-specific gait pattern adopted in response to perceived threats to balance (Maki 1997). A neurologically normal person will adopt this gait pattern on a slippery surface, such as ice, or when walking in the dark. It is a common gait pattern in the clinic because it may be the response to any sensory–motor abnormalities that make the person feel less confident about their balance. Because all gait abnormalities are associated with slowing of walking speed, this gait pattern is also a predecessor of many of the other gait and balance patterns, i.e. cautious gait may progress to marche à petits pas or freezing gait patterns.

Careless gait

This gait does not have any characteristic pattern but is associated with falls. The falls occur because the patient is careless in regard to walking. Carelessness may take the form of attempting to walk in inappropriate clothing and conditions or to inattention to their surroundings. The carelessness may result from impaired attention caused by centrally active drugs or intercurrent illness (such as urinary tract infection (UTI) or upper respiratory infection (URI) or from impaired insight as occurs in dementia. Non-dominant parietal lobe lesions are also predictors of falls (Rapport *et al.* 1993; Ugur *et al.* 2000). In addition to hemisensory deficits and neglect, impulsivity and other behavioral changes may contribute to falls in patients with parietal lobe lesions (Rapport *et al.* 1993; Webster *et al.* 1995).

Psychogenic gait

Psychogenic gaits may assume many patterns, ranging from patterns that imitate hemi-paretic, ataxic, or dystonic gaits to bizarre patterns that defy description (Keane 1989; Lempert *et al.* 1991). The features that are useful for separating other psychogenic neurological signs from genuine neurological disorders are equally useful for suspected psychogenic gait disorders. Distractibility, inconsistency, presence of other psychogenic signs, history of previous psychogenic signs, and history of psychiatric disorders are clues to psychogenic gait disorders.

Higher-level gait (balance) syndromes

Lateral pusher syndrome

The lateral pusher or contraversive pushing syndrome appears to be due to inappropriate postural responses that are associated with disturbed orientation of the body in the gravitational field. Non-dominant parietal lobe lesions can produce the syndrome of the patient actively pushing toward the affected side (contralateral to the lesion)(Perennou *et al.* 1998) and possibly falling as a consequence (Perennou *et al.* 1998; Karnath *et al.* 2000a). This association makes much sense; the posterior parietal lobe is very important for creating spatial maps, although the maps themselves may reside in other areas of the brain (Gross and Graziano 1995). More recently, it has been recognized that thalamic lesions of either hemisphere, but more commonly the non-dominant hemisphere, may be responsible for this syndrome (Karnath *et al.* 2000b). The pusher syndrome is associated with a disturbance of subjective postural verticality with preserved subjective visual verticality (Perennou *et al.* 1998; Karnath *et al.* 2000a,b). The dissociation between subjective postural and visual verticality suggests that two different systems control the orientation of vision and the trunk. The vestibular system is critical for the eyes and vision orientation but postural orientation may depend upon graviceptors in the trunk (Mittelstaedt 1999; Karnath *et al.* 2000b). Because of the misperception of truncal verticality, inappropriate postural strategies are employed, resulting in falls. The relation of the lateral pusher syndrome to other subcortical lesions producing disequilibrium is unclear (Karnath *et al.* 2000b). Table 12.5 presents the disequilibrium syndromes associated with

Table 12.5 Subcortical lesions and disequilibrium

Syndrome	Falls	Subjective visual vertical	Subjective postural vertical
Thalamic astasia	Contralateral and backwards	?	?
Lenticular astasia	Contralateral and backwards	?	?
Thalamic vestibular disequilibrium	Lateral	Abnormal	?
Lateral pusher syndrome	Contralateral	Normal	Abnormal

subcortical lesions and the limited information about their effects on subjective visual vertical and subjective postural vertical. As opposed to the pusher syndrome, thalamic vestibular disequilibrium is associated with a tilt of the visual vertical and is less frequently associated with falls.

Posterior pusher syndrome

A syndrome that has received no attention in the literature is the posterior pusher syndrome. In this syndrome, the patient actively pushes backwards and resists the efforts of the examiner to get their center of mass over their feet. Neither pulling the patient from the front nor pushing from the rear are sufficient to get the patient upright so that they may stand independently. Many of these patients seem to perceive that their center of mass is not over their feet but are unable to voluntarily bring themselves over their feet. As a consequence, these patients are generally unable to stand unaided. This postural pattern is often seen in dementia with diffuse cortical atrophy and subcortical white matter disease. This pattern of disequilibrium is possibly due to faulty body orientation in the anterior–posterior direction, analogous to the pusher syndrome in the lateral direction. It is also possible that it is some form of disinhibited brainstem postural response such as decerebrate posture or, alternatively, that it is a form of *gegenhalten*, i.e. oppositional resistance.

Drifting astasia

Astasia is the inability to stand despite the apparent ability to control the legs. This clinical pattern is characterized by a seeming indifference to postural verticality. Patients may drift sideways or backwards when sitting or standing without any attempt to remain vertically aligned. Sometimes, the patients will make a delayed attempt to realign themselves but they also may drift into a fall with little or no effort to avoid a fall or to break their fall. The resulting falls are often like a 'falling tree' with retained truncal tone throughout the fall. This form of astasia may be seen with vascular lesions of the thalamus (Masdeu and Gorelick 1988) and lenticular nucleus (Labadie *et al.* 1989) and in progressive supranuclear palsy or advanced parkinsonism. This syndrome differs from the pusher syndromes in that there is not active pushing of the body away from verticality but rather a failure to keep the body mass over the support base. Because there seems to be no response to the drifting out of balance, it is tempting to postulate that the thalamic, lenticular, and parkinsonian astasias represent neglect syndromes rather than distortion of spatial information as is believed to underlie the pusher syndromes and thalamic vestibular syndromes. Further studies of patients with drifting astasias are needed to characterize this syndrome.

Balance disorganization

Balance disorganization is a new term that we will use to describe postural synergies that are inappropriate and bizarre and often prohibit independent standing and walking. The term may include gait patterns that have been labeled frontal ataxia (Bruns 1892), gait apraxia(Gerstmann and Schilder 1926; van Bogart and Martin 1929; Bell 1934; Meyer and Barron 1960; Petrovici 1968; Tyrrell 1994; Della *et al.* 2002) and frontal and subcortical disequilibrium syndromes (Nutt *et al.* 1993). This balance pattern is characterized by absence or distortion of normal postural responses. Rolling over and sitting up may be impaired because the patient tries to employ biomechanically impossible strategies. The patient may fail to bring their legs under the chair when trying to rise from the chair and not place their weight over their feet, making rising physically impossible. Strange responses such as crossing the legs when standing or an inability to sit down may be seen. The abnormalities may take many forms and are not stereotyped as are freezing and marche à petits pas syndromes. Disordered and inappropriate stepping, which warrants the description of gait (locomotor) apraxia, is generally seen in the presence of severe imbalance but imbalance overshadows the abnormalities of locomotion. For these reasons, apraxia of balance seems a more appropriate description of the pattern than does apraxia of gait.

It is important to recognize that axial or truncal apraxia that would be most pertinent to locomotion and balance is probably distinct from limb apraxia (Geschwind 1975). That is, axial and limb apraxia arise from different parts of the brain(Geschwind 1975), although other explanations are possible as well (Hanlon *et al.* 1998). Geschwind suggested that limb apraxia may be more closely linked to the pryramidal system while axial apraxia may be associated with other systems (Geschwind and Damasio 1985). This may be analogous to Kuyper's demonstration in monkeys that different descending cerebral and brainstem tracts control distal limb movements and axial movements. Lateral corticospinal tracts controlled fine motor movements of the hands, and anterior-medial descending tracts controlled balance and ability to walk (Kuypers 1981). This suggestion of diffcrent origins of limb and axial apraxia may explain why many investigators find no limb, particularly leg, apraxia accompanying so-called gait and balance apraxias (Estanol 1981; Nutt *et al.* 1993). Further, it would be consistent with the observations that gait and balance disorders are generally not related to dysfunction of a specific hemisphere, unlike limb apraxia which generally arises from lesions in the left hemisphere (Geschwind and Damasio 1985; Hanna-Pladdy *et al.* 2001).

Falls associated with voluntary actions

Anticipatory postural responses are postural adjustments that precede or accompany the voluntary movements to protect balance. A common example is the contraction of the gastrocnemius in a standing person to protect upright balance before the biceps contracts to pull a handle in front of the person (Nashner 1977). Focal frontal lobe lesions have been associated with loss of anticipatory reflexes (Gurfinkel and El'ner 1988; Massion 1992; Palmer *et al.* 1996). What is less clear is whether there is a clinically identifiable syndrome associated with loss of anticipatory responses. Therefore this is a theoretical fall pattern that has not been clearly identified clinically.

Conclusions

A number of higher-level gait patterns are identified by exclusion, if higher-level gait disorders are defined by the absence of lower- and middle-level neurological dysfunction that could explain gait problems. There are two caveats. First, multifactorial causes might not present with sufficient lower- and middle-level neurological signs to be appreciated as lower- and middle-level disorders. Secondly, there may remain lower- and middle-level neurological functions that are crucial to locomotion and balance that are not understood at this time. However, the large number of patients with unexplained abnormal gait patterns and falls suggest that higher-order gait disorders may be relatively common and therefore be worthy of more attention than they have received to date.

Acknowledgements

I thank Mrs Lynn Storey for her assistance in preparing the manuscript. This work was supported in part by Portland Veterans'Administration Parkinson's Disease Research, Education and Clinical Center (PADRECC).

References

Atchison PR, Thompson PD, Frackowiak RSJ, Marsden CD (1993). The syndrome of gait initiation failure: a report of six cases. *Mov Disord*, **8**, 285–92.

Bell A (1934). Apraxia in corpus callosum lesions. *J Neurol Psychopathol*, **15**, 137–46.

Bruns L (1892). Uber Storugen des gleichgewichtes bei Stirnhirntumoren. *Dtsch Med Wochenschr*, **18**, 138–40.

Della SS, Francescani A, Spinnler (2002). Gait apraxia after bilateral supplementary motor area lesion. *J Neurol Neurosurg Psychiatry*, **72**, 77–85.

de Renzi E, Faglioni P, Scarpa M, Crisi G (1986). Limb apraxia in patients with damage confined to the left basal ganglia and thalamus. *J Neurol Neurosurg Psychiatry*, **49**, 1030–8.

Dieterich M, Brandt T (1992). Wallenberg's syndrome: lateropulsion, cyclorotation, and subjective visual vertical in thirty-six patients. *Ann Neurol*, **31**, 399–408.

Elble RJ, Cousins R, Leffler K, Hughes L (1996). Gait initiation by patients with lower-half parkinsonism. *Brain*, **119**, 1705–16.

Estanol BV (1981). Gait apraxia in communicating hydrocephalus. *J Neurol Neurosurg Psychiatry*, **44**, 305–8.

Gerstmann J, Schilder P (1926). Uber eine besondere Gangstorung bei Stirnhirner kranting. *Wien Med Wochenschr*, **76**, 97–107.

Geschwind N (1975). The apraxias: neural mechanisms of disorders of learned movement. *Am Sci*, **63**, 188–95.

Geschwind N, Damasio AR (1985). Apraxia. In AM Freederiks, (ed.) *Clinical Neuropsychology* Vol 1, pp. 423–32. Amsterdam: Elsevier.

Giladi N, McMahon D, Przedborski S, Flaster E, Guillory S, Kostic V, *et al*. (1992). Motor blocks in Parkinson's disease. *Neurology*, **42**, 333–9.

Giladi N, Kao R, Fahn S (1997). Freezing phenomenon in patients with parkinsonian syndromes. *Mov Disord*, **12**, 302–5.

Gross CG, Graziano MSA (1995). Multiple representations of space in the brain. *Neuroscientist*, **1**, 43–50.

Gurfinkel VS, El'ner AM (1988). Contribution of the frontal lobe secondary motor area to organization of postural components in human voluntary movement. *Neurofiziologiya*, **20**, 7–15.

Hanlon RE, Mattson D, Demery JA, Dromerick AW (1998). Axial movements are relatively preserved with respect to limb movements in aphasic patients. *Cortex*, **34**, 731–41.

Hanna-Pladdy B, Heilman KM, Foundas AL (2001). Cortical and subcortical contributions to ideomotor apraxia: analysis of task demands and error types. *Brain*, **124**, 2513–27.

Jackson JH (1932). *Selected Writings of John Hughlings Jackson* Vol 2. London: Hodder and Stoughton.

Karnath HO, Ferber S, Dichgans J (2000a). The origin of contraversive pushing: evidence for a second graviceptive system in humans. *Neurology*, **55**, 1298–1304.

Karnath HO, Ferber S, Dichgans J (2000b). The neural representation of postural control in humans. *Proc Natl Acad Sci USA*, **97**, 13931–6.

Karnath HO, Himmelbach, M, Rorden C (2002). The subcortical anatomy of human spatial neglect: putamen, caudate nucleus and pulvinar. *Brain*, **125**, 350–60.

Keane JR (1989). Hysterical gait disorders: 60 cases. *Neurology*, **39**, 586–9.

Kuypers HGJ (1981). Anatomy of the descending pathways. In VB Brooks, (ed.) *Handbook of Physiology*. Section 1: *The Nervous System*. Vol. 2: *Motor Control* Part 1, pp. 597–666. Bethesda, MD: American Physiological Society.

Labadie EL, Awerbuch GI, Hamilton RH, Rapesak SZ (1989). Falling and postural deficits due to acute unilateral basal ganglia lesions. *Arch Neurol*, **45**, 492–6.

Lempert T, Brandt T, Dieterich M, Huppert D (1991). How to identify psychogenic disorders of stance and gait. *J Neurol*, **238**, 140–6.

Maki BE (1997). Gait changes in older adults: predictors of falls or indicators of fear. *J Am Geriatr Soc*, **45**, 313–20.

Masdeu JC, Gorelick PB (1988). Thalamic astasia: inability to stand after unilateral thalamic lesions. *Ann Neurol*, **23**, 596–603.

Massion J (1992). Movement, posture, and equilibrium: interaction and coordination. *Prog Neurobiol*, **38**, 35–56.

Meyer JS, Barron DW (1960). Apraxia of gait: a clinicophysiological study. *Brain*, **83**, 261–84.

Mittelstaedt H (1999). The role of the otoliths in perception of the vertical and in path integration. *Ann NY Acad Sci*, **871**, 334–43.

Mori S, Takakusaki K (1988). Integration of posture and locomotion. In B Amblard, A Berthoz, F Clarac, (ed.) *Posture and gait: development, adaptation and modulation*, pp. 341–54. Amsterdam: Elsevier.

Nashner LM (1977). Fixed patterns of rapid postural responses among leg muscles during stance. *Exp Brain Res*, **30**, 13–24.

Nutt JG, Marsden CD, Thompson PD (1993). Human walking and higher level gait disorders, particularly in the elderly. *Neurology*, **43**, 268–79.

Palmer E, Downes L, Ashby P (1996). Associated postural adjustments are impaired by a lesion of the cortex. *Neurology*, **46**, 471–5.

Perennou DA, Amblard B, Leblond C, Pelissier J (1998). Biased postural vertical in humans with hemispheric cerebral lesions. *Neurosci Lett*, **252**, 75–8.

Petrovici I (1968). Apraxia of gait and of trunk movements. *J Neurol Sci*, **7**, 229–43.

Rapport LJ, Webster JS, Flemming KL, Lindberg JW, Godlewski MC, Brees JE, *et al.* (1993). Predictors of falls among right-hemisphere stroke patients in the rehabilitation setting. *Arch Phys Med Rehab*, **74**, 621–6.

Tyrrell PJ (1994). Apraxia of gait or higher level gait disorders: review and description of two cases of progressive gait disturbance due to frontal lobe degeneration. *J R Soc Med*, **87**, 454–6.

Ugur C, Gucuyener D, Uzuner N, Ozkan S, Ozdemir G (2000). Characteristics of falling in patients with stroke. *J Neurol Neurosurg Psychiatry*, **69**, 649–51.

van Bogart L, Martin P (1929). Sur deux signes du syndrome de desequilibration frontale: l'apraxie de la marche et l'antonie statique. *Encephale*, **24**, 11–18.

Webster JS, Roades LA, Morrill B, Rapport LJ, Abadee PS, Sowa MV, *et al.* (1995). Rightward orienting bias, wheelchair maneuvering, and fall risk. *Arch Phys Med Rehab*, **76**, 924–8.

Chapter 13

Speech motor control and its disorders

Ray D. Kent

Introduction

This chapter begins with a brief review of the properties of the speech musculature and its neural control. It then proceeds to a discussion of disorders of speech motor control in children and adults. The two primary types of these disorders are dysarthria and apraxia of speech.

Speech motor control: general properties

The motor control of speech is accomplished through widely distributed motor neuron pools in the aerodigestive tract, which consists of the respiratory, laryngeal, and upper airway muscle systems. This complex multi-articulate system includes as many as 100 muscles of several different types, including joint-related muscles (the muscles of the jaw, such as the masseter and the digastrics), sphincteric muscles (the orbicularis oris muscle of the lips and the constrictor muscles of the pharynx), a muscular hydrostat (the intrinsic muscles of the tongue), and muscles specialized for vibration and airway valving (the intrinsic muscles of the larynx). These muscles differ considerably in size, innervation ratio, contraction time, and function. With some exceptions, such as the closing muscles of the jaw, the muscles are specialized for speed rather than force, and they are generally capable of precise coordination in the performance of movement sequences for speech, mastication, deglutition, and other behaviors.

Recent studies show that at least some of these muscles have properties of fatigue resistance or rapid shortening that are relevant to their specialized roles in phonation and articulation. Han *et al.* (1999) described a large number of slow tonic muscle fibers (STFs) in the vocalis muscle compartment of the thyroarytenoid muscle. STFs differ from most muscle fibers in that they do not exhibit a twitch contraction but rather exhibit contractions that are prolonged, stable, precisely controlled, and fatigue resistant. Because STFs have not been observed in the vocal folds of other mammals, Han and coworkers proposed that they 'may be a unique human specialization for speech' (Han *et al.* 1999, p.146). Sciote *et al.* (2002) reported that human laryngeal muscles are comprised of type I, type IIA, type IIX, and tonic myosin heavy chain (MHC) fibers.

Although the first three of these have shortening speeds similar to those of fibers in limb muscles, laryngeal muscles with heterogencous MHC expression have variable shortening speeds, some of which are nearly twice as fast as those of limb muscle fibers. Studies of the rat tongue (Sokoloff 2000) provided evidence of both fatigue resistance and localization of motor unit territory for the intrinsic tongue body. Weijs (1997) reported that the masticatory muscle fibers contain at least four different isoforms of MHC, have a continuous range of contraction speeds, and have a high oxidative capacity and are therefore very fatigue resistant. In summary, the craniofacial and lingual muscles are distinctive in their functional requirements and their molecular phenotypes (Porter *et al.* 2001; Shuler and Dalrymple 2001). McComas (1998), noting structural and functional differences between orofacial and limb muscles, cautioned against extrapolating data from one muscle group to another.

The differences just reviewed are pertinent to the effects of neurologic disease or medical interventions on speech and non-speech motor systems, which may not always demonstrate uniform effects (Kent *et al.* 2001). There are also indications that muscles in humans differ from analogous tissues in mammalian and non-mammalian species, for example, in the case of the inferior pharyngeal constrictor muscle (Mu and Sanders 2001) and vocalis muscle (Han *et al.* 1999). Therefore caution should be observed in selecting animal models of the human speech motor system.

Speech is an unusual motor behavior in other respects. The conversational rate of speech is nearly as fast as its diadochokinetic rate (6–9 syllables/s, or as many as 18 phonemes/s), making speech perhaps the fastest discrete motor behavior in humans. Speech is also precisely controlled, having a temporal precision in the range of 10 ms or less. The rate and precision are accomplished in the face of complexity, given that the speech production system involves more motor fibers than any other human mechanical behavior (Fink 1986).

Speech motor control: neural structures and circuits

The neural control system for speech can be described with respect to lateralization and compartmentalization (Ackermann *et al.*, 2004). The principle structures are the insula, Broca's area, supplementary motor area, premotor cortex, motor cortex, basal ganglia, cerebellum, periaqueductal gray matter, and the brainstem and spinal nuclei of the relevant cranial and spinal nerves. Assigning specific functions to these structures can be difficult, but it is possible to hypothesize general roles that reflect contemporary research.

Lateralization

Lateralization of speech and language has long been established, and it is recognized that 95% of right-handed individuals have a left hemisphere dominance for language (Vikingstad *et al.* 2000). However, the detailed picture of lateralization must take into account, at the minimum, the relationships among gender, brain region, and behavioral task. Males and females may have dissimilar patterns of lateralization, although different conclusions have been drawn on the origin, nature, and significance of these differences (Harasty *et al.* 1997; Amunts *et al.* 1999; Robichon *et al.* 1999; Vikingstad *et al.* 2000; Kansaku and Kitazawa 2001). The relevance of brain structure and task to lateralization can be seen in Table 13.1, which is a summary of selected neuroimaging

Table 13.1 Summary of primary activation regions for various tasks involving oral movements or speaking

	Reference	Frontal operculum	SMA	Insula	Motor cortex	Basal ganglia	Cerebellum
Inner speech	Shergill *et al.* 2001		Bilateral	L			R
Tongue wagging while vocalizing	Bookheimer *et al.* 2000		L		Bilateral		Possible, but weak
Breathing for speech and phonation	Murphy *et al.* 1997		Bilateral		Bilateral	Bilateral, thalamus	*Bilateral*
Syllable sequence	Lotze *et al.* 2000		L		L		
Syllable sequence	Bookheimer *et al.* 2000		L		L		Possible, but weak
Automatic speech	Bookheimer *et al.* 2000		L			L, thalamus	Possible, but weak
Reading words aloud	Raichle 1996		Bilateral	Bilateral	Bilateral		R
Overlearned brief phrase	Murphy *et al.* 1997		Bilateral		Bilateral	R,thalamus caudate	Bilateral
Pledge	Bookheimer *et al.* 2000	L	L	L	Bilateral L > R		R
Prose narrative		L	L		L		
Covert singing	Riecker *et al.* 2000	R			R		L
Overt singing	Riecker *et al.* 2000	Bilateral R > L		R	Bilateral R > L		Bilateral L > R

R, right; L, left

studies on brain activation during speech and related non-speech tasks such as breathing and tongue wagging. Studies were selected for this summary primarily if they used two or more orofacial or speaking tasks and imaged two or more speech-related cortical or subcortical regions. Table 13.1 is by no means exhaustive of the relevant literature, but it is representative. It can be seen that bilateral activation is common across tasks and brain structures, but there is a general pattern of brain activation for speech in which cerebral and basal ganglia activity is predominantly on the left and cerebellar activity is mostly right-sided. In contrast, the general pattern for singing is one of predominantly right activation for the cerebrum and basal ganglia, and predominantly left activation for the cerebellum. This opposing pattern of neural organization between speaking and singing can help to explain non-parallel deficits in these behaviors in some individuals with neurologic disease or damage.

Although the muscles of speech production are commonly regarded as axial or midline, lateralization is easily demonstrated, for example, by transcranial magnetic stimulation of the primary motor cortex of the lips (Liscic and Zidar 1998), tongue (Muellbacher *et al.* 2001), and jaw (Butler *et al.* 2001). The contralateral pathway is prepotent, but the ipsilateral pathway cannot be neglected, especially in its potential to compensate for damage to the contralateral projections. The dominance of the contralateral corticobulbar pathway has a rather subtle manifestation in the form of oral asymmetries during speech production in healthy subjects (Hausmann *et al.* 1998). This normal asymmetry, which appears to be gender and task dependent, should be recognized when considering minor asymmetries in clinical populations.

Compartmentalization

The use of neuroimaging procedures such as positron emission tomography (PET), electromyography (EMG), and functional magnetic resonance imaging (fMRI) have added much to the understanding of the neural control of speech, but there are inconsistencies and ambiguities regarding the roles of several structures. At the cortical level, the structures most consistently activated in speech production are Broca's area (especially for complicated tasks), insula, supplementary motor area, premotor cortex, and orofacial motor cortex. Subcortical structures involved in speech production are similar to these involved in motor control generally: thalamus, basal ganglia, cerebellum, and the motor nuclei of the cranial and spinal nerves. It is beyond the scope of this chapter to consider in detail the various proposals that have been made for the neural network of speech motor control, and the reader is referred to recent papers by Ackerman *et al.* (2004), Jurgens (2002), and Kent *et al.* (2000b, 2001). The following summary identifies the major structures along with hypotheses concerning their roles in speech motor control.

One way of identifying the critical components of the neural control network for speech is to consider the lesions of the nervous system that lead to isolated or pure dysarthria. These cases, although rare, provide an opportunity to identify neural lesions that are apparently restricted to the control pathway for speech. The responsible lesions are distributed along a pathway that includes the cerebral cortex, corona radiata, internal capsule, basal ganglia, and pons (Kent *et al.* 2001) This pathway is complemented by a number of other structures, especially the cerebellum and the basal ganglia.

The cerebral cortex is usually thought to be the site of motor programming for speech, and it appears that major areas contributing to this role are the insula, lateral premotor cortex, supplementary motor area, and Broca's area. Only rather recently has the insula been recognized as having an important role in speech production. The insula is multiply connected with other structures, including regions that serve auditory (superior temporal sulcus) and motor (lateral premotor cortex, supplementary motor area) functions in speech. Wise *et al.* (1999) concluded that the articulatory plan is formulated in the left anterior insula and lateral premotor cortex. By virtue of its connections with the insula, the supplementary motor area may initiate and control sequential movement plans that activate muscle-specific regions of primary motor cortex. It is also possible that the supplementary motor area is involved in the retrieval of information from an articulatory buffer, perhaps the insula. The role of Broca's area is under reconsideration, especially because neuroimaging studies have shown that is not consistently activated in a variety of speaking tasks, as would be the case if it is a motor programming center for speech. Broca's area is activated especially for tasks that require analysis of hierarchical structure (e.g. sentences) or complex sequences (e.g. extracting and manipulating phonetic segments). Broca's area is only minimally activated in the production of single words, which may mean that isolated words are controlled through automatized motor plans that do not rely on this cortical area. Interestingly, it has been proposed that Broca's area is the location of a 'mirror system' that matches observation and execution of gestures (Rizzolatti and Arbib 1998). Skoyles (1998) proposed that speech phones are a 'replication code' between auditory stimuli and speech motor patterns. By this reasoning, Broca's area selects gestures that match or replicate gestures that are seen, heard, or both. Information from these cortical areas is sent to the primay motor cortex, which selects the activation of individual muscles in accord with the motor plan.

Given that lesions to the cerebellum and basal ganglia result in dysarthria, it is clear that these structures participate in the neural control of speech, probably in ways similar to their involvement in skeletal motor control. The cerebellum has several cortical connections, and one of its roles may be to insure that speech movements are performed with requisite precision, using various forms of sensory information. Evidence also indicates that the cerebellum is a primary neural site for a time computation used by sensory, motor, and cognitive systems. This time computation may be a modular function, which is consistent with recently expanded interpretations of cerebellar function. The basal ganglia also participate in sensory and motor processing, perhaps by preparing sensory templates that guide movement execution. Much recent attention has been given to the idea that internal models guide the control of speech movements, and both the cerebellum and basal ganglia could contribute to the formation and revision of such models.

Motor speech disorders in adults

The motor speech disorders appearing in adults as acquired conditions are of two major types, dysarthria and apraxia of speech (also known as verbal apraxia or dyspraxia). Dysarthria is a disorder of speech associated with lesions to the central nervous system, peripheral nervous system, or both, and is typically accompanied by motor signs of weakness, paralysis, or incoordination. The acquired dysarthrias in adults are subclassified into seven major types identified through their auditory-perceptual features and interpreted in terms of classical neurology (Darley *et al.* 1969a,b). Apraxia of speech is more controversial in its definition, especially because descriptions of the disorder often emphasize either phonological or motoric aspects. Duffy (1995) defines apraxia of speech as 'a neurogenic speech disorder resulting from impairment of the capacity to program sensorimotor commands for the positioning and movement of muscles for the volitional production of speech' (Duffy 1995, p. 5). He goes on to state that this disorder 'can occur without significant weakness or neuro-muscular slowness, and in the absence of disturbances of conscious thought or language' (Duffy 1995, p. 5). With some risk of oversimplification, dysarthria can be considered a disorder of motor execution (with an essentially intact motor program) and apraxia of speech a disorder of motor programming or sequencing (with an essentially intact motor execution).

Other terms have been used in reference to motor disorders of speech (e.g. anarthria, aphemia, phonetic disintegration, mutism). However, with the exception of mutism, these terms are not used as often or as consistently, at least in the United States, as are the terms dysarthria and apraxia of speech.

Dysarthria

Dysarthria is identified and described primarily through auditory-perceptual methods, although acoustic and physiologic studies are increasingly important in recent research. The seminal work of Darley *et al.* (1969a,b) identified the seven perceptual types of dysarthria summarized in Table 13.2. This table is much simplified from the original descriptions which used 38 perceptual dimensions to characterize the speech disorder. Table 13.2 shows the perceptual dimensions that ranked in approximately the top 10 (most severe) of judged abnormality for each dysarthria type. These dimensions represent the most salient abnormal features, although they are not necessarily equally useful in differential diagnosis. All seven perceptual types of dysarthria are associated with monotone, harsh voice, and imprecise consonants, and most of them also have the attribute of monoloudness. The other features listed in the table are not as uniform in their occurrence across dysarthria types and these hold value for differential diagnosis. These perceptual types do not necessarily occur in isolation, and it is often the case that an individual patient will be described as having a mixed dysarthria or an undetermined form of dysarthria. In addition, some additional types have been suggested that were not included in Darley's classification; these include unilateral upper motor neuron dysarthria and rhythmic hyperkinetic (tremulous) dysarthria.

Darley and coworkers concluded that the nature of the speech disorder was consistent with classical neurologic descriptions of the pertinent disease (in their words, 'Speech follows neurology'). Although this statement may be generally true, it has sometimes been difficult to confirm the hypothesized pathophysiology with

Table 13.2 Classification of dysarthria types by the most severely abnormal features

	Ataxic	Flaccid	Hypo-kinetic	Hyper-kinetic, chorea	Hyper-kinetic, dystonia	Spastic	Spastic-flaccid (ALS)
Monopitch	X	X	X	X	X	X	X
Harsh voice	X	X	X	X	X	X	X
Imprecise consonants	X	X	X	X	X	X	X
Monoloud	X	X	X		X	X	X
Distorted vowels	X			X	X		
Slow rate	X					X	X
Short phrases		X				X	X
Hypernasal		X				X	X
Prolonged intervals	X			X			X
Low pitch			X			X	X
Inappropriate silences			X	X	X		
Variable rate			X	X			
Breathy voice		X	X				
Strain-strangled voice					X	X	
Irregular breakdowns	X				X		
Excess and equal stress	X						X
Reduced stress			X				
Short rushes			X				

Based on data reported by Darley *et al*. 1969a,b.

physiological methods (Kent and Rosen, 2004). Possibly, this difficulty reflects differences in the neuromotor regulation of speech and non-speech behaviors. This is not to say that neurologic observations of non-speech motor systems have no bearing on the understanding of neurogenic speech disorders, but rather that the relationship is more complicated than was once thought. The relationship between dysarthria type and neurologic lesion or disease is summarized in Table 13.3 (following Darley *et al.* 1969a,b).

The functional disturbances and pathophysiology associated with a particular type of dysarthria (whether classified by auditory–perceptual features or by etiology) can vary with age and gender. An age–gender interaction is not surprising, given that the anatomy and physiology of speech production is sexually dimorphic and that the effects of aging can be gender dependent. Gender differences have been described for the dysarthrias associated with Parkinson's disease, cerebellar disease, and amyotrophic lateral sclerosis among others (Kent *et al.* 1992, 1998, 2000a; Hertrich *et al.* 1998; Luschei *et al.* 1999; Stelzig *et al.* 1999; Holmes *et al.* 2000).

Apraxia of speech

Apraxia of speech has been variously described as a lexical disorder, phonologic disorder, motor disorder, combined phonologic–motor disorder, and even as a misleading and inappropriate term (Ballard *et al.* 2001; Rosenbek 2001; Varley and Whiteside 2001). Presumably, apraxia of speech is an isolated disorder of speech production in which the sequencing or patterning of movements is impaired, in the absence of motoric deficiencies in non-speech movements performed by the same musculature. However, this description may be modified in view of reports showing that the speech impairment is accompanied by impairments of non-speech movements of the oral structures (Ballard *et al.* 2000). The responsible lesion is nearly always in the language-dominant hemisphere, especially in the frontal or parietal lobes, and more

Table 13.3 Clinico-anatomic relationships in dysarthria

Type of dysarthria	Typical lesion(s) and selected associated diseases
Ataxic	Damage to the cerebellum or its outflow tracts.
Flaccid	Damage to the motor neuron.
Hypokinetic	Damage to nigrostriatal pathway
Hyperkinetic (chorea)	Damage to basal ganglia.
Hyperkinetic (dystonia)	Damage to basal ganglia
Spastic	Bilateral damage to the pyramidal motor system.
Spastic-flaccid	Damage to pyramidal tract and ventral horn of spinal cord; upper and lower motor neuron damage

rarely in subcortical regions (Duffy 1995). Cortical lesions have been identified in Broca's area, supplementary motor area, parietal cortex, and the insula, but no one of these is invariably involved. Possibly, the condition results from damage to a cortical network that is specialized for the planning of complex sequential movements related to linguistic structure. This network would include Broca's area and the supplementary motor area in the frontal lobe, sensory association areas in the parietal lobe, and the insula (especially anterior part) in the parietal–temporal junction. The variable involvement of non-speech movements in apraxia of speech may be attributable to differences in lesion location and size, and perhaps to individual differences in the cortical representation of motor patterns.

Motor speech disorders in children

The research literature on these disorders is not extensive, especially on the subject of childhood dysarthria that is not related to cerebral palsy. This paucity is regrettable, particularly because acquired childhood dysarthria is not necessarily a rare disorder (van Mourik *et al.* 1998). Published studies pertain mostly to dysarthria after cerebellar tumor resection (van Mourik *et al.* 1997, 1998). These studies indicated that cerebellar lesions did not have the same speech consequences in children as in adults, and that the severity of the speech disorder in children did not mirror the motor impairment in the limbs and trunk.

Developmental apraxia of speech (also known as developmental verbal apraxia or childhood apraxia of speech) was first described by Yoss and Darley (1974). This disorder has become controversial, with disagreement on whether the disorder can be distinguished from more general speech impairments in children (Hall *et al.*1993; Ozanne 1995; Davis *et al.* 1998; McCabe *et al.* 1998). Although this question has not been completely resolved, recent articles have focused on characteristics of the disorder that hold potential as diagnostic markers. The characteristics include: limitations in maximum performance tasks (Murdoch *et al.* 1995; Thoonen *et al.* 1997, 1999), distinctive patterns of segmental errors (Groenen *et al.* 1996; Forrest and Morrisette 1999), impaired perception or production of rhyme (Marion *et al.* 1993), and inappropriate patterns of stress (Shriberg *et al.* 1997a,b; Skinder *et al.* 1999). The search for consensus has been frustrated by the small numbers of subjects in most studies and by differences in criteria used in subject selection.

Conclusion

The motor speech disorders are becoming better understood as the classical syndromes are investigated with more sophisticated methods. To be sure, these disorders are challenging for both clinical and research purposes. They are complex disorders that result from a variety of neurologic disturbances and that can affect a widely distributed muscular system.

References

Ackermann H, Riecker A, Wildgruber D (2004). Cerebral organization of speech motor control. In B Maassen, W Hultsijn, RD Kent, HFM Peters, PHMM van Lieshout, (ed.) *Speech Motor Control in Normal and Disordered Speech*, pp. 85–121. Oxford: Oxford University Press.

Amunts K, Schleicher A, Burgel U, Mohlberg H, Uylings HBM, Zilles K (1999). Broca's region revisited: cytoarchitecture and intersubject variability. *J Comp Neurol*, **412**, 319–41.

Ballard KJ, Granier JP, Robin DA (2000). Understanding the nature of apraxia of speech: theory, analysis, and treatment. *Aphasiology*, **14**, 969–95.

Ballard KJ, Barlow JA, Robin DA (2001). The underlying nature of apraxia of speech: a critical evaluation of Varley and Whiteside's dual route speech encoding hypothesis. *Aphasiology*, **15**, 50–8.

Bookheimer SY, Zeffiro TA, Blaxton TA, Gaillard PW, Theodore WH (2000). Activation of language cortex with automatic speech tasks. *Neurology*, **55**, 1151–7.

Butler SL, Miles TS, Thompson PD, Nordstrom MA (2001). Task-dependent control of human masseter musles from ipsilateral and contralateral motor cortex. *Exp Brain Res*, **137**, 65–70.

Darley FL, Aronson AE, Brown JR (1969a). Differential diagnostic patterns of dysarthria. *J Speech Hear Res*, **12**, 249–69.

Darley FL, Aronson AE, Brown JR (1969b). Clusters of deviant speech dimensions in the dysarthrias. *J Speech Hear Res*, **12**, 462–96.

Davis BL, Jakielski KJ, Marquardt TP (1998). Developmental apraxia of speech-determiners of differential diagnosis. *Clin Linguist Phonet*, **12**, 25–45.

Duffy JR (1995). *Motor Speech Disorders: Substrates, Differential Diagnosis, and Management*. St Louis, MO: Mosby–Year Book.

Fink BR (1986). Complexity. *Science*, **231**, 319.

Forrest K, Morrisette ML (1999). Feature analysis of segmental errors in children with phonological disorders. *J Speech Lang Hear Res*, **42**, 187–94.

Groenen P, Maassen B, Crul T, Thoonen G (1996). The specific relation between perception and production errors for place of articulation in developmental apraxia of speech. *J Speech Hear Res*, **39**, 468–82.

Hall PK, Jordan LS, Robin DA (1993). *Developmental Apraxia of Speech : Theory and Clinical Practice*. Austin, TX, Pro-Ed.

Han YS, Wang J, Fischman DA, Biller HF, Sanders I (1999). Slow tonic muscle fibers in the thyroarytenoid muscles of human vocal folds: a possible specialization for speech. *Anat Rec*, **256**, 146–57.

Harasty J, Double KL, Halliday GM, Kril JJ, McRitchie DA (1997). Language-associated cortical regions are proportionally larger in the female brain. *Arch Neurol*, **54**, 171–6.

Hausmann M, Behrendt-Korbitz S, Kautz H, Lamm C, Radelt F, Gunturkun O (1998). Sex differences in oral asymmetries during word repetition. *Neuropsychologia*, **36**, 1397–1402.

Hertrich I, Spieker S, Ackermann H (1998). Gender-specific phonatory dysfunctions in disorders of the basal ganglia and the cerebellum: acoustic and perceptual characteristics. In W Ziegler, K Deger, (ed.) *Clinical Phonetics and Linguistics*. London: Whurr, 448–457.

Holmes RJ, Oates JM, Phyland DJ, Hughes AJ (2000). Voice characteristics in the progression of Parkinson's disease. *Int J Lang Commun Disord*, **35**, 407–418.

Jurgens U (2002). Neural pathways underlying vocal behavior. *NeurosciBiobehav Rev*, **26**, 235–58.

Kansaku K, Kitazawa S (2001). Imaging studies on sex differences in the lateralization of language. *Neurosci Res*, **41**, 333–7.

Kent RD, Rosen K (2004). Motor control perspectives on motor speech disorders. In B Maassen, W Hultsijn, RD Kent, HFM Peters, PHMM van Lieshout, (ed.) *Speech Motor Control in Normal and Disordered Speech*, pp. 283–311. Oxford: Oxford University Press.

Kent RD, Kent JF, Duffy JR, Weismer G (1998). The dysarthrias : Speech-voice profiles, related dysfunctions and neuropathologies. *J Med Speech-Lang Pathol*, **6**, 165–211.

Kent RD, Kent JF, Duffy JR, Thomas JE, Weismer G, Stuntebeck S (2000a). Ataxic dysarthria. *J Speech Lang Hear Res*, **43**, 1275–89.

Kent RD, Kent JF, Weismer G, Duffy JR (2000b). What dysarthrias can tell us about the neural control of speech. *J Phonet*, **28**, 273–302.

Kent RD, Duffy JR, Slama A, Kent JF, Clift A (2001). Clinico-anatomic studies in dysarthria: A review, critique, and directions for research. *J Speech Lang Hear Res*, **44**, 535–51.

Liscic RM, Zidar J (1998). Functional organization of the facial motor system in man. *Colleg Antropol*, **22**, 545–50.

Lotze M, Seggewies G, Erb M, Grodd W, Birbaumer N (2000). The representation of articulation in the primary sensorimotor cortex. *NeuroReport*, **11**, 2958–89.

Luschei ES, Ramig LO, Baker KL, Smith ME (1999). Discharge characteristics of laryngeal single motor units during phonation in young and older adults and in persons with parkinson disease. *J Neurophysiol*, **81**, 2131–9.

McCabe P, Rosenthal JB, McLeod S (1998). Features of developmental dyspraxia in the general speech-impaired population. *Clin Linguist Phonet*, **12**, 105–26.

McComas AJ (1998). Oro-facial muscles: internal structure, function and ageing. *Gerodontology*, **15**, 3–14.

Marion M, Sussman H, Marquardt T (1993). The perception and production of rhyme in normal and developmentally apraxic children. *J Commun Disord*, **26**, 129–60.

Mu L, Sanders I (2001). Neuromuscular compartments and fiber-type regionalization in the human pharyngeal constrictor muscle. *Anat Rec*, **264**, 367–77.

Muellbacher W, Boroojerdi B, Ziemannu, Hallett M (2001). Analogous corticocortical inhibition and facilitation in ipsilateral and contralateral human motor cortex representations of the tongue. *Clin Neurophysiol*, **18**, 550–8.

Murdoch BE, Attard MD, Ozanne AE, Stokes PD (1995). Impaired tongue strength and endurance in developmental verbal apraxia: a physiologic analysis. *Eur J Disord Commun*, **30**, 51–64.

Murphy K, Corfield DR, Guz A, Fink GR, Wise RJ, Harrison J, *et al.* (1997). Cerebral areas associated with motor control of speech in humans. *J Appl Physiol*, **83**, 1438–47.

Ozanne A (1995). The search for developmental verbal dyspraxia. In B Dodd (ed.), *Differential Diagnosis and Treatment of Children with Speech Disorder*, 91–109. San Diego, CA: Singular Publishing Group.

Porter JD, Khanna S, Kaminski MJ, Rao JS, Merriam AP, Richmonds CR, *et al.* (2001). Extraocular muscle is defined by a fundamentally distinct gene expression profile. *Proc Natl Acad Sci USA*, **98**, 12062–7.

Raichle ME (1996). What words are telling us about the brain. *Cold Spring Harb Symp Quant Biol*, **59**, 9–14.

Riecker A, Ackermann H, Wildgruber D, Dogil G, Grodd W (2000). Opposite hemispheric lateralization effects during speaking and singing at motor cortex, insula and cerebellum. *NeuroReport*, **11**, 1997–2000.

Rizzolatti G, Arbib MA (1998). Language within our grasp. *Trends Neurosci*, **21**, 188–94.

Robichon R, Giraud K, Berbon M, Habib, M. (1999). Sexual dimorphism in anterior speech regions: an MRI study of cortical asymmetry and callosal size. *Brain Cogn*, **40**, 241–6.

Rosenbek JC (2001). Darley and apraxia of speech in adults. *Aphasiology*, **15**, 261–73.

Sciote JJ, Morris TJ, Brandon CA, Horton MJ, Rosen C (2002). Unloaded shortening velocity and myosin heavy chain variations in human laryngeal muscles. *Ann Otol Rhinol Laryngol*, **111**, 120–7.

Shergill SS, Bullmore ET, Brammer MJ, Williams SCR, Murray RM, McGuire PK (2001). A functional study of auditory verbal imagery. *Psychol Med*, **31**, 241–53.

Shriberg LD, Aram DM, Kwiatkowski J (1997a). Developmental apraxia of speech: II. Toward a diagnostic marker. *J Speech Lang Hear Res*, **40**, 286–312.

Shriberg LD, Aram DM, Kwiatkowski J (1997b). Developmental apraxia of speech: III. A subtype marked by inappropriate stress. *J Speech Lang Hear Res*, **40**, 313–37.

Shuler CF, Dalrymple KR (2001). Molecular regulation of tongue and craniofacial muscle differentiation. *Crit Rev Oral Biol Med*, **12**, 3–17.

Skinder A, Strand EA, Mignerey M (1999). Perceptual and acoustic analysis of lexical and sentential stress in children with developmental apraxia of speech. *J Med Speech-Lang Pathol*, **7**, 133–44.

Skoyles JR (1998). Speech phones are a replication code. *Med Hypotheses*, **50**, 167–73.

Sokoloff AJ (2000). Localization and contractile properties of intrinsic longitudinal motor units of the rat tongue. *J Neurophysiol*, **84**, 827–35.

Thoonen G, Maassen B, Gabreels F, Schreuder R, de Swart B (1997). Towards a standardised assessment procedure for developmental apraxia of speech. *Eur J Disord Commun*, **32**, 37–60.

Thoonen G, Maassen B, Gabreels F, Schreuder R (1999). Validity of maximum performance tasks to diagnose motor speech disorders in children. *Clin Linguist Phonet*, **13**, 1–23.

van Mourik M, Catsman-Berrevoets CE, Paquier PF, Yousef-Bak E, van Dongen HR (1997). Acquired childhood dysarthria—review of its clinical presentation. *Pediatr Neurol*, **17**, 299–307.

van Mourik M, Catsman-Berrevoets CE, Yousef-Bak E, Paquier PF, van Dongen HR (1998). Dysarthria in children with cerebellar or brainstem tumors. *Pediatr Neurol*, **18**, 411–14.

Varley R, Whiteside SP (2001). What is the underlying impairment in acquired apraxia of speech? *Aphasiology*, **15**, 39–49.

Vikingstad EM, George KP, Johnson AF, Cao Y (2000). Cortical language lateralization in right handed normal subjects using functional magnetic resonance imaging. *J Neurol Sci*, **175**, 17–27.

Weijs WA (1997). Masticatory muscles. Part II. Functional properties of the masticatory muscle fibers. *Ned Tijdschr Tandheelkde*, **104**, 210–13 (in Dutch).

Wise RJS, Greene J, Buchel C, Scott SK (1999). Brain regions involved in articulation. *Lancet*, **353**, 1057–61.

Yoss KA, Darley FL (1974). Developmental apraxia of speech in children with defective articulation. *J Speech Hear Res*, **17**, 399–416.

Chapter 14

Disorders of body schema

Patrick Haggard and Daniel M. Wolpert

Introduction

The brain contains multiple representations of the body. First, afferent inputs from the skin and proprioceptive receptors project to maps of the body surface and body segments, respectively, in the primary somatosensory cortex (Penfield and Rasmussen 1950). These somatotopic maps reflect the distribution of sensory receptors within the body and underpin somatic sensation (Romo *et al.* 1998). For example, area 3b contains a distorted 'homunculus', with enlarged lips and hands. Neuroanatomical, neuropsychological, and neurophysiological evidence all suggest that this primary information is further processed to construct higher-order, more cognitive representations of the body. These representations differ from primary maps in providing a supramodal coherent scheme for body representation and skilled action. These higher-order representations form the focus of this chapter.

At the cognitive level, a fundamental distinction can be made between two different higher-order body representations which have been called body schema and body image (Paillard 1999). Body schema refers to a representation of the positions of body parts in space, which is updated during body movement. This typically does not enter into awareness, and is primarily used for spatial organization of action. Therefore the body schema is a central representation of the body's spatial properties, including the length of limb segments, their hierarchical arrangement, the configuration of the segments in space, and the shape of the body surface.

Body image refers to a conscious visual representation of the way the body appears from the outside, typically in a canonical position. The scientific concept corresponds roughly to the everyday use of the term. This chapter is not primarily concerned with body image, since there is little evidence of any special connection between disorders of body image (e.g. in anorexia) and movement control. We will not discuss pure disorders of body image, but we will discuss the many cases where abnormalities of body schema lead to altered body image.

Sir Henry Head first introduced the term body schema in discussing disordered spatial representation of the body following parietal lobe damage (Head and Holmes 1911). His original description covers many different aspects of sensorimotor function, but has at its core the representation in the brain of 'organized models of ourselves'

(Head and Holmes 1911, p.189). Moreover, the term 'schema' has other uses in cognitive science. Therefore we prefer the more neutral term body scheme. By this, we mean a neural representation of the body used for spatial sensorimotor processing. We exclude representations for primary sensory input and motor execution. In this chapter we first define the body scheme by describing several properties based on research with normal human and animal subjects. Then, we show how various neurological and neuropsychological conditions can be explained as pathologies of the body scheme.

Properties of the body scheme

Human and animal studies have consistently shown the following seven fundamental properties of body representation.

Spatially coded

The body scheme represents the position and configuration of the body as a volumetric object in space. Crucially, the body scheme integrates tactile information from the body surface with proprioceptive information about the configuration of the limbs in space (Head and Holmes 1911). This integration means that a stimulus on the body can be localized in external space. For example, combining a tactile sensation on the left hand with information about the joint angles of my left arm allows me to program a rapid movement of my right arm to swat a fly. Thus tactile sensations are obligatorily transformed from body surface locations to locations in external space, suggesting that body scheme representations dominate primary representations in normal human behaviour (Yamamoto and Kitazawa 2001). For example, a visual stimulus on the right side facilitates processing of a subsequent tactile stimulus on whichever hand is adjacent to the visual event. In a normal posture, the right hand shows this facilitation, but if the hands are crossed then the left hand shows a comparable benefit (Spence *et al.* 2000).

Modular

Body postures might, in principle, be stored as individual entries in a database, with each entry describing the entire body configuration and body surface stimuli. However, the evidence suggests that the brain represents different body parts in different neural modules, using the resulting modular network to represent all postures.

Therefore the body scheme comprises body parts or segments which bear spatial and categorical relations to each other (e.g. fingers are elements of hands, which form the ends of arms) (Tessari and Rumiati 2002). For example, Reed and Farah (1995) investigated the effects of moving the legs or arms on visual perceptual judgments. They found facilitation effects for judgements about visual body stimuli, but not for non-body stimuli. These effects were further specific to the body part that the observer was actively controlling, suggesting a division between upper and lower body within the body scheme.

Updated with movement

Any body representation which is used for action must continuously track the positions of our body parts as we move. Head's definition of the body scheme emphasized automatic updating of the positions of body parts in space during voluntary movement: 'every new posture or movement is recorded on this plastic schema, and the activity of the cortex brings every fresh group of sensations evoked by altered posture into relation with it' (Head and Holmes 1911, p.187). The updating process may underlie the finding that the visual receptive fields of many parietal neurons follow the hand when the hand moves (Graziano and Gross 1993). This mechanism would allow the body scheme to modulate perceptual processing of objects according to their position in peripersonal space. This would be essential for control of grasping or avoidance movement.

Adaptable

The body scheme must adapt to allow for gradual changes in the spatial properties of the body. For example, the absolute and relative sizes of body parts change over the lifespan. In addition, the body scheme can change on a shorter timescale to incorporate additional objects as new segments of the body representation. In tool use, for example, visual receptive fields of bimodal neurons previously linked to hand position may move towards the tip of the tool, or towards the visual representation of the tool on a video monitor (Iriki *et al.* 1996, 2001). These plastic changes may occur as gradual extensions to an existing scheme, or as rapid switches between several alternative coexisting schemes (Braun *et al.* 2001).

Supramodal

The body scheme receives multiple sensory inputs. By definition, the body scheme integrates body surface information and proprioception to describe the body as a volumetric object in external space. In addition, however, visual information can be in the same representation. Thus a visual stimulus and a tactile stimulus at the same location on the body surface may form a joint representation within the body scheme (Rorden *et al.* 1999). This may involve transforming primary representations of vision, proprioception, and touch either into a single sensory modality or into an abstract amodal code (Lackner 1988).

Coherent

The brain maintains a coherent spatial organization of the body scheme across space and time. This ensures a continuity of body experience which may play a major role in individual self-consciousness. A basic principle of body scheme coherence is the resolution of intersensory discrepancies. For example, the visual and proprioceptive representations of hand position each have characteristic biases and variabilities, yet we perceive our hand in a single location because the brain optimally combines these sources of information (van Beers *et al.* 2002). These discrepancies can be exaggerated by experimental manipulations which put the modalities into stark conflict. For example, if the forearm is held at a fixed extension angle and the biceps tendon vibrated an illusory extension of the forearm is experienced. If a blindfolded subject holds his nose during this procedure, the nose is perceived to grow in length as the forearm is felt to extend. In this case, the proprioceptive information from the arm, and the tactile information about the contact between the fingers and nose, are preserved and made coherent by adapting the perceived size of another body part (the nose). Thus the overall coherence of the body scheme is preserved by altering the representation of a single body segment (Lackner 1988).

Interpersonal

A common body scheme is used to represent both one's own body and the bodies of others. For example, Reed and Farah (1995) showed that participants could better perceive changes in a model's body posture if they simultaneously moved their own corresponding body part. In a related experiment, Tessari and Rumiati (2002) found that memory for observed actions was facilitated when subjects concurrently moved the congruent body part, but not an incongruent body part. These results imply that the observed and self-generated actions were co-represented within a single modular body scheme. An interpersonal function necessarily implies a supramodal body scheme, since information about others' bodies is generally visual, while information from one's own body is generally tactile or proprioceptive.

Disorders of body scheme

The conceptual framework described above can be used to classify many of the neurological disorders of body representation. Since each of these disorders has previously been discussed extensively in the literature, we focus on how comparisons across several disorders can clarify the structure of the body scheme in the human brain, rather than on detailed aetiology or presentation. We have classified the disorders according to functional deficits. These disorders typically occur after damage to the parietal lobe, particularly its inferior part. However, the specific neural modules subserving the various properties of the body scheme described above are not clearly understood. In particular, few studies have focused on groups of lesion patients (but see Cutting 1978). Therefore it has been difficult to dissociate the neural modules subserving the different aspects of body scheme. Thus, single case studies suggest that both interpersonal body representation (Bottini *et al.* 2002) and updating of the body scheme with movement (Wolpert *et al.* 1998) may occur after parietal damage. However, the specific of locus of these functions has not been clearly shown. We speculate that group lesion studies in this area would make an important contribution to future research.

Pathologies of sensory input

Deafferentation

The most straightforward pathology of body representation occurs in conditions where sensory input from the body is reduced or absent. Peripheral deafferentation is the best studied of these. Gallagher and Cole (1995) describe IW, who became completely deafferented below the neck for touch and proprioception following a viral illness. Although he was not paralysed, it took him many months to learn to control his movement and to walk. Over time he has achieved a remarkable degree of control which is heavily reliant on visual feedback. This control is achieved at the cost of a large attentional demand. Whereas normal subjects can easily perform motor acts while concentrating on other things, IW finds it hard to perform such dual tasks. He requires constant vision of his body to know where his body parts are and how to move them. This demonstrates the primacy of proprioceptive and tactile inputs within the body scheme. In contrast, blind people can achieve accurate sensorimotor control without such an attentional cost. This contrast suggests that the proprioceptive updating of the body scheme is essentially automatic, while the visual input may be less so. Moreover, the automatic proprioceptive updating is a continuous background process: IW's movements becomes increasingly inaccurate in the absence of vision of his body.

Pathologies of bodily spatial organization

Studies of patients with central lesions have shown that the brain circuits for localization of a stimulus on the body surface are separate from those involved in processing tactile form. Thus patients may be able to perceive a tactile stimulus while not correctly locating it, or may be able to locate it without being able to describe it (Paillard 1999). These dissociations have been taken as evidence for separate pathways for 'what' and 'where' processing in tactile perception. However, they have additional implications for body representation. In particular, patients with somatosensory lesions may show changes in the implied spatial organization of the body. Rapp *et al.* (2002) asked patients to report where on the hand they had just been touched. The resulting map of localization errors revealed a systematic distortion of the normal hand shape. Although the patients can detect the tactile stimuli, they have a distorted representation of the body surface, perhaps reflecting changes in neural somatosensory maps induced by the lesion.

Macrosomatognosias and microsomatognosias

Spatial distortions of body size may also occur as a result of specific psychiatric and neural conditions. These are classified as macrosomatognosias or microsomato-gnosias, according to whether subjective body size is increased or decreased. They are typically tested by asking the patient to draw themselves, or match their own body to a visual image. Microsomatognosias typically present as a general underestimation of whole-body size, and may belong more properly in a discussion of body image (Leker *et al.* 1996). In contrast, macrosomatognosias can be specific to some body parts, and therefore may reflect a distortion of an underlying neural representation of the body. Migraine aura has been associated with an increase in the perceived size of the hands and face (Podoll and Robinson 2000). This body-part-specific effect is consistent with human experimental work in which anaesthetizing the thumb induced a perceived enlargement of both the thumb and its primary somatosensory neighbour, the lips (Gandevia and Phegan 1999). Interestingly, the inverse pattern is seen in some psychotic patients. Their somatic delusions may overestimate the size of midline structures, notably the trunk, genitals, and head (Hay 1970). These conditions suggest that the processing chain between primary body surface representation and a higher-level representation of the spatial body configuration can be selectively disrupted. However, the neural site within the processing chain at which these disorders arise is not clear.

Pathologies of segmentation

Autotopagnosia

Autotopagnosia is a disorder of the body scheme typically seen after left parietal lesions. These patients make mislocalization errors when asked to point to specific body parts. The pattern of errors generally implies confusion between adjacent body parts (e.g. pointing to shoulder when asked to point to the elbow). Thus the relative positions of body parts appear disorganized. The disorder involves a higher-level cognitive body scheme rather than a primary sensorimotor representation, because localization on both the patient's own body and on other bodies may be affected (Sirigu *et al.* 1991). Moreover, naming of body parts pointed to by the examiner may be preserved (Ogden 1985). Taken together, these findings suggest that knowledge about body part categories is preserved, but that the position of these categorical elements within the overall spatial organization of the body is lost. The spatial unity of the body is incorrectly segmented into its modular parts.

Finger agnosia

Finger agnosia is a somewhat similar disorder which specifically affects finger segmentation. Like autotopagnosia, it is associated with lesions of the left parietal lobe, and more specifically with the angular gyrus (Kinsbourne and Warrington 1962). When the examiner touches one of the patient's fingers in the absence of vision, the patient is unable to identify which one is touched. The primary deficit appears to involve individuating the fingers; it is as if the patient's fingers become collectively fused and undifferentiated. Because finger agnosia can be found without autotopagnosia for other body parts, the concept of a distinct 'finger schema' has been proposed (Benton 1959). The important evolutionary changes in primate finger dexterity may have driven evolution of a separate abstract representation of the digits. A developmental literature has focused on Gerstmann's syndrome, in which finger agnosia may coexist with a range of deficits including dyscalculia, left–right confusion, and agraphia (Gerstmann 1942). The association with arithmetic suggests that the modular nature of body representations may be an important precursor of categorical and symbolic representations in general.

Pathologies of extent

Phantom limb

When all or part of a limb is amputated many patients still feel its presence (Ramachandran and Hirstein 1998). Stimulation of the skin on areas such as the face can even cause sensation in a phantom (Ramachandra *et al.* 1992; Aglioti *et al.* 1997; Kew *et al.* 1997). This is thought to arise from the reorganization of the deafferented region of the cortex after amputation. This marked neural plasticity means that other parts of the body surface project to a cortical area that previously represented the phantom limb.

More strikingly, patients may feel they can move their phantom immediately after amputation, but lose this ability over time (Ramachandran 1993). The ability to move the phantom voluntarily may rely on efferent signals that normally update the body scheme (Wolpert *et al.* 1995). An efferent copy of motor commands may be processed normally and used to estimate and update the configuration of the limb. This efferent signal is sufficient to cause the sensation of movement in the phantom. This demonstrates that efferent commands can contribute to the body scheme. However, this percept based on the efferent command is not corroborated by appropriate sensory feedback from the limb. As the body scheme is adaptable, over time the system may learn that the efferent commands are ineffective. Such adaptation could explain why, as the efferent signal no longer predicts a change in configuration, patients eventually come to feel that the phantom is 'paralysed'. However, if the patient is given visual feedback via a mirror box suggesting that the efferent command does move the phantom, this rapidly leads to the perception that they are now able to move the phantom limb again (Ramachandran and Rogers-Ramachandran 1996).

Pathology of updating

Supernumerary limbs

Whereas phantom patients must adapt the body scheme to reflect loss of a limb, some patients report experiencing supernumerary limbs (Vuilleumier *et al.* 1997). Hari *et al.* (1998) reported a patient with congenital abnormality of the corpus callosum who suffered a subarachnoid haemorrhage leading to an infarction in the right frontal lobe, including damage to the most anterior region of the right supplementary motor area. This patient experienced an additional left arm that occupied the position vacated by the real left arm a minute or so previously.

Since the estimated position of a limb is based on integrating information from motor commands and sensory feedback (Wolpert *et al.* 1995), a failure to integrate these two sources of information could lead to the experience of two limbs rather than one. In the absence of movement, these two sources of information coincide, and indeed the patient does not experience the ghost limb. However, when she moves her arm, the representation of the estimated position is not updated by the motor commands. Therefore sensory and motor information become discrepant. The normal coherence of the body scheme is lost, and the perceived shape of the body is altered by adding a supernumerary limb to accommodate the discrepancy.

Fading limbs

The inverse situation involves a resting limb fading out of consciousness. Wolpert *et al.* (1998) describe patient PJ, who had a large cyst in the left parietal lobe. She reported that the position and presence of her right limbs faded away over a few seconds if she could not see them. Her experience of a constant tactile stimulus or a weight also faded away, but changes in such sensations could be detected. Slow reaching movements to peripheral targets with the right hand were inaccurate, but reaching movements made at a normal pace were unimpaired. In this case there seemed to be a circumscribed problem with the representation of the current limb position in that it could not be maintained in the absence of changing stimulation.

Pathologies of bodily coherence

Anosognosia

Patients with right-hemisphere damage leading to paralysis (or weakness) on the left side may develop the false belief that there is nothing wrong with the paralysed limb. The motor system in these patients may fail to register discrepancies between the actual and predicted states of the system (Frith *et al.* 2000). These patients perceive their body scheme to be coherent, despite the impairment.

Somatoparaphrenia

In other cases, the patient is clearly aware of the abnormal sensorimotor status of the limb, but the attitude towards the affected limb is clearly abnormal. Such patients often also suffer from neglect, but the relation between the two conditions remain unclear. The patient may have delusions that the affected limb belongs to another person (Bisiach *et al.* 1991) or even to an animal (Halligan *et al.* 1995). The attitude to the exiled limb is generally hostile. These patients present with a quite psychotic account of their deficit, but the delusion is highly specific, being confined to their attitude to the affected limb. The patient does not see any impairment in their own body, but may attribute the deficit to another individual. By reassigning ownership of the limb, the patient may be preserving a coherence of their own body scheme despite the loss of sensation and movement.

Pathologies of interpersonal body representation

Several lines of evidence show that a common neural body scheme is used inter-personally to represent both one's own body and others' bodies. This implies a mapping function linking the codes for specific body parts across people. A patient reported by Bottini *et al.* (2002) showed a tactile neglect that was sensitive to the interpersonal level of body representation. The patient had a profound hemianaesthesia, and in addition a delusional belief that her left hand belonged to her niece. The patient neglected tactile stimuli when asked to respond to touch on her left hand, but reliably detected identical stimuli when asked to respond to touches on her 'niece's hand'. This case appears to demonstrate a complex interplay between primary somatosensory maps and a much more cognitive level of body representation, in which body parts are grouped in a coherent way to be assigned to the 'self' or to another person. Therefore the personal level of body representation may modulate primary tactile processing.

Heterotopagnosia

In some pathological cases, the interpersonal mapping function can be specifically damaged, leaving other aspects of the body scheme, such as its spatial organization, unaffected. Heterotopagnosia, which may follow left parietal damage, offers one example of this interpersonal function, and may be a pure pathology of interpersonal body representation (Degos and Bachoud-Levi 1998). When asked to point to the examiner's own nose, these patients repeatedly point to their own nose. The localization within the body map is correct, but the body representation is transposed from another person to the self. Therefore this disorder seems to involve selective damage to the processing stage at which body parts are assigned to persons.

Conclusion

In this chapter, we have argued from behavioural and neurophysiological data that the human brain contains a cognitive representation of the body. We have shown that this body scheme has the essential properties required for multisensory integration and coordinated sensorimotor action. From an understanding of these normal functions, we have shown that several sensory and motor disorders can be explained by reference to damage to one or more of these essential properties. Interestingly, many disorders of body scheme have both neurological and psychiatric aspects, which suggests that a coherent neural representation of the body is a key element of self-consciousness. Finally, a perhaps surprising but fascinating feature of the brain's body scheme is the commonality between the representation of one's own body and the body of other individuals. This suggests that the body scheme could also form a basis for social cognition.

Acknowledgements

We are grateful to Louise Whiteley for assistance. PH was supported by a Leverhulme Trust Research Fellowship. This work was supported by the Wellcome Trust, ESRC, HFSP, and the McDonnell Foundation.

References

Aglioti S, Smania N, Atzei A, Berlucchi G (1997). Spatio-temporal properties of the pattern of evoked phantom sensations in a left index amputee patient. *Behav Neurosci*, **111**(5), 867–72.

Benton AL (1959). *Right–Left Discrimination and Finger Localization: Development and Pathology*. New York: Hoeber-Harper.

Bisiach E, Rusconi ML, Vallar G (1991). Remission of somatoparaphrenic delusion through vestibular stimulation. *Neuropsychologia*, **29**, 1029–31.

Bottini G, Bisiach E, Sterzi R, Vallar G (2002). Feeling touches in someone else's hand. *NeuroReport*, **13**, 249–52.

Braun C, Heinz U, Schweizer R, Wiech K, Birbaumer N, Topka H (2001). Dynamic organization of the somatosensory cortex induced by motor activity. *Brain*, **125**, 2259–67.

Cutting J (1978) Study of anosognosia. *J Neurol Neurosurg Psychiatry*, **41**, 548–55.

Degos JD, Bachoud-Levi AC (1998). La designation et son objet. Pour une neuropsychologie de l'objectivation. *Rev Neurol (Paris)*, **154**, 283–90.

Frith CD, Blakemore SJ, Wolpert DM (2000). Abnormalities in the awareness and control of action. *Philos Trans R Soc Lond B Biol Sci*, **355**, 1771–88.

Gallagher S, Cole J (1995). Body image and body schema in a deafferented subject. *J Mind Behav*, **16**, 369–89.

Gandevia SC, Phegan CML (1999). Perceptual distortions of the human body image produced by local anaesthesia, pain and cutaneous stimulation. *J Physiol*, **514**, 609–16.

Gerstmann, J (1942). Problem of imperception of disease and of impaired body territories with organic lesions: relation to body scheme and its disorders. *Arch Neurol Psychiatry*, **48**, 890–913.

Graziano MSA, Gross J (1993). A bimodal map of space—somatosensory receptive fields in the macaque putamen with corresponding visual receptive fields. *Exp Brain Res*, **97**, 96–109.

Halligan PW, Marshall JC., Wade DT (1995). Unilateral somatoparaphrenia after right hemisphere stroke: a case description. *Cortex*, **31**, 173–82.

Hari R, Hänninen R, Mäkinen T, Jousmaki V, Forss N, Seppa M, *et al.* (1998). Three hands: fragmentation of human bodily awareness. *Neurosci Lett*, **240**, 131–4.

Hay GG (1970). Dismorphophobia. *Br J Psychiatry*, **533**, 399–406.

Head H, Holmes G (1911). Sensory disturbances in cerebral lesions. *Brain*, **34**, 102–254.

Iriki A, Tanaka M, Iwamura Y (1996). Coding of modified body schema during tool use by macaque postcentral neurons. *NeuroReport*, **7**, 2325–30.

Iriki A, Tanaka M, Obayashi S, Iwamura Y (2001). Self-images in the video monitor coded by monkey intraparietal neurons. *Neurosci Res*, **40**, 163–73.

Kew JJM, Halligan PW, Marshall JC, Passingham RE, Rothwell JC, Ridding MC, *et al.* (1997). Abnormal access of axial vibrotactile input to deafferented somatosensory cortex in human upper limb amputees. *J Neurophysiol*, **77**, 2753–64.

Kinsbourne M, Warrington EK (1962). A study of finger agnosia. *Brain*, **85**, 47–66.

Lackner JR (1988). Some proprioceptive influences on the perceptual representation of body shape and orientation. *Brain*, **111**, 281–97.

Leker RR, Karni A, River Y (1996). Microsomatognosia: whole body schema illusion as part of an epileptic aura. *Acta Neurol Scand*, **94**, 383–5.

Ogden JA (1985). Autotopagnosia: occurrence in a patient without nominal aphasia and with an intact ability to point to parts of animals and objects. *Brain*, **108**, 1009–22.

Paillard J (1999). Body schema and body image—a double dissociation in deafferented patients. In GN Gantchev, S Mori, J Massion, (ed.) *Motor Control: Today and Tomorrow*, pp. 197–214. Sofia, Bulgaria: Academic Publishing House.

Penfield W, Rasmussen TL (1950). *The Cerebral Cortex of Man: A Clinical Study of Localization of Function.* New York: Macmillan.

Podoll K, Robinson D (2000). Macrosomatognosia and microsomatognosia in migraine art. *Acta Neurol Scand*, **101**, 413–16.

Ramachandran VS (1993). Filling in gaps in perception: II. Scotomas and phantom limbs. *Curr Dir Psychol Sci*, **2**, 56–65.

Ramachandran VS, Hirstein W (1998). The perception of phantom limbs: The DO Hebb lecture. *Brain*, **121**, 1603–30.

Ramachandran, VS, Rogers-Ramachandran D (1996). Synaesthesia in phantom limbs induced with mirrors. *Proc R Soc Lond B Biol Sci*, **263**, 377–86.

Ramachandran VS, Stewart M, Rogers-Ramachandran DC (1992). Perceptual correlates of massive cortical reorganization. *NeuroReport*, **3**, 583–6.

Rapp B, Hendel SK, Medina J (2002). Remodeling of somatosensory hand representations following cerebral lesions in humans. *NeuroReport*, **13**, 207–11.

Reed CL, Farah MJ (1995). The psychological reality of the body schema: a test with normal participants, *J Exp Psychol Hum Percept Perform*, **21**, 334–43.

Romo R, Hernandez A, Zainos A, Salinas E (1998). Somatosensory discrimination based on cortical microstimulation. *Nature*, **392**, 387–90.

Rorden C, Heutink J, Greenfield E, Robertson IH (1999). When a rubber hand 'feels' what the real hand cannot. *NeuroReport*, **10**, 135–8.

Sirigu A, Grafman J, Bressler K (1991). Multiple representations contribute to body knowledge processing: evidence from a case of autotopagnosia. *Brain*, **114**, 629–42.

Spence C, Pavani F, Driver J (2000). Crossmodal links between vision and touch in covert endogenous spatial attention. *J Exp Psychol Hum Percept Perform*, **26**, 1298–1319.

Tessari A, Rumiati RI (2002). Motor distal component and pragmatic representation of objects. *Cogn Brain Res*, **14**, 218–27.

van Beers RJ, Wolpert DM, Haggard P (2002). When feeling is more important than seeing in sensorimotor adaptation. *Curr Biol*, **12**, 834–7.

Vuilleumier P, Reverdin A, Landis T (1997). Four legs—illusory reduplication of the lower limbs after bilateral parietal lobe damage. *Arch Neurol*, **54**, 1543–7

Wolpert DM, Ghahramani Z, Jordan MI (1995). An internal model for sensorimotor integration. *Science*, **269**, 1880–2.

Wolpert DM, Goodbody SJ, Husain M (1998). Maintaining internal representations: the role of the human superior parietal lobe. *Nat Neurosci*, **1**, 529–33.

Yamamoto S, Kitazawa S (2001). Reversal of subjective temporal order due to arm crossing. *Nat Neurosci*, **4**, 1265.

Chapter 15

Motor aspects of unilateral neglect and related disorders

Gereon R. Fink and John C. Marshall

Introduction

Many patients who survive brain damage (due to stroke or traumatic brain injury, for example) are left with a variety of cognitive impairments which adversely affect their treatment, management, and subsequent recovery. Unilateral neglect is one such cognitive deficit which severely limits the effectiveness of rehabilitation and curtails many aspects of everyday life (Halligan and Cockburn 1993). Neglect is not a well-defined syndrome but rather a family of different behavioural manifestations characterized by the patient's failure to spontaneously report, respond, or even orient to objects and events in the hemispace contralateral to a brain lesion, and which cannot be attributed to either primary sensory or motor deficits (Heilman *et al.* 1993).

Symptoms of unilateral neglect can be provoked by damage to many brain regions, including thalamus, basal ganglia, white matter, the parahippocampal region, and the frontal, parietal, and temporal cortices (Doricchi and Tomaiuolo 2003). The lesion site most consistently implicated in chronic unilateral spatial neglect is the right temporoparietal junction (Halligan *et al.* 2003; Mort *et al.* 2003). Although many manifestations of neglect can be explained in terms of a failure to attend to or perceive objects located in contralesional space (i.e. perceptual neglect), neuropsychological evidence also suggests that neglect can result from response problems (i.e. disorders of action), which in the neglect literature are often referred to as 'motor' and 'premotor' neglect. Thus, while perceptual neglect is primarily considered a problem of input processing, motor and premotor forms of neglect result from an output problem (Poppelreuter 1917). Accordingly, unilateral neglect is not a unitary disorder; rather, it comprises a number of discrete deficits which may occur conjointly or independently of one another in dissociated forms. Table 15.1 shows a taxonomy of the syndrome according to Vallar (2001), which draws a basic distinction between defective and productive manifestations.

Table 15.1 An interim taxonomy of the clinical syndrome of unilateral spatial neglect (USN)

	Extrapersonal space	**Personal/bodily space**
Defective manifestations		
Dimension	Variety	
Input–output	Perceptual USN[a]	Hemiasomatognosia[b]
	Premotor/intentional USN, directional hypokinesia[c]	Anosognosia[d]
		Motor neglect[e]
Sectors of space (with reference to the body)	Lateral external USN[f]	
	Lateral internal (imaginal) USN	
	Altitudinal[g]	
Reference frames	Egocentric USN[h]	
	Allocentric/object-based USN	
Sensory modality[i]	Visual USN (pseudo-hemianopia)	Somatosensory USN
	Auditory USN	
	Olfactory USN	
Processing domain (material-specific forms of neglect)	Facial USN	
	Neglect dyslexia	
Productive manifestations		
Avoidance[j]		Somatoparaphrenia[k]
Hyper-attention, magnetic attraction (towards ipsilesional targets)		
Perseveration		

[a] Defective awareness of targets in the neglected sector of space.

[b] Defective awareness of the contralesional side of the body.

[c] Defective programming of movements of the ipsilesional limbs toward targets in the neglected contralesional sector of space.

[d] Defective awareness or denial of contralesional motor, somatosensory, and visual half-field deficits.

[e] Failure to move the contralesional limbs, in the absence of primary motor impairment (hemiparesis or hemiplegia).

[f] Along a left–right axis: near, far.

[g] Along a vertical axis: upper, lower.

[h] With reference to the head, trunk, and limbs.

[i] Defective awareness of sensory input in a particular sensory modality.

[j] Active withdrawal from contralesional targets.

[k] Delusional beliefs concerning the contralesional side of the body.

The relationship between spatial cognition and the action system

Liepmann (1908) was one of the first to emphasize the close relationship between spatial cognition and the action system when pointing out that the spatial control of praxis (i.e. what Liepmann referred to as the 'space–time plan') draws upon the left parietal cortex. Lesions of this area can cause a range of disturbed movements (which cannot be explained by primary sensorimotor loss) of both the right and the left arm (henceforth referred to as 'apraxia') (see Chapter 17, this volume). Nearly 100 years later, functional neuroimaging supported Liepmann's conjecture. The integration of temporal and spatial information is a left inferior parietal cortex function (Assmus *et al.* 2003). By contrast, based on his classic case with a large glioma in right occipito-temporo-parietal cortex (extending into the hippocampus) and severe impairments of topographical memory and learning, face recognition, and reading, Hughlings Jackson had conjectured that the 'right posterior lobe' is the 'leading' brain region for 'visual ideation' (Jackson 1876). Balint (1909) described a syndrome where spatial and motor symptoms overlap: Following bilateral posterior parietal lobe damage, patients may show a triad of simultanagnosia (i.e. the patient's field of vision seems to be restricted so that only one object can be attended to at a time), optic ataxia (i.e. the patient cannot point to or grasp an object under direct visual guidance), and ocular apraxia (i.e. the patient's ability to saccade directly to objects is grossly impaired). Although often neglected by the examiner, the patient's ability to attend to left space is usually also impaired in patients suffering from Balint's triad, suggesting the additional presence of spatial neglect.

The issue of the relationship between spatial cognition and the action system is further complicated by reports of dissociations of neglect symptoms depending on the space in which the patient operates: Brain (1941) noted that 'patients with a massive lesion of the right parieto-occipital region exhibit a tendency to neglect the left half of external space and in consequence when following a familiar route to turn to the right instead of the left in error'. Neglect of external space, he argued, resembles 'the amnesia for the left half of the body which may also follow a lesion of the right parietal lobe' (Brain 1941). He also distinguished within 'external' space between near (peripersonal) and far (extrapersonal) space when one of his patients who suffered from a meningioma affecting the right parietal lobe showed an 'inability to localize distant objects' but strikingly was able to 'judge the relative distance of two objects held within a yard of him'. By contrast, another patient suffering from a glioblastoma affecting the right hemisphere showed 'defective localization' that was 'limited to objects within arm's reach'. This double dissociation between near and far space has been replicated using line bisection (Halligan and Marshall 1991; Vuilleumier *et al.* 1998), and neurophysiological data obtained from both the macaque (Rizzolatti *et al.* 1997a) and humans (Weiss *et al.* 2000, 2003; Bjoertomt *et al.* 2002) have shown differential neural mechanisms representing near and far space. Finally, it is important to note that there also exist separate representations of visual space for perception and visually guided behaviour: This provides further evidence that spatial perception, spatial cognition in the service of object perception, and spatial cognition in the service of action need to be differentiated (Bridgeman 1999).

Motor neglect or pure motor negligence

Motor neglect refers to the non-use or diminished spontaneous use of the contralesional but non-hemiplegic hand, arm, or leg despite preserved force and coordination. Crucially, the deficit is in part reversible with visual, sensory, or auditory stimulation by the examiner or, to a certain degree, also by the patient him- or herself when directing attention/volition of the affected limb (Laplane and Degos 1983): Patients need to make an extra voluntary effort to make their affected limb comply with their intentions or the task demands at hand. In the most severe and striking cases, the affected limb may appear paralytic but can be moved readily on command. Likewise, distracting the patient (i.e. drawing away the patient's attention from the limb) may enhance the behavioural deficit: Patients with mild paresis of a leg who can stand or walk may nonetheless fall when their attention is distracted from their walking by, for example, simultaneous manual activity or external distractors. Castaigne *et al.* (1970, 1972) established the following clinical criteria to diagnose motor neglect: absence of paresis, absence of muscle tone changes, absence of pyramidal signs, absence of spontaneous limb movements on the affected side, limb movements of the affected side in response to encouragement by touch, absence of withdrawal of the affected limb from an uncomfortable position, normal sensation, and normal rapid alternating movements.

Motor extinction

A milder form of motor neglect is 'motor extinction', originally described by Critchley (1953). Patients with motor extinction may show unimpaired contralesional hand use in isolation but impaired contralesional hand use during bilateral simultaneous movements. For example, some patients who can move their contralesional limb on its own have difficulty initiating movement of this limb at the same time as they are starting to move the ipsilesional limb (Valenstein and Heilman 1981). The affected arm may not swing normally during walking, and simultaneous movement of the ipsilesional limb may increase the symptoms of motor neglect (Viader *et al.* 1982).

Clinical diagnosis of motor neglect

Motor neglect is comparatively easy to detect by comparing the patient's spontaneous motor behaviour with the results of explicit testing of motor function: it affects the contralesional hand/arm or leg, and the use of the neglected limb may be augmented by the allocation of attention to it (Ghika *et al.* 1998), resembling in this respect the beneficial sensorimotor cueing effects in perceptual neglect (Robertson and North 1992; Robertson and Marshall 1993; Vallar *et al.* 1997; Robertson and Halligan 1999). However, when motor neglect coexists with perceptual neglect and/or a sensory deficit, it may be necessary to resort to the cross-response task originally devised by Watson *et al.* (1978) who studied non-sensory neglect in monkeys. In this task, patients are requested to respond with their ipsilesional arm to a contralesional stimulus and with their contralesional arm to an ipsilesional stimulus. When the patient fails to respond to a contralesional stimulus using the ipsilesional arm, he or she is considered to have perceptual neglect and/or a sensory defect. However, if the patient neither moves the contralesional limb spontaneously nor responds with that limb to an ipsilesional stimulus, then he or she is considered to suffer from motor neglect.

That motor neglect is not the result of a primary sensorimotor deficit or a perceptual problem can also be demonstrated by the use of somatosensory and motor evoked potentials; both electrophysiological tests have been shown to be normal in patients with motor neglect (von Giesen *et al.* 1994). Furthermore, Classen *et al.* (1997) observed a prolonged 'silent period' in the electromyogram of small hand muscles in patients with motor neglect after transcranial magnetic stimulation; the exaggerated inhibition within the primary motor cortex that is structurally intact may constitute a neurophysiological basis underlying motor neglect. A positron emission tomography (PET) study (von Giesen *et al.* 1994) of patients with motor neglect due to subcortical and cortical lesions disclosed widespread depression of regional cerebral glucose metabolism, which exceeded the areas of structural damage. The metabolic abnormalities involved the prefrontal, premotor, cingulate, and parietal cortices, as well as the thalamus, but were restricted to the structurally affected hemisphere. Furthermore, the motor cortical output system was spared from the functional depression, suggesting that an intact output system may be deprived of the voluntary excitation from premotor etc. areas required for movement execution.

Intentional or 'premotor' neglect

More difficult to detect, and hence often neglected by the examiner, is a second type of deficient motor behaviour observed in neglect patients which has also often been called 'motor inattention' or 'premotor' neglect. The condition is characterized by a failure to move the ipsilesional hand, arm, or leg into contralesional space (hemispatial akinesia). Similarly, the patients may fail or be impaired in moving the head or eyes in a contralesional direction (directional akinesia or hypokinesia). The term directional hypokinesia or premotor neglect encompasses a group of manifestations resulting from a disorder of action space, including lack of (akinesia) or delayed (hypokinesia) initiation, slow execution (bradykinesia), reduced amplitude (hypometria), and incompleteness or impersistence of motor activity in a specific spatial direction, usually towards the side opposite the brain lesion (Heilman *et al.* 1985, 2000; Bisiach *et al.* 1990, 1995, 1998; Bisiach 1994; Mattingley *et al.* 1994, 1998; Mattingley and Driver 1997). These phenomena are related to the side of space, rather than to the side of the body. That is, they are apparent even when the patients perform movements with their ipsilesional (i.e. unaffected) arm. Directional hypokinesia of an arm or leg is often associated with delayed and hypometric (Girotti *et al.* 1983) saccadic eye movements to contralesional hemispace, and the pattern of visual search is shifted to the ipsilesional hemispace (Chédru *et al.* 1973; Ishiai *et al.* 1987; Hornak 1992).

Clinical diagnosis of intentional or 'premotor' neglect

In hemispatial hypokinesia, an arm that fails to move into or exhibits decreased movements in contralesional space will move better in the ipsilesional hemispace (Chédru *et al.* 1973; Meador *et al.* 1986, 2000; Ishiai *et al.* 1987; Hornak 1992); thus, hemispatial hypokinesia is direction dependent. A bedside test for a directional bias of an arm consists in asking the patient to point (with eyes closed) with the index finger to a point in space perpendicular to his or her sternum (i.e. the midsagittal plane); patients with hemispatial hypokinesia will mispoint towards the ipsilesional side (Heilman *et al.* 1983). A modification of the De Renzi task (De Renzi *et al.* 1970; De Renzi 1982) consists in requesting the blindfolded patient to search with the hand for small objects (e.g. coins) randomly scattered on both hemifields of a table (Heilman 2004). Patients with directional hypokinesia of the arm fail to explore for objects in the contralesional hemispace. To test for hypometria, one can also ask the patient to move a certain distance into ipsi- and contralesional space and then assess whether he or she undershot the distance on the contralesional side. Prior to all these tasks, however, one must make sure that the patient is able to detect the relevant landmarks (coins etc.), i.e. that the patient does not suffer from perceptual neglect. For example, when a patient is asked to saccade to a target, first of all one needs to ensure that the patient is aware of the target (e.g. by reporting its presence verbally). Only thereafter can the fact that the patient takes multiple small saccades to reach the target be taken as evidence for directional hypometria of the eyes (Heilman *et al.* 2000).

Dissociating perceptual and motor components in tasks involving the processing of spatial information for action

To decouple the direction of visual attention from the direction of action in space (e.g. a hand movement), other tasks can also be applied. For example, Halligan and Marshall (1989) developed versions of the line bisection task such that one could separate perceptual from motor components of the task. The test devised by Halligan and Marshall (1989) required their patient to bisect horizontal lines displayed on a computer video display unit (VDU). On each trial, the computer mouse was used to indicate where the patient considered the midline (i.e. the transsection mark) to be by moving a marker on the VDU. In the congruent condition (i.e. congruent direction of visual attention and hand movement), the mouse and cursor always moved in the same direction. In the incongruent condition (i.e. incongruent direction of visual attention and hand movement), the mouse and cursor moved in opposite directions. Thus the effects of distinguishing the direction of the motor movement from the perceived visual direction allowed the investigators to assess whether motor problems were playing a role in the bisection error.

The neuroanatomy of motor/intentional neglect

A similar task was used by Bisiach *et al.* (1990) in a group study. In the congruent condition, patients were required to indicate the centre of the line by moving a pointer from either end of the line. In the incongruent condition, the pointer was indirectly moved by pulling a string to which it was fixed. In the latter condition, deviation of the pointer to the left or right was achieved by a hand movement in the opposite direction. The hypothesis underlying the experimental set-up was that in the congruent condition patients with perceptual neglect would demonstrate the usual rightward deviation. Likewise, in the incongruent condition patients with perceptual neglect would show the same directionality and magnitude of error. By contrast, patients with premotor neglect would show the opposite directionality of the error. The predictions were confirmed and lesion analysis showed that patients with premotor neglect had strokes that mainly involved the frontal lobes or basal ganglia (Bisiach *et al.* 1990). These studies have been replicated using mirrors with cancellation tasks (Tegner and Levander 1991) and further variants of the line bisection task in which perceptual judgements of pre-transected lines were compared with the patient's own performance (Marshall and Halligan 1995).

Na *et al.* (1998) confirmed and extended these original studies by using both the line bisection task and a cancellation task on the same patients. Both tasks are frequently used to test for spatial neglect but are considered to tap into different domains of spatial behaviour: rightward bisection error and the omission of targets on the left side of an array correlate poorly (Halligan and Marshall 1992), and the line bisection task may be more sensitive to perceptual (attentional) disorders, while the cancellation task may be more sensitive to motor (intentional) disorders (Na *et al.* 1998). Na and coworkers confirmed the association of frontal or exclusively subcortical brain lesions with motor (intentional) neglect, and of brain injury outside the frontal region with perceptual (attentional) neglect, thus supporting the argument for an anatomical–functional segregation within the attentional system. However, they also stressed that the designation of perceptual-attentional versus motor-intentional neglect depends, in part, on the specific task demands: among the nine patients in whom an attentional or intentional classification was possible, only six exhibited the same form of neglect with line bisection as they did with cancellation. Another three patients who showed motor-intentional neglect on the line bisection task also showed a predominance of sensory-attentional neglect using the cancellation task.

Taken together, the neurological data demonstrate that some patients with neglect have problems attending to objects in the contralesional space (perceptual neglect), while others have difficulties in their limb- or eye-directed movements towards contralesional space (directional hypokinesia or premotor neglect) or in the use of their contralesional extremities (motor neglect). Lesion analysis suggests that frontal or exclusively subcortical brain structures are associated with motor aspects of neglect, while posterior brain regions are associated with perceptual aspects of neglect. However, such a dichotomy is relative rather than absolute: First, many patients with extensive lesions within the territory of the middle cerebral artery often show both perceptual and motor aspects of neglect. Secondly, Mattingley and coworkers clearly demonstrated a specific motor initiation deficit with a delayed initiation of leftward movements to targets in left hemispace in patients with inferior parietal lobe lesions (Mattingley *et al.* 1998; see also Heilman *et al.* 1985). This impairment was observed in addition to the patients' perceptual difficulties. The latter finding is further evidence for the notion that the human posterior parietal cortex acts as a sensorimotor interface for visual, tactile, and auditory information (Bremmer *et al.* 2001b; Grefkes *et al.* 2002), rather than having exclusively perceptual functions. Also, one should keep in mind the extensive anatomical connections between the human posterior parietal cortex and premotor cortex (Doricchi and Tomaiuolo 2003).

Neural mechanisms underlying motor aspects of neglect

The neural mechanisms underlying the diverse motor aspects of neglect are still under debate. Divergent views have stated that neglect may result from a defect of attention (Watson *et al.* 1978), from an arousal–attentional mechanism (Heilman and Valenstein 1979; Heilman *et al.* 2000), or from a neural representation deficit which induces attentional disturbances as secondary phenomena. In all accounts, the damage is typically to the right cerebral hemisphere (Rizzolatti and Berti 1990; Rizzolatti *et al.* 1997b; Bisiach and Vallar 2000). Based on anatomical and clinical studies, Mesulam (1981,1990, 1994) proposed the broader conception that the diverse manifestations of hemineglect result from a disruption of a large-scale cognitive network subserving directed attention. This network is made up essentially of three distinct but interacting representations of the extrapersonal world. According to this model, the perceptual representation is centred upon the posterior parietal cortex but also involves other sensory association areas and the thalamus (in particular the pulvinar and lateroposterior nuclei). The motor representation lies in the frontal cortex (frontal eye field), striatum, and superior colliculus. These areas may contain a motor map for the distribution of orienting and exploratory movements within extrapersonal space. A third representation, perhaps centred on the cingulate cortex, may contain a map for the assessment of expectancy and relevance. Each of these representations is non-specifically activated through the ascending reticular activating system and the intralaminar thalamic nuclei. Since the proposal was originally made, both macaque electrophysiology (Andersen *et al.* 1997, 1998, 1999; Andersen and Buneo 2002) and human functional neuroimaging (Bremmer *et al.* 2001a,b; Fink *et al.* 2003) have demonstrated that the human parietal cortex contains multiple sensory and motor maps in both egocentric and allocentric frames of reference (Vogeley and Fink 2003), which are continuously updated for integrating sensory information for action in space. Furthermore, all these areas maintain extensive interconnections with other cortical and subcortical areas, thus contributing to a network which keeps us appropriately oriented and ready for action in three-dimensional space, according to whichever reference frame is most apt (Marshall and Fink 2001; Pouget and Sejnowski 2001).

Heilman *et al.* (2000) proposed that intentional neglect may result from a lesion-induced reduced capacity of the brain to prepare for and trigger action, and that the process by which the brain evaluates the urgency and order of actions ('intention' to act) would hence be impaired. Failure of this triage (intentional) system would cause an inability to initiate a movement (akinesia) or a delay in the initiation of the movement (hypokinesia) (Heilman *et al.* 2000). Owing to its connectivity, these workers suggested that the dorsolateral frontal lobe would play an important role in intention, consistent with electrophysiological evidence (Boussaoud *et al.* 1996; Boussaoud 2001) for the involvement of premotor and prefrontal areas in movement initiation. To test this putative role of the frontal lobes in intentional neglect, Watson *et al.* (1978) trained monkeys in a cross-response paradigm (described above). In this task, monkeys were trained to respond with their right arm when stimulated on the left and with their left arm when stimulated on the right. Following unilateral dorsolateral frontal lobe lesions, the monkeys responded with their ipsilesional arm to contralesional stimuli but failed to respond to ipsilesional stimuli with their contralesional arm (Watson *et al.* 1978). Because the motor areas were not damaged and there was no evidence of hemiparesis in the animals, the results were taken as evidence that the frontal lobes play a critical role in the intentional systems (Watson *et al.* 1978; Heilman *et al.* 2000). The latter account is consistent with many human neuropsychological studies on premotor neglect (see above).

By contrast, Rizzolatti and Berti (1990) suggested that neglect is basically a representational deficit subsequent to damage to the neural representation(s) of space, which is the final result of the activity of several maps, each processing partial aspects of space in parallel. A coexistent but secondary factor, which frequently aggravates the symptoms, would be the release of circuits controlling motor programmes towards contralateral space. Abnormal activation of these circuits would produce an attentional imbalance between opposite spatial sectors (Kinsbourne 1993).

Nevertheless, the attentional and intentional systems have to be interactive, especially for tasks that involve action in space (e.g. exploration tasks). Furthermore, diverse mechanisms may not only underlie different forms of neglect but also left and right unilateral neglect, given the hemispheric biases for action (left) and spatial cognition (right). Whereas in right-brain-damaged patients there may be a double dissociation between motor disorders and left perceptual neglect, patients with left brain damage and signs of right unilateral perceptual neglect seem to show consistent slowing of rightward-directed movements (Bartolomeo *et al.* 2001). These discrepancies led Bartolomeo and coworkers to speculate that right neglect resulting from left-hemisphere lesions might be related more closely to action-related processing stages. This hypothesis is consistent with the notion of left-hemisphere dominance for action selection, motor preparation, and motor attention.

Motor impersistence

Fisher (1956) introduced the term motor impersistence to describe the inability to sustain a movement or posture such as closing the eyes, protruding the tongue, keeping the mouth open, or keeping an arm extended. When testing for impersistence, the examiner may ask the patient to maintain a posture for a given period of time. Although motor impersistence is frequently observed with bihemispheric or diffuse brain damage, it has also been associated with the right hemisphere (Kertesz *et al.* 1985). Patients with acute right-sided focal stroke lesions showed significantly more signs of motor impersistence than did those with left-sided lesions. The most discriminating tests were eye closure, mouth opening, tongue protrusion, and gaze to the left. In particular, right central and frontal lesions seem to be responsible for motor impersistence, and Kertesz *et al.* (1985) suggested that the phenomenon might be related to mechanisms of directed attention that are necessary to sustain motor activity. Since motor impersistence, like hypokinesia, may also be directional (Kertesz *et al.* 1985) or hemispatial (Roeltgen *et al.* 1989), it is essential to test the patient's ability to maintain motor activation (e.g. eyes towards left or right for a period of 20 s) in the contralesional and ipsilesional direction, as well as to test each limb separately (e.g. keep the arm extended for 20 s) in ipsi- and contralateral space.

If patients successfully sustain a single act, they have to be further evaluated for their capacity to perform two acts simultaneously. If they are unable to do so, they may suffer from simultapraxia, which has been considered a subset of motor impersistence and attributed to right hemispheric lesions involving BA 6 and 8 (Sakai *et al.* 2000).

Defective response inhibition

According to Heilman (2004), defective response inhibition is defined as responding when either no response or a response of the opposite limb is called for. There are three forms of defective response inhibition.

1 Motor (limb or directional) allochiria (Jones 1907) is a defect characterized by a movement of the ipsilesional limb when the correct response would be a movement of the contralesional limb.

2 Hyperkinesia is a term applied to characterize a situation where the contralesional limb moves incorrectly or in an improper contralesional direction when there should either be no movement or the movement should be in an ipsilesional direction.

3 Echopraxia is characterized by the patient imitating the movement or posture performed by the examiner.

Before testing for defective response inhibition it is crucial to establish that the patient does not have a sensory or perceptual disorder which may preclude the correct detection of the relevant stimuli to which to respond. The clinical examination consists in instructing the patient to lift the contralateral arm when a hand is stroked downward, and to lift the ipsilateral arm when the hand is stroked upward. If the patient moves the ipsilesional arm when the contralesional hand is brushed upward, he or she has motor allochiria. If the patient moves the contralesional arm (instead of the ipsilesional) arm when the contralesional hand is brushed downward, he or she has contralesional limb hyperkinesia. Finally, if the response involves both arms, the patient has bilateral hyperkinesia (Heilman 2004).

The GO–NO GO tasks described by Luria (1966) can also be useful to evaluate patients with defective response inhibition. The patient is instructed to put up two fingers when the examiner shows one finger, and to put up no fingers when the examiner shows two fingers. If the patient mimics the examiner, he or she has echopraxia; however, if the patient responds when the examiner puts up two fingers, he or she exhibits limb hyperkinesia.

Finally, 'utilization behaviour' in which patients seem compelled to grasp and use any object in front of them is often seen after frontal lesions (Lhermitte 1983).

Attention versus intention: can they be separated?

Some sort of a motor bias towards ipsilesional space is observed not only in most cases of motor/intentional neglect but also in perceptual neglect. Thus the question may be asked as to what extent the disturbed motor behaviour results from a distorted representation of personal and extrapersonal space (Jackson 2001). Or, put the other away around: Are attentional and intentional accounts of neglect behaviour truly separable entities?

There is strong evidence to suggest that attentional and intentional systems can indeed operate separately and hence may rely on differential neural circuits. First, according to the 'two visual systems' account (Goodale and Milner 1993) lesion-induced perceptual distortions and misjudgments should have little or no effect on visuomotor actions. This dissociation is indeed found in some patients (Goodale and Milner 1993).

Second, behaviourally, it appears that attention can influence intention and vice versa. Verfaellie and coworkers (Verfaellie *et al.* 1988a,b; Verfaellie and Heilman 1990) studied right- and left-hand reaction times in normal individuals to stimuli presented in either right or left hemispace. Prior to presenting the imperative stimulus (to which subjects had to react), subjects were given either motor intentional or sensory attentional cues. How these cues influenced reaction times was then measured. Verfaellie and coworkers hypothesized that when a cue directed attention to one side of space, the attentional systems of the hemisphere contralateral to the cue would be activated, and that the activated attentional systems might in turn activate the motor preparatory systems of either one or both hemispheres. Differences in reaction times between the two hands when attention is directed to the right versus left side by an attentional cue would then reveal asymmetric activation of the intentional ystems of the right and left hemispheres. Likewise, when an intentional cue (which gave advance warning as to which hand was likely to be called upon to move) prepared either the left or right hand to respond, the intentional systems of the corresponding hemisphere might in turn activate the attentional systems of the same or both hemispheres.

Verfaellie and coworkers (Verfaellie *et al.* 1988a,b; Verfaellie and Heilman 1990) found that directing attention to the right side of space resulted in faster reaction times for the right hand than the left hand, and they suggested that their data show that the attentional systems of the left hemisphere primarily activate the intentional systems of the left hemisphere. No differences between hands were observed when attention was directed towards the left hemispace, suggesting that the attentional systems of the right hemisphere activated the intentional systems of both hemispheres. In contrast, when the right hand was prepared to respond by the intentional cue, there were no differences in reaction times between responses to stimuli in left versus right hemispace. However, when the left hand was prepared to respond, the responses were more rapid to stimuli presented in the left than in the right hemispace. These findings suggest that the intentional systems of the right hemisphere primarily activate the attentional systems of the right hemisphere, whereas the intentional systems of the left hemisphere activate the attentional systems of both hemispheres. Overall, these attentional and intentional asymmetries reflect the asymmetric pattern of hemispheric specialization suggested for apraxia and neglect: while the right hemisphere is biased for attention to space, the left hemisphere seems to be biased for intention to action.

Finally, functional neuroimaging studies and studies using transcranial magnetic stimulation (TMS) to provoke virtual (functional) lesions confirm the differential involvement of parietal and frontal cortex in the representations of space, movement preparation, motor intention, and action. For example, using functional lesions induced by TMS and neurological patients with structural lesions confined to the left or right parietal cortex, Rushworth *et al.* (1997) demonstrated that some parietal regions, particularly in the right hemisphere, are concerned with covert orienting and the redirecting of covert orienting, as originally shown by Posner *et al.* (1984). In contrast, left parietal regions (and the anterior inferior parietal cortex in particular) are concerned with covertly preparing and switching ('reprogramming') intended movements. This neurological and behavioural evidence has been confirmed (Castiello and Paine 2002) and corresponds well to electrophysiological data from the macaque. The results strongly imply that the left anterior inferior parietal cortex is implicated in redirecting motor attention (Rushworth *et al.* 2001), a role which has also been confirmed using functional imaging (Rushworth *et al.* 2003). It has sometimes been argued that covert motor attention, and covert orienting of spatial attention, is more of an experimental artefact than a functionally significant process. However, left or right parietal TMS has little effect on movements or orienting in space, respectively. They are executed as initially intended, despite TMS (Desmurget *et al.* 1999; Rushworth *et al.* 2001). However, it is important to note that this latter account of motor attention is different from the account previously given for the interpretation of motor intentional neglect; motor attention as discussed by Rushworth and coworkers refers solely to the execution of specific movements made and the redirection thereof. Thus the account (and in fact the underlying lesions) differs from the motor intentional account provided in the context of motor/premotor neglect. Nevertheless, the data provide further evidence for the neurophysiological separateness of the neural mechanisms underlying attentional and intentional processes. A critical review of the functional imaging literature relevant to motor intention, preparation and attention is clearly beyond the scope of this chapter, and the reader is referred to Chapter 4 of this volume.

Therapy of motor/intentional neglect

The therapy of motor neglect is in its infancy. There is no evidence-based treatment yet available, and no trials that have recruited sufficient numbers of patients to assess the efficacy of treatment. Nevertheless, frequent reminders to use the neglected limb should be integrated into physiotherapy and occupational therapy as well as into all activities of daily living on the ward. The efficacy of constraining the good arm to force the patient to use the impaired arm, although theoretically reasonable, remains to be proven. Likewise, whether or not any of the therapy strategies currently employed for the remediation of perceptual neglect are efficacious in motor neglect needs further investigation.

Conclusion

Many neglect behaviours are likely to result from an impairment in the ability to construct an appropriate representation of personal, peripersonal, and extrapersonal space or are a consequence of an attentional bias which favours the processing of ipsilesional stimuli. Nonetheless, some neglect patients show behavioural deficits that are best characterized as a disorder of motor intention, i.e. a difficulty in initiating and performing movements towards targets presented contralesionally (premotor neglect) or a reduced use of the contralesional limbs (motor neglect).

Acknowledgements

GRF is supported by the Deutsche Forschungsgemeinschaft (DFG-KFO 112). JCM was supported by the Medical Research Council (MRC), United Kingdom. Additional support from the VolkswagenStiftung and the Bundesministerium für Bildung und Forschung (BMBF) is gratefully acknowledged.

References

Andersen RA, Buneo CA (2002). Intentional maps in posterior parietal cortex. *Annu Rev Neurosci*, 25, 189–230.

Andersen RA, Snyder LH, Bradlet DC, Xing J (1997). Multimodal representation of space in the posterior parietal cortex and its use in planning movements. *Annu Rev Neurosci*, 20, 300–30.

Andersen RA, Snyder LH, Batista AP, Buneo CA, Cohen YE (1998). Posterior parietal areas specialized for eye movements (LIP) and reach (PRR) using a common coordinate frame. *Novartis Found Symp*, **218**, 109–22.

Andersen RA, Shenoy KV, Snyder LH, Bradley DC, Crowell JA (1999). The contributions of vestibular signals to the representations of space in the posterior parietal cortex. *Ann NY Acad Sci*, **871**, 282–92.

Assmus A, Marshall JC, Ritzl A, Noth J, Zilles K, Fink GR (2003). Left inferior parietal cortex integrates time and space during collision judgments. *Neuroimage*, **20**, S82–8.

Balint R (1909). Seelenlähmung des Schauens, optische Ataxie, räumliche Störung der Aufmerksamkeit. *Monatssch Psychiatrie Neurol*, **25**, 51–81.

Bartolomeo P, Chokron S, Gainotti G (2001). Laterally directed arm movements and right unilateral neglect after left hemisphere damage. *Neuropsychologia*, **39**, 1013–21.

Bisiach E (1994). Perception and action in space representation: evidence from unilateral neglect. In G d'Ydewalle, P Eele, P Bertelson, (ed.) *International Perspectives on Psychological Science*, pp. 51–66. Hove, UK: Erlbaum.

Bisiach E, Vallar G (2000). Unilateral neglect in humans. In F Boller, J Grafman, G Rizzolatti, (ed.) *Handbook of Neuropsychology*. Amsterdam: Elsevier, 459–502.

Bisiach E, Geminiani G, Berti A, Rusconi ML (1990). Perceptual and premotor factors of unilateral neglect. *Neurology*, **40**, 1278–81.

Bisiach E, Tegner R, Ladavas E, Rusconi ML, Mijovic D, Hjaltason H (1995). Dissociation of ophthalmokinetic and melokinetic attention in unilateral neglect. *Cereb Cortex*, **5**, 439–47.

Bisiach E, Ricci R, Lualdi M, Colombo MR (1998). Perceptual and response bias in unilateral neglect. *Brain Cogn*, **37**, 369–86.

Bjoertomt O, Cowey A, Walsh V (2002). Spatial neglect in near and far space investigated by repetitive transcranial magnetic stimulation. *Brain*, **125**, 2012–22.

Boussaoud D (2001). Attention versus intention in the primate premotor cortex. *Neuroimage*, **14**, S40–5.

Boussaoud D, di Pellegrino G, Wise SP (1996). Frontal lobe mechanisms subserving vision-for-action versus vision-for-perception. *Behav Brain Res*, **72**, 1–15.

Brain WR (1941). Visual disorientation with special reference to lesions of the right hemisphere. *Brain*, **64**, 244–72.

Bremmer F, Schlack A, Duhamel J-R, Graf W, Fink GR (2001a). Space coding in primate posterior parietal cortex. *Neuroimage* **14**, S46–51.

Bremmer F, Schlack A, Shah NJ, Zafiris O, Kubischik M, Hoffman K, *et al.* (2001b). Polymodal motion processing in posterior parietal and premotor cortex: a human fMRI study strongly implies equivalencies between humans and monkeys. *Neuron*, **29**, 287–96.

Bridgeman B (1999). Separate representations of visual space for perception and visually guided behavior. In G Aschersleben, T Bachmann, J Müsseler, (ed.) *Cognitive Contributions to the Perception of Spatial and Temporal Events*. Amsterdam: Elsevier.

Castaigne P, Laplane D, Degos JD (1970). Trois cas de négligence notrice par lesion rétrorolandique. *Rev Neurol (Paris)*, **122**, 234–42.

Castaigne P, Laplane D, Degos JD (1972). Trois cas de négligence motrice par lésion frontale pré-rolandique. *Rev Neurol (Paris)*, **126**, 5–15.

Castiello U, Paine M (2002). Effects of left parietal injury on covert orienting of attention. *J Neurol Neurosurg Psychiatr*, **72**, 73–6.

Chédru F, Léblanc M, Lhermitte F (1973). Visual searching in normal and brain damaged subjects: contributions to the study of unilateral inattention. *Cortex*, **9**, 94–111.

Classen J, Schnitzler A, Binkofski F, Werhahn KJ, Kim YS, Kessler KR, *et al.* (1997). The motor syndrome associated with exaggerated inhibition within primary motor cortex. *Brain*, **120**, 605–19.

Critchley M (1953). *The Parietal Lobes*. New York: Hafner.

De Renzi E (1982). *Disorders of Space Exploration and Cognition*. New York: Wiley.

De Renzi E, Faglioni P, Scotti G (1970). Hemispheric contribution to exploration of space through the visual and tactile modality. *Cortex*, **6**, 191–203.

Desmurget M, Epstein CM, Turner RS, Prablanc C, Alexander GE, Grafton ST (1999). Role of the posterior parietal cortex in updating reaching movements to a visual target. *Nat Neurosci*, **2**, 563–7.

Doricchi F, Tomaiuolo F (2003). The anatomy of neglect without hemianopia: a key role for parietal-frontal disconnection. *NeuroReport*, **14**, 2239–43.

Fink GR, Marshall JC, Weiss PH, Stephan T, Gretkes C, Shah NJ, *et al.* (2003). Performing allocentric visuospatial judgments with induced distortion of the egocentric reference frame: an fMRI study with clinical implications. *Neuroimage*, **20**, 1505–17.

Fisher CM (1956). Left hemiplagia and motor impersistence. *J Neuro Ment Dis*, **123**, 201.

Ghika J, Ghika-Schmid F, Bogousslavski J (1998). Parietal motor syndrome: a clinical description in 32 patients in the acute phase of pure parietal strokes studied prospectively. *Clin Neurol Neurosurg*, **100**, 271–81.

Girotti F, Casazza M, Musicco M, Avanzini G (1983). Oculomotor disorders in cortical lesions in man: the role of unilateral neglect. *Neuropsychologia*, **21**, 543–53.

Goodale MA, Milner AD (1993). Separate visual pathways for perception and action. *Trends Neurosci*, **15**, 20–5.

Grefkes C, Weiss PH, Zilles K, Fink GR (2002). Crossmodal processing of object features in human anterior intraparietal cortex. An fMRI study implies equivalencies between humans and monkeys. *Neuron*, **35**, 173–84.

Halligan PW, Cockburn J (1993). Cognitive sequelae of stroke: visuospatial and memory disorders. *Crit Rev Phys Rehab Med*, **5**, 57–81.

Halligan PW, Marshall JC (1989). Percepual cueing and perceptuo-motor compatibility in visuo-spatial neglect: a single case study. *Cogn Neuropsychol*, **6**, 423–35.

Halligan PW, Marshall JC (1991). Left neglect for near but not far space in man. *Nature*, **350**, 498–500.

Halligan PW, Marshall JC (1992). Left visuospatial neglect: a meaningless entity? *Cortex*, **28**, 525–35.

Halligan PW, Fink GR, Marshall JC, Vallar G (2003). Spatial cognition: evidence from visual neglect. *Trends Cogn Sci*, **7**, 125–33.

Heilman KM (2004). Intentional neglect. *Frontiers in Bioscience*, **9**, 694–705.

Heilman KM, Valenstein E (1979). Mechanisms underlying hemispatial neglect. *Ann Neurol*, **5**, 166–70.

Heilman KM, Bowers D, Watson RT (1983). Performance on hemispatial pointing task by patients with neglect syndrome. *Neurology*, **33**, 661–4.

Heilman KM, Bowers D, Coslett HB, Whelan H, Watson RT (1985). Directional hypokinesia: prolonged reaction times for leftward movements in patients with right hemisphere lesions and neglect. *Neurology*, **35**, 855–9.

Heilman KM, Watson RT, Valenstein E (1993). Neglect and related disorders. In KM Heilman, E Valenstein, (ed.) *Clinical Neuropsychology*. New York: Oxford University Press, 279–336.

Heilman KM, Valenstein E, Watson RT (2000). Neglect and related disorders. *Semin Neurol*, **20**, 463–70.

Hornak J (1992). Ocular exploration in the dark by patients with visual neglect. *Neuropsychologia*, **30**, 547–52.

Ishiai S, Furukawa T, Tsukagoshi H (1987). Eye-fixation patterns in homonymous hemianopia and unilateral spatial neglect. *Neuropsychologia*, **25**, 675–9.

Jackson JH (1876). Case of rare cerebral tumour without optic neuritis and with left hemiplegia and imperception. *R Lond Ophthalmic Hosp Rep.*, **8**, 434–44.

Jackson SR (2001). Motor aspects of hemispatial neglect. *Behav Neurol*, **13**, 1–2.

Jones E (1907). The precise diagnostic value of allochiria. *Brain*, **30**, 490–532.

Kertesz A, Nicholson I, Cancelliere A, Kassa K, Black SE (1985). Motor impersistence: a right-hemisphere syndrome. *Neurology*, **35**, 662–6.

Kinsbourne M (1993). Orientational bias model of unilateral neglect: evidence from attentional gradients within hemispace. In IH Robertson, JC Marshall, (ed.) *Unilateral Neglect: Clinical and Experimental Findings*, pp. 63–86. Hove, UK: Erlbaum.

Laplane D, Degos JD (1983). Motor neglect. *J Neurol Neurosurg Psychiatry*, **46**, 152–8.

Lhermitte F (1983). 'Utilisation behaviour' and its relation to the frontal lobes. *Brain*, **106**, 237–55.

Liepmann H (1908). *Drei Aufsätze aus dem Apraxiegebiet.* Berlin: Karger.

Luria AR (1966). *Higher Cortical Functions in Man.* New York: Basic Books and Plenum Press.

Marshall JC, Fink GR (2001). Spatial cognition: where we were and where we are. *Neuroimage*, **14**, S2–7.

Marshall JC, Halligan PW (1995). Within- and between-task dissociations in visuo-spatial neglect: a case study. *Cortex*, **31**, 367–76.

Mattingley JB, Driver J (1997). Distinguishing sensory and motor deficits after parietal damage: An evaluation of response selection biases in unilateral neglect. In P Thier, H-O Karnath, (ed.) *Parietal Contributions to Orientation in 3D Space*, pp. 309–38, eds. Heidelberg: Springer.

Mattingley JB, Bradshaw JL, Bradshaw JA, Nettleton NC (1994). Recovery from directional hypokinesia and bradykinesia in unilateral neglect. *J Clin Exp Neuropsychol*, **16**, 861–76.

Mattingley JB, Husain M, Rorden C, Kennard C, Driver J (1998). Motor role of human inferior parietal lobe revealed in unilateral neglect patients. *Nature*, **392**, 179–82.

Meador KJ, Watson RT, Bowers D, Heilman KM (1986). Hypometria with hemispatial and limb motor neglect. *Brain*, **109**, 293–305.

Meador KJ, Moore EE, Martin RC, Loring DW, Hess DC, Heilman KM (2000). Limb and hemispatial hypometria. *J Int Neuropsychol Soc*, **6**, 71–5.

Mesulam MM (1981). A cortical network for directed attention and unilateral neglect. *Ann Neurol*, **10**, 309–25.

Mesulam MM (1990). Large-scale neurocognitive networks and distributed processing for attention, language, and memory. *Ann Neurol*, **28**, 597–613.

Mesulam MM (1994). The multiplicity of neglect phenomena. *Neuropsychol Rehab*, **4**, 173–6.

Mort DJ, Malhotra P, Mannan SK, Rorden C, Pambakian A, Kennard C, *et al.* (2003). The anatomy of visual neglect. *Brain*, **126**, 1986–97.

Na LD, Adair JC, Williamson DJ, Schwartz RL, Haws B, Heilman KM (1998). Dissociation of sensory-attentional from motor-intentional neglect. *J Neurol Neurosurg Psychiatr*, **64**, 331–8.

Poppelreuter W (1917). *Die psychischen Schädigungen durch Kopfschuß im Kriege 1914/16.* Leipzig: Leopold Voss.

Posner MI, Walker JA, Friedrich FJ, Rafal R (1984). Effects of parietal injury on covert orienting of attention. *J Neurosci*, **4**, 1863–74.

Pouget A, Sejnowski TJ (2001). Simulating a lesion in a basis function model of spatial representations: comparison with hemineglect. *Psychol Rev*, **108**, 653–73.

Rizzolatti G, Berti A (1990). Neglect as a neural representation deficit. *Rev Neurol*, **146**, 626–34.

Rizzolatti G, Fadiga L, Fogassi L, Gallese V (1997a). The space around us. *Science*, **277**, 190–1.

Rizzolatti G, Fogassi L, Gallese V (1997b). Parietal cortex: from sight to action. *Curr Opin Neurobiol*, **7**, 562–7.

Robertson IH, Halligan PW (1999). *Spatial Neglect: A Clinical Handbook for Diagnosis and Treatment*. Hove, UK: Psychology Press.

Robertson IH, Marshall JC, (ed.) (1993). *Unilateral Neglect: Clinical and Experimental Findings*. Hove, UK: Erlbaum.

Robertson IH, North N (1992). Spatio-motor cueing in unilateral neglect: the role of hemispace, hand and motor activation. *Neuropsychologia*, **30**, 553–63.

Roeltgen MG, Roeltgen DP, Heilman KM (1989). Unilateral motor impersistence and hemispatial neglect from a striatal lesion. *Neuropsychiatry Neuropsychol Behav Neurol*, **2**, 125–35.

Rushworth MF, Nixon PD, Renowden S, Wade DT, Passingham RE (1997). The left parietal cortex and motor attention. *Neuropsychologia*, **35**, 1261–73.

Rushworth MF, Ellison A, Walsh V (2001). Complementary localization and lateralization of orienting and motor attention. *Nat Neurosci*, **4**, 656–61.

Rushworth MFS, Johansen-Berg H, Gobel SMG, Devlin JT (2003). The left parietal and premotor cortices: motor attention and selection. *Neuroimage*, **20** (Suppl 1), 89–100.

Sakai Y, Nakamura T, Sakurai A, Yamaguchi H, Hirai S (2000). Right frontal areas 6 and 8 are associated with simultanapraxia, a subset of motor impersistence. *Neurology*, **54**, 522–4.

Tegner R, Levander M (1991). Through a looking glass: a new technique to demonstrate directional hypokinesia in unilateral neglect. *Brain*, **114**, 1943–51.

Valenstein E, Heilman KM (1981). Unilateral hypokinesia and motor extinction. *Neurology*, **31**, 445–8.

Vallar G (2001). Extrapersonal visual unilateral spatial neglect and its neuroanatomy. *Neuroimage*, **14**, S52–8.

Vallar G, Guariglia C, Rusconi ML (1997). Modulation of the neglect syndrome by sensory stimulation. In P Thier, H-O Karnath, (ed.) *Parietal Lobe Contributions to Orientation in 3D Space*, pp. 555–78, Heidelberg: Springer-Verlag.

Verfaellie M, Heilman KM (1990). Hemispheric asymmetries in attentional control: implications for hand preference in sensorimotor tasks. *Brain Cogn*, **14**, 70–80.

Verfaellie M, Bowers D, Heilman KM (1988a). Attentional factors in the occurence of stimulus–response compatibility effects. *Neuropsychologia*, **26**, 435–44.

Verfaellie M, Bowers D, Heilman KM (1988b). Hemispheric asymmetries in mediating intention, but not selective attention. *Neuropsychologia*, **26**, 521–31.

Viader F, Cambier J, Pariser P (1982). Left motor extinction due to an ischemic lesion of the anterior limb of the internal capsule. *Rev Neurol (Paris)*, **138**, 213–17.

Vogeley K, Fink GR (2003). Neural correlates of the first-person perspective. *Trends Cogn Sci*, **7**, 38–42.

von Giesen HJ, Schlaug G, Steinmetz H, Benecke R, Freund H-J, Seitz RJ (1994). Cerebral network underlying unilateral motor neglect: evidence from positron emission tomography. *J Neurol Sci*, **125**, 29–38.

Vuilleumier P, Valenza N, Mayer E, Reverdin A, Landis T (1998). Near and far visual space in unilateral neglect. *Ann Neurol*, **43**, 406–10.

Watson RT, Miller B, Heilman KM (1978). Nonsensory neglect. *Ann Neurol*, **3**, 505–8.

Weiss PH, Marshall JC, Wunderlich G, Tellmann L, Halligan PW, Freund HJ, *et al.* (2000). Neural consequences of acting in near versus far space: a physiological basis for clinical dissociations. *Brain*, **123**, 2531–41.

Weiss PH, Marshall JC, Zilles K, Fink GR (2003). Are action and perception in near and far space additive or interactive factors? *Neuroimage*, **18**, 837–46.

Chapter 16

Anarchic hand

Sergio Della Sala and Clelia Marchetti

'Consciousness is a disease' Unamuno says . . .
John Updike (1989) *Self Consciousness*

Definition

Anarchic hand (AH) is one of the most intriguing phenomena in neurology. It defines the occurrence of complex movements of one hand that are apparently directed to a goal and are smoothly executed, i.e. the movements are not ballistic nor apraxic; however, according to the affected people they are unintended. These unwanted movements might interfere with the desired actions carried out by the other (healthy) hand. The patients are aware of the bizarre and potentially hazardous behaviour of their hand but cannot inhibit it. They often refer to the feeling that one of their hands behaves as if it has a will of its own, but never deny that this capricious hand is part of their own body. The bewilderment comes from the surprising and unwanted actions, not from a sensation of the hand not belonging to them.

Examples of anarchic hand

One evening Mrs GP was having dinner with her family when, out of the blue, much to her dismay her left hand took some left-over fish-bones and put them into her mouth. She was abashed by what she did, although a little later, while she was begging her hand not to embarrass her anymore, her mischievous hand grabbed the ice-cream that her brother was licking. Her right hand immediately intervened to put things in place and as a result of the fighting the dessert dropped on the floor. She apologized profusely for this behaviour that she attributed to her hand's disobedience. Indeed, she claimed that her hand had a mind of its own and often did whatever 'pleased it' (Della Sala *et al.* 1994). A second patient, Mrs GC, often complained that her hand did what it wanted to do, and she tried to control its wayward behaviour by hitting it violently or talking to it in anger and frustration (Della Sala *et al.* 1991). Another such patient had problems in choosing television channels, because 'no sooner had the right hand selected one station, the left hand would press another button' (Parkin 1996).

The issue of agency

We tend to take for granted that what we do is the result of a choice. After all, we can inhibit whatever gesture, action, or behaviour we are about to undertake. Sometimes people can perform actions for which they are not technically responsible, for example, if harassed by a threat or if affected by a severe psychiatric condition. However, even if stalwartness fades, one can still make a choice and when acting under a schizophrenic urge one does not experience the conflict between desired action and performed action. On the contrary, people with AH have no choice but to perform actions that they do not want to carry out, and often should not be carrying out. This condition seems to demonstrate that self-ownership of actions can be separated from awareness of actions. Indeed, Spence and Frith (1999) demonstrated with an elegant neuroimaging experiment that 'action' and 'agency' implicate distinct brain networks. The patients affected by AH are aware of the 'actions' of their anarchic hand, which they know to be their hand and not a robotic counterfeit, and yet they disown these actions.

Differential diagnosis

Anarchic hand is often referred to in the literature as 'alien hand'. The confusion arose due to a misinterpretation of a paper in French where alien hand was labelled *main étrangère* (foreign hand, or strange hand, as the authors themselves translated it in the English abstract of their paper) and this continued in subsequent scientific reports [see Marchetti and Della Sala (1998) for a full account of this conundrum]. The sign was described as the failure to recognize the ownership of one's left limb, when this is held by the right hand out of visual control. They reported this 'alien hand' sign in four patients, three affected by a tumour in the posterior part of the corpus callosum and the fourth presenting a left posterior paracallosal angioma. However, the term prevailed and alien hand began to mean very different things for different authors. AH, which is characterized by unwanted goal-directed actions, should be differentiated from the feeling of non-belonging of an arm, which characterizes alien hand (see Box 16.1). Therefore, alien hand, originally reported after posterior lesions of the corpus callosum probably encroaching upon the parietal cortex (Brion and Jedynak 1972), should be thought of as a partial hemisomatognosia, i.e. a unilateral loss of the knowledge or sense of one's own body. Alien hand is a sensory deficit, not a motor deficit (Ay *et al.* 1998; Rohde *et al.* 2002). Clinical pictures similar to those observed by Brion and Jedynak have been reported in patients affected by different diseases; for example, Ventura *et al.* (1995) described the feeling of non-belonging of her left arm in a patient with a right capsulothalamic haemorrhage with mesencephalic extension, and Kaufer *et al.* (1996) reported the case of a man presenting features of a diffuse leucodystrophy showing left alien arm. In many instances the term alien hand has been used as a misnomer to identify clinical signs that have little in common with either of the two phenomena defined above. For instance, alien hand has been used to describe

Box 16.1 Original description of alien hand

The patients reported by Brion and Jedynak (1972, 1974) did not present with any involuntary movement; they felt their left hand as a foreign body, which they failed to recognize. Their description of the symptom is compelling:

> Le patient qui se tient ses mains l'une dans l'autre derriére le dos, ne reconnaìt pas l'appartenance de la main gauche ... le déficit ne porte pas sur la reconnaissance tactile de la main, mais sur la reconnaissance de son appartenance (Brion and Jedynak 1972, p. 262).

Translation: The patient who holds his hands one within the other behind his back does not recognize the left hand as his own ... The sign does not consist in the lack of tactile recognition of the hand as such, but in the lack of recognition of the hand as one's own.

involuntary movements shown by patients suffering from corticobasal degeneration (Gibb *et al.* 1989) or other degenerative diseases such as Alzheimer's disease (Ball *et al.* 1993). The pathological hand of these patients is seen to wander involuntarily and to perform purposeless movements with a tendency to levitate and wave the fingers like tentacles (Rinne *et al.* 1994); complete actions are seldom reported.

Other syndromes to consider when making the diagnosis of AH are listed in Table 16.1. Basically, AH is the only such syndrome characterized by full-blown actions carried out by the mischievous hand apparently at odds with the patient's stated will. However, the labels given to the various syndromes are sometimes confusing. For example, agonistic dyspraxia (Lavados *et al.* 2002) is meant to be different from diagonistic dyspraxia, which in turn could be considered a synonym of intermanual conflict (Tanaka *et al.* 1996).

Anatomical site of lesion

Goldstein (1908) reported the first case of AH. His patient HM stated that she felt as if there were two personalities (*zweierlei Menschen*): the hand and herself. Goldstein's paper has been largely overlooked (Della Sala *et al.* 1994). He performed a post-mortem on his patient HM, and maintained that the lesion responsible for the *Spontanbewengungen* (spontaneous movements) his patient had shown was a lesion in the gyrus fornicatus, largely corresponding to the current supplementary motor area (SMA), coupled with a lesion in the corpus callosum. Indeed, for many years a section of the corpus callosum, either surgical or due to a pathological process, has been held solely responsible for the phenomenon. AH has been interpreted as the result of the disconnection between the right hemisphere motor cortex (governing the left hand)

Table 16.1 Syndromes to be considered when making a diagnosis of anarchic hand

Syndrome	Main feature	Difference from AH	Lesion site
Optic ataxia (Balint's syndrome)	Difficulty grasping objects at sight	Movements match patient's intention	Posterior parietal lobe
Magnetic misreaching (Carey *et al.* 1997)	Slavishly reaching to the foveal fixation point	Misdirected movements compensated by fixation	Parietal lobe
Intermanual conflict (diagonistic dyspraxia) (Tanaka *et al.* 1996)	Interference of one hand with movements performed by the other hand	Non-persistent left-hand (in right-handers), intrusive actions	Corpus callosum
Supernumerary hands (Halligan *et al.* 1993)	Sensation of having more than two hands	No motor abnormalities	Right basal ganglia/parietal lobe
Agonistic dyspraxia (Lavados *et al.* 2002)	Action on verbal commands performed by the non-requested hand	No conflict of intention	Corpus callosum
Phantom limb (Ramachandran and Hirstein 1998)	Feeling presence of limb which does not exist	Somatoagnosic illusion	Deafferentation of projection areas
Mirror movements (Hermsdörfer *et al.* 1995)	Associated movements in Symmetric muscles on opposite side	Non-goal-directed mirrored activity which accompany voluntary activity	Genetic basis
Compulsive grasping hand syndrome (Kumral 2001)	Compulsive, involuntary left hand grasp reaction to the right hand as a consequence of right hand purposeful movements	No finalized actions	Corpus callosum
Mirror ataxia (Binkoski *et al.* 2000)	Directional errors in reaching objects seen through a mirror	Misreaching through mirrors	Areas around the post-central sulcus in the parietal lobe
Conflict of intentions (Nishikawa *et al.* 2001)	Inability to perform intended whole-body actions due to another intention interference	Whole body	Corpus callosum

and the left hemisphere areas devoted to planning and the correct execution of complex motor activities. However, the callosal hypothesis is slippery on more than one ground. If the isolated lesion of the corpus callosum suffices to elicit the sign, the anarchic hand must always be ipsilateral to the hemisphere dominant for praxis (i.e. the left hand in right-handers). This assumption has been disputed by the observation of right-handed patients with a right anarchic hand (Goldberg 1985; Della Sala *et al.* 1991). In a review of 39 detailed cases reported in the literature (Della Sala *et al.* 1994), it appeared that most of the patients showing AH had a lesion encroaching upon the medial wall of the frontal lobe contralateral to the wayward hand. In particular, lesions seem to be centred on the corpus callosum and the SMA. However, cases of patients with clear signs of AH have been reported where no lesion to the corpus callosum was observed (McNabb *et al.* 1988; Leiguarda *et al.* 1993; Trojano *et al.* 1993; Marchetti and Della Sala 1998). Therefore a lesion to the corpus callosum cannot be solely responsible for the emergence of AH.

Anarchic hand as a sign of intrafrontal disconnection

AH could be interpreted (Goldberg 1985; Boccardi *et al.* 2002) as an imbalance between the damaged premotor medial system, centred on the SMA proper ((Lüders 1996; see also Chapter 1 of this volume;), and the spared lateral motor system centred on a region sometimes referred to as premotor cortex (PMC) (Fig. 16.1). These two systems carry different functions and have different phylogenetic origin: the medial system originates from the hippocampal archicortex, while the lateral system stems from the pyriform paleocortex. The medial system is believed to be responsible for inner-driven actions and for the inhibition of automatic responses. The lateral system is considered to be responsible for the so-called 'responsive movements', which are generated in response to external stimuli (Goldberg 1985; Passingham 1993; Cunnington *et al.* 1996; Gazzaniga *et al.* 2002). Although the theory is not universally accepted, several experiments indicate that the control of movements may vary as a function of whether the action is internally or externally guided (Frith *et al.* 1991; Halsband *et al.* 1993).

A single-cell animal experiment by Mushiake *et al.* (1991) is particularly relevant to this account. Monkeys were trained to press buttons in a given sequence. In one condition, the 'external condition', lights told the monkeys which button to press (it was a visually guided sequence). In the other condition the monkeys performed the sequence from memory with no external cues; this was the 'internal condition'. The movements made by the monkeys were identical. However, the SMA neurons were more active during the internal condition and the PMC neurons were more active during the external visually guided condition. This and other similar experiments indicate that the control of movements may vary as a function of whether the action is internally or externally guided (Eslinger 2002). The medial portion of area 6, the SMA proper

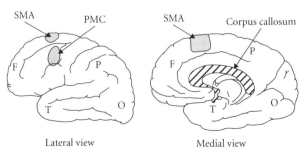

SMA PMC SMA Corpus callosum

Lateral view Medial view

Fig. 16.1 An anatomical sketch of the localizations of the premotor cortex (PMC) and the supplementary motor area (SMA) in the lateral and medial view of the left hemisphere of the human.

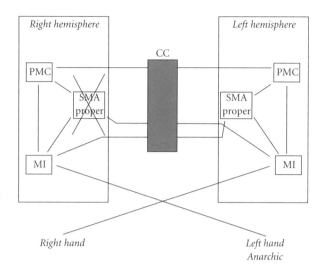

Fig. 16.2 Mechanisms for anarchic hand to emerge after a lesion of the contralateral SMA:CC, corpus callosum; MI, primary motor cortex; PMC, premotor cortex; SMA, supplementary motor area.

(Rizzolatti *et al.* 1996), which is thought to be responsible for action monitoring (Gentilucci *et al.* 2000; Luu *et al.* 2000) dominates when the task is internally guided. In contrast, the lateral region becomes more relevant when the task is triggered by the environment (Goldberg 1992).

An account of AH could be given as a phenomenon resulting from the imbalance of this complex mechanism; a lesion of the medial system would leave the contralateral hand at the mercy of external stimuli that operate through the premotor lateral system (Boccardi *et al.* 2002). The damaged medial system would be unable to inhibit the automatic provoked responses. Therefore this hand would show 'anarchic' behaviour (Fig. 16.2). However, patients will feel dismayed by the rivalry between their two hands in performing an action and by their inability to inhibit the actions of the anarchic hand—actions that they do not wish to carry out. Whether the lesion to the SMA is responsible per se for the occurrence of AH, or whether this is due to the interruption of the flow of information coming from the anterior cingulate, which may have a distinctive role in the intention to act, is still a matter of debate (Frith and Dolan 1997).

A caveat to this interpretation is the observation of mischievous actions performed by the AH, such as the fish-bone example given at the beginning of this chapter. Why the wayward hand should carry out actions potentially hazardous for the patient is still puzzling.

Bilateral SMA lesion

Whose will are the actions of the anarchic hand responding to? It would be possible to maintain that this epistemological problem springs from the conflict between stated will and performed action. Let us consider another sign of frontal dysinhibition known as 'utilization behaviour' (see Chapter 20 of this volume), in which patients show a compulsive urge to utilize objects at sight with either hand (Lhermitte 1983). Boccardi *et al.* (2002) recently reported on the case of patient CU who presented with severe utilization behaviour.

CU suffered from a bilateral stroke within the territory of the anterior cerebral artery that damaged both SMA, sparing the lateral regions, including the premotor cortices, the corpus callosum, and the gyri cinguli. The hypothesis that intrafrontal disconnection would account for utilization behaviour as well as for AH was put forward. In this frame, utilization behaviour should be conceived as a double anarchic hand, and its interpretation should rest on the damaged balance between the premotor cortices, responsive to environmental triggers, and the SMAs, which modulate actions and inhibit them. The imbalance due to the lesion would result in the patient's being left at the mercy of environmental stimuli, unable to inhibit inappropriate actions. Damage to one SMA results in AH; damage to both will elicit utilization behaviour. In both cases the affected patient will perform inappropriate actions and will utilize objects at sight. However, patients with utilization behaviour are not aware that their behaviour is inappropriate, or show any conflict between wanted and unwanted actions.

A cognitive account

Shallice *et al.* (1989) have interpreted utilization behaviour in terms of a derangement of the supervisory attentional system within the action control model (Norman and Shallice 1980) [for a computational model see Cooper and Shallice (2000)]. In the absence of a working supervisory system, they argued, perceptual input alone can lead to activation of more automatic action schemata which are triggered by environmental stimuli (see also Chapter 9, this volume). This is precisely what we have seen happening in patients with utilization behaviour, but also, on one side only, in patients with AH. The two syndromes are phenomenologically different (Table 16.2). Notwithstanding these differences, AH can still be accounted for in terms of an impaired supervisory attentional system, if we assume that within its fractionation one considers the possibility of unilateral symptoms. In AH it may well be that the part of the system which is not under the control of the supervisory system acts automatically at the mercy of environmental triggers, yet the functioning half of the supervisory system allows the patients to be aware that what they are doing is inappropriate. It may well be that the lack of awareness observed in patients with utilization behaviour comes from complete impairment of the medial system, wheres patients with AH still have some access to their inner 'supervisor' through the spared half of the system, although sometimes affordances, environmental or sensorial stimuli, may elude its control. This may also explain why instances of AH, as opposed to instances of utilization behaviour, are so rare in the affected patients.

Table 16.2 Similarities and differences between anarchic hand and utilization behaviour

Features of the movements	Anarchic hand	Utilization behaviour
Bilateral	No	Yes
Responsive	Yes	Yes
Unwanted	Yes	No
Disowned	Yes	No
Frequent instances	No	Yes
Long-lasting syndrome	Yes	Yes
Interference	Yes	No
Self-restriction as remedy	Yes	No
Awareness	Yes	Yes
Distress	Yes	No
Affordance	Yes	No?
Control	No	No
Ownership of hands	Yes	Yes

Experimental approach to anarchic hand

Riddoch *et al.* (1998) proposed studying whether visual affordances direct actions. They demonstrated that a patient with AH showed manual interference responses in a series of laboratory tasks whereby she was asked to reach for, pick up, and point to objects (cups on the right or on the left space, with the handle on the right or on the left) or non-objects (cup-like blocks) with either her left or her right hand. The results demonstrated that interfering motor responses were prompted by stimulus familiarity (cup versus blocks), by orientation, and in particular by visual affordances (object–hand compatibility). However, the patient, who was fully aware of her inappropriate actions in real life, was not aware of her mistakes in the laboratory. Riddoch and coworkers postulated that perhaps AH patients are aware of the consequences of their actions rather than of their actions per se.

In a recent experiment Kritikos *et al.* (2001) investigated the issue of the influence of the presence of cues and of non-relevant information on goal-directed actions in a patient with a left-sided AH and on his ability to carry out bimanual tasks. The results demonstrated that left-hand movements were slower than those with the right hand and confirmed the role of affordances in eliciting unwanted actions. Moreover, the internally generated movements of the left AH took longer to initiate than externally generated movements and were more prone to distraction than right-hand movements, and bilateral movements were scaled down to the velocity and efficiency of those performed by the left AH. The authors interpreted their findings within the framework of the motor control system postulated by Frith *et al.* (2000) (reviewed by Blakemore *et al.* 2002). Within this framework, AH would be conceived as an inappropriate activation of object representation; the sight of an object would be sufficient to elicit an action even if this is at odds with the patient's stated general goal. Sensory information provided by affordances would automatically trigger anarchic movements that can no longer be inhibited.

Free 'won't' rather than free will

Anarchic Hand seems to indicate that the conscious will can only veto some undesired actions. The only control we have over our actions is negative—the possibility of inhibiting them. In the case of AH or utilization behaviour one should then talk of 'intentionless actions' (Marcel, 2003). To achieve the (desired?) aim, the motor system makes non-stop refinements, of which we are usually unaware (reviewed by Libet *et al.* 1999; Blakemore *et al.* 2002; Wegner 2002). These include inhibition of actions triggered by environmental affordances. AH is the result of the lack of such inhibition due to a lesion of the mainly inner-driven medial-frontal motor system, the SMA proper or the anterior cingulate.

References

Ay H, Buonanno FS, Price BH, Le DA, Koroshetz WJ (1998). Sensory alien hand syndrome: case report and review of the literature. *J Neurol Neurosurg Psychiatry*, **65**, 366–9.

Ball J, Lantos PL, Jackson M, Marsden CD, Scadding JW, Rossor MN (1993). Alien hand sign in association with Alzheimer's histopathology. *J Neurol Neurosurg Psychiatry*, **56**, 1020–3.

Binkoski F, Buccino G, Dohle C, Seitz RJ, Freund HJ (2000). Mirror agnosia and mirror ataxia constitute different parietal lobe disorders. *Ann Neurol*, **47**, 553–4.

Blakemore S-J, Wolpert DM, Frith CD (2002). Abnormalities in awareness of action. *Trends Cogn Sci*, **6**, 237–42.

Boccardi E, Della Sala S, Motto C, Spinnler H (2002). Utilisation behaviour consequent to bilateral SMA softening. *Cortex*, **38**, 289–308.

Brion S, Jedynak CP (1972). Trouble du transfert interhémisphérique à propos de trois observations de tumeurs du corps calleux: le signe de la main étrangère. *Rev Neurol (Paris)*, **136**, 257–66.

Brion S, Jedynak CP (1974). Séméiologie calleuse dans les tumeurs et les malformations vasculaires. In F Michel, B Schott, (ed.) *Les Syndromes de Disconnexion Calleuse Chez l'Homme*, pp. 253–64. Colloque International de Lyon.

Carey DP, Coleman RJ, Della Sala S (1997). Magnetic misreaching. *Cortex*, **33**, 639–52.

Cooper R, Shallice T (2000). Contention scheduling and the control of routine activities. *Cogn Neuropsychol*, **17**, 297–338.

Cunnington R, Bradshaw JL, Iansek R (1996). The role of the supplementary motor area in the control of voluntary movement. *Hum Mov Sci*, **15**, 627–47.

Della Sala S, Marchetti C, Spinnler H (1991). Right-sided anarchic (alien) hand: a longitudinal study. *Neuropsychologia*, **29**, 1113–27.

Della Sala S, Marchetti C, Spinnler H (1994). The anarchic hand: a fronto-mesial sign. In F Boller, J Grafman, (ed.), *Handbook of Neuropsychology*, Vol 9, pp. 233–55. Amsterdam: Elsevier.

Eslinger PJ (2002). The anatomic basis of utilisation behaviour: a shift from frontal-parietal to intra-frontal mechanisms. *Cortex*, **38**, 273–6.

Frith CD, Dolan RJ (1997). Higher cognitive processes. In RSJ Frackowiack, KJ Friston, CD Frith, RJ Dolan, JC Mazziotta, (ed.) *Human Brain Function*, pp. 329–66. London: Academic Press.

Frith CD, Friston K, Liddle PF, Frackowiak RSJ (1991). Willed action and the prefrontal cortex in man: a study with PET. *Proc R Soc Lond B Biol Sci*, **244**, 241–6.

Frith CD, Blakemore S-J, Wolpert DM (2000). Abnormalities in the awareness and control of action. *Philos Trans R Soc Lond B Biol Sci*, **355**, 1771–88.

Gazzaniga MS, Ivry RB, Mangun GR (2002). *Cognitive Neuroscience. The Biology of the Mind*. New York: Norton, 499–536.

Gentilucci M, Bertolani L, Benuzzi F, Negrotti A, Pavesi G, Gangitano M (2000). Impaired control of an action after supplementary motor area lesion: a case study. *Neuropsychologia*, **38**, 1398–404.

Gibb WRG, Luthert PJ, Marsden CD (1989). Corticobasal degeneration. *Brain*, **112**, 1171–92.

Goldberg G (1985). Supplementary motor area structure and function. Review and hypotheses. *Behav Brain Sci*, **8**, 567–616.

Goldberg G (1992). Premotor system, attention to action and behavioural choice. In CR McCrohan, W Winlow, (ed.) *Neurobiology of Motor Programme Selection*, pp. 225–49. Oxford: Pergamon Press.

Goldstein K (1908). Zur Lehre von der motorisschen Apraxie. *Z Physiol Neurol*, **11**, 169–87.

Halligan PW, Marshall JC, Wade DT (1993). Three arms: a case study of supernumerary phantom limb after right hemisphere stroke. *J Neurol Neurosurg Psychiatry*, **65**, 159–66.

Halsband U, Ito N, Tanji J, Freund H-J (1993). The role of premotor cortex and the supplementary motor area in the temporal control of movement in man. *Brain*, **116**, 243–66.

Hermsdörfer J, Danek A, Winter T, Marquardt C (1995). Persistent mirror movements: force and timing of 'mirroring' are task-dependent. *Exp Brain Res*, **104**, 126–34.

Kaufer D, Mendez MF, Mischel PS, Verity MA, Benson DF (1996). Alien hand syndrome in adult-onset orthochromatic leukodystrophy. Disconnection of a limb from supplementary motor areas. *Behav Neurol*, **9**, 5–10

Kritikos A, Mattingley JB, Breen N (2001). Anarchic hand syndrome: bimanual co-ordination and sensitivity to irrelevant information in unimanual reaches (abstract). *Aust J Psychol*, **53** (Suppl), 194.

Kumral E (2001). Compulsive grasping hand syndrome: a variant of anarchic hand. *Neurology* **57**, 2143–4.

Lavados M, Carrasco X, Pea M, Zaidel E, Zaidel D, Aboitiz F (2002). A new sign of callosal disconnection syndrome: agonistic dyspraxia. A case study. *Neurocase*, **8**, 480–3.

Leiguarda R, Starkstein S, Nogues M, Berthier M, Arbelaiz R (1993). Paroxysmal alien hand syndrome. *J Neurol Neurosurg Psychiatry*, **56**, 788–92.

Libet B, Freeman A, Sutherland K (1999). *The Volitional Brain*. Thorverton: Imprinting Academic.

Lhermitte F (1983). 'Utilisation behaviour' and its relation to lesions of the frontal lobes. *Brain*, **106**, 237–55.

Lüders HO (ed.) (1996). *Supplementary Sensormotor Area*. Philadephia, PA: Lippincott–Raven.

Luu P, Flaisch T, Tucker DM (2000). Medial frontal cortex in action monitoring. *J Neurosci*, **20**, 464–9.

McNabb AW, Carroll WM, Mastaglia FL (1988). 'Alien hand' and loss of bimanual coordination after dominant anterior cerebral artery territory infarction. *J Neurol Neurosurg Psychiatry*, **51**, 218–22.

Marcel A (**2003**). The sense of agency. In J Roessler, N Elian, (ed.) *Agency and Self-Awareness*, pp. 48–93. Oxford: Oxford University Press.

Marchetti C, Della Sala S (1998). Disentangling the alien and anarchic hand. *Cognitive Neuropsychiatry*, **3**, 191–207.

Mushiake H, Masahiko I, Tanji J (1991). Neuronal activity in the primate premotor, supplementary, and precentral motor cortex during visually guided and internally determined sequential movements. *J Neurophysiol*, **66**, 705–18.

Nishikawa T, Okuda J, Mizuta I, Ohno K, Tanase H, Takeda M (2001). Conflict of intentions due to callosal disconnection. *J Neurol Neurosurg Psychiatry*, **71**, 462–71.

Norman DA, Shallice T (1980). *Attention in action: willed and automatic control of behaviour*. Chip Report 99, University of California, San Diego, CA.

Parkin AJ (1996). The alien hand. In PW Halligan, JC Marshall, (ed.) *Method in Madness: Case Studies in Cognitive Neuropsychiatry*, pp. 173–83. Hove, UK: Psychology Press.

Passingham R (1993). *The Frontal Lobes and Voluntary Action*. New York: Oxford University Press.

Ramachandran VS, Hirstein W (1998). The perception of phantom limbs. *Brain*, **121**, 1603–30.

Riddoch MJ, Edwards MG, Humprheys GW, West R, Heafield T (1998). Visual affordances direct action: neuropsychological evidence from manual interference. *Cogn Neuropsychol*, **15**, 645–83.

Rinne JO, Lee MS, Thomson PD, Marsden CD (1994). Corticobasal degeneration. A clinical study of 36 cases. *Brain*, **117**, 1183–96.

Rizzolatti G, Matelli M, Pavesi G (1996). The classic supplementary motor area is formed by two independent areas. In HO Lüders, (ed.) *Supplementary Sensorimotor Area*, pp. 45–56. Philadelphia, PA: Lippincott–Raven.

Rohde S, Weidauer S, Lanfermann H, Zanella F (2002). Posterior alien hand syndrome: case report. *Neuroradiology*, **44**, 921–3.

Shallice T, Burgess PW, Shon F, Boxter DM (1989). The origins of utilization behaviour. *Brain*, **112**, 1587–98.

Spence SA, Frith CD (1999). Towards a functional anatomy of volition. *J Conscious Stud*, **6**, 11–29.

Tanaka Y, Yoshida A, Kawahata N, Hashimoto R, Obayashi T (1996). Diagonistic dyspraxia. Clinical characteristics, responsible lesion and possible underlying mechanism. *Brain*, **119**, 859–73.

Trojano L, Cresci C, Lanzillo B, Elefante R, Caruso G (1993). How many alien hand syndromes? Follow-up study of a case. *Neurology*, **43**, 2710–12.

Ventura MG, Goldman S, Hildebrand J (1995). Alien hand syndrome without a corpus callosum lesion. *J Neurol Neurosurg Psychiatry*, **58**, 735–7.

Wegner DM (2002). *The Illusion of Conscious Will*. Cambridge, MA: MIT Press.

Chapter 17

Apraxias as traditionally defined

Ramón Leiguarda

Introduction

Apraxia is a term used to denote a wide spectrum of higher-order motor disorders due to acquired brain disease affecting the performance of skilled learned movements with or without preservation of the ability to perform the same movement outside the clinical setting in the appropriate situation or environment. The disturbance of purposive movements cannot be termed apraxia, however, if it results from a language comprehension disorder or from dementia, or if the patient suffers from any elementary motor or sensory deficit (i.e. paresis, dystonia, ataxia) which could fully explain the abnormal motor behaviour (Heilman and Rothi 1985; Roy and Square 1985; De Renzi 1989). Nevertheless, praxic errors are at present much better defined clinically and kinematically, and can be distinguished from other non-apractic motor disturbances, although it should be taken into account that the spectrum of motor dysfunction may be continuous rather than qualitatively divided into different categories (Poizner *et al.* 1990, 1995; Rothi *et al.* 1997; Leiguarda *et al.* 2003).

De Renzi *et al.* (1982) and Geschwind and Damasio (1985) emphasized the significance of the stimulus by means of which the learned movement is normally elicited, since earliest observations had already noticed that impairment could be seen under some performance conditions but not others (Liepmann 1908). Therefore they suggested the following operational definition: (i) failure to produce the correct movement to verbal command, or (ii) failure to imitate correctly a movement, or (iii) failure to perform a movement correctly in response to a seen object, or (iv) failure to use an object correctly (Geschwind and Damasio 1985).

Apraxias are common, but poorly recognized, disorders that can result from a wide variety of focal (i.e. stroke, trauma) or diffuse (i.e. corticobasal degeneration, Alzheimer's disease) brain damage (Heilman and Rothi 1985; Freund 1992; Leiguarda 2003). There are two main reasons why apraxia may go unrecognized. First, many patients with apraxia, particularly ideomotor apraxia, show a voluntary-automatic dissociation, which means that they do not complain about the deficit because the execution of the movement in the natural context is relatively well preserved, and the deficit appears mainly in the clinical setting when the patient is required to represent explicitly the content of the action outside the situational props.

Secondly, although in apraxic and aphasic patients specific functions are selectively affected, language and praxic disturbances frequently coexist and the former may interfere with the proper evaluation of the latter (Freund 1992).

Praxic disorders may affect various body parts such as the eyes, face, trunk, or limbs, and may involve both sides of the body (i.e. ideational and ideomotor apraxias), one side preferentially (i.e. limb-kinetic apraxia), or interlimb coordination (i.e. apraxia of gait). The present chapter will be devoted mainly to limb apraxia, although a brief description of apraxia affecting the face and trunk will be presented at the end. Gait and speech apraxias are described in Chapters 12 and 13, respectively.

Limb apraxias

Although the original definition of apraxia goes back to Steinthal (1871), contemporary ideas stem from the classical works of Liepmann (Liepmann 1900, 1905, 1908, 1920). He posited that the idea of the action, or movement formula, containing the space–time picture of the movement, was stored in the left parietal lobe. In order to carry out a skilled movement, the space–time plan has to be retrieved and associated via cortical connections with the innervatory pattern stored in the left sensorimotorium that conveys the information on formula to the left primary motor areas. When the left limb performs the movement, the information has to be transmitted from the left to the right sensorimotorium through the corpus callosum to activate the right motor cortex. Liepmann conceived ideational apraxia (IA) as a disruption of the space–time plan or its proper activation, so that it was impossible to construct the idea of the movement; the patient does not know what to do. In contrast, in ideomotor apraxia (IMA), the space–time plan is intact but it can no longer guide the innervatory engrams that implement the movement because it is disconnected from them; the patient knows what to do, but not how to do it. Finally, limb-kinetic apraxia (LKA) appears when the disruption of the innervatory engrams interferes with the selection of the required muscle synergies to perform the skilled movement.

Since Liepmann's time, the classification of limb praxic disorders has been subject to multiple modifications and is still under debate. Roy and Square (1985) initially argued that apraxia might result from a disruption in a conceptual system and/or a production system. Later, Roy (1996) expanded this model to account for three differ-ent patterns of limb apraxia. Apraxia when pantomiming to command but not on imi-tation would reflect dysfunction of the conceptual system, affecting knowledge of tool function or knowledge of actions, or in the early stage of the production system involv-ing image generation or response selection. Apraxia in the imitation condition alone would reflect a disruption in the ability to analyse visual gestural information or in the translation of this information into movements. Finally, apraxia in both conditions would reflect a selective disruption at a later stage of gestural performance involving movement execution. An influential cognitive neuropsychological model was advanced by Rothi *et al.* (1991), mapped onto the model of language processing. They proposed separating input pathways for verbal and visual stimuli to explain the dissociation between the ability to perform an action on command versus on imitation, separating semantic and non-semantic pathways to account for dissociations in the ability to represent meaningful versus meaningless actions, and separating input and output lexicons to allow for differences in the ability to conceptualize actions and to perform them.

More recently, Cubelli *et al.* (2000) and Buxbaum *et al.* (2000) modified the Rothi *et al.* model (1991) to account for patterns of IMA not explained by this cognitive neuropsychological model. Cubelli *et al.* introduced a visuomotor conversion mechanism, to transcode visual analysis into a motor program in order to account for isolated impairment of action imitation. The model outlined by Buxbaum *et al.* (2000) provided a different approach to meaningful and meaningless action relationships, since they proposed an interplay between a dynamic body-centred representation of actions and a stored representation of learned actions. Notwithstanding the clear advances in understanding apraxia that these models accomplished, neurological and physiological data still require to be brought together within a coherent framework. In a recent review, we attempted to approach in this way, though with partial success, the different types of limb praxic deficit (Leiguarda and Marsden 2000). Since then, further advances in functional neuroimaging and behavioural motor neurophysiology in non-human primates, together with more refined clinical studies, have allowed a better neurophysiological and cognitive approach to the neural processes underlying normal and impaired praxis.

Evaluation of limb praxis

A systematic evaluation of limb praxis is critical in order (i) to identify the presence of apraxia, (ii) to classify correctly the nature of limb praxis deficit according to the errors committed by the patient and the modality through which these errors are elicited, and (iii) to gain an insight into the underlying mechanism of the patient's abnormal motor behaviour (Table 17.1).

Patients' performance should be assessed in both forelimbs if an elementary motor-sensory deficit does not preclude testing the limb contralateral to the damaged hemisphere. Intransitive and transitive movements should be evaluated. The sample of intransitive gestures tested has to include movements performed towards or on the body (salute, crazy) versus away from the body (okay sign, wave goodbye), and repetitive (beckon, go away) or non-repetitive (sign of victory), since the dimensions of spatial location relative to the body and repetitiveness contribute to the overall complexity of the task and may be differentially influenced by the disorder (Roy *et al.* 1998). Likewise, several types of transitive movements have to be evaluated, since it is not an uncommon finding that apraxic patients perform some but not all movements

Table 17.1 Assessment of limb praxis

Intransitive movements	Non-representational (e.g. touch your nose, wriggle your fingers)
	Representational (e.g. wave good-bye, hitch-hike)
Transitive movements	For example, use a hammer or a screwdriver) under verbal, visual, and tactile modalities
Imitation of meaningful and meaningless movements, postures and sequences	
Tool[a] selection tasks	Select the appropriate tool to complete a task, such as a hammer for a partially driven nail
Alternative tool selection tasks	Select an alternative tool such as pliers to complete a task such as pounding a nail, when the appropriate tool (i.e. hammer) is not available
Mechanical problem-solving tasks	For example, select the appropriate one of three novel tools for lifting a wooden cylinder out of a socket
Multiple step tasks	For example, prepare a letter for mailing
Gesture recognition and discrimination tasks	To assess the capacity to comprehend gestures, either verbally (name gestures performed by the examiner) or non-verbally (match a gesture performed by the examiner with cards depicting the tool/object[b] corresponding to the pantomime), and to assess the ability to discriminate a correctly performed from a wrongly performed gesture.

[a] Tool: implement with which an action is performed (e.g. hammer, screwdriver).

[b] Object: the recipient of the action (e.g. nail, screw).

Sources: De Renzi 1989; Rothi *et al*. 1997; Goldenberg and Hagmann 1998.

in a particularly abnormal fashion and/or that individual differences appear in some but not all components of a given movement. Therefore the dissimilar complexity and features of transitive movements should be considered in order to analyse and interpret praxic errors accurately. For instance, (i) movements may or may not be repetitive in nature (e.g. hammering versus using a bottle opener to remove the cap), (ii) an action may be composed of sequential movements (e.g. to reach for a glass and take it to the lips in drinking), (iii) a movement may primarily reflect proximal limb control (transport) such as transporting the wrist when carving a turkey; proximal and distal limb control such as reaching and grasping a glass of water, or primarily distal control as when the patient is asked to manipulate a pair of scissors, and (iv) movements may be performed in the peripersonal space (e.g. carving a turkey) or in body-centred space (e.g. tooth-brushing), or may require the integration of both, such as the drinking action.

Transitive movements should be assessed under different modalities, including verbal, visual (seeing the tool or the object upon which the tool works), and tactile (using actual tools and/or objects) as well as on imitation, since impairment can be seen under some performance conditions but not others. Nevertheless, the most sensitive test for apraxia is asking patients to pantomime to verbal commands because this test provides the least cues and is almost entirely dependent on stored movement representations (see below). In addition to the specific praxis assessment tasks listed in Table 17.1, it is important to evaluate other cognitive functions, since they may contribute to understanding the neural mechanisms of some praxic deficits. Thus the evaluation of conceptual tool and object knowledge, such as correct naming, descriptions, or correct associative semantic judgement, may help to discern the specific nature of an object/tool use deficit. Knowledge about body part (body semantics) and body structural description as well as the evaluation of the processes coding the dynamic position of the body parts relative to one another, i.e. the body schema, may provide clues to elucidating the neural mechanisms underlying deficits in gesture imitation (Buxbaum *et al.* 2000).

Analysis of a patient's performance is based on both accuracy and error patterns (Table 17.2). One problem with many investigations of apraxia is that the analysis of gestural performance may be insensitive to subtle apraxic deficits, which may have led to an uncorrected estimation about the frequency and degree of apraxia (Roy *et al.* 2000). Therefore detailed error analysis is crucial to unveil and to classify properly an apraxic disorder. The patient with IA has difficulty mainly in sequencing actions (e.g. making coffee) and exhibits content errors or semantic parapraxias (e.g. mimicking a hammer use when requested to use a knife). Ideomotor apraxia patients show primarily temporal and spatial errors, which are more evident when they perform transitive than intransitive movements. Errors in LKA represent slowness, coarseness, and fragmentation of finger and hand movements.

Three-dimensional analysis of different types of movements has provided a better and more accurate method of capturing objectively the nature of the praxis errors observed in clinical examination. Patients with IMA due to focal left-hemisphere lesions (Clark *et al.* 1994; Poizner *et al.* 1995), different asymmetric cortical degenerative syndromes, and basal ganglion disease (Leiguarda and Starkstein 1998; Leiguarda *et al.* 2000a) have shown several kinematic abnormalities of dissimilar complexity such as slow and hesitant build-up of hand velocity, irregular and non-sinusoidal velocity profiles, abnormal amplitudes, alterations in the plane of motion and in the direction and shapes of wrist trajectories, decoupling of hand speed and trajectory curvature, and loss of interjoint coordination. All these studies have evaluated gestures, such as carving a turkey or slicing a loaf of bread, which mainly explore the transport or reaching phase of the movement. However, the majority of transitive gestures included in most apraxia batteries include prehension (reaching and grasping) movements that reflect proximal (transport) as well as distal (grasping) limb control. The kinematic analysis of aiming movements in apraxic patients has demonstrated spatial deficits, in particular when visual feedback is not available (Haaland *et al.* 1999), whereas the analysis of prehension movements has shown disruption of both the transport

Table 17.2 Types of praxis errors

Temporal		
S	Sequencing	Some pantomimes require multiple positionings that are performed in a characteristic sequence. Sequencing errors involve any perturbation of this sequence including addition, deletion, or transposition of movement elements as long as the overall movement structure remains recognizable
T	Timing	This error reflects any alterations from the typical timing or speed of a pantomime and may include abnormally increased, decreased, or irregular rate of production, or searching or groping behaviour
O	Occurrence	Pantomimes may involve either single (i.e. unlocking a door with a key) or repetitive (i.e. screwing in a screw with a screwdriver) movement cycles. This error type reflects any multiplication of single cycles or reduction of a repetitive cycle to a single event.
Spatial		
A	Amplitude	Any amplification, reduction, or irregularity of the characteristic amplitude of a target pantomime
IC	Internal configuration	When pantomiming, the fingers and hand must be in specific spatial relation to one another to reflect recognition and respect for the imagined tool. This error type reflects any abnormality of the required finger/hand posture and its relationship to the target tool. For example, when asked to pretend to brush teeth, the subject's hand may close tightly into a fist with no space allowed for the imagined toothbrush handle
BPO	Body part as object	The subject uses his or /her finger, hand, or arm as the imagined tool of the pantomime. For example, when asked to smoke a cigarette, the subject might puff on his or her index finger
ECO	External configuration orientation	When pantomiming, the fingers/hand/arm and the imagined tool must be in a specific relationship to the 'object' receiving the action.Errors of this type involve difficulties orienting to the 'object' or in placing the 'object' in space. For example, the subject might pantomime brushing teeth by holding his hand next to his mouth without reflecting the distance necessary to accommodate an imagined toothbrush. Another example would be when asked to hammer a nail. The subject might hammer in differing locations in space reflecting difficulty in placing the imagined nail in a stable orientation or in a proper plane of motion (abnormal planar orientation of the movement)
M	Movement	When acting on an object with a tool, a movement characteristic of the action and necessary to accomplish the goal is required. Any disturbance of the characteristic movement reflects a movement error. For example, a subject, when asked to pantomime using a screwdriver, may orient the imagined screwdriver correctly to the imagined screw but instead of stabilizing the shoulder and wrist and twisting at the elbow, the subject stabilizes the elbow and twists at the wrist or shoulder.

Table 17.2 *(Continued)*

Content		
P	Perseverative	The subject produces a response that includes all or part of a previously produced pantomime
R	Related	The pantomime is an accurately produced pantomime associated in content with the target. For example, the subject might pantomime playing a trombone for a target of a bugle
N	Non-related	The pantomime is an accurately produced pantomime not associated in content with the target. For example, the subject might pantomime playing a trombone for a target of shaving
H		The patient performs the action without benefit of a real or imagined tool. For example, when asked to cut a piece of paper with scissors, he or she pretends to rip the paper
Other		
C	Concretization	The patient performs a transitive pantomime not on an imagined object but on a real object not normally used in the task. For example, when asked to pantomime sawing wood, the patient pantomimes sawing on his or her leg
NR	No response	
UR	Unrecognizable response	The response shares no temporal or spatial features of the target

Source: Rothi *et al.* 1997.

and grasp phases of the movements as well as transport–grasping uncoupling (Caselli *et al.* 1999; Leiguarda *et al.* 2000a). Furthermore, the study of manipulating finger movements in patients with LKA has disclosed severe abnormalities unveiling the nature of the motor deficit. The workspace is highly irregular and of variable amplitude, there is breakdown of the temporal profiles of the scanning movements, and, overall, severe interfinger incoordination has been found (Leiguarda *et al.* 2003). Thus exploration of the kinematics of reaching, grasping, and manipulating may provide useful information regarding the specific neural subsystems involved in patients with different types of limb praxic disorders.

Lateralization of motor functions

Apraxia as tested by the imitation of gestures and object use pantomime has been found in about 50% of patients with left-hemisphere damage and in less than 10% of those with right-hemisphere damage (De Renzi 1989). However, considerable variability in these figures is found across studies because of the use of different tasks to assess limb praxis, lack of adequate matching of patients with similar lesion location and extension, and variation in criteria for diagnosing the different praxic disorders. Nevertheless, most of the errors exhibited by IMA patients are seen equally in left-hemisphere-damaged (LHD) or right-hemisphere-damaged (RHD) patients when they pantomime non-representative and representative/intransitive gestures, but are observed predominantly in LHD patients when they pantomime transitive movements, because it is this action which is performed outside the natural context (Haaland and Flaherty 1984; Schnider *et al.* 1997). Moreover, it has been suggested that, whereas either hemisphere would be able to process intransitive movements as well as transitive movements using tools/objects, the left hemisphere would be dominant not only for the 'abstract' performance (pantomiming to verbal command) of transitive movements, but also for learning and reproducing novel movements such as meaningless movements and sequences (Rapcsak *et al.* 1993; Weiss *et al.* 2001; Goldenberg and Strauss 2002). Recent clinical and functional magnetic resonance imaging (fMRI) studies support these views. Roy *et al.* (2000) studied 99 patients with a single unilateral hemispheric stroke and found that LHD patients were more likely to be impaired at pantomiming the use of tools to verbal command than RHD patients, whereas a comparable proportion of patients in both groups were apraxic when imitating the same transitive movements performed by the examiner. Hanna-Pladdy *et al.* (2001a) evaluated the types of errors committed by left- and right-hemisphere stroke patients and demonstrated that the LHD group made significantly more qualitative errors than the RHD group; specifically, they committed a wide range of spatiotemporal and conceptual errors for both transitive and intransitive gestures, whereas the RHD group exhibited specific spatial (e.g. external configuration) and temporal errors mainly when performing transitive movements. In relating with intransitive movements the results of this study are at odds with those of Heath *et al.* (2001). These authors evaluated 57 left-hemisphere and 62 right-hemisphere stroke patients; analysis of pantomime and imitation performance on intransitive movements revealed an equal percentage of apraxic patients in each stroke group.

Pantomiming tool-use gestures, regardless of which hand is used, activates different parietofrontal areas predominantly in the left hemisphere (Moll *et al.* 2000; Choi *et al.* 2001; Fridman *et al.*, unpublished data). Imitation of meaningless hand movements is associated with activation mainly of the left occipitotemporal region and left Brodmann's area (BA) 40, whereas imitation of meaningless finger postures produces additional activations in the right intraparietal sulcus (IPS) and supramarginal gyrus (Hermsdörfer *et al.* 2001). Sequential finger movements performed with the right and left hand mainly activate the left premotor cortex (Hlustik *et al.* 2002), whereas learning both finger and timing sequences increases rCBF in the left intraparietal cortex (Sakai *et al.* 2002). Lastly, short-term action planning using script events is associated with activation of distinct regions in the left frontal and parietal cortices (Ruby *et al.* 2002) (see below).

The left hemisphere also seems to be dominant for the selection of learned actions (Rushworth *et al.* 1998b), motor preparation (Krams *et al.* 1998), and motor attention (Rushworth *et al.* 1997a, 2001). Schluter *et al.* (2001) demonstrated with positron emission tomography (PET) that the selection of finger movements with the right and left hands activated the left hemisphere (intraparietal, premotor, and prefrontal regions); when the left hand was used activation of the right hemisphere was also found, in agreement with previous studies which showed that activations are more widespread, the less automated a task may be (Jenkins *et al.* 1994). Whereas the term motor preparation encompasses any of the cognitive processes preceding the initiation of movement, motor attention refers to the process of directing attention and preparing for a particular limb movement. Motor preparation and motor attention activate the left supramarginal gyrus (BA 40), whereas the latter also activates the adjacent part of the IPS and the premotor ventral cortex (PMv), together with premotor dorsal (PMd) and dorsolateral prefrontal (DLPF) cortices (BA 46) (Krams *et al.* 1998; Rushworth *et al.* 2001). Furthermore, Coull *et al.* (2000) have shown increased rCBF in similar regions in the left hemisphere, in particular the inferior parietal cortex (BA 40) and inferior premotor/prefrontal cortices when subjects prepare to move a finger within a specific time ('temporal orienting').

The left hemisphere also seems to be specialized for the selection of object-oriented actions (Rushworth *et al.* 1998b). Moreover, the perception of objects activates cortical areas in the left hemisphere involved in motor representation, indicating that objects automatically afford actions that can be made towards them (Grèzes and Decety 2002), and the retrieval of action knowledge in general, including knowledge related to tools, involves the left hemisphere, in particular the posterior middle temporal area (MT) (see below).

Thus it seems likely that interhemispheric differences in the control of actions largely depend on the context in which the movement is performed and on the cognitive requirements of the task; that is, when a single and/or sequence of object-oriented movements are performed outside the usual context and/or require different cognitive abilities, such as action selection, motor attention and/or action orientation in time, the left hemisphere emerges as more dominant than the right (Leiguarda and Marsden 2000).

Types of limb apraxia

Limb-kinetic apraxia

In 1907, Kleist wrote:

> Theoretically, we can advance a third form of apraxia together with the motor (ideomotor) and ideatory (ideational) apraxias, which would be due to a lesion of the sensorimotor territory rather than to a separation of the sensorimotor world from the rest of the brain.

He called it 'innervatory apraxia' and attributed it to a lesion of area 6 (premotor area) in the region that corresponds to the arm (Kleist 1931).

The clinical features of innervatory apraxia were then described as follows:

> There was a loss of hand and finger ability. We found slowness and stiffness of movements, increased difficulty with isolated movements, and a tendency for generalized and associated movements, as well as loss of fine and composed structure of movements in which the

simultaneous and sequential actions of several individual movements have suffered. Errors in innervatory apraxia represent a coarseness and fragmentation of the model. It may also occur as a digital disorder, limited to individual fingers. Perhaps, it should not be called apraxia at all. Nonetheless, it is different from paresis. Motility is not weakened, or only slightly, but even when there is slight weakness, this does not explain the uniqueness of the disorder. What is lacking or defective are functions which lie above the innervations: the ability to connect and isolate individual innervations. The greater the innervatory complexity of hand functions, the greater the disorder. (Kleist 1907)

Based on an early observation by Westphal of a patient with loss of 'limb-kinetic concepts', Liepmann considered this type of praxic deficit as the most motor of all the limb apraxias, and later called it limb-kinetic (Liepmann 1905, 1908, 1920).

Even simple and practiced movements for which we have purely kinetic memory are always coarse and mutilated. The virtuosity given to movement by practice is lost. Movements are at best those of someone who is unpractised, rough and awkward; a starting point cannot even be found for many movements, or the movements become amorphous (formless). (Liepmann 1905)

According to Liepmann, the kinetic engrams lie in the sensorimotorium, a region comprising the pre- and post-central gyri and the pes of the superior, middle, and inferior frontal convolutions. Partial damage to this area by an elective process, such as senile atrophy or progressive paralysis, can disrupt the engrams without causing paralysis; thus the movable extremities exhibit apraxic symptoms, along with possible cortical ataxia due to loss of sense impressions.

Recently, a reviewed interest in LKA has arisen mainly from the study of patients with corticobasal degeneration. The deficit in LKA is mainly confined to finger and hand movements contralateral to the lesion, regardless of its hemispheric side, with preservation of power and sensation. Manipulatory finger movements are predominantly affected, but in most cases all movements, either complex or routine, are involved independently of the modality to evoke them. There is a delay in the initiation and slowing of movements, but what is specially striking is the temporal disordering of cooperative muscle action and loss of selective muscle activation; the fingers no longer act in concert and there is lack of interfinger coordination. Simultaneous and sequential actions of individual fingers are distorted, and the movement becomes coarse, fragmented, and mutilated. Fruitless attempts usually precede wrong movements, which in turn are frequently contaminated by extraneous movements. Imitation of finger postures is also abnormal, and some patients use the less affected or normal hand to reproduce the requested posture. The severity of the deficit is consistent, exhibiting the same degree in everyday activities as in the clinical setting; thus there is no voluntary-automatic dissociation (Liepmann 1908; Faglioni and Basso 1985; Leiguarda *et al.* 2003).

Performance with the limb-kinetic apraxic hand may superficially resemble tactile apraxia due to posterior parietal lesions, since both are finger and hand apraxias with gross disturbances of object exploration and manipulation. However, intransitive and expressive movements are preserved and imitation of hand and finger movements is normal in tactile apraxia. In addition, patients with tactile apraxia may exhibit complex somatosensory disturbances (see Chapter 18).

Ideomotor apraxia

Ideomotor apraxia has been defined as 'an impairment in the timing, sequencing and spatial organization of gestural movements' (Rothi *et al.* 1991). Patients with IMA exhibit mainly temporal and spatial errors (Table 17.2). The movements are incorrectly produced but the goal of the action can usually be recognized. Occasionally, however, the performance is so severely deranged that the examiner cannot recognize the movement. Transitive movements are more affected than intransitive ones on pantomiming to commands, and patients usually improve on imitation when performance is compared with responses to verbal commands (Heilman and Rothi 1985). Acting with tools/objects is carried out better than pantomiming their use but, even so, movements may not be entirely normal. IMA is commonly associated with damage to the parietal association areas, less frequently with lesions of the PM cortex and supplementary motor area (SMA), and usually with disruption of the intrahemispheric white matter bundles which interconnect them (Leiguarda and Marsden 2000). Although small lesions of the basal ganglia and thalamus may cause IMA, in the majority of patients the pathology extends to the internal capsule and periventricular and peristriatal white matter (Pramstaller and Marsden 1996). Most studies examining possible clinico-anatomical correlation for IMA have found a strong association of apraxia with large cortico-subcortical lesions in the suprasylvian perirolandic region of the left dominant hemisphere, but no specific lesion site which correlated with apraxia (Kertesz and Ferro 1984; Alexander *et al.* 1992; Schnider *et al.* 1997). However, a recent study using quantitative structural image analysis to determine the location and greatest lesion overlap in patients with left-hemisphere stroke and IMA, as determined by assessing spatiotemporal errors on imitating meaningful and meaningless gestures, found that damage to the left middle frontal gyrus (BA 46, 9, 8, and 6) and left superior and inferior parietal cortex surrounding the IPS (BA 7, 39, and 40) more commonly produce IMA than damage to other areas (Haaland *et al.* 2000). The authors found target errors more commonly with parietal- than frontal-lobe-damaged apraxic patients. Hanna-Pladdy *et al.* (2001b) compared praxis performance on a variety of tasks (transitive and intransitive communicative gestures on verbal command and imitation) in patients with left-hemisphere cortical and subcortical lesions. They found that patients with cortical lesions exhibited deficits in the production of transitive and intransitive gestures to verbal command and imitation, whereas the subcortical group demonstrated milder deficits, though only when performing transitive gestures to verbal commands. These findings are in agreement with the pattern of praxic deficits found in patients with basal ganglion diseases (Leiguarda *et al.* 1997; Hamilton *et al.* 2003).

IMA may coexist with LKA; nevertheless, both types of apraxia can be clinically distinguished on the basis of the following aspects. First, IMA, though asymmetric, is invariably bilateral, whereas LKA is found contralateral to the affected hemisphere. Secondly, all movements in LKA, whether symbolic or non-symbolic, intransitive or transitive, are affected irrespective of the modality (i.e. verbal, visual, tactile) through which they are evoked, whereas in IMA intransitive movements are less compromised than transitive movements and these are unequally involved depending on the modality under which they are tested. Thirdly, finger and hand movements and posture errors typical of LKA are readily distinguished from temporospatial errors (i.e. external configuration, movement trajectory) exhibited by patients with IMA, which predominantly involve the arm and hand rather than the fingers, although internal configuration types of error may be common to both disorders; however, such errors in IMA are usually characterized by abnormal postures and movements of the whole hand but fail to reflect the severe distortion of individual finger movements and the interfinger incoordination so typical of LKA.

Ideational or conceptual apraxia

There has been a great deal of confusion about the term ideational apraxia. Liepmann (1908) defined IA as an impairment of tasks requiring a sequence of several acts with tools and objects (e.g. preparing a letter for mailing). However, other authors use the term to denote a failure to use single tools appropriately (De Renzi 1989). To overcome this confusion, Ochipa *et al.* (1992) have suggested restricting the term IA to a failure to conceive a series of acts leading to an action goal, and introduced the term conceptual apraxia (CA) to denote deficits in the different types of tool-action knowledge as proposed by Roy and Square (1985). However, a strict difference between IA and CA is not always feasible, since patients with IA not only fail on tests of multiple object use, but may also perform abnormally when using a single object (De Renzi and Lucchelli 1988). Thus, according to Freund (1992) and following Liepmann (1920), IA could be defined as a deficit in the conception of the movement so that the patient does not know what to do.

Patients with IA or CA exhibit primarily content errors or semantic parapraxias (e.g. use a comb as a toothbrush) in the performance of transitive movements (Table 17.2). They are unable to associate tools with the objects that receive their action; thus, when a partially driven nail is shown, the patient may select a pair of scissors rather than a hammer from an array of tools to complete the action, and may also fail to describe a function of a tool or point to a tool when the function is described by the examiner. In addition, patients may have difficulties in matching objects for shared purposes; for example, when they are asked to complete an action and the appropriate tool is not available (e.g. a hammer to drive a nail), they may not select the most adequate tool for that action (e.g. a wrench), but rather one which is inadequate (e.g. a screwdriver), as well as being unable to solve novel mechanical problems (Ochipa *et al.* 1992; Heilman *et al.* 1997). However, selection and application of novel tools seem to rely on the direct influence of structure on function, which in turn would depend upon a parietal-lobe-based system of non-semantic sensorimotor representation that may be triggered by object affordance (see below) (Hodges *et al.* 1999). Patients with IA are impaired in the sequencing of tool/object use, exhibiting many types of errors including deletion, addition, omission, misuse, substitution, and perseveration (Pick 1905; Liepmann 1920; Poeck 1983; De Renzi and Luchelli 1988). Patients with IA or CA are disabled in everyday life, because they use tools/objects improperly, they misselect tools/objects for an intended activity, perform a complex sequential activity (e.g. make espresso coffee) in a mistaken order, or do not complete the task at all (Foundas *et al.* 1995). IA has been traditionally allocated to the left parieto-occipital and parietotemporal regions (Liepmann 1920), although left frontal and frontotemporal lesions may also cause IA (De Renzi and Lucchelli 1988) or CA (Heilman *et al.* 1997). Nevertheless, semantic or conceptual errors are particularly observed in patients with temporal lobe pathology (e.g. semantic dementia) (Hodges *et al.* 2000) (see below).

Modality-specific or dissociation apraxias

The modality-specific (De Renzi *et al.* 1982) or dissociation apraxias (Rothi *et al.* 1991) refer to those types of praxic deficits exhibited by patients who commit errors only, or predominantly, when the movement is evoked by one but not all modalities. Thus the impairment of patients who perform abnormally only under verbal commands has been attributed to a left-hemispheric lesion most likely located in the parietal lobe, disrupting the lexicomotor transformation process (Heilman 1973; De Renzi *et al.* 1982; Ruby *et al.* 2002), or in the corpus callosum (Geschwind and Kaplan 1962). Patients who performed poorly to seen objects, but performed much better when given object visual and tactile input and when asked to gesture to the name of the object, have also been reported (Pilgrim and Humphreys 1991). On occasion, praxic deficits may be predominantly confined to the tactile modality (De Renzi *et al.* 1982). Finally, patients have been reported who, unlike those with IMA who improved on imitation, were more impaired when imitating than when pantomiming to command (conduction apraxia) (Ochipa *et al.* 1994), or could not imitate but performed flawlessly under other modalities (visuoimitative apraxia) (Merians *et al.* 1997). Deficits may be restricted solely to the imitation of meaningless gestures with preserved imitation to meaningful gestures (see below) (Mehler 1987; Goldenberg and Hagmann 1997; Peigneux *et al.* 2000a).

Callosal apraxia

Patients with damage to the body of the corpus callosum with or without genu involvement (Liepmann and Maas 1907; Watson and Heilman 1983; Graff-Radford *et al.* 1987; Leiguarda *et al.* 1989) may develop unilateral apraxia of the non-dominant limb whose characteristics vary according to the type of test given and the lateralization pattern of praxic skills in each patient. Some patients could not correctly pantomime to verbal commands with their left hand, but performed normally on imitation and object use (Geschwind and Kaplan 1962), whereas others could not use their left hand on command, by imitation or while holding the object (Watson and Heilman 1983; Leiguarda *et al.* 1989). Moreover, a few patients could not pantomime to verbal commands and while holding the object, but performed fairly well on imitation (Graff-Radford *et al.* 1987), or improved over time on imitation and object use (Watson and Heilman 1983). Thus the most enduring callosal type of praxic defect is demonstrated when verbal–motor tasks, such as pantomiming to command, are used (Graff-Radford *et al.* 1987).

Neural processes underlying limb praxis

As described in a previous section, the various types of limb apraxia may be observed with lesions affecting several distinct brain structures, i.e. predominantly the premotor cortex of either hemisphere in LKA, premotor and parietal association cortices with their corresponding subcortical (basal ganglia and thalamus) connections, in particular of the left hemisphere, in IMA, and mainly the left parietotemporal region in IA. Therefore it seems clear that the neural components subserving the multiple processes involved in limb praxis are distributed over a large network of neural structures, both cortical and subcortical, made up by many interrelated systems pertaining to dissimilar levels of action representation. Partial or complete damage to one or more of these systems, depending on the location and extension of the pathological process, would explain the different types of apractic disorders, as well as the commonly observed clinical dissociations.

The selection of learned actions

Neurophysiological, neuroimaging, and clinical studies have allowed delineating at least two distributed neural systems essential for learning the selection of limb-movement responses and for learning the relation of object-oriented responses (Halsband and Freund 1990; Kurata and Hoffman 1994; Passingham 1993; Rushworth *et al.* 1998b; Schluter *et al.* 2001). The system consisting of the lateral premotor (BA 6) and parietal cortices, basal ganglia, thalamus, and white matter fascicles would participate in the selection of limb-movement responses, whereas an adjacent system made up by lateral area 8 and interconnected parietal regions, thalamus, striatum, and white matter fascicles would be concerned with the selection of object-oriented responses (Rushworth *et al.* 1998b; Schluter *et al.* 2001).

The striatum seems to play some role in context-dependent response selection. The corticostriatal circuit architecture, in which virtually the entire cortex projects onto the striatum, which then projects onto the pallidum before returning via the thalamus to select cortical regions (see Chapter 23), strongly suggests that some form of selection/modification process is occurring within the circuitry. Furthermore, it seems likely that different corticostriatal circuits may govern response selection in different domains. Context-relevant information processing would allow the striatum to instruct cortical areas as to which sensory input or patterns of motor output are behaviourally significant in a given context; that is, the striatum would modify coarsely coded cortical representations of motor intentions/plans into representations which are context appropriate (Beiser *et al.* 1997; Lawrence *et al.* 1999).

Rushworth *et al.* (1998b) found that damage to the left frontoparietal cortices, striatum, thalamus, and white matter fascicles impaired the selection of both limb-movement responses and object-oriented responses; by using PET they showed activation of the prefrontal (within the inferior frontal gyrus) dorsal premotor and intraparietal cortices on the left hemisphere when the subject selects moving one or two fingers depending on the cue presented (Schluter *et al.* 2001). Furthermore, the inhibition of competing motor memories has been shown to activate the ventrolateral prefrontal cortex as well as the caudate nucleus (Shadmehr and Holcomb 1999). However, successful motor selection requires not only making the appropriate motor response but also doing it at the right time (timing adjustment). Using fMRI, Sakai *et al.* (2000) found that the selection of a motor response activates the pre-SMA and rCMA, as well as the posterior part of the cerebellum, which was related to timing adjustment; although partially separated, both processes were functionally integrated in the IPS and the lateral PM cortex to generate a final motor schema.

Neural representation of gestures

Transitive gestures

Skilful tool/object use and competent conventional use of objects and tools requires a normal prehension system, intact representations of functional actions for an adequate utilization behaviour, and an intact semantic knowledge.

Visually guided reaching, grasping, and object manipulation are paramount components in any task-related movement. Such object-oriented action implies a cerebral interface set up to align sensory information concerning position and shape of both object and limb, with specific motor commands encoding distance, velocity, direction, and grip (Sakata *et al.* 1995; Kalaska *et al.* 1997). Research on primates has identified a series of segregated parietofrontal circuits, working in parallel, each involved in a specific sensorimotor transformation process. The proposed functions of the main parietofrontal circuits are as follows: (i) visual and somatosensory transformation for reaching; (ii) somatosensory transformation for posture and transformation of body part location data into information required to control body part movements; (iii) visuomotor transformation for grasping and manipulation; (iv) coding peripersonal space for limb and neck movements; (v) internal representation of actions; (vi) visual transformation for eye movements (Rizzolatti *et al.* 1998) (see Chapters 2 and 3). The parietal areas reciprocally interconnected with those areas in the motor cortex making up the parietofrontal circuits send extensive projections to the basal ganglia. Yeterian and Pandya (1993) have suggested that connections between the caudal superior parietal lobule and the dorsal putamen and dorsolateral caudate nucleus may play a role in the preparation and kinematic coding of movements as well as in reaching. Individual neurons within the putamen exhibit either preparatory (set related) or movement-related responses similar to those found in the SMA and the premotor and primary motor cortices. Some neurons in the globus pallidus and substantia nigra pars reticulata have been shown to increase their discharge frequency in relation to the amplitude and peak velocity of movements (Georgopoulos *et al.* 1983), whereas other pallidal as well as putaminal cells discharge in relation to the direction of arm movements (Mitchell *et al.* 1987). Orientation-related neurons have also been found in the caudate nucleus; these neurons discharge not only in relation to the direction and amplitude of the orientation, but also depending on the sequence in which the orientation is executed (Kemardi and Joseph 1995). Moreover, Burnod *et al.* (1999) have suggested, in relation to reaching, that the basal ganglia could provide the cortex with gating signals that can trigger the sequence of movements at the appropriate time and in the appropriate order when several outputs are possible for a given task and when the decision has to be made between concurrent tasks.

Several functional brain-imaging studies on reaching, grasping, and manipulation in humans have demonstrated activation of the parietal and frontal areas corresponding to those involved in the circuits described in monkeys. In particular, activation has been observed bilaterally in the superior (BA 7) and inferior (BA 39 and 40) parietal lobules, PMd and PMv cortices, and SMA, as well as in the primary sensorimotor cortex. In addition, activation has been documented in the caudate and putamen, globus pallidus, thalamus, and cerebellum (Grafton *et al.* 1996; Matsumura *et al.* 1996; Rizzolatti *et al.* 1996; Faillenot *et al.* 1997). Grasping specifically activates the lateral bank of the anterior IPs (Binkofski *et al.* 1998), whereas during grasping and manipulation the PMv cortex and second somatosensory area (S_{II}) and dorsal part of area 5 (Pe) are also involved; the last two areas participate in tactile and prioprioceptive control of manipulation, respectively (Binkofski *et al.* 1999).

It has also been demonstrated that viewing and naming man-made tools or objects activate the left PMd and PMv areas, as well as the left posterior parietal (BA 40) cortex, demonstrating a close link between objects capable of manipulation and information about activations associated with their use (Grafton *et al.* 1997; Chao and Martin 2000). Grèzes and Decety (2002) found that the perception of an object was associated with increased rCBF in a common set of cortical regions in the left hemisphere, such as the occipitotemporal junction, inferior parietal lobule, SMA, pars triangularis in the inferior frontal gyrus, and the dorsal and ventral precentral gyrus, all of which are involved in motor representations, thus providing neurophysiological evidence that the perception of objects automatically affords actions requiring their use.

However, the competent conventional use of objects and tools depends primarily on an intact semantic knowledge. Two possible models of semantic system functioning have been posited. The model advocated by McCarthy and Warrington (1988) is based on a multimodal distributed semantic architecture in which objects of all types, animate as well as inanimate, are represented by visual, tactile, and motor/proprioceptive nodes in proportion to the degree to which these various sensory and motor system(s) became involved as the representation was acquired and elaborated; in the case of tools and body parts, the dominant 'channel' of experience involves sensorimotor (i.e. how the tool is held and used/manipulated) and functional information (i.e. knowing the usage context). The second model implies that a verbal propositional semantic system operates by 'reading' the sensorimotor representations or gestural engrams (Hodges *et al.* 1999, 2000). Milner and Goodale (1995) have suggested that skilled and appropriate object use requires the combination of dorsal stream processing ('how' system) with the product of ventral pathway processing which provides access to semantics, a proposal supported by functional imaging studies in normal subjects (Passingham and Toni 2001).

A common brain region activated throughout most studies investigating tool and action knowledge has been the left posterior MT area (BA 21) (Perani *et al.* 1995; Martin *et al.* 1996; Phillips *et al.* 2002). The left posterior MT area is usually activated together with neural systems associated with semantic retrieval [left inferior and middle temporal gyri (BA 20 and 21)], left inferior frontal cortex (BA 47, 45 and 44), left premotor cortex, and left frontomarginal gyrus (BA 10/12). The left posterior MT area is involved when stimuli show or imply human movements i.e. when body parts (e.g. hand) or manipulable objects (e.g. tools) are involved in the gesture (Martin *et al.* 1995; Decety *et al.* 1997; Grèzes *et al.* 1999; Phillips *et al.* 2002b), when a gestural/manipulative movement is implied (e.g. static image of hand gesturing, object falling) (Kourtzi and Kanwisher 2000; Peigneux *et al.* 2000b), or when an action is verbally planned (e.g. action-word generation) (Martin *et al.* 1995; Warburton *et al.* 1996). The generation of action verbs related to tool/object use also activates the left angular gyrus, indicating that the system mediating access to verbs is anatomically close to those that support concepts of movements and space–time relationships (Grèzes and Decety 2002).

Functional brain imaging of tool-use

In normal subjects, the sole brain region activated during manipulation with a tool, compared with the finger, was the lateral edge of the IPS (Inoue *et al.* 2001). Activation of the IPS most likely represents its involvement in mental (or introspective) processes to locate and update the body's representation so as to manipulate ongoing tool acts purposefully (Inoue *et al.* 2001). Thus the tool is incorporated into the body's representation, becoming a part or an extension of the arm (Iriki *et al.* 1996; Obayashi *et al.* 2001). So far, only two fMRI studies of pantomiming tool-use gestures have been published (Moll *et al.* 2000; Choi *et al.* 2001). Both demonstrated activation predominantly in the left hemisphere regardless of the hand used; however, whereas Moll *et al.* (2000) found activation only in the IPS and dorsolateral frontal area, Choi *et al.* (2001) documented a larger extent of activation, including the superior parietal lobule, more than the supramarginal gyrus,

SMA and PMd cortex, putamen, and cerebellum. We performed fMRI investigations of normal subjects while pantomiming transitive versus intransitive representational gestures with the right hand and found activation restricted to the PMv cortex and inferior parietal lobule (IPL) on the left hemisphere. In a further study, we evaluated normal subjects while pantomiming tool use involving distal movements (e.g. using scissors) as well as more proximal movements (e.g. screw-driving. We found (i) predominance of left-hemisphere activation with distal more than with proximal movements, even when the left hand was used, (ii) activation of the superior and inferior parietal lobule around the IPS and the basal ganglia irrespetive of the type of movement, and (iii) activation mainly of the PMv cortex with distal transitive gestures and predominantly of the PMd with more proximal transitive gestures (Fridman *et al.*, unpublished data).

   In conclusion, skilful and competent use of tool/object depends upon tool/object-specific conceptual knowledge and specific sensorimotor transformation circuits involved in reaching, grasping, and manipulation, and therefore subserved by a extensive temporo-parietofrontal system which integrates tool/object knowledge with the ideation and generation of actions (Milner and Goodale 1995; Hodges *et al.* 2000). A putative temporoparietal route may constitute an intermediary and necessary step to integrate the functional properties of objects into adequate movement patterns such as those required for utilization behaviour.

Intransitive gestures

Since Morlass (1928) originally suggested that transitive and intransitive gestures could be selectively impaired in apraxia, plentiful evidence has accumulated indicating that these different gesture types might be processed by different systems. Intransitive gestures are usually much less complex than transitive movements, are geared to sociocultural contexts, and are stimulated by environmental cues (e.g. salute), rather than constrained by the shape and function of tools/objects as in the case of transitive movements. Furthermore, since intransitive movements and postures are used with communicative intent, their representations are more frequently and fully activated by speech or by seeing someone else's gesture than by transitive movements. Therefore it has been suggested that intransitive movements and postures are subserved by a more widely and differently distributed intrahemispheric network and/or that they are bilaterally represented (Cubelli *et al.* 2000; Heath *et al.* 2001; Mozaz *et al.* 2002).

Physiopathology of limb apraxia
Limb-kinetic type of praxic deficit

Proper grasping and manipulation require the integrity of the corresponding sensorimotor transformation circuit, the capacity to generate independent finger movements, and a delicate somatosensory control process (Jeannerod *et al.* 1995).

On the basis of the anatomical connections and functional properties of the F5 and anterior intraparietal (AIP) areas, a sensorimotor circuit for grasping has been proposed whereby the AIP neurons represent the entire hand action and frontal neurons encode particular segments of the action (Jeannerod *et al.* 1995) (see Chapter 3).

Direct corticomotoneural projection systems underpin the ability to perform relatively independent finger movements. However, movements of an individual digit require activation of a complex set of muscles; as well as moving the required digit, muscular activity must also stabilize the bony chain and prevent unwanted digit movements. Both cortical and corticospinal inhibition seem to be essential for the selection and control of hand muscle activity (Lemon 1997). Injection of the γ-aminobutyric acid antagonist bicuculline in the primary motor and post-arcuate premotor cortices in monkeys caused disturbed manual dexterity in the raising pick-up test due to disinhibition of neuronal activity in the cortex (Matsumura *et al.* 1991).

Finally, when the object is adequately grasped, a delicate somatosensory control of finger movement is necessary for precise manipulation to be performed. During actual manipulation, discrete mechanical events are encoded in the spatiotemporal pattern of signals in parallel sensory channels, particularly tactile (Johansson and Cole 1992). We have proposed that the most typical examples of LKA, such as those seen in cortico-basal degeneration, are due to disruption of the frontoparietal circuits devoted to grasping and manipulation, combined with impaired generation and control of independent finger movements due to disruption of intracortical inhibitory circuits, as well as to dysfunction of somatosensory control of manipulation (Leiguarda *et al.* 2003). However, because patients with corticobasal degeneration and LKA have neither clinical signs of corticospinal deficit nor involvement of fast-conducting corticomoto-neural projections as evaluated with transcranial magnetic stimulation, and a defect in somaesthesis may not be present, this distinctive apractic disorder may basically result from dysfunction of the non-primary cortical motor areas, as previously suggested (Blasi *et al.* 1999; Fogassi *et al.* 2001; Leiguarda *et al.* 2003).

Limb-kinetic apraxia has been scantily reported with focal lesions (Faglioni and Basso 1985, Shiota and Kawamura 1994). There are two potential explanation. First, most PM lesions also involve the precentral cortex, and therefore the contralateral paresis or paralysis precludes the expression of the praxic deficit. Secondly, bilateral activation of the PM cortex is often observed with unilateral hand movements, and bilateral activation of this region has been demonstrated when subjects manipulate complex objects (Binkofski *et al.* 1999); thus a unilateral lesion would not be enough for an overt deficit, since bilateral involvement would most likely be necessary. In fact, all recently pathologically confirmed cases of LKA suffered a degenerative process such as corticobasal degeneration and Pick's disease, involving frontal and parietal cortices or, predominantly, the PM cortex (Leiguarda *et al.* 2003).

Ideomotor types of praxic deficits
Dysfunction of frontoparietal circuits involved in sensorimotor transformation

A subgroup of patients with IMA usually commit spatial and temporal errors when performing transitive as well as intransitive symbolic or communicative movements under all modalities of elicitation (i.e. verbal command, imitation, seeing and handling the object), although performance usually improves on imitation and with object use. These patients also exhibit errors when imitating meaningless postures and novel motor sequences. It was originally suggested that the crucial underlying neural mechanism in this group of IMA patients was a disruption of the parietofrontal circuits and their subcortical connections, subserving the computations required to translate an action goal into movements by integrating sensory input with central representation of actions based on prior experience (Haaland *et al.* 2000; Leiguarda and Marsden 2000). Whereas damage to specific circuits will cause unimodal deficit (see Chapter 18), involvement of several circuits by a larger lesion or disruption of their integration in supramodal reference frames will cause IMA. Thus damage to circuits devoted to sensorimotor transformation for grasping, reaching, and posture, for transformation of body-part location into information required to control body-part movements, and for coding extrapersonal space would produce incorrect finger and hand posture and abnormal orientation of the tool/object, inappropriate arm configuration, and faulty movement orientation (with respect to both the body and the target of the movement in extrapersonal space), as well as movement trajectory abnormalities. Several lines of evidence support our proposal.

1 The spatiotemporal errors made by some patients with IMA are similar to those seen in patients with isolated reaching and grasping deficits, and conversely some IMA patients themselves made errors when reaching and grasping (reviewed by Leiguarda 2003).

2 Monkeys with lesions or inactivation in regions of the parietal and premotor cortices, which are involved in sensorimotor transformation circuits, show almost identical kinematic, spatial, and interjoint coordination deficits (Kurata and Hoffman 1994; Rushworth *et al.* 1997b, 1998).

3 The spatial, temporal, and interjoint coordination deficits during performance of a transitive movement are observed along all types of instruction modalities (i.e. verbal command, imitation, seeing and handling the object) (Clark *et al.* 1994), and it has been shown that the temporal organization of object-oriented action remains stable under all such instruction modalities, which suggests that there is a level within action representation where all modalities converge (Weiss *et al.* 2000).

Therefore damage to the circuits involved in different sensorimotor transformation processes subserving the representation of object-oriented action or pragmatic representations most likely causes this type of IMA. Involvement of body representations in the posterior parietal lobe (Lacquaniti *et al.* 1995) would contribute to the praxic deficit, in particular to the disruption of meaningless and meaningful gestures imitation (see below) and perhaps also to the performance of intransitive movements. Patients correctly select movements but have difficulties in translating the selected response into action due to an 'execution' disturbance; the on-line guidance of movements may be defective and they may complain of disability in everyday activities. According to Roy *et al.* (2000), disruption at the movement-execution stage of gesture performance is the most common mechanism of IMA.

Disruption of the subcortical connection of the parietofrontal circuits devoted to the sensorimotor transformation processes, including the one coding the representation of peripersonal space somatotopically (Graziano and Gross 1998), may be one of the mechanisms involved in some of the ideomotor types of praxic deficits observed in patients with some basal ganglia diseases (e.g. Parkinson's disease, progressive supranuclear palsy) since they exhibit similar kinematic abnormalities, although less severe, as these patients with IMA due to parietal lesions (Leiguarda *et al.* 2000b). In support, putaminal lesions (in marmosets) cause inaccurate reaching (Kendall *et al.* 2000), whereas inactivation of GPi (in monkeys) leads to impaired reaching and grasping (Wenger *et al.* 1999). Moreover, studies of reaching and grasping in patients with Parkinson's disease have also shown several abnormalities (Jackson *et al.* 1995; Majsak *et al.* 1998).

Disruption of skilled learned body postures

Some patients with ideomotor type of apraxia have deficits in forming hand configuration only when appropriate for object use; i.e. they show inadequate hand grasp when the object has to be manipulated with the intention to use it, but neither during visually guided (on-line) reaching and grasping movements (Sirigu *et al.* 1995a), nor when grasping novel objects (Buxbaum *et al.* 2003). These patients can correctly name and recognize fingers and objects and verbally define their functions, but are unable to discriminate between normal and abnormal hand postures and exhibit deficits in the perception of self-generated movements (Sirigu *et al.* 1999) and in mentally simulating hand gestures (Sirigu *et al.* 1995b). These types of deficits have been associated with left inferior parietal cortex lesion; damage to these regions may degrade the storing or interrupt the access to representations of learned body postures and/or movement associated with familiar objects (Heilman and Rothi 1985; see also Chapter 19). Rushworth *et al.* (2003) have suggested that a failure to update motor attention, as it is defined as the updating of the representation of the hand and arm, may underlie the errors of some patients with left-parietal lesions when using tool/objects; these patients would fail when a body part has to effectively change and accommodate to the addition of a tool/object.

Disruption of action selection

Another subgroup of patients with IMA exhibit spatial and temporal errors predominantly when pantomiming to verbal command with either hand, i.e. outside the appropriate context. They improve on imitation, and performance may normalize when handling the object. These patients do not complain of difficulties in everyday activities; there is an automatic–voluntary dissociation. The on-line guidance of movements is normal and they have no pointing and/or grasping deficits (Ietswaart *et al.* 2001). Thus the pragmatic representations for object-oriented actions are not directly affected, as it is a higher-level deficit involving a premovement neural process. The deficits arise when the subject has to shift from a strategy where object-oriented actions are processed automatically to a more cognitive mode due to inability to select the appropriate motor schemas from stored motor representations to be organized into purposive action. They might also have deficits in mentally evoking (imaging) the action (Jeannerod 1997). It has been argued that movement simulation may actually be involved in the refinement and selection of a premovement plan (Johnson *et al.* 2002). Furthermore, it has been postulated that the internal manipulation of the body image underlies the generation of motor imagery; updated and maintained spatial hand-image representation would allow for the simulation of continuous spatiotemporal trajectories of the hand path for most efficient tool use (Obayashi *et al.* 2001). Imaging a left- or right-hand movement causes bilateral activation in the prefrontal premotor, SMA, and superior and inferior parietal lobules, and predominantly left-hemisphere activation of the IPL and caudate nucleus (Gerardin *et al.* 2000; Grèzes and Decety 2001), and both real and imagined tool-use pantomiming activate the same intraparietal region (Moll *et al.* 2000). Most of these regions closely correspond to those involved in the neural system subserving action selection, which are lateralized to the left hemisphere (Schluter *et al.* 2001). In the study conducted by Rushworth *et al.* (1998b), all patients with deficits in the selection of learned actions and apraxia had lesions in the left hemisphere located predominantly in the parietal lobe, but many also had lesions involving the lateral PM cortex, as well as interconnecting white matter fascicles and basal ganglia and thalamus. When the corticostriatal circuits are damaged, apraxia may specifically result from an inability to gate competing motor schemas or programmes effectively, which then overwhelm the system with competing response options and lead to disruption of the organized production of purposeful movements. Therefore patients with impaired performance predominantly when pantomiming to verbal commands may be those with lesions involving systems subserving movement selection, with preservation of circuits devoted to sensorimotor transformation. In fact, in monkeys it has been possible to dissociate an impairment in movement selection from an impairment in kinematics (Kurata and Hoffman 1994). The dramatic improvement shown by this subgroup of IMA patients when imitating transitive gestures may be explained in several ways: (i) the contribution of the right hemisphere to gesture imitation; (ii) the influence that the presentation of the model, such as the motor configuration of the limb, may exert on knowledge about manual interaction with objects (Jeannerod 1997); (iii) the use of the undamaged temporofrontal component of the putative system subserving imitation of meaningful gestures in the left hemisphere when the lesion is restricted to the parietal lobe (Carey *et al.* 1997). The normal performance that this subgroup of patients also shows when seeing and handling the object may be explained by the affordance provided by the visual/ tactile cues emanating from the tool/object, which in addition provides a 'more natural context' and facilitates the correct hand/limb position for the gesture (Leiguarda and Marsden 2000).

An alternative explanation for a restricted deficit in pantomiming to verbal command observed in IMA patients with limb apraxia may be ascribed to a disruption of the lexicomotor transformation process due to a parietal lesion which spares the parietal node devoted to visuo(graphic)motor transformation (Ruby *et al.* 2002), although these patients seem to exhibit content rather than temporospatial errors (Heilman 1973).

Inability to infer function from structure

Numerous neuropsychological studies have described patients with impaired use of familiar objects and impaired performance of tasks requiring selection and use of novel tools, but with preserved semantic knowledge of object functions (Goldenberg and Hagmann 1998; Hodges *et al.* 1999; Spatt *et al.* 2002). Most patients with difficulties in mechanical problem-solving (novel tool selection), which unveil the incapacity to infer function from structure, fail also on pantomime of object use and commit errors on actual use of familiar tools, so that they are disabled in everyday life. Errors are mainly of the spatiotemporal type, usually characterized by marked abnormal hand postures but without semantic parapraxias (Hodges *et al.* 1999).

However, selection of novel tools can dissociate from pantomime of tool use, which is another demonstration that different manifestations of apraxia can occur independently of each other. For example, patients with left frontal lobe damage may be defective only when pantomiming tool use, whereas left parietal lobe lesions may specifically disrupt novel tool selection. In fact, defective tool selection is particularly seen in patients with parietal damage (Goldenberg and Hagmann 1998). Thus this type of apractic deficit may be ascribed to the disruption of a parietal-lobe base system specialized for visuomotor interaction with the environment, which may be triggered by visual and perhaps tactile object affordance (Hodges *et al.* 1999).

Ideational or conceptual types of praxic deficits

The syndrome of semantic dementia provides an ideal testing ground for investigating the role of conceptual knowledge in the ability to use familiar objects. Structural and functional imaging in semantic dementia reveals bilateral though asymmetrical atrophy and hypometabolism in polar and inferolateral temporal regions, thus mainly affecting the ventral or 'what' pathway (Milner and Goodale 1995). It has been demonstrated that patients with semantic dementia are impaired in the use of objects for which they have lost conceptual knowledge; in other words, they are no longer able to use familiar objects in the conventionally correct and conceptually determined fashion (Hodges *et al.* 1999, 2000). They exhibit many types of semantic or conceptual errors, such as omission or lack of response (e.g. soap treated as if it were an ornament), incorrect (e.g. using a potato peeler as a knife), or partially incorrect (e.g. opening and closing arms on corkscrew) and ill-defined (e.g. moving whisk from side to side). However, performance in the selection and use of novel tools is usually normal (Hodges *et al.* 2000). The preserved ability to use some objects normally that these patients may exhibit was ascribed to degraded but partially retained conceptual knowledge about such objects, enhanced by sensorimotor information (Buxbaum *et al.* 1997), or, more precisely, on reliance upon visual/tactile affordance jointly with good problem-solving skills, since patients efficiently manipulate novel tools (Hodges *et al.* 2000). Patients with temporal lesions of the dominant hemisphere are also affected in their ability to recognize gestures (see Chapter 19).

Imitation of meaningful and meaningless actions

Converging evidence from neuropsychological, neurophysiological, behavioural, and brain-imaging data support the assumption that there is a close relationship between action observation and action execution; i.e. the direct matching account of imitative behaviour (see Chapters 8 and 19). Cognitive studies have demonstrated that imitating a movement is an easier task than responding to a symbolic stimulus like a verbal command (Brass *et al.* 2000), suggesting that distinct mechanisms mediate action imitation and response to symbolic instructions. It has also been shown that well-learnt meaningful (MF) actions are imitated more efficiently than novel meaningless (ML) actions (Rumiati and Tessari 2002). These differences can be predicted on the basis of a cognitive imitation model, which postulates disparate processing routes to the motor system. Imitation of ML actions/postures would be processed through a non-semantic route from visual analysis, including mental transformation of another person's body part, and temporary holding in working/short-term memory of the observed movement/posture, to the motor system for actual execution. Imitation of MF actions/postures, in turn, can be imitated using either a non-semantic or a semantic route through a long-term/semantic memory station. Neuroimaging and neuropsychological data support the existence of at least two partly independent routes (Mehler 1987; Decety *et al.* 1997; Goldenberg and Hagmann 1997; Grèzes *et al.* 1999; Peigneux *et al.* 2000b; Hermsdörfer *et al.* 2001).

1 The perception of an MF action/posture with the aim to be imitated activates the dorsal pathway extending to the dorsolateral premotor cortex from MT/V5 (BA 18/19), always involving the IPL and with the additional participation of the semantic route (temporal cortex).

2 In turn, imitation of an ML action/posture involves predominantly the dorsal pathway, with predominant activation of the left IPL (BA 40) for hand gestures,

and the right IPS and medial visual association areas (BA 8/19) for finger gestures. The lateral occipitotemporal junction is activated by both hand and finger postures (Decety *et al.* 1997; Grèzes *et al.* 1999; Peigneux *et al.* 2000; Hermsdörfer *et al.* 2001).

Thus, imitation seems to be body-part specific; the gesture's visual appearance is mentally transformed into categories of body part relationships mainly in the left IPL when hand postures are to be imitated, and the addition of the right occipitoparietal cortex for precise perceptual analysis and spatial attention for finger gesture imitation (Peigneux *et al.* 2000b; Hermsdörfer *et al.* 2001; Goldenberg and Strauss 2002).

Defective performance on gesture imitation has been found in patients with lesions in several cortical regions (i.e. frontal, parietal, and even temporal) (De Renzi *et al.* 1983; Hermsdörfer *et al.* 1996). Haaland *et al.* (2000) studied patients with left-hemisphere stroke and IMA, as disclosed by spatial errors while imitating gestures, and identified a middle frontal-intraparietal network as the crucial one involved in the representation of goal-directed movements. Interestingly, these patients exhibited more errors when imitating transitive than intransitive and meaningless movements (Haaland *et al.* 2000). Furthermore, patients with left parietal lobe damage seem to have more difficulties when imitating meaningful transitive gestures on their own bodies than when imitating movements with reference to external object use, a finding that may suggest that the basic deficit in these subjects concerns the ability to code movements in relation to their body schema (Halsband *et al.* 2001).

Imitation of meaningless foot, hand, and finger postures discloses differential susceptibility to right- and left-brain damage. Left-brain-damaged patients have more difficulties imitating foot and hand than finger postures, whereas right-brain-damaged patients commit more errors with finger postures (Goldenberg 1999). Therefore it seems that the left hemisphere is mainly responsible for coding gestures with reference to knowledge concerning body parts, but needs the contribution of the right hemisphere when demands are made on perceptual analysis of the demonstrated gesture (Goldenberg and Strauss 2002).

Schwoebel *et al.* (2004) studied distinct types of body representation underlying the production and imitation of meaningful and meaningless movements. Their findings support the 'two routes' model for action imitation since performance on body semantics (knowledge about body parts) and body schema (dynamic mapping of the current positions of one body part relative to another) were predictive of meaningful gesture performance, whereas body schema measure alone predicted imitation of meaningless movements.

Representation of sequential movements and actions

Functional brain imaging has shown that different neural systems are actively engaged in planning and executing sequential movements depending on whether the sequence has been prelearned or is a new one, and contingent upon the complexity of the movement sequence. The SMA, primary sensorimotor cortex, mid-posterior putamen, and cerebellum are mainly involved in the execution of automatic overlearned sequential movements, whereas the prefrontal, premotor, and parietal association cortices and the anterior part of the caudate/putamen are particularly recruited, in addition to such areas engaged in the execution of simple movement sequences, when a complex or newly learned sequence, which requires attention, integration of multimodal information, and working memory processing for its appropriate selection and monitoring, has to be performed (Jenkins *et al.* 1994; Catalan *et al.* 1998; Harrington *et al.* 2000). Furthermore, when a specific sequence of finger movements is learned at a specific timing, there is enhanced activation in the left IPS, as well as in the mid-dorsolateral prefrontal and premotor cortices. These areas may integrate effectors and temporal information of the sequence, and implement an action-oriented representation so as to perform a motor sequence accurately and in timely fashion (Sakai *et al.* 2002) (see below).

Harrington *et al.* (2000) have demonstrated that the complexity of a sequential action can be defined in many ways, including the surface structures of the sequences (perceptual, i.e. number of movements and motoric effectors such as fingers) and the abstract or cognitive structures (relations between movements such as repetitions or alternations), and that each structure of sequential movements can be distinguished by distinct distributed systems that support their underlying mental operations. The number of different finger movements contained within a sequence (surface structure) correlated with activation of anterior BA 7 and the cerebellum, both involved in the kinematic and sensorimotor representation of movements, respectively, whereas, the abstract structure (increased number of finger transitions) activated the angular gyrus, caudal area BA 40 and the PMd cortex, as well as the superior temporal cortex and middle frontal gyrus. While the temporofrontal interconnecting pathways may subserve working memory processes, the inferior parietal cortex most likely encodes sequence-specific information, which may be retrieved and programmed for execution in the PMd cortex (Harrington *et al.* 2000).

Patients with IMA may exhibit several types of errors such as omissions, deletions, additions, transpositions, and perseverations (De Renzi *et al.* 1983) when performing sequencing limb movements (Roy and Square 1985; Rothi and Heilman 1997), and they have been found to be particularly impaired in planning and implementing sequences of various hand movements (Harrington and Haaland 1992). Abnormalities in movement sequencing have been reported more commonly in patients with left parietal lobe lesions, but also with left frontal and basal ganglion involvement (Kimura and Archibald 1974; Luria 1980; De Renzi *et al.* 1983; Benecke *et al.* 1987; Harrington and Haaland 1992; Halsband *et al.* 1993). Weiss *et al.* (2001) kinematically studied the execution and imitation of meaningless arm movement sequences in patients with parietal lesions, and found that patients with left parietal lesions, some with clinically apparent apraxia, showed more temporal and spatial errors than those with right parietal lesions, whereas additions and omissions of movement components occurred almost equally in both groups. The study demonstrated that the cumulative effects of the disturbances of spatial and temporal aspects already existing at the level of simple movements compromised the production of more complex motor behaviour. Therefore the apractic deficit is at least in part a result of the derangement of constituent elements that may be compounded by cognitive deficits.

In turn, patients with unilateral lesions of the frontal lobe involving the SMA and PM cortex were found to have deficits in the generation of motor sequences from memory that fit into a precise timing plan (Halsband *et al.* 1993). Lastly, Rushworth *et al.* (1997a) have suggested that left-hemisphere-damaged patients exhibit abnormalities in the sequencing of movements owing to inability to constantly redirect motor attention from one movement to the next. These patients may find not only sequences but also multiple component movements and posture transitions particularly difficult because they fail to predictively remap representations of the hand as it moves (Rushworth *et al.* 2003).

Thus different neural systems would be engaged depending on the characteristics of movement sequences requested to be executed during the evaluation of praxis. Most of the sequences used to test praxis are new (e.g. sequencing of movements in the movement imitation test), or the content of an otherwise well-learned sequence has to be represented explicitly. In any case, the system made up by the prefrontal, premotor, and parietal cortices as well as the caudate would be specifically engaged. When the sequence is well known, automated, or overlearned, the SMA–putamen would be preferentially recruited. Interestingly, activation shifted back to the caudate–anterior putamen when attention was paid to the overlearned action (Jueptner and Weiller 1998). In addition, it might be possible that, within this system, there are many different subsystems subserving functionally separate cognitive computations involved in motor sequencing (i.e. working memory, timing, motor attention, selection of limb movements) which may be selectively damaged by the pathological process and so produce different types of sequencing impairment in apractic patients (Harrington and Haaland 1992; Roy and Square 1994; Rushworth *et al.* 1997a, 2003).

The sequential organization of actions, rather than movements, has been studied using script event ordering to address the cognitive activity which occurs during action planning at covert level (Ruby *et al.* 2002). A script consists of a goal-oriented sequence of events that typically occur in a specific and systematic order. Functional imaging studies have shown that short-term scripts, such as those used when testing IA (e.g. peeling, opening and eating an orange), cause activation in the left hemisphere of the dorsolateral prefrontal cortex, supramarginal gyrus, inferior temporal, and middle occipital gyrus. The IPS is involved in short-term script only in the graphic modality, whereas the supramarginal gyrus (BA 39) is also activated by short-term scripts but irrespective of the presentation modality (graphic or lexical). Under the verbal modality, the angular gyrus (BA 40) is also activated (Ruby *et al.* 2002). Patients with ideational apraxia due to lesions damaging the left inferior parietal lobule failed in tests requiring a sequential structuring of common everyday actions (short-term script ordering) (e.g. making coffee) (Pick 1905; Poeck 1983).

Distribution of the apraxias in other body parts

Since its original description (Jackson 1879), face apraxia has been generally equated with oral non-verbal apraxia (Roy and Square 1985; De Renzi 1989), i.e. the inability to perform skilled movements of the lips, cheeks, and tongue. However, early reports of patients with facial apraxia have described eye and/or eyebrow movement deficits (see Bizzozero *et al.* 2000). Therefore face apraxia should refer to a disturbance of upper and lower face movements not explained by elementary motor or sensory deficits. Patients exhibit spatial and temporal errors of similar quality to those observed in limb and speech apraxia when performing representational and non-representational movements such as sticking out the tongue, blowing out a match, smiling, blowing a kiss, showing the teeth, blinking the left or right eye, looking down, or sucking on a straw. Although lower face or buccofacial apraxia often coexists with Broca's aphasia, and thus is more frequently observed with left-hemisphere lesions, in particular involving the frontal and central operculum, insula, centrum semiovale, and basal ganglia (Raade *et al.* 1991), it can also be seen with lesions confined to left posterior cortical regions as well as with right-hemisphere damage. A recent study showed that 46% and 68% of left-hemisphere-damaged patients had upper and lower face apraxia, respectively, whereas 44% and 38% of right-hemisphere-damaged patients exhibited upper and lower face apraxia, respectively, so that a distributed neuroanatomical network in both hemispheres also appears to be involved in face apraxia (Bizzozero *et al.* 2000).

Truncal or whole-body apraxia is a disorder of axial movements attributable to neither elementary motor (e.g. extrapyramidal) or sensory deficit nor to dementia. Patients experience difficulties in dancing or turning around, and may even be unable to adapt the body to the furniture; they have difficulty sitting down in a chair, showing hesitation, sitting in the wrong position (e.g. on the edge of the chair), and in incorrect directions (e.g. facing the back of the chair). When lying in bed, their body is not aligned parallel to the major axis of the bed and they place the pillow in an unusual position. Patients may have minimal or no difficulty in standing or getting up, in contrast with features of some basal ganglion disorders such as parkinsonism. Truncal apraxia is particularly seen with bilateral hemispheric damage involving the parietal or parietotemporal cortex or affecting parietofrontal connections; it is most often observed in cortical degenerative syndromes such as progressive apraxia and corticobasal degeneration (Okuda *et al.* 2001). Truncal apraxia is commonly found associated with other apractic disorders such as limb apraxia.

References

Alexander MP, Baker E, Naeser MA, Kaplan E, Palumbo C (1992). Neuropsychological and neuroanatomical dimensions of ideomotor apraxia. *Brain*, **115**, 87–107.

Beiser DG, Hua SE, Houk JC (1997). Network models of the basal ganglia. *Curr Opin Neurobiol*, **7**, 185–90.

Benecke R, Rothwell JC, Dick JPR, Day BL, Marsden CD (1987). Disturbance of sequential movements in patients with Parkinson disease. *Brain*, **110**, 361–79.

Binkofski F, Dohle C, Posse S, Stephan KM, Heffer H, Seitz RJ, *et al.* (1998) Human anterior intra-parietal area subserves prehension: a combined lesion and functional MRI activation study. *Neurology*, **50**,1253–9.

Binkofski F, Buccino G, Posse S, Seitz RJ, Rizzolatti G, Freund HJ (1999). A fronto-parietal circuit for object manipulation in man: evidence from an fMRI study. *Eur J Neurosci*, **11**, 3276–86.

Bizzozero I, Costato D, Della Sala S, Papagno C, Spinnler H, Venneri A (2000). Upper and lower face apraxia: role of the right hemisphere. *Brain*, **123**, 2213–30.

Blasi V, Labruna L, Soricelli A, Carlomagno S (1999). Limb-kinetic apraxia: a neuropsychological description. *Neurocase*, **5**, 201–11.

Brass M, Bekkering H, Wohlschläger A, Prinz W (2000). Compatibility between observed and executed finger movements: comparing symbolic, spatial and imitative cues. *Brain Cogn*, **44**, 124–43.

Burnod Y, Baraduc P, Battaglia-Mayer A, Guigon E, Koechlin E, Ferraina S, *et al.* (1999) Parieto-frontal coding of reaching: an integrated framework. *Exp Brain Res*, **129**, 325–46.

Buxbaum LJ, Schwartz MF, Carew TG (1997). The role of semantic memory in object use. *Cogn Neuropsychol*, **14**, 219–54.

Buxbaum LJ, Giovannetti, Libon D (2000). The role of the dynamic body schema in praxis: evidence from primary progressive apraxia. *Brain Cogn*, **44**, 166–91.

Buxbaum LJ, Sirigu A, Schwartz MA, Klatzby R (2003). Cognitive representation of hand posture in ideomotor apraxia. *Neuropsychologia*, **41**, 1091–113.

Carey DP, Perrett D, Oram M (1997). Recognizing, understanding and reproducing action. In F Boller, J Grafman, (ed.) *Handbook of Neuropsychology* Vol 11, pp. 111–29. Amsterdam: Elsevier.

Caselli RJ, Stelmach GE, Caviness JV, Timmann D, Royer T, Boeve BF, *et al.* (1999) A kinematic study of progressive apraxia with and without dementia. *Mov Disord*, **14**, 276–87.

Catalan MJ, Honda M, Weeks R, Cohen L, Hallett M (1998). The functional neuroanatomy of simple and complex sequential finger movements: a PET study. *Brain*, **121**, 253–64.

Chao LL, Martin A (2000). Representation of manipulable man-made objects in the dorsal stream. *Neuroimage*, **12**, 478–84.

Choi SH, Na DL, Kang E, Lee KM, Lee, SW, Na DG (2001). Functional magnetic resonance imaging during pantomiming tool-use gestures. *Exp Brain Res*, **139**, 311–17.

Clark MA, Merians AS, Kothari A, Poizner H, Macauley B, Gonzalez Rothi LJ, *et al.* (1994). Spatial planning deficits in limb apraxia. *Brain*, **117**, 1093–106.

Coull JT, Frith CD, Büchel C, Nobre AC (2000). Orienting attention in time: behavioural and neuroanatomical distinction between exogenous and endogenous shifts. *Neuropsychologia*, **38**, 808–19.

Cubelli R, Marchetti C, Boscolo G, Della Sala S (2000). Cognition in action: testing a model of limb apraxia. *Brain Cogn*, **44**, 144–65.

De Renzi E (1989). Apraxia. In F Boller, J Grafman, (ed.) *Handbook of Neuropsychology* Vol 2, pp. 245–63. Amsterdam: Elsevier.

De Renzi E, Lucchelli F (1988). Ideational apraxia. *Brain*, **113**,1173–88.

De Renzi E, Faglioni P, Sorgato P (1982). Modality-specific and supramodal mechanisms of apraxia. *Brain*, **105**, 301–12.

De Renzi E, Faglioni P, Lodesani M, Vecchi A (1983). Performance of left brain-damaged patients on imitation of single movements and motor sequences. Frontal and parietal-injured patients compared. *Cortex*, **19**, 333–43.

Decety J, Grezes J, Costes N, Perani D, Jeannerod M, Procyk E, *et al.* (1997). Brain activity during observation of action. Influence of action content and subject¥s strategy. *Brain*, **120**, 1763–77.

Faglioni P, Basso A (1985). Historical perspectives on neuroanatomical correlates of limb apraxia. In Roy EA, ed. *Neuropsychological Studies of Apraxia and Related Disorders*. Amsterdam: North-Holland, 3–44.

Faillenot I, Toni I, Decety J, Grégorie M, Jeannerod M (1997). Visual pathways for object-oriented action and object recognition: functional anatomy with PET. *Cereb Cortex*, **7**, 77–85.

Fogassi L, Gallese V, Buccino G, Craighero L, Fadiga L, Rizzolatti G (2001). Cortical mechanism for the visual guidance of hand grasping movements in the monkey: a reversible inactivation study. *Brain*, **124**, 571–86.

Foundas A, Macauley BL, Raymer AM, Maher LM, Heilman KM, Rothi LJG (1995). Ecological implications of limb apraxia: evidence from mealtime behavior. *J Int Neuropsychol Soc*, **1**, 62–6.

Freund HJ (1992). The apraxias. In AK Asbury, GM McKhann, WJ McDonald, (ed.) *Diseases of the Nervous System. Clinical Neurobiology*, 2nd edn. pp. 751–67, Philadelphia, PA: WB Saunders.

Georgopoulos AP, DeLong MR, Crutcher ML (1983). Relations between parameters of step-tracking movements and single cell discharge in the globus pallidus and subthalamic nucleus of the behaving monkey. *J Neurosci*, **3**, 1586–98.

Gerardin E, Sirigu A, Lehéricy S, Poline JB, Gaymard B, Marsault C, *et al.* (2000). Partially overlapping neural networks for real and imagined hand movements. *Cereb Cortex*, **10**, 1093–1104.

Geschwind N, Damasio A (1985). Apraxia. In JA Frederiks, (ed.) *Handbook of Clinical Neurology*, pp. 423–32. New York: Elsevier Science.

Geschwind N, Kaplan E (1962). A human cerebral disconnection syndrome. *Neurology*, **12**, 675–85.

Goldenberg G (1999). Matching and imitation of hand and finger postures in patients with damage in the left or right hemispheres. *Neuropsychologia*, **37**, 559–66.

Goldenberg G, Hagmann S (1997). The meaning of meaningless gestures: a study of visuo-imitative apraxia. *Neuropsychologia*, **35**, 333–41.

Goldenberg G, Hagmann S (1998). Tool use and mechanical problem solving in apraxia. *Neuropsychologia*, **36**, 581–9.

Goldenberg G, Straus S (2002). Hemisphere asymmetries for imitation of novel gestures. *Neurology*, **59**, 893–7.

Graff-Radford NR, Welsh K, Godersky J (1987). Callosal apraxia. *Neurology*, **37**, 100–5.

Grafton ST, Arbid MA, Fadiga L, Rizzolatti G (1996). Localization of grasp representation in humans by PET: 2 Observation compared with imagination. *Exp Brain Res*, **112**, 103–11.

Grafton ST, Fadiga L, Arbib MA, Rizzolatti G (1997). Premotor cortex activation during observation and naming of familiar tools. *Neuroimage*, **6**, 231–6.

Graziano MS, Gross CG (1998). Spatial maps for the control of movement (review). *Curr Opin Neurobiol*, **8**, 195–201.

Grèzes J, Decety J (2001). Functional anatomy of execution, mental simulation, observation, and verb generation of actions: a meta-analysis. *Hum Brain Mapping*, **12**, 1–19.

Grèzes J, Decety J (2002). Does visual perception of object afford action? Evidence from a neuroimaging study. *Neuropsychologia*, **40**, 212–22.

Grèzes J, Costes N, Decety J (1999). The effects of learning and intention on the neural network involved in the perception of meaningless actions. *Brain*, **122**, 1875–87.

Haaland KY, Flaherty D (1984). The different types of limb apraxia errors made by patients with left vs. right hemisphere damage. *Brain Cogn*, **3**, 370–84.

Haaland KY, Harrington DL, Knight RT (1999). Spatial deficits in ideomotor limb apraxia. A kinematic analysis of aiming movements. *Brain*, **122**, 1169–82.

Haaland KY, Harrington DL, Knight RT (2000). Neural representations of skilled movement. *Brain*, **123**, 2306–13.

Halsband U, Freund HJ (1990). Premotor cortex and conditional motor learning in man. *Brain*, **113**, 207–22.

Halsband U, Ito N, Tanji J, Freund HJ (1993). The role of premotor cortex and the supplementary motor area in the temporal control of movement in man. *Brain*, **116**, 243–66.

Halsband U, Schmitt J, Weyers M, Binkofski F, Grützner G, Freund H-J (2001). Recognition and imitation of pantomimed motor acts after unilateral parietal and premotor lesions: a perspective on apraxia. *Neuropsychologia*, **39**, 200–16.

Hamilton JM, Haaland KY, Adair JC, Brandt J (2003). Ideomotor limb apraxia in Huntington's disease: implication for corticostriatal involvement. *Neuropsychologia*, **41**, 614–21.

Hanna-Pladdy B, Daniels SK, Fieselman MA, Thompson K, Vasterling JJ, Heilman KM, *et al.* (2001a). Praxis lateralization: errors in right and left hemisphere stroke. *Cortex*, **37**, 219–30.

Hanna-Pladdy B, Heilman KM, Foundas AL (2001b). Cortical and subcortical contributions to ideomotor apraxia. Analysis of task demands and error types. *Brain*, **124**, 2513–27.

Harrington DL, Haaland KY (1992). Motor sequencing with left hemisphere damage. Are some cognitive deficits specific to limb apraxia? *Brain*, **115**, 857–74.

Harrington DL, Rao SM, Haaland KY, Bobholz JA, Mayer AR, Binderx JR, *et al.* (2000). Specialized neural systems underlying representations of sequential movements. *J Cogn Neurosci*, **12**, 56–77.

Heath M, Roy EA, Black SE, Westwood DA (2001). Intransitive limb gestures and apraxia following unilateral stroke. *J Clin Exp Neuropsychol*, **23**, 628–42.

Heilman KM (1973). Ideational apraxia—a re-definition. *Brain*, **96**, 861–4.

Heilman KM, Rothi LJG (1985). Apraxia. In KM Heilman, E Valenstein, (ed.) *Clinical Neuropsychology*, pp. 131–50. New York: Oxford University Press.

Heilman KM, Maher LH, Greenwald L, Rothi LJ (1997). Conceptual apraxia from lateralized lesions. *Neurology*, **49**, 457–64.

Hermsdörfer J, Mai N, Spatt J, Marquardt C, Veltkamp R, Goldenberg G (1996). Kinematic analysis of movement imitation in apraxia. *Brain*, **119**, 1575–86.

Hermsdörfer J, Goldenberg G, Wachsmuth C, Conrad B, Ceballos-Baumann AO, Bartenstein P, *et al.* (2001). Cortical correlates of gesture processing: clues to the cerebral mechanisms underlying apraxia during the imitation of meaningless gestures. *Neuroimage*, **14**, 149–61.

Hlustik P, Solodkin A, Gullapalli RP, Noll DC, Small SL (2002). Functional lateralization of the human premotor cortex during sequential movements. *Brain Cogn*, **49**, 54–62.

Hodges JR, Spatt J, Patterson K (1999). 'What' and 'how': evidence for the dissociation of object knowledge and mechanical problem-solving skills in the human brain. *Proc Natl Acad Sci USA*, **96**, 9444–8.

Hodges J, Bozeat S, Lambon RM, Patterson K, Spatt J (2000). The role of conceptual knowledge in object use evidence from semantic dementia. *Brain*, **123**, 1913–25.

Ietswaart M, Carey DP, Della Sala S, Dijkhuizen RS (2001). Memory-driven movements in limb apraxia: is there evidence for impaired communication between the dorsal and the ventral streams? *Neuropsychologia*, **39**, 950–61.

Inoue K, Kawashima R, Sugiura M, Ogawa A, Schormann T, Zilles K, *et al.* (2001) Activation in the ipsilateral posterior parietal cortex during tool use: a PET study. *Neuroimage*, **14**, 1469–75.

Iriki A, Tanaka M, Iwamura Y (1996). Coding of modified body schema during tool use by macaque postcentral neurons. *NeuroReport*, **7**, 2325–30.

Jackson JH (1879). On affection of speech from diseases of the brain. *Brain*, **1**, 304–30.

Jackson SR, Jackson GM, Harrison J, Henderson L, Kennard C (1995). The internal control of action and Parkinson's disease: a kinematic analysis of visually-guided and memory-guided prehension movements. *Exp Brain Res*, **105**, 147–62.

Jeannerod M (1997). *The Cognitive Neuroscience of Action.* Oxford: Blackwell.

Jeannerod M, Arbid MA, Rizzolatti G, Sakata H (1995). Grasping objects: the cortical mechanisms of visuomotor transformation. *Trends Neurosci*, **18**, 314–20.

Jenkins IH, Brooks DJ, Nixon PD, Frackowiak RSJ, Passingham RE (1994). Motor sequence learning: a study with positron emission tomography. *J Neurosci*, **14**, 3775–90.

Johansson RS, Cole KJ (1992). Sensory–motor coordination during grasping and manipulatory actions. *Curr Opin Neurobiol*, **2**, 815–23.

Johnson SH, Rotte M, Grafton ST, Hinrichs H, Gazzaniga MS, Heinze H-J (2002). Selective activation of a parietofrontal circuit during implicitly imagined prehension. *Neuroimage*, **17**, 1693–704.

Jueptner M, Weiller C (1998). A review of differences between basal ganglia and cerebellar control of movements as revealed by functional brain imaging. *Brain*, **121**, 1437–49.

Kalaska JF, Stephen HS, Cisek P, Sergio L (1997). Cortical control of reaching movements. *Curr Opin Neurobiol* **7**, 849–59.

Kendall AL, David F, Rayment G, Torres EM, Annett LE, Dunnett SB (2000). The influence of excitotoxic basal ganglia lesions on motor performance in the common marmoset. *Brain*, **123**, 1442–58.

Kemardi I, Joseph JP (1995). Activity in the caudate nucleus of monkey during spatial sequencing. *J Neurophysiol*, **74**, 911–33.

Kertesz A, Ferro JM (1984). Lesion size and location in ideomotor apraxia. *Brain*, **107**, 921–33.

Kimura D, Archibald Y (1974). Motor functions of the left hemisphere. *Brain*, **97**, 337–50.

Kleist K (1907). Kortikale (innervatorische) Apraxie. *Jahrb Psychiatrie Neurol*, **28**, 46–112.

Kleist K (1931). Gehirnpathologische und lokalisatorische Ergebnisse: das Stirnhirn im engeren Sinne und seine Störungen. *Z Neurol Psychiatrie*, **131**, 442–8.

Kourtzi Z, Kanwisher N (2000). Activation in human MT/MST by static images with implied motion. *J Cogn Neurosci*, **12**, 48–55.

Krams M, Rushworth M, Deiber M, Frackowiak R, Passingham R (1998). The preparation, execution and suppression of copied movements in the human brain. *Exp Brain Res*, **120**, 386–98.

Kurata K, Hoffman DS (1994). Differential effects of muscimol microinjection into dorsal and ventral aspects of the premotor cortex of monkeys. *J Neurophysiol*, **71**, 1151–64.

Lacquaniti F, Guigon E, Bianchi L, Ferraina S, Caminiti R (1995). Representing spatial information for limb movement: role of area 5 in the monkey. *Cereb Cortex*, **5**, 391–409.

Lawrence AD, Sahabian BJ, Rogers RD, Hodges JR, Robbins TW (1999). Discrimination, reversal and shift learning in Huntington's disease: mechanisms of impaired response selection. *Neuropsychologia*, **37**, 1359–74.

Leiguarda R (2003). Apraxias and the lateralization of motor functions in the human parietal lobe. In AM Siegel, RA Andersen, HJ Freund, DD Spencer, (ed.) *The Parietal Lobes. Advances in Neurology* Vol 93, pp. 235–48. Philadelphia, PA: Lippincott–Williams & Wilkins.

Leiguarda R, Marsden CD (2000). Limb apraxias: higher-order disorders of sensorimotor integration. *Brain*, **123**, 860–79.

Leiguarda R, Starkstein S (1998). Apraxia in the syndromes of Pick complex. In A Kertesz, DG Muñoz, (ed.) *Pick's Disease and Pick Complex*, pp. 129–43. New York: Wiley–Liss.

Leiguarda R, Starkstein S, Berthier M (1989). Anterior callosal haemorrhage. A partial interhemispheric disconnection syndrome. *Brain*, **112**, 1019–37.

Leiguarda R, Pramstaller P, Merello M, Starkstein S, Lees AJ, Marsden CD (1997). Apraxia in Parkinson's disease, progressive supranuclear palsy, multiple system atrophy, and neuroleptic induced parkinsonism. *Brain*, **120**, 75–90.

Leiguarda R, Merello M, Balej J (2000a). Apraxia in corticobasal degeneration. In I Litvan, C Goetz, A Lang, (ed.) *Corticobasal Degeneration and Related Disorders.Advances in Neurology* Vol 82, pp. 103–21. Philadelphia, PA: Lippincott–Williams & Wilkins.

Leiguarda R, Merello M, Balej J, Starkstein S, Nogués M, Marsden CD (2000b). Disruption of spatial organization and interjoint coordination in Parkinson's disease, progressive supranuclear palsy, and múltiple system atrophy. *Mov Disord*, **15**, 627–40.

Leiguarda R, Merello M, Nouzeilles MI, Balej J, Rivero A, Nogués M (2003). Limb-kinetic apraxia in corticobasal degeneration: clinical and kinematic findings. *Mov Disord*, **18**, 49–59.

Lemon RN (1997). Mechanisms of cortical control of hand function. *Neuroscientist*, **3**, 389–98.

Liepmann H (1905). Der weitere Krankheitsverlauf bei dem einseitig Apraktischen und der Gehirnbefund auf Grund von Serienschnitten. *Monatsschr Psychiatrie Neurol*, **17**, 289–311.

Liepmann H (1908). Drei Aufsätze aus dem Apraxiegebiet. Berlin: Karger.

Liepmann H (1920). Apraxie. *Ergeb Gesamt Med*, **1**, 516–43.

Liepmann H, Maas O (1907). Eie Fall von linksseitiger Agraphie und Apraxie bei rechtsseitiger Lähmung. *Monatsschr Psychiatrie Neurol*, **10**, 214–27.

Luria AR (1980). *Higher Cortical Function in Man*, 2nd edn. New York: Basic Books.

McCarthy RA, Warrington EK (1988). Evidence for modality specific meaning systems in the brain. *Nature*, **334**, 428–30.

Majsak MJ, Kaminski T, Gentile A, Flanagan J (1998). The reaching movements of patients with Parkinson's disease under self-determined maximal speed and visually cued conditions. *Brain*, **121**, 755–66.

Martin A, Haxby JV, Lalonde FM, Wiggs CL, Ungerleider LG (1995). Discrete cortical regions associated with knowledge of color and knowledge of action. *Science*, **270**, 102–5.

Martin A, Wiggs CL. Ungerleider LG, Haxby JV (1996). Neural correlates of category-specific knowledge. *Nature*, **379**, 649–52.

Matsumura M, Sawaguchi T, Oishi T, Veki K, Kubota K (1991). Behavioral deficits induced by local injection of bicuculline and muscimol into the primate motor and premotor cortex. *J Neurophysiol*, **65**, 1542–53.

Matsumura M, Kawashima R, Naito E, Satoh K, Takahashi T, Yanagisawa T, *et al.* (1996) Changes in rCBF during grasping in humans examined by PET. *NeuroReport*, 749–52.

Mehler MF (1987). Visuo-imitative apraxia (abstract). *Neurology*, **34** (Suppl 1), 129.

Merians AS, Clark M, Poizner H, Macauley B, Rothi LJ, Heilman KM (1997). Visual-imitative dissociation apraxia. *Neuropsychologia*, **35**, 1483–90.

Milner AD, Goodale MA (1995). *The Visual Brain in Action*. Oxford: Oxford University Press.

Mitchell SJ, Richardson RT, Baker FH, DeLong MR (1987). The primate globus pallidus: Neuronal activity related to direction of movement. *Exp Brain Res*, **68**, 491–505.

Moll J, de Oliveira-Souza R, Passman LJ, Cimini Cunha F, Souza-Lima F, Andreiuolo PA (2000). Functional MRI correlates of real and imagined tool-use pantomimes. *Neurology*, **54**, 1331–6.

Morlass J (1928). *Contribution á l'Etude de l'Apraxie*. Paris: Amédée, Legrand.

Mozaz M, Gonzalez Rothi L, Anderson J, Crucian G, Heilman K (2002). Postural knowledge of transitive pantomimes and intransitive gestures. *J Int Neuropsychol Soc*, **8**, 958–62.

Obayashi S, Suhara T, Kawabe K, Okauchi T, Maeda J, Akine Y, *et al.* (2001). Functional brain mapping of monkey tool use. *Neuroimage*, **14**, 853–61.

Ochipa C, Rothi LJG, Heilman KM (1992). Conceptual apraxia in Alzheimer's disease. *Brain*, **115**, 1061–71.

Ochipa C, Rothi LJ, Heilman KM (1994). Conduction apraxia. *J Neurol Neurosurg Psychiatry*, **57**, 1241–4.

Okuda B, Tanaka H, Kawabata K, Tachibana H, Sugita M (2001). Truncal and limb apraxia in corticobasal degeneration. *Mov Disord*, **16**, 760–2.

Passingham RE (1993). *The Frontal Lobes and Voluntary Action*. Oxford Psychology Series 21. Oxford: Oxford University Press.

Passingham RE, Toni I (2001). Contrasting the dorsal and ventral visual systems: guidance of movements versus decising making. *Neuroimage*, **14**, S125–31.

Peigneux Ph, Van Der Linden M, Andres-Benito P, Sadzot B, Franck G, Salmon E (2000a). Exploration neuropsychologique et par imagerie fonctionnalle cérébrale d'une apraxia visuo-imitative. *Rev Neurol (Paris)*, **156**, 459–72.

Peigneux P, Salmon E, van der Linden M, Garraux G, Aerts J, Delfiore G, *et al.* (2000b). The role of lateral occipitotemporal junction and area MT/V5 in the visual analysis of upper-limb postures. *Neuroimage*, **11**, 644–55.

Perani D, Cappa SF, Bettinardi V, Bressi S, Gorno-Tempini M, Matarrese M, *et al.* (1995). Different neural systems for the recognition of animals and man-made tools. *NeuroReport*, **6**, 1637–41.

Phillips JA, Noppeney U, Humphreys GW, Price CJ (2002). Can segregation within the semantic system account for category-specific deficits? *Brain*, **125**, 2067–80.

Pick A (1905). *Studien ü ber Motorische Apraxie und ihre Mahestenhende Erscheinungen: ihre Bedeutung in der Symptomatologie Psychopathologischer Symptomenkomplexe*. Leipzig: Deuticke.

Pilgrim E, Humphreys GW (1991). Impairment of action to visual objects in a case of ideomotor apraxia. *Cogn Neuropsychol*, **8**, 459–73.

Poeck K (1983). Ideational apraxia. *J Neurol*, **230**, 1–5.

Poizner H, Mack L, Verfaellie M, Rothi LJG, Heilman KM (1990). Three-dimensional computergraphic analysis of apraxia. *Brain*, **113**, 85–101.

Poizner H, Clark MA, Merians AS, Macauley B, Rothi LJG, Heilman KM (1995). Joint coordination deficits in limb apraxia. *Brain*, **118**, 227–42.

Pramstaller P, Marsden CD (1996). The basal ganglia and apraxia. *Brain*, **119**, 319–41.

Raade AS, Rothi LJG, Heilman KM (1991). The relationship between buccofacial and limb apraxia. *Brain Cogn*, **16**, 130–46.

Rapcsak SZ, Ochipa C, Beeson P, Rubens A (1993). Praxis and the right hemisphere. *Brain Cogn*, **23**, 181–202.

Rizzolatti G, Fadiga L, Matelli M, Bettinardi V, Paulesu E, Perani D (1996). Localization of grasp representations in humans by positron emission tomography. 1. Observation versus execution. *Exp Brain Res*, **111**, 246–52.

Rizzolatti G, Luppino G, Matelli M (1998). The organization of the cortical motor system: new concepts. *Electroencephalogr Clin Neurophysiol*, **106**, 283–96.

Rothi LJG, Ochipa C, Heilman KM (1991). A cognitive neuropsychological model of limb praxis. *Cogn Neuropsychol*, **8**, 443–58.

Rothi LJG, Raimer AN, Heilman KM (1997). Evaluation of praxis. In LJG Rothi, KM Heilman, (ed.) *Apraxia: the Neuropsychology of Action*, pp. 61–74. Hove, UK: Psychology Press.

Roy EA (1996). Hand preference, manual asymmetries, and limb apraxia. In D Elliot, EA Roy, (ed.) *Manual Asymmetries in Motor Control*, pp. 215–36. Boca Raton, FL: CRC Press.

Roy EA, Square PA (1985). Common considerations in the study of limb, verbal, and oral apraxia. In EA Roy, (ed.) *Neuropsychological Studies of Apraxia and Related Disorders*, pp. 111–61. Amsterdam: North-Holland.

Roy EA, Square PA (1994). Neuropsychology of movement sequencing disorders and apraxia. In DW Zaidel, (ed.) *Neuropsychology*, pp. 183–218. London: Academic Press.

Roy EA, Black SE, Blair N, Dimeck PT (1998). Analysis of deficits in gestural pantomime. *J Clin Exp Neuropsychol*, **20**, 628–43.

Roy EA, Heath M, Westwood D, Schweizer TA, Dixon MJ, Black SE, *et al.* (2000). Task demands and limb apraxia in stroke. *Brain Cogn*, **44**, 253–79.

Ruby P, Sirigu A, Decety J (2002). Distinct areas in the parietal cortex involved in long-term and short-term action planning: a PET investigation. *Cortex*, **38**, 321–39.

Rumiati R, Tessari A (2002). Imitation of novel and well-known actions: the role of short-term memory. *Exp Brain Res*, **142**, 425–33.

Rushworth MFS, Nixon PD, Renowden S, Wade DT, Passingham RE (1997a). The parietal cortex and motor attention. *Neuropsychologia*, **35**, 1261–73.

Rushworth MFS, Nixon PD, Passingham RE (1997b). Parietal cortex and movement. II. Spatial representation. *Exp Brain Res*, **117**, 311–23.

Rushworth MFS, Johansen-Berg H, Young SA (1998a). Parietal cortex and spatial-postural transformation during arm movements. *J Neurophysiol*, **79**, 478–82.

Rushworth MFS, Nixon PD, Wade DT, Renowden S, Passingham RE (1998b). The left hemisphere and the selection of learned actions. *Neuropsychologia*, **36**, 11–24.

Rushworth MFS, Krams M, Passingham RE (2001). The attentional role of the left parietal cortex: the distinct lateralization and localization of motor attention in the human brain. *J Cogn Neurosci*, **13**, 698–710.

Rushworth MFS, Johansen-Berg H, Göbel SM, Deulin JT (2003). The left parietal and premotor cortices: motor attention and selection. *Neuroimage*, **20**, S89–100.

Sakai K, Hokosaka O, Takino R, Miyauchi S, Nielsen M, Tamada T (2000). What and when: parallel and convergence processing on motor control. *J Neurosci*, **20**, 2691–700.

Sakai K, Ramnani N, Passingham RE (2002). Learning of sequences of finger movements and timing: frontal lobe and action-oriented representation. *J Neurophysiol*, **88**, 2035–46.

Sakata H, Taira M, Murata A, Mine S (1995). Neural mechanisms of visual guidance of hand action in the parietal cortex of the monkey. *Cereb Cortex*, **5**, 429–38.

Schluter ND, Krams M, Rushworth M, Passingham R (2001). Cerebral dominance for action in the human brain: the selection of actions. *Neuropsychologia*, **39**, 105–13.

Schnider A, Hanlon RE, Alexander DN, Benson F (1997). Ideomotor apraxia: behavioural dimensions and neuroanatomical basis. *Brain Lang*, **58**, 125–36.

Schwoebel J, Buxbaum L, Coslett B (2004). Representations of the human body in the production and imitation of complex movements. *Cogn Neuropsychol*, **21**, 285–98.

Shadmehr R, Holcomb HH (1999). Inhibitory control of competing motor memories. *Exp Brain Res*, **126**, 235–51.

Shiota J, Kawamura M (1994). Symptomatological study of limb-kinetic apraxia. *Shinkei Kenkyu No Shimpo (Adv Neurol Sci)*, **38**, 597–605.

Sirigu A, Cohen L, Duhamel JR, Pillon B, Dubois B, Agid Y (1995a). A selective impairment of hand posture for objects utilization in apraxia. *Cortex*, **31, 41**–55.

Sirigu A, Cohen L, Duhamel JR, Pillon B, Dubois B, Agid Y, *et al.* (1995b) Congruent unilateral impairments for real and imagined hand movements. *NeuroReport*, **6**, 997–1001.

Sirigu A, Daprati E, Pradat-Diehl P, Franck N, Jeannerod M (1999). Perception of self-generated movement following left parietal lesion. *Brain*, **122**, 1867–74.

Spatt J, Bak T, Bozeat S, Patterson K, Hodges JR (2002). Apraxia, mechanical problem solving and semantic knowledge. Contributions to object usage in corticobasal degeneration. *J Neurol*, **249**, 601–8.

Steinthal P (1871). *Abriss der Sprachwissenschaft*. Berlin.

Warburton E, Wise RJ, Price CJ, Weiller C, Hadar U, Ramsay S, *et al.* (1996). Noun and verb retrieval by normal subjects. Studies with PET (review). *Brain*, **119**, 159–79.

Watson RT, Heilman KM (1983). Callosal apraxia. *Brain*, **106**, 391–403.

Weiss PH, Jeannerod M, Paulignan Y, Freund HJ (2000). Is the organization of goal-directed action modality specific? A common temporal structure. *Neuropsychologia*, **38**, 1136–43.

Weiss PH, Dohle C, Binkofski F, Schnitzler A, Freund H-J, Hefter H (2001). Motor impairment in patients with parietal lesions: disturbances of meaningless arm movement sequences. *Neuropsychologia*, **39**, 397–405.

Wenger KK, Musch KL, Mink JW (1999). Impaired reaching and grasping after focal inactivation of globus pallidus pars interna in the monkey. *J Neurophysiol*, **82**, 2049–60.

Yeterian EH, Pandya DN (1993). Striatal connections of the parietal association cortices in rhesus monkeys. *J Comp Neurol*, **332**, 175–97.

Chapter 18

Unimodal sensory–motor transformation disorders

Hans-Joachim Freund

Introduction

The act of reaching and grasping (reviewed in Chapters 2 and 3) is one of the most thoroughly examined motor behaviours in both monkeys and humans. It is particularly suitable for disentangling the different facets of the sensory–motor transformations required for the adjustment of separate eye-, head-, body- and world-referenced coordinate systems. Experimentally, different neural repertoires involved in specific aspects of this multistage process have been identified by microrecordings of monkey behaviour. They are implicated in the spatial transformations based on the dynamic remapping of receptive fields by means of the convergence of sensory and efference copy signals and in the coordinate transformations converting target location into arm-centred motor commands (Andersen and Bueno 2003). The neural aggregates involved in these transformations lie in closely adjacent areas along the intraparietal sulcus (Jeannerod *et al.* 1995; Sakata *et al.* 1995). The control of eye movement plays an important role in these sensory–motor processes linking sensation and action and in the rapid update mechanisms underlying the integration of the reference frames required for the interactions between the body, head, and eyes in relation to the external world.

The pivotal role of the posterior parietal lobe for this set of functions revealed in the experimental studies has been complemented by clinical data revealing specific disturbances of reaching and grasping behaviour in patients with posterior parietal lesions. Patients with lesions of the anterior part of the intraparietal sulcus (AIP) show a highly selective disturbance of grasping with preservation of other hand motor skills (Binkofski *et al.* 1998) closely resembling the situation in the monkey after muscimol injections in the AIP (Sakata *et al.* 1995). Conversely, functional activation of this gesture in normal subjects shows activation of the same area, emphasizing its key role in tactile exploration and manipulation. The noteworthy difference is that the activations are bilateral whereas the deficit is purely contralesional.

This chapter deals with selective disturbances of motor behaviour of the arm and hand, concentrating on those dysfunctions that are strictly confined to movements guided by and acting on one particular sensory modality. Two examples are discussed: disturbances of somatosensory–motor transformation, and a specific impairment of visuomotor behaviour that is selectively induced by the use of mirrors. Both are characterized by the fact that motor behaviour is impaired only if it relates to the respective modality. This is a principal difference to the apraxias as traditionally defined. They interfere with the conception of purposive movements of both sides of the body at a supramodal level, irrespective of the modality involved (see Chapter 17). The specific unimodal somatomotor and visuomotor sensory–motor transformation disorders illustrate that unimodal information processing can be affected before integration into these supramodal reference frames occurs.

Patients with unimodal sensory–motor transformation disorders are special in several respects. First, they reveal a class of sensory–motor deficits with a relatively homogeneous pathophysiology—a disturbance of sensory–motor transformation for only one particular modality. Secondly, they have topological significance since they indicate damage of the posterior parietal lobe or its fibre connections. Thirdly, the frequent association with sensory disturbances reveals that the sensory and motor processing modules are coextensive or closely adjacent. Lastly, information gained from functional imaging studies provides complementary evidence for parietal lobe involvement in a set of tasks mirroring the deficits ensuing from the lesions.

The clinical symptomatology of the somatosensory–motor and visuomotor transformation disorders representing a cortical synthetic dysfunction is sometimes similar to the ataxic disturbances seen in deafferented patients. This shows that the lack of sensory information required for the elaboration of motor programs and the impairment at the processing level may have similar consequences for motor behaviour. This makes the clinical distinction between the two conditions difficult. Terminology reflects this difficulty, as some of the disturbances are designated as ataxic, and some as apractic or even agnostic. In the following sections, the two unimodal sensory–motor transformation disorders will be discussed, beginning with the somatomotor functions.

Ataxia due to deficient somatosensory information

Neurosurgical cases with well-documented excisions of the postcentral gyrus (Foerster 1936) demonstrate very clearly that sensorimotor transformations can obviously not be accomplished if the required sensory information is not available. The clinical picture characterizing damage of the input stages in the anterior parietal lobe closely resembles that of patients with diffuse peripheral or spinal deafferentation. Loss of elementary sensation compromises the elaboration of more complex stimulus attributes such as the form and surface texture of tactile objects. On the motor side, deafferentation interferes with motor behaviour insofar as it relies on the deprived sensory information. Ataxia is the inevitable consequence. The motor deficits can be partially compensated by visual guidance.

The situation is different in patients with lesions restricted to the posterior superior parietal lobule. The hallmark is the preferential disturbance of higher-order cortical somatosensory and sensory–motor processing along with a relative preservation of elementary sensation (Pause *et al.* 1989). The impairment of 'epicritic' sensibility along with stereoagnosia may be similar to that seen after dorsal column lesions. However, according to the modular organization of the parietal cortex, virtually every aspect of feature extraction and elaboration can be selectively disturbed: discrimination of object size, weight, surface texture, form, spatial attributes, and object identity. Thus tactile recognition can be compromised on the basis of the combination of these dysfunctions or by sensory loss, but can also be disturbed in isolation.

Tactile apraxia as a model of disordered sensory–motor transformation

The motor deficits seen in patients with damage of the posterior parietal lobule are often apractic rather than ataxic in nature. They are characterized by a specific inability to use tactile feedback to generate the exploratory procedures necessary for tactile shape recognition, although somatosensory functions may be normal or only moderately disturbed. The dissolution of the purposive character of movements represents an essential feature of apraxia as defined by Liepmann (1900, 1920). The extension of this concept from the three apraxias originally described (ideational, ideomotor, and limb-kinetic apraxias) to a selective disturbance of tactile exploration was first established by Klein (1931). He adopted the term tactile apraxia for a purely contralesional disturbance of active touch in a case who could not engender adequate finger movements required for the exploration of objects put into his hand. However, when he could see an object placed in front of him, a correct reaching for grasping movement was initiated. The unimodal nature of this dysfunction was emphasized by the fact that there was no apraxia when the patient saw the object, but there was apraxia when he was blindfolded and then started active touching. His intransitive and expressive movements were well preserved.

The breakdown of the finely tuned exploratory patterns of the fingers in active touch or of the ocular scan paths during visual search reveals that the essence of these dysfunctions lies in the impairment of the purposive nature of those movements necessary to shape the required sensory input. This in turn further amplifies the coexisting deficient sensory control of movement.

The interdependence between perception and action is exemplified by microneurographic recordings from the median nerve together with the movement trajectories of the exploring fingers. Figure 18.1 illustrates the activation of mechanoreceptors recorded from the finger pads of a normal subject during active touch. The activation pattern depends on the type of receptor and the kinetics of the digital palpation scans.

What is not shown here is the activity of proprioceptive afferents. However, the use of the hand as a sense organ entails the synthesis of exteroceptive information received

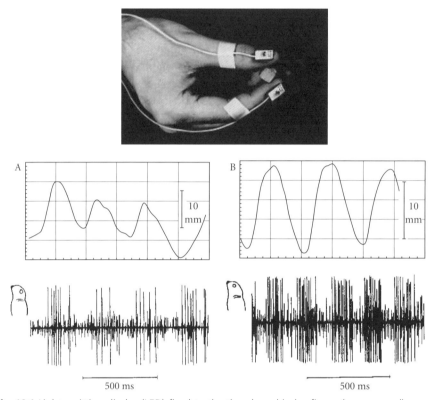

Fig. 18.1 Light emitting diodes (LED) fixed to the thumb and index finger (upper panel) provide time histories of their distance (middle panel) during tactile exploration of a cube. The lower panel shows the discharge of a microneurographic recording of a slowly adapting (SA I, A) and a rapidly adapting (RA I, B) mechanoreceptive unit during this movement. Receptive field locations are indicated on the left of the lower panels. Whereas the SA I unit is only activated during movements in one direction, the SA I unit responds bidirectionally. Modified from Kunesch *et al.* 1994.

from the skin and the proprioceptive input, thus specifying the difference between touching and being touched (Gibson 1962). Active touch elaborates the unity, stability, plasticity, and shape of phenomenal objects. When a single object is grasped with several fingers, the subject perceives one object only although several cutaneous receptor sheets are engaged. The percept is object form, not skin form, and obviously not the continuous feedback from the finger movements.

   Thus effective grasping and object manipulation rely on the ability to transform sensory information concerning the object to be grasped into an appropriate hand configuration and a sophisticated somatosensory control of finger movements (Jeannerod *et al.* 1995). However, the formation of adequate hand apertures and digital palpation patterns also require stored object representations in order to generate knowledge-driven preprogrammed exploratory hand movements (Lederman and

Klatzky 1987). Thus normal exploratory manipulation depends on the integrity of both constituents: the ongoing sensory–motor transformations and the ability to mentally evoke actions from stored motor representations. Their interplay allows the continuous adaptation of the highly overlearned repertoire of automated hand motor skills to the on-line fine tuning of the object guided and consciously monitored digital palpations. Damage of these circuits can preferentially interfere with either of these mechanisms or with their integration.

This is illustrated by the various combinations of sensorimotor deficits in patients with parietal lobe damage. Tactile apraxia is often associated with tactile agnosia. Although the relative impairment varies between cases, their frequent association reveals the intricate interdependence between processes linking perception to action and the anatomical proximity of their processing modules (Freund 1987). However, cases with isolated somatosensory deficits affecting different levels of complexity demonstrate that the respective modules can function separately. Patients with tactile apraxia without astereognosia (Yamadori 1982) or the reverse condition, a near-normal exploratory manual pattern but severe disturbances of tactile recognition (Reed *et al.* 1996), reveal the selective impairment of the processes required for the elaboration of motor concept formation or of the cognitive aspects of object recognition. Obviously, some patients with tactile apraxia can learn to assume a different strategy by moving the hand as a whole and composing object features from passive touch. Cases with tactile apraxia without astereognosis argue against the view that the motor deficit is secondary to the disturbance of complex somatosensory processing. They also show that the sensory–motor transformations required for the elaboration of motor concepts engage different neural repertoires.

The frequent occurrence of the concomitant disturbance of cognitive and motor functions in cases with damage of the posterior parietal lobule makes another important point. It emphasizes a principal difference between visual and somatosensory information flow. In contrast to the dichotomy into a pragmatic parietal and a cognitive temporal route shown for the visual channel, both aspects of somatosensory processing are mediated in closely adjacent and interleaved circuitries within the parietal lobe.

The impact of kinematic recordings

The clinical spectrum of disturbances seen in cases with damage of the parietal lobe covers motor disturbances ranging from ataxia to apraxia with various transitional forms. Their characteristic features have become clearer through quantitative analyses of movement trajectories from patients with different types of motor disturbances. The changes in the digital palpation pattern in patients whose finger movements are hampered by executive motor deficits such as paresis, bradykinesia, or tremor have little effect on tactile cognition. As shown by kinematic recordings, they compromise the amplitude, speed, or regularity of the finger movements, whereas the configuration of the explorative pattern remains preserved (Binkofski *et al.* 2001). In contrast,

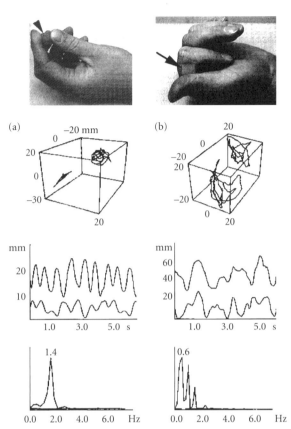

Fig. 18.2 Exploratory finger movements. Top left panel shows a typical position of the thumb and the fingers of a healthy volunteer during tactile exploration of a small object. Top right panel shows the inadequate position of the patient's fingers in relation to the object.
(a) Kinematic analysis of exploratory finger movements in a normal subject, (b) in a patient with a posteroparietal lesion. The analysis includes a 3D reconstruction of thumb (upper right part within the cube) and forefinger (lower left part) movement trajectories, the time histories of the thumb and index finger (middle panels) and the frequency distribution of the thumb movements (lower panels).

kinematic analysis of apractic cases shows that the spatial aspects of the trajectories are affected as well as their sequential organization. Figure 18.2 shows the derangement of the digital trajectories along with a breakdown of their spatial–temporal exploratory patterns.

In the case of whole-limb movements, kinematic recordings in patients with limb apraxia have demonstrated that the derangement of the spatial–temporal pattern is different from the disruption of interjoint coordination that characterizes the failure to control the interactive forces arising among limb segments during multijoint movements in deafferented patients (Sainburg *et al.* 1993).

Together with the inadequate posturing of the arm and hand and the decomposition of movement organization, these apractic characteristics represent a distinctive feature of the ataxic pointing or reaching behaviour seen in blind or sensory-deprived subjects. The latter miss the target because of their lack of sensory information, but they can remember target location from previous trials and learn to adapt their trajectories. They can also learn to substitute the missing channel by complementary information provided by other cues or modalities.

Is the level of complexity a determinant of apraxic dysfunction?

The kinematic patterns of patients with somatosensory–motor transformation complement the clinical examination, document the results for longitudinal evaluation, and may help to clarify the classification. However, there is another aspect of movement recordings. This relates to the question of whether their role is restricted to such confirmatory or illustrative aspects, thus showing in detail what is known in principle, or whether they also provide new information that escapes clinical detection.

A suitable example for illustrating this point is an investigation of five meaningless whole-limb movement sequences of increasing complexity that had to be performed by imitation or on verbal command by patients with parietal lesions (Weiss *et al.* 2001). The movement sequences were combinations of horizontal, vertical, and circular arm movements. Performance errors were classified as omission or addition of movement components, and as spatial or temporal errors.

The kinematic recordings showed that instruction modality had no influence on performance and that both arms were equally affected irrespective of the side of the lesion. Patients with left parietal damage were different in two respects: they showed an increase of error rate with task complexity, and they produced more temporal and spatial errors than those with right parietal lesions, whereas additions and omissions occurred about equally in both groups.

The consistent impairment of the performance of meaningless movement sequences in patients with parietal damage with and without apraxia demonstrate that the disturbance of spatial and temporal movement characteristics already exists at the level of sequences of simple straight or circular movements. They also show that the derangement of elementary movement occurs much more frequently than the clinically apparent apraxias. Further, they suggest that these disturbances at more elementary levels also represent constitutive elements of the apractic disorder. Thus quantitative movement recordings provide crucial information that is critical for the understanding of higher-order motor disturbances and their pathophysiology.

These data do not support the existence of a 'complexity threshold', leaving movements below intact and affecting what is above. Rather, there is a complexity gradient. Therefore apraxia may be at least partly due to the derangement of its constituent elements that may or may not be complemented by cognitive deficits that in turn produce disturbed motor behaviour. The kinematic data also show the more severe effects in left-hemisphere-damaged patients; only these patients showed a cumulative effect of errors in the production of more complex movement sequences. Interestingly, this was seen also in those patients who scored as non-apractic. Thus these data provide evidence that laterality effects already exist at the level of the organization of elementary motion sequences.

Is the level of complexity a determinant for the lateralization of motor functions?

The association of left-hemisphere damage and apraxia led Liepmann (1920) to conclude that the major hemisphere is dominant not only for language, but also for praxis. What the above mentioned results by Weiss *et al.* (2001) show is that the superiority of the left hemisphere obviously applies not only to the complex aspects of motor concept formation and action semantics, but also to the performance of elementary non-representational movements.

Asymmetries of executive motor areas have already been established for the hand area in the primary motor cortex in monkeys (Nudo *et al.* 1992) and humans (Amunts *et al.* 1996). In the monkey the distal forelimb representations on the hemisphere opposite the preferred hand generally were greater in number, larger in total area, displayed a longer total boundary length, and showed a greater index of spatial complexity. In humans, *in vivo* magnetic resonance morphometry revealed a significant deeper central sulcus on the left hemisphere than on the right in male consistent right-handers.

These neural–behavioural correlates of handedness in primary motor cortex are obviously associated with even more pronounced asymmetries in areas upstream of the motor cortex. It is interesting that this aspect of the functional organization of motor behaviour did not emerge from experimental studies in non-human primates, but from clinical observations in the human. As pointed out by Ettlinger (1969), there is no experimental model of apraxia.

The superiority of the language-dominant hemisphere for praxis is not easy to understand, because investigation of split-brain patients reveals that the right hemisphere of right-handers is perfectly able to organize even the most complex aspects of motor behaviour flawlessly, provided that it receives the required sensory input. So why can the right hemisphere not function this way after left parietal lesions? Freeman (1984) suggested that this 'paradox of the left hemisphere' may be due to a priority of action control exerted by the dominant hemisphere. How this is instrumented in terms of interhemispheric interactions is an unresolved issue. However, the asymmetries at the level of non-representational motor behaviour and of simple sensory–motor transformations make an important point, since they show that hemisphere dominance is not restricted to language-related motor behaviour at the symbolic level.

Sensory–motor transformation disorders in the visual system

The discussion of the somatomotor dysfunctions has shown that it is often difficult to distinguish between the effects of disruption of afferent information and of damage of the subsequent cortical processing stages involved in the sensory–motor transformations.

A similar situation exists for visuomotor disturbances. A typical example is optic ataxia (Balint 1909), which is a disorder of visuomotor behaviour characterized by misreaching and false gaze direction, leaving visual cognitive functions less affected. Rondot *et al.* (1997) proposed the term visuomotor ataxia for this condition and pointed out that the occipitoparietal lesions are often large and bilateral. Despite this, the functional deficit is often confined to visually guided movements. In this respect it is similar to the ataxia–tactile apraxia complex as it represents a strictly unimodal sensory–motor dysfunction. What is also similar is that some of the case reports address the ataxic and others the apractic features of the respective cases, a difference that can be unveiled by kinematic analysis (Classen *et al.* 1995). However, also clinically, most of the cases reported are different from motor behaviour in blind people.

An experimental model of optic ataxia was established by undercutting the long occipito-parietofrontal association fibres in the monkey (Haaxma and Kuypers 1975). The impairment produced by this selective fibre damage resembled the deficits observed in human patients, thus supporting the view of a visuomotor disconnection syndrome (Geschwind 1965). However, these long cortico-cortical fibre bundles are not the only major connection mediating visuomotor functions. A severe visuomotor deficit was also observed after subcortical damage of the descending parietopontine projections well below the level of the occipito-parietofrontal association fibres (Classen *et al.* 1995). This projection is known to convey visual information into the brainstem and cerebellar circuitries, where they are integrated with vestibular and proprioceptive inputs (Glickstein 1980). Their back projections towards the frontal motor areas represent a second pathway subserving visuomotor functions in addition to the parietofrontal association fibres. This connectivity may be the reason that visuomotor ataxia is typically seen in those cases where the occipitoparietal lesions are large and mostly bilateral, probably damaging not only direct cortico-cortical fibres but also descending fibres. Fibre imaging by diffusion-weighed tensor imaging may help to disentangle the effects of the selective impairment of either of these tracts in future studies.

These 'direct' visuomotor dysfunctions are more thoroughly discussed in Chapter 2. In this chapter we focus on a specific impairment of sensorimotor transformation that has recently been described. This is a selective visuospatial and visuomotor disturbance affecting only mirror-related motor behaviour leaving direct visuomotor functions unaffected. Patients can reach and grasp flawlessly towards what they see, but when the targets are viewed through a mirror, these movements are grossly disturbed.

Mirror transformation disorders

A special case of a unimodal sensorimotor transformation disorder: mirror agnosia and ataxia

Performing goal-directed actions while looking in a mirror requires additional transformations of images in more than one frame of reference in order to combine what we perceive as a reflection in mirror space with what we know is present in real space. Therefore there is a distinction between passively using a mirror to perceive objects, and using mirrors to actively guide our movements using an object's reflected image. This difference is reflected by the deficits seen in patients with mirror agnosia. The affected patients are fully aware of the purpose of a mirror and they recognize the objects shown by the mirror. What they cannot accomplish is to infer the position of the real object while looking in the image reflected in the mirror. The disturbance is characterized by the fact that, when seeing an object through a mirror, the patients believe that the object is actually in the mirror and keep grasping there without being able to learn from other cues that the real object is somewhere else.

This new category of unimodal sensory–motor transformation disorders has been introduced by reports on cases with damage of the posterior parietal lobe and a selective dysfunction of motor behaviour involving the use of mirrors. Ramachandran *et al.* (1997) reported four patients with right-hemisphere lesions and left-sided hemineglect who could not distinguish between a real object and its mirror image. When a mirror was placed on their right side, they reached towards the mirror rather than to the real object in the neglected left hemifield. This right-hemisphere deficit was regarded as either reflecting the neglect or a disturbance of spatial abilities. It was termed mirror agnosia because the patients were convinced that the object was in the mirror.

Binkofski *et al.* (1997, 1999) reported a similar disturbance, but at variance to the above cases in patients without neglect and with lesions of the posterior parietal lobe of either side. When a vertical mirror (Fig. 18.3) adjusted to the body midline was used, there was no left–right inversion so that the misreaching could not be due to laterality effects. As illustrated in Fig. 18.3 the common denominator in all cases was that the patients mistook the mirror image of an object for the real image and continuously searched for the object in the mirror.

Although the patients could understand and explain the purpose of a mirror, they were unaware of the mirror-induced alterations of the spatial relationships of the objects. Thus this disorder is characterized by a dissociation between the intact recognition and identification of both the meaning of a mirror and of the spatial attributes of the objects viewed in the mirror, and the false spatial allocation of the target with concomitant misreaching. The 'agnostic' features only relate to spatial localization and its use for the guidance of movements. The distinction between spatial cognition in the service of object identification and spatial cognition in the service of action is further evidence for separate representations of visual space for perception and for motor control (Bridgeman *et al.* 1979; Bard *et al.* 1995).

Another remarkable aspect of the disturbance is that it is context dependent and confined to specific aspects of mirror-related motor behaviour. On the one hand, proprioceptive feedback was not helpful for the patients, so that repeated passive guidance of the arm could not correct the wrong direction of the trajectory. The patients were

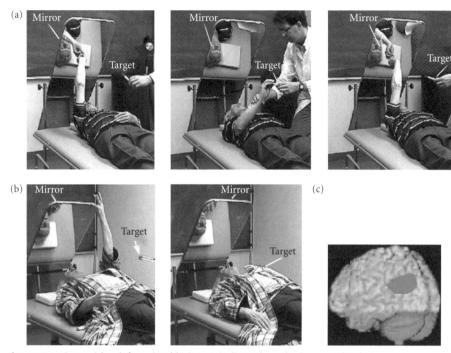

Fig. 18.3 Patient with a left parietal lesion as indicated on the lower right during various visuomotor pointing tasks. Upper left: the patient views the target through a vertical mirror. When asked to point to the target he points straight towards the virtual image in the mirror. Upper middle: the patient views the target through a vertical mirror while his arm is passively guided to the real position of the target. Further, the error of his former trial is explained to him and he is asked to remember the real position. This procedure is repeated several times. Upper right: the next trial goes like the first. Lower left: mispointing with the left arm is different as the arm is not directed to the virtual target but somewhere near the 'attractor' mirror space. Lower right: When the target seen through the mirror is placed somewhere at or very near his body, he points there flawlessly.

not capable of changing their behaviour even after repeated guidance of their arm to the previously seen position of the real object. However, the patients reached towards the mirror images instead of the real images only when the mirror images alone were visible to them. When they could see both the real object and its mirror image, most of them looked and reached towards the real object. Consequently, only actions towards objects seen in the mirror that could not be simultaneously monitored in the periphery of the visual field were misguided.

The dissociation between mirror reaching in personal and peripersonal space

Another context-specific feature of mirror agnosia was that the patients exhibited the deficits in reaching for targets presented through a mirror only when these were localized in their peripersonal space. When they were required to reach towards their own body parts viewed through a mirror, their reaching performance was flawless (Binkofski *et al.* 2003). This implies a dissociation between personal space, defined as the space confined directly to the body, and peripersonal space, defined as the space localized within reaching distance (Rizzolatti *et al.* 1983, 1997a; Graziano 1999).

The dissociation between flawless reaching in personal space but misreaching in peripersonal space is of interest in the light of the old concept that 'visual perception within and without arm's reach may be subserved by different neural mechanisms' (Paterson and Zangwill 1944). This view, derived from clinical observations, was further supported by an imaging study where subjects had to bisect horizontal lines either in extrapersonal 'far space' or in near 'peripersonal space' by means of a laser pointer (Weiss *et al.* 2000). Whereas task performance in far space activated the ventral occipital cortex bilaterally and the right medial temporal cortex, the near-space task recruited the left dorsal occipital, left intraparietal, and ventral premotor cortex. The differential involvement of the two processing streams in tasks performed in the two spaces led to the conclusion that the visual world surrounding us seems to be represented not only as visual space but also as a motor space, representing a space for actions within reaching distance and a space beyond.

The intact mirror reaching towards the own body may be the reason that the patients themselves were not aware of the deficit. Despite this gross misreaching towards external objects viewed through a mirror, movements targeting their own body parts like shaving and combing were not affected. Obviously, grasping for external objects shown by a mirror is a rarely employed visuomotor behaviour so that its disturbance escapes the patient's attention. Therefore the situation is different from visuomotor and tactile apraxia where the disturbance of object-related motor behaviour is clinically apparent. The impairment of mirror-related visuomotor transformation disorders needs to be disclosed by special tests.

The contrast between the normal pointing movements in personal and peripersonal space indicates a highly selective disturbance of the mirror-induced coordinate transformations mediating the spatial relation between the body and objects within reaching distance. Thus mirror agnosia may originate from a dissociation between the representations of body schema and peripersonal space, whereas objects located on the body surface remain integrated into the body schema.

However, it is not just the complex set of coordinate transformations that is required by the use of mirrors that is disturbed in these patients. Other aspects of the formation of the body image and the ongoing update about its relation to external objects is also compromised in many cases. This became apparent by the examination of the subjective vertical (Binkofski *et al.* 1999). When the patients were asked to demarcate their body midline by drawing a vertical line in the air with their hand, they were accurate as long as the head and eyes looked forward. However, when the head was turned to the right or the left all patients reoriented the subjective midsagittal plane in relation to the head. The poor performance on the Benton line orientation test on mirror writing and mental rotation tasks in most patients further demonstrates the close association between the performance in mirror actions and other coordinate transformation tasks.

A pure agnosia for mirror stimuli was reported for a patient with a highly selective deficit in tasks requiring mirror-stimulus discrimination or misalignment of the object's coordinates with respect to the body (Priftis *et al.* 2003). This was regarded as indicating a disorder of the discrimination of mirror stimuli defined in object-based coordinates and a failure in processing the directionality of an object's intrinsic *x*-axis.

Mirror ataxia

A second group of patients in the series reported by Binkofski *et al.* (1999) showed a distinct clinical picture. They could distinguish real from mirror space, but they also produced mirror-induced directional errors in contrast with their otherwise normal reaching under direct view. This condition was called mirror ataxia. Although some of the patients first pointed towards the mirror, they could learn to redirect their movements to the real object. Kinematic recordings make the differences between the mirror-agnostic and mirror-atactic patients clearer. A typical recording of the movement trajectory is shown in Fig. 18.4 for a patient with mirror ataxia. The deranged velocity profile shows a variable and hesitating performance with frequent corrections of the spatial coordinates of the trajectory. In contrast, the movement trajectory of a patient with mirror agnosia shows normal kinematic features. Thus mirror agnosia is characterized by correct movement trajectories that are performed straightforwardly to the wrong target, and mirror ataxia is characterized by an ataxic movement aiming for the correct target. As Fig. 18.4 shows, these differences are reflected by both the directional features of the trajectories and the velocity profiles.

An analysis of lesion sites showed different clusters of the common zone of overlap in the two conditions. In the cases with mirror agnosia the lesions scattered in the inferior posterior parietal lobule, sometimes extending into the superior temporal gyrus. Therefore it is unclear at present whether this disorder represents a selective parietal lobe dysfunction. The lesions in the mirror ataxia group overlapped more anteriorly around the anterior part of the intraparietal sulcus.

Since we reported our first series of patients, we have encountered more than 30 cases, a surprisingly high incidence amongst patients with parietal lobe lesions. This indicates that mirror transformation disorders are much more frequent than the clinically apparent visuomotor ataxia that is mostly seen in patients with large and often bilateral parietotemporo-occipital damage. The high incidence of mirror agnosia and mirror ataxia after parietal lobe damage suggests that the complex sensory–motor transformations required for actions in mirror space and entrained later in life are more vulnerable than the more robust direct visuomotor processes. Therefore disorders of mirror transformation may reflect the greater liability to disturbance of a more widely distributed functional network rather than the selective clustering of

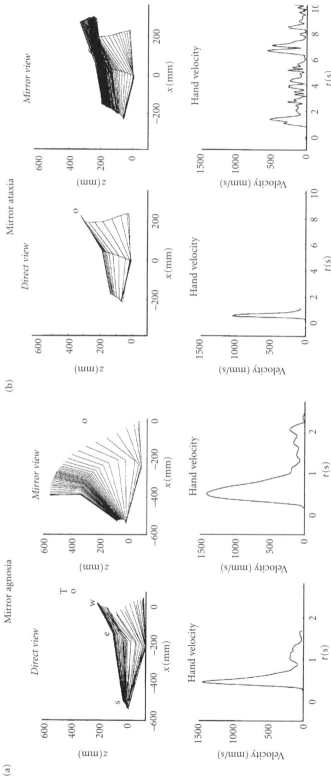

Fig. 18.4 Kinematic recordings of reaching movements of the right arms of a patient with (a) mirror agnosia and (b) mirror ataxia (a) The stick figures representing the position of the wrist (w), elbow (e), and shoulder (s) show the different movement paths toward the object (T) under direct visual control and towards the mirror when the object is presented through the mirror. The velocity profiles show that both movements were performed with normal peak velocities and without additional corrections (b). The stick figures show that the object was approached under direct view and when presented through the mirror. However, the movement path shows many corrections as can also be seen from the deranged velocity profile and the multiple velocity peaks.

lesions at a 'mirror transformation locus'. Perturbations of the distributed network required for such complex transformations disclose their lower redundancy but leave direct visuomotor behaviour unaffected. In view of the close interactions between parietal and premotor cortex, it is noteworthy that at present there is no evidence for similar dysfunctions in cases with premotor lesions.

The pathophysiology of the mirror transformation disorders

Regarding terminology, mirror apraxia would be one possibility of qualifying the selectively action-related nature of mirror agnosia and the preservation of the cognitive and semantic aspects of the perception of mirror images. Another feature of the disturbance is its context dependence, which has repeatedly been emphasized as a hallmark of apraxia (Geschwind 1965). However, the kinematic recordings demonstrate unambiguously that the movement trajectories are correct. What is wrong is the patient's inference about the spatial location of the target—the patient's belief that the object is in the mirror. This false spatial localization of the real objects guides the movement towards the virtual image in the mirror. The perfectly normal movement paths and the flawless hit of the goal indicates that is not impairment of the ability to organize actions in space. The core feature of the dysfunction lies in the spatial cognitive domain—mistaking the reflected image in the mirror for the real image. In this respect the disorder meets the criteria of an agnosia. The difficulty of disentangling agnostic and apractic features of a disturbance led Grünbaum (1930) to coin the term 'apractognosia' for designating this complexity.

Taking a similar perspective for the cases with mirror ataxia, there is another ambiguity regarding the nature of the disturbance. In this condition patients finally reach to the real object and learn to improve their performance in repeated trials. What is wrong here is the movement itself. Looking at the trajectories (Fig. 18.4) shows the typical paths seen in ataxia with frequent deviations from and corrections towards the intended course. This may reflect continuous error correction on the basis of feedback mechanisms during a misconducted movement, a typical attribute of ataxia. However, there is one feature that may need an alternative explanation. This is the frequent change of direction of the trajectory between the location of the mirror and the real object, in particular during the first trials—almost like a flip-flop between the two. This may well reflect an ongoing rivalry between the real and the mirror image. If so, the disorder would represent a minor version of mirror agnosia characterized by an intermittent rather than a persistent failure in localization. In this case the different locations of the centres of overlap of the lesions would be disturbing, but this issue needs clarification by future studies.

Activation studies on mirror transformation

The prominent role of the parietal lobe for direct visuomotor behaviour not involving the use of mirrors was shown by a number of imaging studies elaborating the various facets of visuomotor performances involved in reaching or pointing to directly viewed objects. The activations seen in these tasks delineate a right dorsal occipito-parietofrontal network of areas involved in visuospatial analysis and visuomotor transformations (Decety *et al.* 1992; Grafton *et al.* 1992, 1996; Kertzman *et al.* 1997; Binkofski *et al.* 2003; Desmurget *et al.* 2001). The areas identified in these studies reveal close homologies to several areas in the macaque inferior parietal cortex where neurons code for different aspects of action in space (Andersen *et al.* 1997; Rizzolatti *et al.* 1997b; Caminiti *et al.* 1998).

The data derived from observations of patients with mirror agnosia and mirror ataxia do not provide any cues allowing isolation of the effects of the mirror itself and the transformations imposed by inferring the location of a real object from its mirror image. However, functional imaging can single out these different processes and specify their effects. Binkofski *et al.* (2003) studied the cerebral activation pattern during reaching to objects presented through a mirror in the peripersonal space in healthy subjects. The results showed increased neural activity in the anterior part of the intraparietal sulcus and in the dorsal premotor cortex when transformation of the target position from the mirror space to real space was required. In contrast, the activity related to object localization in the mirror occurred at the parieto-occipital junction. These results demonstrate that acting through a mirror involves spatial and mirror-related coordinate transformations that are processed in segregate neural clusters along the dorsal stream.

The contribution of the unimodal sensory-motor transformation deficits to the understanding of the higher-order motor disorders

In terms of mechanism, mirror agnosia and mirror ataxia represent a disturbance of the transformations required to allocate external objects viewed in a mirror correctly in space and to organize motor behaviour towards them accordingly. The core deficit in this disorder seems to consist of the inability of patients with inferior parietal lesions to relocate the position of an object from the virtual mirror space into the real space for action. The mirror disorders illustrate how much the conception of the movement plan is determined by the specific requirements of a particular action, in this case of the spatial target attributes with respect to the subject's own body. Along with the somatosensory–motor transformation disorders, they further illustrate the close interlacing of the sensory and motor processes or, in more general terms, of action and perception.

This makes the assignation of these recently described disorders to any of the traditional categories, such as agnosia, apraxia, and ataxia, somewhat arbitrary and ambiguous. Nevertheless, clinical neurology is providing a diversity of terms that can be combined to describe partial deficits of action and perception.

The attribution of these disturbances to distinct pathophysiologies is less biased. The advantage of such an approach is that it can be adapted to the new data and concepts.

For the topics discussed here, the term unimodal sensorimotor transformation disorders seems adequate to designate the specifity of the disturbances (Freund 1992). In contrast with the more general apractic conditions affecting polymodal integration, they specify the restriction of the dysfunction to only one modality.

The sensorimotor transformation disorders raise some intriguing questions about the relationship between the cognitive and action-related aspects of sensorimotor information processing. Regarding motor cognition, it has been demonstrated that covert actions and overtly executed actions represent a continuum in the sense that the state where an action is simulated necessarily precedes execution of that action (see Chapters 5 and 9). Both evoke concomitant activations of overlapping neural repertoires upstream motor cortex. These premotor–parietal activations have been shown not only during motor imagery but also during action observation (see Chapter 8). The discharges of mirror neurons during both the observation and performance of the same gesture (di Pellegrino *et al.* 1992) showed that this dual coding can even be accomplished by the same neurons.

How these new concepts derived from the field of motor cognition and neurophysiology relate to the executional aspects of motor behaviour and the involvement of sensorimotor transformations is unclear. The precision of the estimated movement parameters during mental imagery experiments, revealing the same temporal characteristics for both the covert and overt conditions, favours the view that covert motor behaviour also involves the spatial–temporal transformations engaged in the actual performance. What is different between these transformations and cognitive processing is their accessibility to conscious awareness. The performance theory of voluntary action suggests that voluntary actions are represented in terms of their behavioural goals and the percepts they generate (see Chapter 5). We are aware of the effects of our actions in the environment, but not of the kinematics and dynamics determining the biomechanics that are automatically adjusted and obviously processed subconsciously.

Since both the mirror neuron system and the neuronal aggregates subserving the multiple sensorimotor transformations are embedded in the parietal–premotor circuitry, damage could interfere with both the performance and the recognition of representational motor behaviour. Comparing the comprehension of the symbolic content and the imitation of gestures in apractic patients with parietal lobe damage revealed that only imitation was disturbed (Halsband *et al.* 2001). The preservation of the understanding of the meaning conveyed by purposive goal-directed actions suggests that parietal damage interferes with the pragmatic aspects of dorsal route processing.

The mirror transformation disorders provide a further example for this visual processing dichotomy. They show that movements requiring specific spatial transformations are compromised as are the respective spatial inferences about objects. But the meaning of the objects or of the purpose of a mirror, their cognitive appreciation remains preserved.

This type of organization is obviously different for the somatosensory system where both, the recognition of tactile objects and the elaboration of the motor programs required for active touch are compromised in patients with damage restricted to the parietal lobe.

References

Amunts K, Schlaug G, Schleicher A, Steinmetz H, Dabringhaus A, Roland PE, *et al.* (1996). Asymmetry in the human motor cortex an handedness. *Neuroimage*, **4**, 216–22.

Andersen RA, Bueno CA (2003). Sensorimotor integration in posterior parietal cortex. In AM Siegel, RA Andersen, HJ Freund, D Spencer (ed.) *The Parietal Lobes : Advances in Neurology*, pp. 159–77. Philadelphia, PA: Lippincott, Williams and Wilkins.

Andersen RA, Synder LH, Bradley DC, Xing J (1997). Multimodal representation of space in the posterior parietal cortex and its use in planning movements. *Annu Rev Neurosci*, **20**, 303–30.

Balint R (1909). Seelenlähmung des Schauens, optische Ataxie, räumliche Störung der Aufmerksamkeit. *Monatsschr Psychiatrie Neurol*, **25**, 51–81.

Bard C, Fleury M, Teasdale N, Paillard J, Nougier V (1995). Contribution of proprioception for calibrating and updating the motor space. *Can J Physiol Pharmacol*, **73(2)**, 246–54.

Binkofski F, Seitz RJ, Dohle C, *et al.* (1997). Dissociation of retinotopic space and proprioceptive body scheme: characterization of parietal lesion. *Soc Neurosci Abstr*, **23**, 1374.

Binkofski F, Dohle C, Posse S, Hefter H, Seitz RJ, Freund H-J (1998). Human anterior intraparietal area subserves prehension: a combined lesion and fMRI study. *Neurology*, **50**, 1253–9.

Binkofski F, Buccino G, Dohle C, Seitz RJ, Freund H-J (1999). Mirror agnosia and mirror ataxia constitute different parietal lobe disorders. *Ann Neurol*, **46**, 51–61.

Binkofski F, Kunesch E, Classen J, Seitz RJ, Freund H-J (2001). Tactile apraxia: unimodal apractic disorder of tactile object exploration associated with parietal lobe lesions. *Brain*, **124**, 132–44.

Binkofski F, Butler A, Buccino G, Heide W, Fink G, Freund H-J, *et al.* (2003). Mirror apraxia affects the peripersonal mirror space. A combined lesion and cerebral activation study. *Exp Brain Res*, **153**, 210–19.

Bridgeman B, Lewis S, Heit G, Nagle M (1979). A relation between cognitive and motor-oriented systems of visual position perception. *J Exp Psychol Hum Percept Perform*, **5**, 692–700.

Caminiti R, Ferraina S, Mayer AB (1998). Visuomotor transformations: early cortical mechanisms of reaching. *Curr Opin Neurobiol*, **8**, 753–61.

Classen J, Kunesch E, Binkofski F, Hilperath F, Schlang G, Seitz RJ, *et al.* (1995). Subcortical origin of visuomotor apraxia. *Brain*, **118**, 1365–74.

Decety J, Kawashima R, Gulyas B, Roland PE (1992). Preparation for reaching: a PET study of the participating structures in the human brain. *NeuroReport*, **3**, 761–4.

di Pellegrino G, Falliga L, Fogassi L, Gallese V, Rizzollatti G (1992). Understanding motor events: a neurophysiological study. *Exp Brain Res*, **91**, 176–80.

Desmurget M, Grea H, Grethe JS, Prablanc C, Alexander GE, Grafton ST (2001). Functional anatomy of nonvisual feedback loops during reaching: a positron emission tomography study. *J Neurosci*, **21**, 2919–28.

Ettlinger G (1969). Apraxia considered as a disorder of movements that are language-dependent: evidence from cases of brain bisection. *Cortex*, **5**, 285–9.

Foerster O (1936). Motor cortex in man in the light of Hughlings Jackson's doctrines. *Brain*, **59**, 135–9.

Freeman RB (1984). The apraxias, purposeful motor behavior, and left-hemisphere function. In W Prinz, AF Sanders, (ed.) *Cognition and Motor Processes*, pp. 29–50. Berlin: Springer-Verlag.

Freund H-J (1987). Abnormalities of motor behaviour after cortical lesions in humans. In F Plum, (ed.) *Handbook of Physiology*. Section 1 *The Nervous System*. Vol. 5. *Higher Functions of the Brain*, Part 2, pp. 763–810. Baltimore, MD: Williams & Wilkins.

Freund H-J (1992). The apraxias. In AK Asbury, GM McKhann, WI McDonald, (ed.) *Diseases of the Nervous System. Clinical Neurobiology* Vol. 2, pp. 751–67. Chichester: Wiley.

Geschwind N (1965). Disconnexion syndromes in animals and man. I. *Brain*, **88**, 237–94.

Gibson JJ (1962). Observations on active touch. *Psychol Rev*, **69**, 477–91.

Glickstein M, Cohen JL, Dixon C, Gibson A, Hollins M, Labossiere E, *et al.* (1980). Corticopontine visual projections in macaque monkeys. *J Comp Neurol*, **190**, 209–29.

Grafton ST, Mazziotta JC, Woods RP, Phelps ME (1992). Human functional anatomy of visually guided finger movements. *Brain*, **115**, 565–87.

Grafton ST, Fagg AH, Woods RP, Arbib MA (1996). Functional anatomy of pointing and grasping in humans. *Cerebral Cortex*, **6**, 226–37.

Graziano MS (1999). Where is my arm? The relative role of vision and proprioception in the neuronal representation of limb position. *Proceedings of the National Academy of Sciences USA* **96**, 10418–21.

Grünbaum AA (1930). Aphasie und Motorik Zeitschrift für die gesamte Neurologie und Psychiatrie **130**, 385–412.

Haaxma R, Kuypers HGJM (1975). Intrahemispheric cortical connections and visual guidance of hand an finger movements in the rhesus monkey. *Brain*, **98**, 239–60.

Halsband U, Schmitt J, Weyers M, Binkofski F, Grutzner G, Freund HJ (2001). Recognition and imitation of pantomimed motor acts after unilateral parietal and premotor lesions: a perspective on apraxia. *Neuropsychologia*, **39**, 200–16.

Jeannerod M, Arbib MA, Rizzolatti G, Sakata H (1995). Grasping objects: the cortical mechanisms of visuomotor transformation (Review). *Trends Neurosci*, **18**, 314–20.

Jeannerod M, Decety J (1995). Mental motor imagery: a window into the representational stages of action. *Current Opinion in Neurobiology*, **5**, 727–32.

Kertzman C, Schwarz U, Zeffiro TA, Hallett M (1997). The role of posterior parietal cortex in visually guided reaching movements in humans. *Exp Brain Res*, **114**, 170–83.

Klein R (1931). Zur Symptomatologie des Parietallappens. *Zeitschrift für die Gesamte Neurologie und Psychiatrie*, **135**, 589–608.

Kunesch E (1994). Neurophysiologische Untersuchungen zur sensomotorischen Interaktion der menschlichen Hand. Habilitationschrift der Medizinischen Fakultät der Heinrich-Heine Universität Düsseldorf.

Lederman SJ, Klatzky RL (1997). Hand movements: a window into haptic object recognition. *Cognitive Psychology*, **19**, 342–68.

Liepmann H (1900). Das Krankheitsbild der Apraxie ("motorische Asymbolie"), auf Grund eines Falles von einseitiger Apraxie. *Monatsschrift für Psychiatrie und Neurologie*, **8**, 182–197.

Liepmann H (1920). Apraxie. In: Brugsch's Ergebnisse der Gesamten Medizin. pp. 518–543. Berlin: Urban & Schwarzenberg.

Nudo RJ, Jenkins WM, Merzenich MM, Prejean T, Grenda R (1992). Neurophysiological correlates of hand preference in primary motor cortex of adult squirrel monkeys. *J Neurosci*, **12**, 2918–4.

Paterson A, Zangwill OL (1944). Disorders of visual space perception associated with lesions of the right cerebral hemisphere. *Brain*, **67**, 331–58.

Pause M, Kunesch E, Binkofski F, Freund H-J (1989). Sensorimotor disturbances in patients with lesions of the parietal cortex. *Brain*, **112**, 1599–625.

Priftis K, Rusconi E, Umilta C, Zorzi M. (2003). Pure agnosia for mirror stimuli after right inferior parietal lesion. *Brain*, **126**, 908–19.

Ramachandran VS, Altschuler EL, Hillyer S (1997). Mirror agnosia. *Proceedings of the Royal Society London B*, **264**, 645–7.

Reed CL, Caselli RJ, Farah MJ (1996). Tactile agnosia: Underlying impairment and implications for normal tactile object recognition. *Brain*, **119**, 875–88.

Rizzolatti G, Fadiga L, Fogassi L, Gallese V (1997a). The space around us [see comments]. *Science*, **277**, 190–1.

Rizzolatti G, Fogassi L, Gallese V (1997b). Parietal cortex: from sight to action. *Current Opinion in Neurobiology*, **7**, 562–7.

Rizzolatti G, Matelli M, Pavesi G (1983). Deficits in attention and movement following the removal of postarcuate (area 6) and prearcuate (area 8) cortex in macaque monkeys. *Brain*, **43**, 118–36.

Rondot P, de Recondo J, Ribadeau Dumas JL (1997). Visuomotor ataxia. *Brain*, **100**, 355–76.

Sainburg RL, Poizner H, Ghez C (1993). Loss of proprioception produces deficits in interjoint coordination. *Journal of Neurophysiology*, **70**, 2136–47.

Sakata H, Taira M, Murata A, Mine S (1995). Neural mechanisms of visual guidance of hand action in the parietal cortex of the monkey. *Cerebral Cortex*, **5**, 429–38.

Weiss PH, Marshall JC, Wunderlich G, Tellmann L, Halligan PW, Freund H-J, Zilles K, Fink GR (2000). Neural consequences of acting in near versus far space: a physiological basis for clinical dissociations. *Brain*, **123**, 2531–41.

Weiss PH, Dohle C, Binkofski F, Schnitzler A, Freund H-J, Hefter H (2001). Motor impairment in patients with parietal lesions: disturbances of meaningless arm movement sequences. *Neuropsychologia*, **39**, 397–405.

Wise SP, Boussaoud D, Johnson PB, Caminiti R (1997). Premotor and parietal cortex: corticocortical connectivity and combinatorial computations. *Annual Reviews of Neuroscience*, **20**, 25–42.

Yamadori A (1982). Palpatory apraxia. European *Neurology*, **21**, 277–83.

Chapter 19

Action recognition disorders following parietal damage

Elena Daprati and Angela Sirigu

From the moment of our birth, we act in the world. Despite such a large motor experience, we have a poor subjective knowledge of the entire set of processes that underlie our motor skills. Interestingly, even if we remain largely unaware of the contents of our actions, we are usually good at judging whether an action has originated from ourselves or not. In the present chapter, we will review the putative mechanisms responsible for recognition of self-generated actions. We will suggest that the ability of an individual to perceive and visually recognize a given movement as his or her own (i.e. his or her motor awareness) relies on the opportunity to process anticipatory information on motor production as well as on the capacity to monitor motor execution on-line. Moreover, we will emphasize the necessity of mapping the acting limb correctly on a reliable body representation. Evidence for this hypothesis will be drawn from the study of brain-damaged subjects.

Introduction

The ability to construct and manipulate mental representations is probably a unique human capability; it enables us to create an internal image of ourselves and the environment we act upon, and to anticipate the consequences of our behavior. Although we frequently refer to this ability for creating second-order representations, i.e. to access our own thoughts, this competence is deeply embedded in our most elementary behaviors. The immediate feeling of recognition when looking at ourselves in a mirror as well as the extremely natural sense of ownership we perceive when observing our movements are rather familiar examples. As an elementary function, self-perception appears early in human development. Infants as young as 2 months recognize themselves in the different auditory traces of their own actions. In an interesting experience, Rochat and Striano (1999) showed that babies modulate their oral activity on a dummy pacifier in order to obtain a contingent sound, which is released only when the infant sucks above a certain pressure. Similarly, by 3 months, infants become sensitive to spatial invariants related to self-generated movements; for example, when perceiving that they move their legs in a given direction, infants expect to see their legs moving in that direction (Rochat and Morgan 1995). In other words, long before mirror self-recognition (which usually develops by 18 months), babies already show an early sense of self and they seem to be able to perceive their own body as an agent in the environment.

Thus, it is perfectly clear that whenever pathology disrupts such a basic system, consequences can be dramatic; abnormalities in the control and awareness of actions have been largely described in both the neuropsychological and neuropsychiatric literature. For instance, following mesiofrontal and/or callosal damage, patients may present with an alien hand syndrome. These patients apparently lose control of the motor behavior of their contralesional arm, which seems to act independently of the patient's will; for example, the alien hand might undo buttons that have just been done up, or open a door that has just been closed. In the most extreme cases, the patient may even deny ownership of the alien hand and report a lack of recognition of the arm as his or her own (Feinberg *et al.* 1992; Geschwind *et al.* 1995; Chan and Ross 1997; Chan and Liu 1999). Similarly, following right parietal damage, subjects may develop bizarre attitudes toward the contralesional limbs, including feeling of non-belonging or complex productive delusions (somatoparaphrenia) (Gerstman 1942; Hècaen and Ajuriaguerra 1952; Weinstein and Kahn 1955; Bisiach and Geminiani 1991). Interestingly, in the most severe forms of somatoparaphrenia, these patients may even claim that the contralesional limb belongs to someone else (Cutting 1978; Halligan *et al.* 1995). Finally, in schizophrenia, patients may experience 'passivity' phenomena, namely they may report that thoughts are made up for them by some other person or that their action are controlled by some external force (Mellor 1970).

Overall, the disorders mentioned above represent the consequences of the loss, at different levels, of the elementary ability to perceive one part of the body as our own and to recognize a given act as the product of our own motor activity. In this chapter, we will briefly review the mechanisms involved in action observation and recognition and then focus on defining the mechanisms that enable us to attribute an action to the correct agent, and accordingly to recognize a movement as our own.

Observing actions

Visual perception of biological motion has been widely investigated. A primitive point-light display of a walking human is known to be sufficiently informative to convey a vivid image of a moving subject, and may even allow detection of the sex and other details of the walker (Johansson 1973; Kozlowski and Cutting 1977; Mather and Murdoch 1994). By means of a similar display, recent neuroimaging reports have suggested that perception of biological motion may be subserved by a specific neural network. By contrasting biological motion with random dot motion, activation was found in the human homologue of monkey area V5/MT, an area typically involved in motion perception, and bilaterally in the superior temporal sulcus (STS) (Howard *et al.* 1996). More recently, a similar positron emission tomography (PET) study confirmed how biological motion is effective in specifically activating the posterior portion of the STS and the left anterior portion of the intraparietal sulcus (Grèzes *et al.* 2001). These observations are further supported by a neuropsychological dissociation showing preserved perception of biological motion in a patient who had lost the ability to perceive the motion of objects, following a V5 lesion (Vaina *et al.* 1990). Moreover, robust monkey data demonstrate the specific involvement of STS neurons in observation of body movements (reviewed by Puce and Perrett 2003). Further PET studies on healthy humans have detailed differential cortical involvement in the perception of meaningful actions versus observation of meaningless movements (Decety *et al.* 1997). Interestingly, observation of pantomimes was found to activate the left frontal and temporal regions (i.e. the ventral visual pathway), while meaningless actions involved mainly the right occipitoparietal (dorsal) pathway (Milner and Goodale 1995).

Even more noticeably, monkey studies have shown that neurons responding to action are found also in area F5, in the ventral premotor cortex (see also Chapter 8, this volume). In contrast with STS neurons, these neurons typically discharge both when the monkey performs a given action and when it observes a similar action performed by the experimenter. Accordingly, these so-called 'mirror neurons' (di Pellegrino *et al.* 1992; Gallese *et al.* 1996) have been proposed as being part of a system for matching observation and execution of motor actions, which might provide a neural substrate for action recognition. This hypothesis finds support in humans from the distribution of activity found by Rizzolatti *et al.* (1996) in a PET study contrasting observation of an actor grasping an object with grasping execution and passive object observation. Observation of a person performing a goal-directed action produced a significant increase in blood flow in the temporal cortex, including the STS. Moreover, the caudal part of the left inferior frontal gyrus, namely Brodmann's area 45, was also activated. This latter area is suggested to be a functional homologue of monkey frontal area F5.

In strict agreement with this hypothesis, observing an action for the later purpose of imitating it has been found to activate regions involved in the planning and generation of actions, namely the dorsolateral prefrontal cortex on both sides and the pre-supplementary motor area (Decety *et al.* 1997), thus supporting the idea that an observed action can be understood and imitated whenever it becomes the source of a representation of the same action within the observer. This observation was further extended by the finding that observation of object-related actions also activates the posterior parietal lobe (Buccino *et al.* 2001).

Parietal involvement in action imitation and recognition is a well-known finding in the apraxia literature. Recent neuropsychological studies have explored the ability to imitate gestures in patients with lesions in the parietal cortex of both hemispheres (Halsband *et al.* 2001). Interestingly, it was shown that when lesions affected the left parietal cortex, sparing temporal lobe structures, action imitation but not recognition was severely impaired. This dissociation is in agreement with the hypothesis of a dorsal visual stream processing action-related information and of a ventral stream processing more 'scmantic' information on observed actions.

Recognizing oneself

In 1943, Wolff claimed that, despite a consistent difficulty in recognizing photographs of their own hands, normal subjects are 100% accurate in recognizing something that they had never seen before: a film of themselves walking, with face and bodily appearance disguised. This interesting observation was pursued further in the 1960s when Nielsen (1963) devised a paradigm that allowed direct investigation of recognition of one's own motion. By means of an optical apparatus, Nielsen asked subjects to distinguish their moving hand from an alien hand that appeared in the same location. As predicted by Wolff's observation, subjects could recognize their movements, although they frequently defined the alien hand as theirs, eventually reporting a feeling of strangeness towards it, as if they had lost control of their movements. Nielsen's study suggests that in an ambiguous situation, normal subjects select movement-related visual information in preference to signals arising from kinesthetic feedback (thus accepting an alien hand as theirs). Namely, conscious access to the contents of motor activity seem to be extremely limited. More recently, a similar observation was reported by Fourneret and Jeannerod (1998) who examined which signals normal subjects use to monitor voluntary actions. The authors asked normal volunteers to draw a straight line over a digital tablet. Subjects could see the result of their strokes on a computer screen that, in some trials, allowed introduction of a bias in the output of the digital tablet. Namely, the line shown on the screen could deviate from the sagittal direction by a given angle, to either the right or the left. Results showed that subjects consistently corrected their tracing for the bias. However, when interviewed on the corrections, they largely underestimated their hand deviation, mostly reporting a direction close to straight ahead, i.e. corresponding to the line they saw on the screen. Moreover, when asked in which direction they had moved, one group of subjects reported that they had deviated in the direction of the bias, thus relying on movement-related visual information rather than on their actual kinesthetic feedback. In other words, normal subjects have poor access to the actual correction movements they perform, confirming that they remain largely unaware of the relevant components of motor control.

Despite such poor access, both Wolff's (1943) and Nielsen's (1963) remarks were correct: normal subjects can recognize their own motion with reliable accuracy. In a pilot study, Daprati et al. (1997) adapted Nielsen's paradigm in order to recreate an experimental situation where an action is executed and visually monitored, but its origin is ambiguous. Thirty normal subjects (19 males and 11 females, mean age 28.8 years) were requested to produce, on verbal command, a particular gesture with their unseen hand. Simultaneously, the image of a moving hand was presented on a screen in front of the subjects, who were asked to judge whether the movement they observed on the screen belonged to them or not. Ambiguity was introduced by capturing movement of the subject's hand as well as that of the hand of a hidden actor by two different cameras (Fig 19.1(a)). By operating a switch, either hand could be displayed on the screen in front of the subject. As gross hand morphology was hidden by a glove, subjects were forced to use movement as a cue to recognizing their own hand. In each trial, both the actor and the subject performed a particular gesture on verbal command (e.g. stretch thumb, stretch fingers one and two, etc); however, on some trials the actor produced a movement which departed from the instruction. As a result, the subject randomly saw on the screen either his or her own hand (Subject's Hand Condition), or the actor's hand performing an identical movement (Experimenter Same Condition) or a different movement (Experimenter Different Condition). At the end of each trial, subjects gave their response verbally, stating whether the hand they had seen was their own. As shown in Fig. 19.1(b), subjects were able to determine whether the moving hand seen on the screen was their own. This was particularly true for the conditions when they actually saw their own hand (Subject's Hand Condition). Similarly, when they saw the actor's hand performing a different movement (Experimenter Different Condition) they easily excluded the possibility that the hand belonged to them. Their performance slightly degraded in those trials where they saw the actor's hand performing a movement identical to the one they were executing (Experimenter Same Condition); in this condition, in agreement with Nielsen's data, they sometimes reported the alien hand as their own, although they could tell the difference in nearly 70% of cases.

One possible mechanism for ensuring such a high proportion of correct answers is based on a theory that was very popular in the 1950s, i.e. the corollary discharge model (Sperry 1950) or efference copy model (Von Holst and Mittelstaedt 1950; see also Chapter 9, this volume). This theory assumes that for each self-generated action, the central nervous system generates a copy of the motor commands sent to the effectors, which is used to anticipate for the consequences of the action. More recently, feedforward models (Wolpert *et al.* 1995; Wolpert 1997; Kawato 1999) have extended this

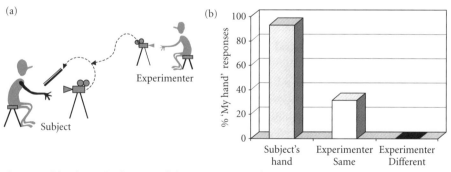

Fig. 19.1 (a) Schematic diagram of the apparatus used in the hand recognition experiment. Adapted from Daprati *et al.* (1997). *Cognition*, **65**, 71–86. (b) Percentage of 'my hand' responses given by normal subjects when seeing their own hand (Subject's Hand Condition) or the experimenter's hand performing an identical (Experimenter Same Condition) or different movement (Experimenter Different Condition).

hypothesis, suggesting that when a voluntary act is performed, a representation of the final desired state is also generated. This anticipatory model includes the reafferences that the motor act itself would produce and permits, prior to execution, a comparison with the initial internal model in order to prevent (by correction) any mismatch. Similarly, in overt motor execution, reafferent signals, such as proprioceptive and visual information, are checked against the desired state and any mismatch is processed for correction. It has been suggested that this mechanism largely operates automatically, i.e. without inducing any subjective experience in the agent. However, one can hypothesize that large discrepancies, such as those occurring when observing someone else's movement, would be beyond capabilities of the automatic level of correction, thus making the contents of the movement conscious. More precisely, it can be suggested that in self-movement recognition, when subjects see someone else's hand, a large mismatch occurs between visual reafferences and proprioceptive information. Accordingly, subjects become aware that the movement on the screen is not the one that they executed.

This interesting framework suggests that integration among several different abilities is required in order to ensure correct attribution of an action to the proper agent. As internal models are most likely involved in the self-recognition process, the ability to construct and manipulate internal images plays a major role in providing the tools necessary to produce an attribution judgment. Support for this hypothesis comes from results drawn from the application of a paradigm similar to that described by Nielsen (1963) and Daprati *et al.* (1997) to a sample of parietal patients suffering from ideomotor apraxia.

Evidence from apraxia

It has been widely demonstrated that the parietal cortex plays a leading role in monitoring internal representation of actions. For instance, the ability to mentally simulate hand gestures is selectively impaired following lesions to the parietal lobe, and this deficit has been interpreted as a failure to generate and/or monitor an internal model of one's own movement (Sirigu *et al.* 1996). More precisely, apraxia secondary to acute parietal damage, affects the patient's ability to voluntary produce skilled motor actions, disrupting symbolic and meaningless gestures (Liepmann 1920). The deficit may extend to correct tool use, and impair gesture recognition as well as pantomime (Heilman *et al.* 1982; Sirigu *et al.* 1995; De Renzi *et al.* 1966, 1982). Movement can be affected on both spatiotemporal aspects (Poizner *et al.* 1990) and the ability to generate complex hand postures correctly (Sirigu *et al.* 1995).

Using a paradigm similar to the one described above (Daprati *et al.* 1997), Sirigu *et al.* (1999) required three apraxic patients to perform and recognize the origin of two separate categories of movements: simple gestures (i.e. extend thumb, open hand wide) and complex gestures (i.e. cross middle finger on index finger, extend index and little finger). Patients executed gestures on verbal command and could monitor their execution on a screen which could display, at random, either the image of their movements or that of the movement executed by a hidden actor (Fig 19.1(a)). Their task was to decide whether the hand moving on the screen corresponded to their own motor production. The patients (two men and one woman, mean age 61.0 years, range 50–74 years) were all right-handed and had suffered from a unilateral lesion in the parietal area of the left hemisphere. All of them presented impairments in the execution of symbolic gestures on verbal command, imitation of meaningless gestures, and pantomime of object use. Apraxia was most pronounced for the contralesional limb in two patients, and bilateral in the third. None of the patients presented evidence for perceptual or motor deficit, or for cognitive impairment.

As expected, patients were impaired when executing complex gestures which were often clumsy and poorly produced. Interestingly, with respect to their ability to produce attribution judgments, apraxic patients were impaired when they had to discriminate their own movement from that of an actor executing the same gesture (Fig. 19.2). In this condition, patients attributed the actor's hand to themselves in over 70% of trials. This was not the case for a control group of four patients suffering from a right parietal lesion (two men and two women, mean age 49 years, range 42–68 years) who were still able to detect their own movement in 55% of cases when the ipsilesional hand was concerned (unpublished data). Moreover, performance of two patients suffering from a motor lesion and an inferotemporal lesion, respectively (who scored about 100% correct) confirmed that results obtained in apraxics could not be ascribed to either motor disturbance or general cerebral damage. The dramatically poor performance of left parietal patients becomes even more unusual when gesture type is considered; patients were significantly more impaired in the case of complex gestures. More precisely, when patients were required to acquire postures that required movement of multiple digits and/or complex coordination among them, apraxic patients were significantly impaired with respect to controls. Apraxics correctly identified their own ipsilesional (left) hand in approximately 33% of trials, whereas they accepted the actor's

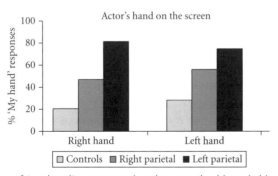

Fig. 19.2 Percentage of 'my hand' responses given by normal subjects (white bars), patients with right parietal lesion (gray bars), and left parietal lesion (black bars) when seeing an actor's hand performing a movement identical to their own. Adapted from Sirigu *et al.* (1999). *Brain*, **122**, 1867–74.

hand as their own in over 90% of cases when the contralesional and more affected hand was concerned. It is noteworthy that the performance of controls in the same trials never dropped below 75% of correct responses. The behavior of the apraxics becomes even more interesting if one considers that, owing to apraxia, patients produced clumsy gestures in about 20% of these trials. In those cases, as the movement presented on the screen (the actor's movement) was correctly executed, an involuntary mismatch was created between performed and viewed movement. The over-attribution reported by apraxics suggests that, rather than using this additional clue to attribute the movement to its proper source, these patients preferentially selected visual information, thus accepting the actor's movement as their own. Interestingly, some of the patients even commented on their improved performance.

As suggested earlier, apraxia severely affects the ability to mentally simulate hand gestures, and this deficit may be ascribed to a failure to generate and/or monitor an internal model of one's own movement (Sirigu *et al.* 2003). The poor performance of apraxic patients, particularly when complex gestures are concerned, suggest that an essential step to producing a correct ownership judgment is an efficient ability to generate and/or access internal images of the on-going motor act. One can speculate that, following left parietal lesion, the internal model of the movement to be produced becomes defective, or alternatively that it cannot be adequately updated on-line during movement execution (Sirigu *et al.* 1996, 1999, 2003). In both cases, patients lose the opportunity to keep trace of their own movement correctly and entirely rely on movement-related visual information to provide their answer, canceling signals arising from their actual kinesthetic feedback.

Role of body representation

In addition to the elementary ability to access an internal model of the motor act, attributing a movement to the correct agent probably requires that subjects have a sound internal representation of their body. Some years ago, Sirigu *et al.* (1991) proposed that body knowledge might reflect multiple representations, for naming and functional description of body parts (propositional representation), for a structural description of the body (visuospatial representation), for providing information on position, and changes in position, of body parts in relation to the external space (emergent body-reference system), and for coordinating body and external space representations (motor representation). It has been postulated that in order to recognize a motor act as the product of our own activity, a necessary piece of information is an efficient dynamic internal representation of one's body (i.e. emergent body-reference system). This prerequisite is strongly suggested by the behavior of a patient recently described by Daprati *et al.* (2000).

PA, a 50-year-old right-handed highly educated man, suffered from a vascular accident that produced a right thalamic/temporoparietal infarction. As is often the case following right parietal lesion, in the acute phase PA showed somatoparaphrenic delusions towards his left upper limb and severe neglect, although he was completely anosognosic for his symptoms. He gradually recovered the voluntary use of his left hand and although neglect for the left hemispace persisted, personal neglect and somatoparaphrenia had disappeared at the time of testing. The patient was recruited to perform the same task previously used for apraxic patients (Fig 19.1(a)) which he correctly understood. Despite a correct motor performance, PA was very inaccurate in judging on the origin of the hand on the screen. This behavior was particularly true for his left hand (Fig 19.3). In a considerable number of these trials, PA complained that no image was provided on the screen or confabulated on the nature of the image shown. In most cases, he refused ownership of the hand presented on the screen, even when it was really his own hand. The performance of PA visibly increased when he was required to recognize his ipsilesional right hand, which he correctly identified in over 80% of trials (Fig 19.3). In other words, denial of ownership as well as the confabulations and somatoparaphrenic delusions were elicited by the task specifically for the contralesional hand, reproducing a condition that the patient experienced in the acute phase of his illness. These results point towards two main issues. On the one hand, they suggest a massive disturbance in the dynamic internal body representation in patient PA, which is consistent with previous evidence suggesting that lesions of the right parietal cortex produce severe disorders of body awareness. Indeed, body schema disorders have frequently been reported in neglect patients (Guariglia and Antonucci 1992; Rode *et al.* 1992; Sellal *et al.* 1996; Coslett 1997). Similarly, sense of nonbelonging towards the contralesional limb has been described following right brain damage (Cutting 1978; Halligan *et al.* 1995). Moreover, abnormal activity in the right parietal cortex have been described in recent PET studies on schizophrenic patients suffering from delusions of alien control (Spence *et al.* 1997). In the present case, the authors suggested that, owing to an abnormal sensorimotor feedback, PA had became more dependent on direct visual control for reconstruction of his own internal body representation. Therefore, in the absence of a direct visual contiguity between arm and hand, as was the case in the device used for the experiment, when moving his hand, the patient could not reconstruct the newly acquired posture nor include it in his dynamic

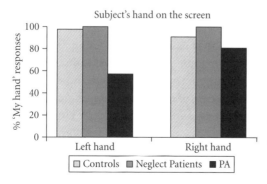

Fig. 19.3 Percentage of 'my hand' responses given by normal subjects (white bars), neglect patients (gray bars), and patient PA (black bars) when seeing their own hand. Adapted from Daprati *et al.* (2000) *Neurocase*, **6**, 477–86.

internal body representation. In other words, the emergent body-reference system, deprived of most of its sources of information, failed in updating any newly acquired hand posture. Accordingly, PA denied ownership of the presented movement.

On the other hand, PA's performance suggests that body awareness is a relevant prerequisite to the mechanisms responsible for recognition of the source of an action. This hypothesis has recently been confirmed by van den Bos and Jeannerod (2002) who directly assessed the effects of bodily cues on self-recognition. These authors adapted the paradigm previously described by Daprati *et al.* (1997) in order to be able to present the hand on the screen in both a first-person and a third-person perspective. Accordingly, in the ambiguous condition, when subjects were shown an actor's hand performing the same movement as their own, the actor's hand could be oriented as if it were part of the participant's body. Similarly, when the subject's hand was presented, this could be seen as if it belonged to the actor's body. By comparing error rates for these different orientations, the authors showed that, in the ambiguous conditions, bodily cues differentially affected the proportion of errors. In particular, errors were most frequent (35%) when the actor's hand orientation was congruent with the participant's body orientation; they diminished (24%) when the orientation of both hands was incongruent with the subject's body orientation, and were lowest (15%) when hand orientation was congruent with the participant's body orientation.

Conclusions

Although the mechanisms that enable us to attribute an action to the correct agent appear very natural, they are far from being trivial and even farther from being entirely understood. The data reviewed here provide some initial evidence about the prerequisites that are crucial to an action-recognition system as well as about their putative neural bases. First, several sources of information are required, including anticipatory information (i.e. intention to move) and reafferent information (i.e. somatosensory and proprioceptive input). This information is currently used to re-actualize an internal motor representation of the ongoing movement. As suggested by data on apraxic patients, loss of the ability to generate and/or internally manipulate motor images strongly affects own-movement recognition, probably by damaging the patient's agency knowledge. Secondly, in order for the self to become aware of its own productions, solid-body knowledge is required; in other words, the activity of the moving limb should be continuously updated within the framework of an internal dynamic body representation. Disruption of a sound body image has its counterpart in a strong decay of the sense of ownership. Localization of the lesions in the neuropsychological studies reviewed, strongly suggest the hypothesis that the parietal cortex provides a relevant role in discrimination of self-generated actions, in agreement with functional magnetic resonance imaging studies (Spence *et al.* 1997; Farrer *et al.* 2003).

References

Bisiach E, Geminiani G (1991). Anosognosia related to hemiplegia and hemianopia. In PG Prigatano, DL Schacter, (ed.) *Awareness of Deficit After Brain Injury*, pp. 17–52. Oxford: Oxford University Press.

Buccino G, Binkofski F, Fink GR, Fadiga L, Fogassi L, Gallese V, *et al.* (2001). Action observation activates premotor and parietal areas in a somatotopic manner: an fMRI study. *Eur J Neurosci*, **13**, 400–4.

Chan JL, Liu AB (1999). Anatomical correlates of alien hand syndromes. *Neuropsychiatry Neuropsychol Behav Neurol*, **12**, 149–55.

Chan JL, Ross ED (1997). Alien hand syndrome: influence of neglect on the clinical presentation of frontal and callosal variants. *Cortex*, **33**, 287–99.

Coslett HB (1997). Evidence for a disturbance of the body schema in neglect. *Brain Cogn*, **37**, 527–44.

Cutting J (1978). Study of anosognosia. *J Neurol Neurosurg Psychiatry*, **51**, 112–15.

Daprati E, Franck N, Georgieff N, Proust J, Pacherie E, Dalery J, *et al.* (1997). Looking for the agent: an investigation into consciousness of action and self-consciousness in schizophrenic patients. *Cognition*, **65**, 71–86.

Daprati E, Sirigu A, Pradat-Dihel P, Franck N, Jeannerod M (2000). Recognition of self-produced movement in a case of severe neglect. *Neurocase*, **6**, 477–86.

Decety J, Grezes J, Costes N, Perani D, Jeannerod M, Procyk E, *et al.* (1997). Brain activity during observation of actions. Influence of action content and subject's strategy. *Brain*, **120**, 1763–77.

De Renzi E, Pieczuro A, Vignolo LA (1966). Ideational apraxia: a quantitative study. *Neuropsychologia*, **6**, 41–52.

De Renzi E, Faglioni P, Sorgato P (1982). Modality-specific and supramodal mechanisms of apraxia. *Brain*, **105**, 301–12.

di Pellegrino G, Fadiga L, Fogassi L, Gallese V, Rizzolatti G (1992). Understanding motor events: a neurophysiological study. *Exp Brain Res*, **91**, 176–80.

Feinberg TE, Schindler RJ, Flanagan NG, Haber LD (1992). Two alien hand syndromes. *Neurology*, **42**, 19–24.

Fourneret P, Jeannerod M (1998). Limited conscious monitoring of motor performance in normal subjects, *Neuropsychologia*, **36**, 1133–40.

Farrer C, Franck N, Georgieff N, Frith CD, Decety J, Jeannerod M (2003). Modulating the experience of agency: a positron emission tomography study. *NeuroImage*, **18**, 324–33.

Gallese V, Fadiga L, Fogassi L, Rizzolatti G (1996). Action recognition in the premotor cortex. *Brain*, **119**, 593–609.

Gerstman J (1942). Problem of imperception of disease and impaired body territories with organic lesions. *Arch Neurol Psychiatry*, **48**, 890–913.

Geschwind DH, Iacoboni M, Mega MS, Zaidel DW, Cloughesy T, Zaidel E (1995). Alien hand syndrome: interhemispheric motor disconnection due to a lesion in the midbody of the corpus callosum. *Neurology*, **45**, 802–8.

Grèzes J, Fonlupt P, Bertenthal B, Delon-Martin C, Segebarth C, Decety J (2001). Does perception of biological motion rely on specific brain regions? *Neuroimage*, **13**, 775–85.

Guariglia C, Antonucci G (1992). Personal and extrapersonal space: a case of neglect dissociation. *Neuropsychologia*, **30**, 1001–9.

Halligan PW, Marshall JC, Wade DT (1995). Unilateral somatoparaphrenia after right hemisphere stroke: a case description. *Cortex*, **31**, 173–82.

Halsband U, Schmitt J, Weyers M, Binkofski F, Grutzner G, Freund HJ (2001). Recognition and imitation of pantomimed motor acts after unilateral parietal and premotor lesions: a perspective on apraxia. *Neuropsychologia*, **39**, 200–16.

Hècaen H, Ajuriaguerra J (1952). *Méconnaissances et Hallucinations Corporelles*. Paris: Masson.

Heilman KM, Rothi LJ, Valenstein E (1982). Two forms of ideo-motor apraxia. *Neurology*, **32**, 342–6.

Howard RJ, Brammer M, Wright I, Woodruff PW, Bullmore ET, Zeki S (1996). A direct demonstration of functional specialization within motion-related visual and auditory cortex of the human brain. *Curr Biol*, **6**, 1015–19.

Johansson G (1973). Visual perception of biological motion and a model for its analysis. *Percept Psychophys*, **14**, 201–11.

Kawato M (1999). Internal models for motor control and trajectory planning. *Curr Opin Neurobiol*, **9**, 718–27.

Kozlowski LT, Cutting JE (1977). Recognizing the sex of a walker from point-lights display. *Percept Psychophys*, **21**, 575–80.

Liepmann H (1920). Apraxie. *Ergeb Gesamt Med*, **1**, 516–43.

Mather G, Murdoch L (1994). Gender discrimination in biological motion displays based on dynamic cues. *Proc R Soc Lond B Biol Sci*, **258**, 273–9.

Mellor CS (1970). First rank symptoms of schizophrenia. *Br J Psychiatry*, **117**, 15–23.

Milner AD, Goodale MA (1995). *The Visual Brain in Action*. Oxford: Oxford University Press.

Nielsen TI (1963). Volition: a new experimental approach. *Scand J Psychol*, **4**, 225–30.

Poizner H, Mack L, Verfaellie M, Rothy LJG, Heilman KM (1990). Three-dimensional computergraphic analysis of apraxia. *Brain*, **113**, 85–101.

Puce A, Perrett D (2003). Electrophysiology and brain imaging of biological motion. *Philos Trans R Soc Lond B Biol Sci*, **358**, 435–45

Rizzolatti G, Fadiga L, Matelli M, Bettinardi V, Paulesu E, Perani D, *et al.* (1996). Localization of grasp representations in humans by PET: 1. Observation versus execution. *Exp Brain Res*, **111**, 246–52.

Rochat P, Morgan R (1995). Spatial determinants in the perception of self-produced leg movements by 3–5 month old infants. *Dev Psychol*, **31**, 626–36.

Rochat P, Striano, T. (1999). Emerging self-exploration by 2-month-old infants. *Dev Sci*, **2**, 206–18.

Rode G, Charles N, Perenin MT, Vighetto A, Trillet M, Aimard G (1992). Partial remission of hemiplegia and somatoparaphrenia through vestibular stimulation in a case of unilateral neglect. *Cortex*, **28**, 203–8.

Sellal F, Renaseau-Leclerc C, Labrecque R (1996). The man with six arms. An analysis of supranumerary phantom limbs after right hemisphere stroke. *Rev Neurol (Paris)*, **152**, 190–5.

Sirigu A, Grafman J, Bressler K, Sunderland T (1991). Multiple representations contribute to body knowledge processing. Evidence from a case of autotopagnosia. *Brain*, **114**, 629–42.

Sirigu A, Cohen L, Duhamel JR, Pillon B, Dubois B, Agid Y (1995). A selective impairment of hand posture for object utilization in apraxia. *Cortex*, **31**, 41–56.

Sirigu A, Duhamel JR, Cohen L, Pillon B, Dubois B, Agid Y (1996). The mental representation of hand movements after parietal cortex damage. *Science*, **273**, 1564–8.

Sirigu A, Daprati E, Pradat-Diehl P, Frank N, Jeannerod M (1999). Perception of self-generated movement following left parietal lesion. *Brain*, **122**, 1867–74.

Sirigu A, Daprati E, Buxbaum LG, Giraux P(2003). How the human brain represents manual gestures: effects of brain damage. In SH Johnson, (ed.) *Cognitive Neuroscience Perspectives on the Problem of Intentional Action*, pp. 167–84. Cambridge, MA: MIT Press.

Spence SA, Brooks DJ, Hirsch SR, Liddle PF, Meehan J, Grasby PM (1997). A PET study of voluntary movement in schizophrenic patients experiencing passivity phenomena (delusions of alien control). *Brain*, **120**, 1997–2011.

Sperry RW (1950). Neural basis of the spontaneous optokinetic response produced by visual inversion. *J Comp Physiol Psychol*, **43**, 482–9.

Vaina LM, Lemay M, Bienfang DC, Choi AY, Nakayaa K (1990). Intact 'biological motion' and 'structure from motion' perception in a patient with impaired motion mechanisms: a case study. *Vis Neurosci*, **5**, 353–69.

van den Bos E, Jeannerod M (2002). Sense of body and sense of action both contribute to self-recognition. *Cognition*, **85**, 177–87.

von Holst E, Mittelstaedt H (1950). Das Reaffernzprinzip. *Naturwissenschaften*, **37**, 464–76.

Weinstein EA, Kahn R (1955). *Denial of Illness: Symbolic and Physiological Aspects*. Springfield, IL: Charles C. Thomas.

Wolff W (1943). *The Expression of Personality*. New York: Harper.

Wolpert DM (1997). Computational approaches to motor control. *Trends Cogn Sci*, **1**, 209–16.

Wolpert DM, Ghahramani Z, Jordan MI (1995). An internal model for sensorimotor integration. *Science*, **269**, 1880–2.

Chapter 20

From the grasping reflex to the environmental dependency syndrome

Bernard Pillon and Bruno Dubois

Introduction

The frontal lobes have been implicated at different levels of motor organization, from the more automatic activities such as walking (Tyrrell 1994) to more elaborate activities such as planning of sequential motor programmes (Luria 1966). In this chapter, we shall consider motor organization from the point of view of environmental adherence, thus emphasizing the role of the frontal lobes in the control of behavioural responses to sensory stimuli. For that purpose, we will analyse behavioural disorders such as forced grasping (Adie and Critchley 1927), prehension and utilization behaviours (Lhermitte 1983), forced collectionism (Volle *et al.* 2002), imitation behaviour (Lhermitte *et al.* 1986), and environmental dependency (Lhermitte 1986). The anatomophysiological basis of the concept of environmental autonomy will be discussed.

Grasping behaviour

Grasping consists of one stereotyped response of flexion–adduction of the patient's hand on the fingers of the examiner, provoked by a distal ascending pressure on the palm. Using a standardized procedure in a large cohort of patients, De Renzi and Barbieri (1992) found grasping behaviour in 8% of brain-damaged patients. Grasping never occurred when the disease was confined to the retro-Rolandic regions. The locus of the lesion was either in the frontal lobe or in the deep nuclei and subcortical white matter. Grasping was found in 70% of patients who had involvement of the frontal medial areas and was always associated with damage to the cingulate gyrus; the supplementary motor cortex was less consistently encroached upon. It also occurred following damage to the lateral motor and premotor areas, but only in 26% of cases. No hemispheric asymmetry was reported. The clinical evaluation showed that the symptom usually affects both hands, even when the lesion is unilateral, and that it does not manifest itself as a forced phenomenon in most patients. It could be modified by will, although it reappeared as soon as the patient's attention was diverted. This demonstrates that two different types of grasping may be observed: 'forced' grasping reflex in which the patient cannot impede the behaviour, and 'non-forced' grasping behaviour that can be modulated by the will of the subject (Bieber 1940). These results were confirmed by a more recent study using the same standardized procedure (Etcharry-Bouyx *et al.* 2000). However, according to these authors, the grasping behaviour would depend more on an associative fasciculus connecting subcortical structures to the anterior cingulate gyrus rather than on the cingulate gyrus itself.

Prehension and utilization behaviours

Denny-Brown (1956, 1958) used the term 'magnetic apraxia' for manual activity in which the patient tries to grasp objects presented by the examiner as tactile and visual stimuli. In most instances, this activity is unilateral. It can be observed after unilateral lesions (Castaigne *et al.* 1961) or bilateral frontal and diffuse lesions of the cerebral cortex (Tissot *et al.* 1975).

Because prehension behaviour is bilateral even in the case of unilateral frontal lobe lesions, it probably depends on a more elaborate level of motor organization (Lhermitte 1983). To test for this behaviour, the examiner first places his hands within the proximity of the patient's hands and then touches both of the patient's palms to see if he will spontaneously take them (see Table 20.1 for the standard procedure). In the case of prehension behaviour, the sight or sensory perception of the examiner's hands compels the patient to grasp them. Some patients even rise, take a few steps, and sit down again, following the examiner's hands. In severe cases, the behaviour may be maintained, even though the patient is asked not to grasp the examiner's hands and is instructed to repeat this command aloud.

To search for utilization behaviour, similar visual–manual stimulations are used with familiar objects (Lhermitte 1983). The examiner places an object, such as a glass, within reach of one of the patient's hands. The patient grasps the object. The examiner

Table 20.1 Manual prehension behaviour

The examiner is seated in front of the patient and places the patient's hands, palms up, on the patient's knees. Without saying anything or looking at the patient's eyes, the examiner brings his hands close to the patient's hands and touches the palms of both of the patient's hands, to see if he will spontaneously take them. If the patient takes the hands, the examiner will try again later after explicitly stating: 'This time, do not take my hands'.

	Score
The patient does not take the examiner's hands	0
The patient hesitates and asks what he has to do	1
The patient takes the hands without hesitation	2
The patient takes the examiner's hand even after he has been explicitly told not to do so	3

then holds a bottle of water within the proximity of the other hand under the same conditions. The patient grasps it as well (see Table 20.2 for the standard procedure). The patient may remain rather puzzled and even ask the examiner what he has to do. At no time does the examiner speak, answer a question, or look at the patient's eyes; his eyes are fixed on the patient's hands or on the objects presented so that he does not influence the patient's behaviour. After a few seconds of hesitation, the patient pours the water from the bottle into the glass, which he raises to his mouth and drinks. The test can be performed with a variety of objects provided that one of them is necessary to use the other (hammer and nail; knife and apple; envelope and sheet of paper). Different stages of the behaviour may be observed: the stage when the patient hesitates and does not use the grasped objects; the stage when, after a moment of hesitation, he uses them; the stage when, without hesitation, he uses them at once. Although utilization behaviour indicates an exaggerated dependence on the physical environment for behavioural cues, it is not a compulsive behaviour but may be partially modulated by the patient's will. For instance, 'if the patient is a smoker, he draws a cigarette from the pack and lights it with a lighter. If he is a non-smoker, he uses neither the pack of cigarettes nor the lighter, but if the examiner brings a cigarette to his own lips, the patient kindly lights it with the lighter that he holds in one hand' (Lhermitte 1983). The normal balance between the patient's will and environmental cues is disturbed. It must be emphasized that the behaviour is exhibited without any internal motivation. Patients eat or drink even when they are saying that they are not hungry or thirsty. If asked by the examiner why they took and used the objects, patients usually answer that the examiner gave them to him and that they thought that they had to use them. Furthermore, in severe cases, even after a patient is repeatedly instructed not to take and use the objects, he will present the utilization behaviour again after a few seconds of delay, during which his attention has been diverted.

Table 20.2 Grasping of objects and utilization behaviour

The examiner is seated in front of the patient. Without saying anything or looking at the patient's eyes, the examiner brings objects (a candle and a semi-opened box of matches, a glass and a bottle of water, a pen and a sheet of paper) close to the patient's hands and touches the palms of both hands with the objects to see if the patient will spontaneously take them and use them. If the patient takes and uses the objects, the examiner will try again later after explicitly stating: 'This time do not take and use the objects'.

	Score
The patient does not take the objects	0
The patient hesitates and asks what he has to do	1
The patient takes and uses the objects without hesitation	2
The patient takes and uses the objects even after he has been explicitly told not to do so	3

Utilization behaviour is bilateral and observed in unilateral frontal lobe lesions whichever hemisphere is impaired (Lhermitte *et al.* 1986). Its frequency is inconsistently reported for patients with frontal lobe lesions. Lhermitte *et al.* (1986) found utilization behaviour in 50% of patients, whereas De Renzi *et al.* (1996) reported it in only 4%. Differences in the sampling of patients and in the methodology used could explain this discrepancy. In the first study all frontal focal lesions were in an acute stage and limited to the frontal lobes, whereas in the second study the lesions were classified as frontal even in case of multiple lesions as long as one of them was located in the frontal lobe. In Lhermitte's procedure, the test begins with the solicitation of manual grasping behaviour, followed by that of prehension behaviour in response to the objects, and only then by that of utilization behaviour, pausing each time the patient is puzzled, without speaking or looking at his eyes. Therefore an induced form of the behaviour is sought. In contrast, De Renzi's procedure searches for an incidental form of the behaviour. In this procedure, the objects are simply placed in front of the patient while the examiner is looking at him directly. Both groups agree that utilization behaviour is never observed in the case of retro-Rolandic lesions. Some patients with temporoparietal lesions may spontaneously use objects, but only to show that they recognize them even though they are not able to name them. In contrast, patients with subcortical lesions may present true prehension and utilization behaviours (Lhermitte *et al.* 1986; Eslinger *et al.* 1991; Hashimoto *et al.* 1995), particularly those with subcorticofrontal degenerative diseases such as progressive supranuclear palsy (Pillon *et al.* 1996; Dubois *et al.* 2000).

Forced collectionism

One consequence of environmental adherence in daily life may be forced collectionism, which is an irrepressible need to seize surrounding objects and store them (hoarding behaviour). This pathological collecting behaviour, although voluntarily irrepressible, may be selective. After the rupture of an aneurysm of the anterior communicating artery, a man who had been working for 10 years as a test driver in a car factory began to borrow cars, not selling them but accumulating them in the vicinity of his house (Cohen *et al.* 1999). Despite a dozen stays in prison and although he was well aware that this was illegal, borrowing cars gave him a kind of pleasurable relief. Following bilateral damage of the orbito- and polar prefrontal cortex, another patient specifically collected household electrical appliances, such as television sets, telephones, refrigerators, washing machines, and videocassette recorders (Volle *et al.* 2002). Unlike the first patient, his behaviour was planned. Twice a month, he roamed the town and brought appliances back home. He stocked them first in the living room (Fig. 20.1), then in his daughter's bedroom, in the corridors, and even in the bathroom, then in three cellars, and finally, as there was no other empty place, in ventilation shafts. Therefore the patient behaved as a true collector, selecting specific items and planning his actions. A lack of involvement of the dorsolateral prefrontal areas may

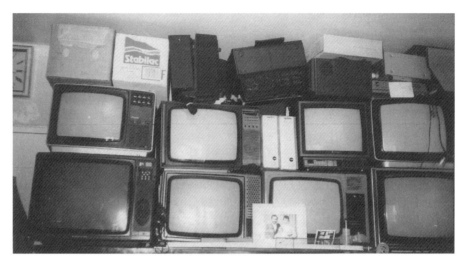

Fig. 20.1 Picture of the living room of a patient with forced collectionism showing the stocking of television sets. Reproduced from Volle *et al.* (2002) *Neurology*, *58*, 488–90.

explain the persistence of planning ability. However, inertia prevented him from attaining the ultimate goal of his behaviour, which was to repair each electrical apparatus. Indifference towards his social environment prevented him from taking into account the discomfort of his family caused by the progressive invasion of electrical appliances throughout the apartment.

Imitation behaviour

Dependence on physical environment is directly implicated in utilization behaviour or forced collectionism, whereas imitation behaviour is related to dependence on the social environment. Patients imitate the gestures and behaviour of the examiner (see Table 20.3 for the standard procedure). Lhermitte *et al.* (1986) reported that patients spontaneously imitated body gestures performed by the examiner, such as scratching the head, resting the chin on the hand, or tapping the leg with the hand in various rhythms. Patients may refuse to imitate some gestures that they consider as ridiculous but agree to imitate others, copy some gestures although verbalizing their disagreement ('it's not fair'), or sometimes even imitate unacceptable gestures such as urinating against a wall in front of many people. Questioned as to the reason for their imitative behaviour, patients replied that because the examiner had made the gesture, they felt that they had to imitate him. This behaviour may be maintained even when the patient is explicitly asked not to imitate the examiner. The fact that patients may be critical of the inadequacy of some gestures and in some cases able to refuse to make them shows that imitation behaviour is different from echopraxia, which is an automatic imitation of other people's gestures (Dromard 1905).

Table 20.3 Imitation behaviour

The examiner is seated in front of the patient. Without saying anything or looking at the patient's eyes, the examiner scratches his head, touches his chin, crosses his arms, and taps the legs with the hands to see if the patient will spontaneously imitate him. If the patient imitates, the examiner will try again later after explicitly stating: 'This time do not imitate what I am doing'.

	Score
The patient does not imitate	0
The patient hesitates and asks what he has to do	1
The patient imitates without hesitation	2
The patient imitates even after he has been explicitly told not to do so	3

Also encountered in unilateral frontal lobe lesions, imitation behaviour is more frequent than utilization behaviour and is the first stage of the environmental dependency syndrome. The incidence of imitation behaviour was 96% for Lhermitte *et al.* (1986), but only 39% for De Renzi *et al.* (1996). As previously emphasized, the sampling of patients was not the same in the two studies. The precise location of the lesion in the frontal lobe is also variable: involvement of the inferior half of the anterior part of one or both frontal lobes (Lhermitte *et al.* 1986), of the dorsolateral prefrontal region (Sarazin *et al.* 1998), or of the upper medial and lateral prefrontal cortex (Degos *et al.* 1993; Fukui *et al.* 1993; De Renzi *et al.* 1996).

A recent event-related functional magnetic resonance imaging study showed the involvement of both frontomedial and frontolateral brain regions in the inhibition of imitative response tendencies in normal subjects (Brass *et al.* 2001). The experiment used a simple response task in which subjects were instructed to execute predefined finger movements in response to an observed congruent or incongruent finger movement. A comparison of brain activation in incongruent and congruent trials revealed strong activation in the dorsolateral prefrontal cortex (middle frontal gyrus)and activation in the right frontopolar cortex. The dorsolateral activation reflects a conflict between two intentions, one internally generated and one externally induced. The frontopolar activation is related to the determination of the agent of the action if the observed action conflicts with the action to be executed. According to the authors, these findings might explain why patients with frontal lobe lesions are not able to defend their action against external response tendencies and do not perceive these tendencies as inappropriate.

Environmental dependency syndrome

Although they can be investigated using standardized conditions in the laboratory, utilization and imitation behaviours may also be spontaneously observed in daily life, as shown by forced collectionism, suggesting that they may be components of a larger environmental dependency syndrome (Lhermitte 1986). Some patients with frontal lobe lesions demonstrate bingeing behaviour as long as they see food in front of them (utilization behaviour), but stop eating without any problems if the food is taken away. A patient described by Shallice *et al.* (1989), if left to him-self, 'would, for instance, continually make tea if he saw tea bags'. Other patients lose their way because they follow people who are going out of the subway, out of the bus, or out of the elevator (imitation behaviour).

According to Lhermitte's (1986) hypothesis, the environmental dependency syndrome will be more frequent when subjects are in environments that are more complex than the examiner–patient situation. On visiting Professor Lhermitte's apartment as if it was a museum, with an appropriate behaviour for any normal museum visitor, a patient saw that a painting was missing from the wall, hammered in a nail, and hung the painting, as if it was in his own house. Later, going into the bedroom, where the bedspread had been taken off and the top sheet had been turned back, he immediately began to get undressed and prepared to go to sleep as if he was in his own bedroom and really wanted to sleep. Therefore the patient did not maintain the contextual information (a visit to a museum) and could not inhibit the influence of environmental cues. These two types of deficits, 'context neglect' and 'environmental adherence', best differentiated patients with frontal lobe lesions from control subjects in script execution, such as 'shopping for groceries and preparing a chocolate cake', an ecological approach to planning dysfunction (Chevignard *et al.* 2000). This observation confirms that the environmental dependency syndrome is not limited to the laboratory, but has clear consequences in daily life. The weakening control of the supervisory attentional system can predispose to environmental capture (Shallice *et al.* 1989).

The concept of human autonomy and its relationship with the prefrontal cortex

Grasping, prehension and utilization behaviours, forced collectionism, imitation behaviour, and environmental dependency all stem from an excessive control of behaviour by external stimuli at the expense of behavioural autonomy. Therefore it seems that all these behaviours may result from a more fundamental dysfunction, the expression of which would vary according to the exact location of the lesion, the type of stimulations proposed by the environment or the examiner, and the previous personality of the patient. What might this fundamental disorder be?

First, we must remember that normal controls never exhibit these behaviours. Questioned about the examiner's stimulations, they generally express perplexity: 'You were probably looking for something, but I do not know what'. In contrast, patients with acute or progressive frontal lobe lesions spontaneously exhibit these behaviours. When asked why, they answer that they grasped the objects or imitated the gestures of the examiner because they thought that the examiner wanted them to do so, although they agree that the examiner gave no explicit order. In severe cases, the patients continue to grasp, utilize, or imitate even when the examiner asked them explicitly not to do so or even while repeating loudly: 'I do not take your hands . . . I do not imitate your gestures . . . '. These data indicate that the patient with frontal lobe lesion can no longer inhibit the spontaneous activation of behavioural patterns in response to sensory stimuli: the sensory stimulation of the palm provokes a motor behaviour of prehension; the sight of the examiner's gestures provoke a motor behaviour of imitation. In other words, the environment drives the behaviour, even if the patient does not want it to. Therefore we can conclude that one of the functions of the frontal lobes is to suspend the cycle stimulus–response to develop a goal-directed and adaptable schema of response, taking into account both the subject's internal state (information from limbic regions processed in the paralimbic orbitofrontal cortex) and environmental contingencies (information from associative sensory areas processed in the dorsolateral prefrontal cortex). The fact that these pathological behaviours result from frontal lobe lesions suggest, in normal conditions, a dynamic interaction between frontal and parietal activation of behavioural sets depending on contextual parameters. In patients with prefrontal lesions, automatic behaviours triggered by parietal cortex stimulation would be released, whereas more specific behaviours taking into account internal (motivation) and external (representation of the situation) contexts would not be elaborated. Evidence in humans suggests that the posterior parietal cortex plays a role in creating multiple space representations to seize or handle objects under visual control (Jeannerod 1994). Conversely, the dorsolateral prefrontal cortex is involved in the behavioural relevance of events and external stimuli, whereas the paralimbic component of the frontal lobe (anterior cingulate gyrus and caudal orbitofrontal regions) should be of crucial importance for channeling drive and emotion to appropriate targets of the environment (Mesulam 1986). Thus the environmental dependency syndrome results from an approach–avoidance disequilibrium due to impaired reciprocal inhibition between prefrontal cortex and posterior parietal network. Prefrontal lesions promote not only an excessive approach to the environment, but also an excessive distance from the intrapsychic processes necessary for foresight and abstraction (Slachevsky et al. 2001). Such an interpretation may explain why environmental adherence may be observed following lesions of the upper medial and lateral prefrontal cortex (deficit of drive and of goal-directed behaviour), the dorsolateral prefrontal region (neglect of the physical context and environmental capture), or the inferior half of the anterior part of one or both frontal lobes (neglect of the social environment and indifference to the consequences of action).

Acknowledgements

We thank Nikki Horne for revising the English. These studies were supported by INSERM and Assistance Publique.

References

Adie WJ, Critchley M (1927). Forced grasping and groping. *Brain*, **50**, 142–70.

Bieber I (1940). Grasping 'forced' and 'non-forced'. *J Nerv Ment Dis*, **91**, 417–21.

Brass M, Zysset S, von Cramon DY (2001). The inhibition of imitative response tendencies. *Neuroimage*, **14**, 1416–23.

Castaigne P, Cambier J, Laplane D, Baumann N (1961). Thrombose distale de la cérébrale antérieure droite avec anomalies du comportement moteur du membre supérieur gauche (apraxie d'aimantation). *Rev Neurol (Paris)*, **104**, 436–8.

Chevignard M, Pillon B, Pradat-Diehl P, Taillefer C, Rousseau S, Le Bras C, *et al.* (2000). An ecological approach to planning dysfunction: script execution. *Cortex*, **36**, 649–69.

Cohen L, Angladette L, Benoit N, Pierrot-Deseilligny C (1999). A man who borrowed cars. *Lancet*, **353**, 34.

Degos JD, Da Fonseca N, Gray F, Cesaro P (1993). Severe frontal syndrome associated with infarcts of the left anterior cingulate gyrus and the head of the right caudate nucleus. A clinico-pathological case. *Brain*, **116**, 1541–8.

Denny-Brown D (1956). Positive and negative aspects of cerebral cortical functions. *N C Med J*, **17**, 295–303.

Denny-Brown D (1958). Nature of apraxia. *J Nerv Ment Dis*, **126**, 9–32.

De Renzi E, Barbieri C (1992). The incidence of the grasp reflex following hemispheric lesion and its relation to frontal damage. *Brain*, **115**, 293–313.

De Renzi E, Cavalleri F, Facchini S (1996). Imitation and utilization behaviour. *J Neurol Neurosurg Psychiatry*, **61**, 396–400.

Dromard G (1905). Etude psychologique et clinique sur l'echopraxie. *J Psychol (Paris)*, **2**, 385–403.

Dubois B, Slachevsky A, Litvan I, Pillon B (2000). The FAB: a frontal assessment battery at bedside. *Neurology*, **55**, 1621–6.

Eslinger PJ, Warner GC, Grattan LM, Easton JD (1991). 'Frontal lobe' utilization behavior associated with paramedian thalamic infarction. *Neurology*, **41**, 450–2.

Etcharry-Bouyx F, Le Gall D, Allain P, Mercier P, Aubin G, Emile J (2000). Incidence of grasping and its relationship to cerebral lesions. *Rev Neurol (Paris)*, **156**, 977–83.

Fukui T, Hasegawa Y, Suguta K, Tsukagoshi H (1993). Utilization behaviour and concomitant motor neglect by bilateral frontal lobe damage. *Eur Neurol*, **33**, 325–330.

Hashimoto R, Yoshida M, Tonaka Y (1995). Utilization behaviour after right thalamic infarction. *Eur Neurol*, **35**, 58–62.

Jeannerod M (1994). The representing brain. Neural correlates of motor intention and imagery. *Behav Brain Sci*, **17**, 187–245.

Lhermitte F (1983). 'Utilization behaviour' and its relation to lesions of the frontal lobes. *Brain*, **106**, 237–55.

Lhermitte F (1986). Human autonomy and the frontal lobes. Part II: Patient behavior in complex and social situations: the 'environmental dependency syndrome'. *Ann Neurol*, **19**, 335–43.

Lhermitte F, Pillon B, Serdaru M (1986). Human autonomy and the frontal lobes. Part I: Imitation and utilization behaviors: a neuropsychological study of 75 patients. *Ann Neurol*, **19**, 326–34.

Luria AR (1966). *Higher Cortical Functions in Man*. New York: Basic Books.

Mesulam MM (1986). Frontal cortex and behavior. *Ann Neurol*, **19**, 320–5.

Pillon B, Dubois B, Agid Y (1996). Testing cognition may contribute to the diagnosis of movement disorders. *Neurology*, **46**, 329–33.

Sarazin M, Pillon B, Giannakopoulos P, Rancurel G, Samson Y, Dubois B (1998). Clinico-metabolic dissociation of cognitive functions and social behaviors in frontal-lobe lesions. *Neurology*, **51**, 142–8.

Shallice T, Burgess PW, Schon F, Baxter DM (1989). The origins of utilization behaviour. *Brain*, **112**, 1587–98.

Slachevsky A, Pillon B, Fourneret P, Pradat-Diehl P, Jeannerod M, Dubois B (2001). Preserved adjustment but impaired awareness in a sensory-motor conflict following prefrontal lesions. *J Cogn Neurosci*, **13**, 332–40.

Tissot R, Constandinidis J, Richard J (1975). *La Maladie de Pick*. Paris: Masson.

Tyrrell PJ (1994). Apraxia of gait or higher level gait disorders: review and description of two cases of progressive gait disturbance due to frontal lobe degeneration. *J R Soc Med*, **87**, 454–6.

Volle E, Beato R, Levy R, Dubois B (2002). Forced collectionism after orbitofrontal damage. *Neurology*, **58**, 488–90.

Chapter 21

Tics and stereotypies

Joseph Jankovic

Tics

Tics are brief and intermittent movements (motor tics) or sounds (vocal or phonic tics). Simple motor tics involve only one group of muscles, causing a brief jerk-like movement. They are usually abrupt in onset and rapid ('clonic tics'), but they may be slower, causing a briefly sustained abnormal posture ('dystonic tics') (Jankovic and Stone 1991)or an isometric contraction ('tonic tics') (Jankovic 1992). Clonic and dystonic tics may occasionally occur in patients with primary dystonia, possibly more frequently than in the general population (Stone and Jankovic 1991; Németh *et al.* 1999).

In order to understand better the categorization of tics and how they fit in the general schema of movement disorders, it might be helpful to provide a simple classification of movements (Jankovic 1992). All movements can be classified into one of four categories.

1 Voluntary: (a) intentional (planned, self-initiated, internally generated); (b) externally triggered in response to some external stimulus (e.g. turning the head toward a loud noise or withdrawing the hand from a hot plate).

2 Semivoluntary (unvoluntary): (a) induced by inner sensory stimulus (e.g. need to 'stretch' a body part); (b) induced by an unwanted feeling or compulsion (e.g. compulsive touching or smelling).

3 Involuntary: (a) non-suppressible (e.g. reflexes, seizures, myoclonus); (b) suppressible (tics, tremor, dystonia, chorea, stereotypy).

4 Automatic (learned motor behaviors performed without conscious effort, such as the act of walking or speaking).

Most tics can be categorized as either semivoluntary (unvoluntary) or involuntary–suppressible, although some tics are truly involuntary–non-suppressible.

In most patients motor tics are preceded by premonitory sensations that are either localized to the body region affected by the tics or are more generalized (Kwak and Jankovic 2002a). Examples of local premonitory sensations include a 'burning feeling' in the eye before an eye blink, 'tension or crick in the neck' relieved by stretching of the neck or jerking of the head, 'feeling of tightness or constriction' relieved by arm or leg extension, 'nasal stuffiness' before a sniff, 'dry or sore throat' before throat clearing or grunting, and 'itching' before a rotatory movement of the scapula. In addition to these local sensations, premonitory phenomenon may be a non-localizable, less specific, and poorly described feeling, such as an urge, anxiety, anger, or other psychic sensation.

In contrast with other hyperkinetic movement disorders, tics are usually intermittent and may be repetitive and stereotypic (Table 21.1). Tics are also typically exacerbated by dopaminergic drugs and central nervous system (CNS) stimulants, including methylphenidate and cocaine (Cardoso and Jankovic 1993). Finally, motor and phonic tics may persist during all stages of sleep (Rothenberger *et al.* 2001; Hanna and Jankovic 2003). Tics, although rarely disabling, can be quite troublesome for Tourette syndrome (TS) patients because they cause embarrassment, interfere with social interactions, and at times can be quite painful or uncomfortable. Rarely, they can cause secondary neurological deficits, such as compressive cervical myelopathy in patients with violent head and neck tics (Krauss and Jankovic 1996).

There are many other causes of tics in addition to TS (Jankovic 2001a)(Table 21.2). Since there is no diagnostic test for TS, the diagnosis is based on clinical history and examination. To aid in the diagnosis of TS, in 1993 the Tourette Syndrome Classification Study Group (TSCSG) formulated criteria for the diagnosis of definite, probable, and possible TS. Several instruments, some based on ratings of videotapes, have been developed to measure and quantitate tics, but they all have some limitations (Goetz and Kampoliti 2001; Goetz *et al.* 2001).

In addition to motor and phonic tics, patients with TS often exhibit a variety of behavioral symptoms, particularly attention deficit–hyperactivity disorder (ADHD) and obsessive–compulsive disorder (OCD), but the discussion of these and other comorbidities as well as the genetics and other pathogenetic mechanisms of TS is beyond the scope of this chapter. The reader is referred to other publications on this topic (Robertson 2000; Jankovic 2001b; Leckman 2002; Stein 2002).

Neurophysiology

Despite the observation that some tics may be, at least in part, voluntary, physiologic studies suggest that tics are not mediated through normal motor pathways utilized for willed movements. Using back-averaging techniques, Obeso *et al.* (1982) observed normal *Bereitschaftspotential* (premovement potential) in six subjects who voluntarily simulated tic-like movements, but no such premovement potential was noted in association with an actual tic. The common absence of premotor potentials in simple motor tics suggests that tics are truly involuntary or that they occur in response to some external cue. However, Karp *et al.* (1996) documented premotor negativity in two of five patients with simple motor tics. Although the investigators could not correlate the presence of *Bereitschaftspotential* with the premonitory sensation, the physiology of the premovement phenomenon requires further study.

Transcranial magnetic stimulation (TMS) studies have demonstrated a shortened cortical silent period and defective intracortical inhibition (determined in a conditioning

Table 21.1 Differential diagnosis of tics

	Differential diagnosis
Classification	
Simple motor tics	
Clonic	Myoclonus
	Chorea
	Seizures
Dystonic	Dystonia
	Athetosis
Tonic	Muscle spasms and cramps
Complex motor tics	Mannerisms
	Stereotypies
	Restless leg
	Seizures
Phenomenology	
Abrupt	Myoclonus
	Chorea
	Hyperekplexia
	Paroxysmal dyskinesia
	Seizures
Sensory phenomenon (urge–relief)	Akathisia-stereotypy
	Restless legs syndrome
	Dystonia
Perceived as voluntary	Akathisia
Suppressibility but less than tics	All hyperkinesias
Decrease with distraction	Akathisia
	Psychogenic movements
Increase with stress	Most hyperkinesias
Increase with relaxation(after a period of stress)	Parkinsonian tremor
Multifocal, migrate	Chorea
	Myoclonus
Fluctuate spontaneously	Paroxysmal dyskinesias
	Seizures
Present during sleep	Myoclonus (segmental)
	Periodic movements
	Painful legs/moving toes
	Other hyperkinesias
	Seizures

test paired-stimulus paradigm) in patients with TS (Ziemann *et al.* 1997) and OCD (Greenberg *et al.* 1998), thus providing a possible explanation for intrusive phenomena. Subsequent studies utilizing the same technique have demonstrated that patients with tic-related OCD have more abnormal motor cortex excitability than OCD patients without tics (Greenberg *et al.* 2000). TMS studies have also demonstrated that TS

Table 21.2 Causes of tics

Primary

Sporadic

    Transient motor or phonic tics ($<$ 1 year)
    Chronic motor or phonic tics ($>$ 1 year)
    Adult-onset (recurrent) tics
    Tourette syndrome
    Primary dystonia

Inherited

    Tourette syndrome
    Huntington disease
    Primary dystonia
    Neuroacanthocytosis
    Hallervorden–Spatz
    Tuberous sclerosis
    Wilson disease
    Duchenne muscular dystrophy

Secondary

Infections	Encephalitis, Creutzfeldt–Jakob disease, neurosyphilis, Sydenham chorea
Drugs	Amphetamines, methylphenidate, pemoline, levodopa, cocaine, carbamazepine, phenytoin, phenobarbital, lamotrigine, antipsychotics, and other dopamine receptor blocking drugs (tardive tics, tardive tourettism)
Toxins	Carbon monoxide
Developmental	Static encephalopathy, mental retardation syndromes, chromosomal abnormalities, autistic spectrum disorders (Asperger syndrome)
Chromosomal disorders	Down syndrome, Kleinfelter syndrome, XYY karyotype, fragile X, triple X, and 9p, mosaicism, partial trisomy 16, 9p monosomy, citrullinemia, Beckwith–Wiedemann syndrome
Other	Hhead trauma, stroke, neurocutaneous syndromes, schizophrenia, neurodegenerative diseases

Related manifestations and disorders

Stereotypies/habits/mannerisms
Self-injurious behaviors
Motor restlessness
Akathisia
Compulsions
Excessive startle
Jumping Frenchman

children have a shorter cortical silent period, but their intracortical inhibition was no different from that of controls, although intracortical inhibition is reduced in children with ADHD (Moll *et al.* 2001; Castellanos and Tannock 2002).

Sleep studies have provided additional evidence that some tics are truly involuntary. Polysomnographic studies in 34 TS patients recorded motor tics in various stages of sleep in 23 and phonic tics in four (Jankovic and Rohaidy 1987). Additional sleep studies have suggested that some patients with TS have alterations of arousal, decreased percentage (up to 30%) of stage 3–4 (slow-wave) sleep, decreased percentage of rapid eye movement sleep, paroxysmal events in stage 4 sleep with sudden intense arousal, disorientation and agitation, restless legs syndrome, periodic leg movement of sleep (Chokroverty and Jankovic 1999), and other sleep-related disorders including sleep apnea, enuresis, sleep-walking and sleep-talking, nightmares, myoclonus, bruxism, and other disturbances (Rothenberger *et al.* 2001; Hanna and Jankovic 2003).

Neuroimaging

Although standard anatomical neuroimaging studies in TS are unremarkable, several interesting findings obtained using special volumetric, metabolic, blood flow, ligand, and functional imaging techniques have been reported that have strong implications for the pathophysiology of TS. Careful volumetric magnetic resonance imaging (MRI) studies have suggested that the normal asymmetry of the basal ganglia is lost in TS (Peterson 2001). In a volumetric MRI study, Frederickson *et al.* (2002) found evidence of smaller gray matter volumes in the left frontal lobes of patients with TS, supporting the previously reported findings of loss of normal left–right asymmetry. Quantitative MRI studies have found subtle, but possibly important, reductions in the volume of caudate nuclei in patients with TS. Functional MRI studies show decreased neuronal activity during periods of suppression in the ventral globus pallidus, putamen, and thalamus, and increased activity in the caudate, frontal cortex, and other cortical areas normally involved in the inhibition of unwanted impulses (prefrontal, parietal, temporal, and cingulated cortical areas) (Peterson 2001). In another study of three patients with TS, functional MRI showed marked reduction or absence of activity in secondary motor areas while the patient attempted to maintain a stable grip force load (Serrien *et al.* 2002).

Positron emission tomography (PET) scanning has shown variable rates of glucose utilization in basal ganglia compared with controls. In one study, [^{18}F]fluorodeoxyglucose (FDG) PET has shown evidence of increased metabolic activity in the lateral premotor and supplementary motor association cortices and in the midbrain (pattern 1), and decreased metabolic activity in the caudate and thalamic areas (limbic basal ganglia–thalamocortical projection system) (pattern 2) (Eidelberg *et al.* 1997). Using event-related [^{15}O]H$_2$O PET combined with time-synchronized audio- and videotaping in six patients with TS, Stern *et al.* (2000) found increased activity in the sensorimotor, language, executive, paralimbic, and frontal-subcortical areas that were temporarily related to the motor and phonic tics and the irresistible urge that precedes these behaviors.

Treatment of tics

Various controlled and open-label trials have found that the dopamine receptor blocking drugs (neuroleptics) are clearly the most effective of the pharmacologic agents used for tic suppression. Haloperidol and pimozide are the only neuroleptics actually approved by the US Food and Drug Administration (FDA) for the treatment of TS, but we prefer fluphenazine (Prolixin) as the first-line anti-tic pharmacotherapy since it appears to have a lower incidence of sedation and other side effects. If fluphenazine fails to control tics adequately, we substitute risperidone or pimozide. Ziprasidone (Geodon), the most recently studied atypical neuroleptic, which is a potent blocker of both D2 and D3 as well as 5-HT_{2A}, 5-HT_{2C}, 5-HT_{1A}, 5-HT_{1D}, and α_1 receptors, was found to decrease tic severity by 35% compared with a 7% change in the placebo group (Sallee *et al.* 2000). Tetrabenazine, a monoamine depleting drug, is a powerful anti-tic drug, but it is not yet readily available in the United States (Jankovic and Beach 1997; Hunter *et al.* 2002). This drug has been found very effective in the treatment of TS and has the advantage over the conventional neuroleptics in that it does not cause tardive dyskinesias. Other drugs used in the treatment of tics include sulpiride, tiapride, metoclopramide, and piquindone (Jimenez-Jimenez and Garcia-Ruiz 2001). Motor tics can be successfully treated with botulinum toxin injections in the affected muscles, and this treatment is emerging as the treatment of choice in patients with focal or segmental tics. Such focal chemodenervation ameliorates not only the involuntary movements but also the premonitory sensory component (Kwak *et al.* 2000; Marras *et al.* 2001).

Surgical treatment of TS is controversial, and the overall experience of stereotactic surgery in the treatment of tics has been rather disappointing. Experience with 17 patients, median age 23 years (range 11–40 years), treated between 1970 and 1998 was reviewed by Babel *et al.* (2001). Unilateral zona incerta and VL/LM lesioning was used, and occasional second surgery on the contralateral side was performed. The authors concluded that the procedures 'sufficiently' reduced both motor and phonic tics. Transient complications were reported in 68% of patients but only one patient suffered permanent complication. Although stereotactic surgery has not been found generally useful in the treatment of tics, a preliminary report of a 42-year-old man with severe motor and phonic tics controlled by high-frequency deep brain stimulation of the thalamus is quite encouraging (Vandewalle *et al.* 1999).

Stereotypies

Stereotypies can be defined as involuntary or unvoluntary, coordinated, patterned, repetitive, rhythmic, and seemingly purposeless movements or utterances (Jankovic 1994). Typical stereotypies include body rocking, head weaving and banging, hand waving, repetitive and sequential finger movements, lipsmacking, chewing movements, grunting, moaning, and humming. Mannerisms, which are gestures peculiar or unique to the individual, may at times seem stereotypical. An example of a stereotypical mannerism is the ritualistic movements performed by a baseball pitcher before he actually pitches the ball. There is no clear anatomical–clinical correlation for stereotypies, although it is believed that both cortical and subcortical structures are involved. Stereotypies have been observed in patients with bilateral lesions of the medial frontoparietal cortices (Sato *et al.* 2001).

There is often an overlap between stereotypies and self-injurious behavior, such as biting, scratching, and hitting (Jankovic *et al.* 1998; Schroeder *et al.* 2001).

The observation that self-biting behavior induced by dopaminergic drugs in 6-hydroxydopamine rats and monkeys with a unilateral lesion in the ventral medial tegmentum can be blocked by the selective D_1 antagonist SCH 23390 suggests that self-injurious behavior is mediated primarily by the D_1 receptors (Schroeder *et al.* 2001). This is in contrast with stereotypies which are presumably mediated by the D_2 receptors. Stereotypical behavior is common in animals in lower species up to and including the primates, and are particularly common in farm and zoo animals housed in restraining environments with low stimulation (Novak 2003). Therefore stereotypy has been viewed as either a self-generating sensory stimulus or a motor expression of underlying tension and anxiety. The repetitive and ritualistic behavior displayed by some animals has been used as an experimental model of OCD (Pitman 1989). Indeed, studies of animal and human stereotypies have provided important insights into relationships between motor function and behavior. It is well known that stereotypies often accompany a variety of behavioral disorders such as anxiety, OCD, TS, schizophrenia, autism, mental retardation, akathisia, and restless legs syndrome. Thus stereotypy is a motor-behavioral disorder found most frequently in patients who are in the borderland between neurology and psychiatry.

Stereotypical movements can be classified as either simple (foot tapping, body rocking) or complex (complicated rituals, sitting down and arising from a chair). Stereotypies can also be described according to distribution of the predominant site of involvement (orolingual, hand, leg, truncal). The term stereotypy should be used to describe a phenomenological, not an etiological, category of hyperkinetic movement disorder. However, recognition of stereotypy as a distinct movement disorder can logically lead from a phenomenological to an etiological diagnosis (Table 21.3).

Physiological stereotypies

Certain stereotypies, such as tapping of the feet, adduction–abduction, and crossing–uncrossing or other repetitive movements of the legs may be part of a repertoire of movements seen in otherwise normal individuals. In infants and children there seems to be a progression of normal stereotypies (Castellanos *et al.* 1996). For example, thumb and hand sucking in infancy is later replaced by body rocking, head banging, and head rolling resembling 'bobble-head doll syndrome' (Hottinger-Blanc *et al.* 2002). Some girls exhibit stereotypic crossing and extending of legs which actually represents a masturbatory behavior (Mink and Neil 1995).

Mental retardation and autism

It is beyond the scope of this chapter to review the current ideas about the clinical features and pathogenesis of mental retardation, but the reader is referred to some recent reviews of this topic (Nokelainen and Flint 2002). In a recent study of 100 individuals with severe or profound intellectual disability randomly selected and followed for 26 years, Thompson and Reid (2002) found that stereotypies, emotional

Table 21.3 Stereotypies

Physiological
Pathological
Mental retardation
Autism (Kanner infantile autism, Asperger syndrome)
Rett syndrome
Neuroacanthocytosis
Schizophrenia
Catatonia
Obsessive–compulsive disorder
Tourette syndrome
Tardive and other dyskinesias
Akathisia
Restless legs syndrome
Epileptic automatism
Psychogenic

abnormalities, eye avoidance, and other behavioral symptoms persist. Although there seems to be an inverse correlation between stereotypies and IQ, stereotypical behavior may be seen even in the mildly retarded.

Autism is a type of pervasive developmental disorder (PDD), sometimes referred to as autistic spectrum disorder, with onset during infancy or childhood, which is characterized by impairment in reciprocal social and interpersonal interactions, impairment in verbal and non-verbal communication, markedly restricted repertoire of activities and interests, and stereotyped movements (Bodfish *et al.* 2000, 2001). Recent epidemiological studies have estimated that the prevalence of autistic disorders and related PDD ranges between 0.3% and 0.6% (Yeargin-Allsopp *et al.* 2003).

There are many causes of autism, including the fragile X syndrome and a variety of eponymically classified types such as Kanner, Heller, Asperger, Down, and Rett syndromes (Ringman and Jankovic 2000). Characterized by social isolation in combination with odd and eccentric behavior, Asperger syndrome shares many features with infantile autism. We studied eight patients with Asperger syndrome and an additional four with other forms of PDD referred to our Movement Disorders Clinic for evaluation of tics (Ringman and Jankovic 2000). All patients exhibited stereotypic movements; in addition seven had tics and six of these met inclusion diagnostic criteria for TS.

One hypothesis about the pathogenesis of autism suggests that in autistic children the normal high brain serotonin synthesis capacity is somehow disrupted during early development (Chugani and Chugani 2000), which may explain the beneficial effects of selective serotonin uptake inhibitors (SSRIs) in some patients with autism (DeLong 1999). Drugs that block postsynaptic dopamine and serotonin receptors, such as risperidone, have been found to be effective in the treatment of tantrums, aggression, and self-injurious behaviors in patients with autistic disorders (Research Units on Pediatric Psychopharmacology Autism Network 2002). Other agents used in the treatment of autistic disorders include CNS stimulants, anticonvulsants, naltrexone, lithium, anxiolytics, and other treatments, but well-controlled double-blind studies are lacking (Owley 2002).

Rett syndrome is an autistic disorder occurring only in girls and manifested clinically by stereotypic movements and other movement disorders (Fitzgerald *et al.* 1990a; Percy 2002). In contrast with infantile autism and mental retardation, Rett patients tend to have normal development until 6–18 months of age; this is then followed by gradual regression of both motor and language skills. Usually between the ages of 9 months and 3 years there is a gradual social withdrawal and psychomotor regression, with loss of acquired communication skills. Acquired finger and hand skills are gradually replaced by stereotypical hand movements, including hand clapping, wringing, clenching, washing, patting, rubbing, picking, and mouthing. Additionally, Rett girls often exhibit body-rocking movements and shifting of weight from one leg to the other. Although most girls with Rett syndrome are able to walk, the gait is usually broad-based and apraxic, and is usually associated with retropulsion and losss of balance. Other motor disturbances include respiratory dysregulation with episodic hyperventilation and breath-holding, bruxism, ocular deviations, dystonia, myoclonus, athetosis, tremor, jerky truncal and gait ataxia, and parkinsonian findings (Fitzgerald *et al.* 1990b).

The major advance in understanding the biology of Rett syndrome has come with the discovery of a gene that is responsible for most cases of the Rett phenotype. Since the initial discovery of the gene in 1999, loss-of-function mutations of the X-linked gene encoding methyl-CpG binding protein 2 (MECP2) have been found to be responsible for more than 80% of Rett cases (Amir *et al* 1999; Akbarian 2003). A broad range of associations with MECP2 mutations involving not only girls and women, but also males, have been described, including a variety of autistic spectrum disorders such as Angelman syndrome, learning disability, mental retardation, and fatal encephalopathy (Percy 2002). We excluded mutations in the *MECP2* gene in our population of patients with TS (Rosa *et al.* 2003).

Neuroacanthocytosis

Neuroacanthocytosis is another disorder manifested by stereotypical and self-injurious behavior (e.g. lip and tongue biting). Symptoms usually begin in the third and fourth decades of life with lip and tongue biting, followed by orolingual ('eating') dystonia, motor and phonic tics, generalized chorea, distal and body stereotypies, parkinsonism, and seizures. Other features include cognitive and personality changes, dysphagia, dysarthria, amyotrophy, areflexia, evidence of axonal neuropathy, and elevated serum creatine kinase without evidence of myopathy. Ueno *et al.* (2001) carried out a linkage-free analysis in the region of chromosome 9q21 in the Japanese population and identified a 260bp deletion in the EST (expressed sequence tags) region K1AA0986 in exon 60, 61 which was homozygous in patients with neuroacanthocytosis and heterozygous in their parents. Further sequencing has identified a polyadenylation site with a protein with 3096 amino acid residues which has been named 'chorein' by the authors. In another study by Rampoldi *et al.* (2001) in European patients a novel gene encoding a 3174 amino acid protein on chromosome 9q21 with 73 exons was identified.

Schizophrenia and catatonia

Various stereotypies were described in schizophrenic patients long before neuroleptics were first introduced for the treatment of psychotic disorders. Although conventionally classified as a subtype of schizophrenia, catatonia is commonly associated with affective disorders and only about 5–10% of catatonics satisfy diagnostic criteria for schizophrenia. Thus catatonia should be viewed as a syndrome caused by a variety of medical, neurological, and psychiatric conditions, with abnormal motor behavior ranging from extreme hyperactivity to akinesia with mutism and stupor. Stereotypies, such as shifting position, maintaining unusual postures, tapping or touching objects, repetitively moving mouth and jaw, performing rituals and mannerisms, repeating phrases and sentences (verbigeration), and repeating the examiner's questions (echolalia) are among the most characteristic motor disorders in catatonia. When catatonia is associated with stereotypies, the diagnosis of mania should be considered and a favorable response to treatment should be expected. When agitated, stereotypic movements such as rocking, hand waving, or complex repeated movements of the face, trunk, or limbs may be seen. Vocalizations include chanting, humming, moaning, and repetitious utterances. A gene locus on chromosome 15q15 has been identified in periodic catatonia (Stober *et al.* 2002). Catatonia has been successfully treated with benzodiazepines, neuroleptics, and anticonvulsants, but electroconvulsive therapy may be required in severe cases. (Ihara *et al.* 2002; see also Chapter 23, this volume).

Obsessive–compulsive disorder

Another psychiatric disorder frequently accompanied be stereotypic movements is OCD. Foot tapping, crossing and uncrossing the legs, tapping fingers on a chair arm, and similar stereotypic behaviors may be associated with obsessive–compulsive symptoms (Niehaus *et al.* 2000). Once considered a rare psychiatric disorder, recent epidemiological studies indicate that the lifetime prevalence of OCD is approximately 2.5% (Snider and Swedo 2000). Compulsions may be difficult to differentiate from stereotypies. In contrast with stereotypies, compulsions are usually preceded by or associated with feelings of inner tension or anxiety and a need to perform the same act repeatedly in the same manner. Examples of compulsions are ritualistic hand washing, repetitively touching the same place, straightening up, and arranging and checking doors, locks, and appliances (see also Chapter 23). Reports of focal striatal lesions giving rise to severe OCD and the frequent association of OCD with basal ganglia disorders such as TS, Parkinson's disease, and Sydenham's chorea provide additional support for the link between abnormal behavior, such as OCD, and extrapyramidal dysfunction (Church *et al.* 2002; Kwak and Jankovic 2002b; Rosario-Campos *et al.* 2003).

Tardive dyskinesia

Repetitive and patterned movements, phenomenologically identical with stereotypy, are characteristically seen in patients with tardive dyskinesia (Jankovic 1995). Because all types of movement disorders, including parkinsonism, chorea, dystonia, tics, myoclonus, and stereotypy, can result from the use of dopamine receptor blocking drugs (neuroleptics), the nosology of the movement disorders in tardive dyskinesia is sometimes problematic and controversial. The most typical form of tardive dyskinesia, the orofacial–lingual–masticatory movement, is one of the best examples of a stereotypic movement disorder. In an analysis of 125 patients referred to the Baylor College of Medicine Movement Disorders Clinic with a drug-induced movement disorder, 79 (63%) had stereotypical movements, originally classified as chorea (Miller and Jankovic 1990; Stacy *et al.* 1993). Other hyperkinetic movement disorders included tardive dystonia, seen in 30 patients (24%) and tardive akathisia in nine patients (7%), and two patients had isolated tardive tremor. More complex stereotypies, such as hair and face rubbing, picking at clothes, crossing and uncrossing of legs, adduction–abduction and up-and-down pumping of legs, arising and sitting down, marching in place, pacing, and shifting weight, often associated with feelings of restlessness, are typically seen in patients with tardive akathisia. Akathisia may be associated with the use of dopamine-receptor blocking or depleting drugs, Parkinson's disease, various forms of mental retardation, and autism, and may be confused with the restless legs syndrome (Chokroverty and Jankovic 1999; Ondo *et al.* 2002). Both disorders exhibit stereotypical movements and motor restlessness, but patients with restless legs seem to complain more of paresthesias, particularly a creeping or crawling sensation in the legs associated with an irresistible urge to keep the limbs in motion. The restless legs syndrome is often worse at night, causing insomnia, and it may be associated with periodic movements of sleep. A variety of stereotypies, such as body rocking and marching in place, occur in these patients even when they are awake.

References

Akbarian S (2003). The neurobiology of Rett syndrome. *Neuroscientist*, **9**, 57–63.

Amir RE, Van den Veyver IB, Wan M, Tran CQ, Francke U, Zoghbi MY, (1999). Rett syndrome is caused by mutations in X-linked MECP2, encoding methyl-CpG-binding protein 2. *Nat Genet*, **23**, 185–8.

Babel TB, Warnke PC, Ostertag CB (2001). Immediate and long term outcome after infrathalamic and thalamic lesioning for intractable Tourette's syndrome. *J Neurol Neurosurg Psychiatry*, **70**, 666–71.

Bodfish JW, Symons FJ, Parker DE, Lewis MH (2000). Varieties of repetitive behavior in autism: comparisons to mental retardation. *J Autism Dev Disord*, **30**, 237–43.

Bodfish JW, Parker DE, Lewis MH, Sprague RL, Newell KM (2001). Stereotypy and motor control: differences in the postural stability dynamics of persons with stereotyped and dyskinetic movement disorders. *Am J Ment Retard*, **106**, 123–34.

Cardoso FEC, Jankovic J (1993). Cocaine related movement disorders. *Mov Disord*, **8**, 175–8.

Castellanos FX, Tannock R (2002). Neuroscience of attention-deficit/hyperactivity disorder: the search for endophenotypes. *Nat Rev Neurosci*, **3**, 617–28.

Castellanos FX, Ritchie GF, Marsh WL, Rapoport JL (1996). DSM-IV stereotypic movement disorder: persistence of stereotypies of infancy in intellectually normal adolescents and adults. *J Clin Psychiatry*, **57**, 116–22.

Chokroverty S, Jankovic J (1999). Restless legs syndrome. A disease in search of identity. *Neurology*, **52**, 907–10.

Chugani DC, Chugani HT (2000). PET: mapping of serotonin synthesis. *Adv Neurol*, **83**, 165–71.

Church AJ, Cardoso F, Dale RC, Lees AJ, Thompson EJ, Giovannoni G (2002). Anti-basal ganglia antibodies in acute and persistent Sydenham's chorea. *Neurology*, **59**, 227–31.

Eidelberg D, Moeller JR, Antonini A, Kazumata K, Dhawan V, Budman C, *et al.* (1997). The metabolic anatomy of Tourette's syndrome. *Neurology*, **48**, 927–34.

Fitzgerald PM, Jankovic J, Glaze DG, Schultz R, Percy AK (1990a). Extrapyramidal involvement in Rett's syndrome. *Neurology*, **40**, 293–5.

Fitzgerald PM, Jankovic J, Percy AK (1990b). Rett syndrome and associated movement disorders. *Mov Disord*, **5**, 195–203.

Frederickson KA, Cutting LE, Kates WR, Mostofsky SH, Singer HS, Cooper KL, *et al.* (2002). Disproportionate increases of white matter in right frontal lobe in Tourette syndrome. *Neurology*, **58**, 85–9.

Goetz CG, Kampoliti K (2001). Rating scales and quantitative asssement of tics. *Adv Neurol*, **85**, 31–42.

Goetz CG, Leurgans S, Chumara TA (2001). Home alone: methods to maximize tic expression for objective videotape assessments in Gilles de la Tourette syndrome. *Mov Disord*, **16**, 693–7.

Greenberg BD, Ziemann U, Cora-Locatelli G, Harmon A, Murphy DL, Keel JC, *et al.* (2000). Altered cortical excitability in obsessive–compulsive disorder. *Neurology*, **54**, 142–7.

Hanna PA, Jankovic J (2003). Sleep and tic disorders. In S Chokroverty, A Hening Walters, (ed.) *Sleep and Movement Disorders*, pp. 464–71. Woburn, MA: Butterworth Heinemann.

Hottinger-Blanc PM, Ziegler AL, Deonna T (2002). A special type of head stereotypies in children with developmental (cerebellar) disorder: description of 8 cases and literature review. *Eur J Paediatr Neurol*, **6**, 143–52

Hunter CB, Wang A, Vuong KD, Jankovic J (2002). Tetrabenazine in the treatment of Tourette syndrome. *Mov Disord*, **17** (Suppl 5), S341.

Ihara M, Kohara N, Urano F, Ichinose H, Takao S, Nishida T, *et al.* (2002) Neuroleptic malignant syndrome with prolonged catatonia in a dopa-responsive dystonia patient. *Neurology*, **59**, 1102–4.

Jankovic J (1992). Diagnosis and classification of tics and Tourette's syndrome. *Adv Neurol*, **58**, 7–14.

Jankovic J (1994). Stereotypies. In CD Marsden, S Fahn, (ed.) *Movement Disorders*, 3rd edn, pp. 503–17. London: Butterworth Heinemann.

Jankovic J (1995). Tardive syndromes and other drug-induced movement disorders. *Clin Neuropharmacol*, **18**, 197–214.

Jankovic J (2001a). Differential diagnosis and etiology of tics. *Adv Neurol*, **85**, 15–29.

Jankovic J (2001b). Tourette's syndrome. *N Engl J Med*, **345**, 1184–92.

Jankovic J, Beach J (1997). Long-term effects of tetrabenazine in hyperkinetic movement disorders. *Neurology*, **48**, 358–62.

Jankovic J, Rohaidy H (1987). Motor, behavioral and pharmacologic findings in Tourette's syndrome. *Can J Neurol Sci*, **14**, 541–6.

Jankovic J, Stone L (1991). Dystonic tics in patients with Tourette's syndrome. *Mov Disord*, **6**, 248–52.

Jankovic J, Sekula SL, Milas D (1998). Dermatological manifestations of Tourette's syndrome and obsessive–compulsive disorder. *Arch Dermatol*, **134**, 113–14.

Jimenez-Jimenez FJ, Garcia-Ruiz PJ (2001). Pharmacological options for the treatment of Tourette's disorder. *Drugs*, **61**, 2207–20.

Karp BI, Porter S, Toro C, Hallett M (1996). Simple motor tics may be preceded by a premotor potential. *J Neurol Neurosug Psychiatry*, **61**, 103–6.

Krauss JK, Jankovic J. (1996) Severe motor tics causing cervical myelopathy in Tourette's syndrome. *Mov Disord*, **11**, 563–6.

Kwak CH, Jankovic J (2002a). Premonitory sensations in tics. *Mov Disord*, **17** (Suppl 5), S339–440.

Kwak C, Jankovic J (2002b). Tourettism and dystonia after subcortical stroke. *Mov Disord*, **17**, 821–5.

Kwak CH, Hanna PA, Jankovic J (2000). Botulinum toxin in the treatment of tics. *Arch Neurol*, **57**, 1190–3.

Leckman JF (2002). Tourette's syndrome. *Lancet*, **360**, 1577–86.

Marras C, Andrews D, Sime EA Lang AE (2001). Botulinum toxin for simple motor tics: a randomized, double-blind, controlled clinical trial. *Neurology*, **56**, 605–10.

Miller LG, Jankovic J (1990). Neurological approach to drug-induced movement disorders: a study of 125 patients. *South Med J*, **83**, 525–35.

Mink JW, Neil JJ (1995). Masturbation mimicking paroxysmal dystonia or dyskinesia in a young girl. *Mov Disord*, **10**, 518–20.

Moll GH, Heinrich H, Troo GE, Wirth S, Bock N, Rothenberger A, (2001) Children with comorbid attention-deficit–hyperactivity disorder and tic disorder: Evidence for additive inhibitory deficits with the motor systems. *Ann Neurol*, **49**, 393–6.

Németh AH, Mills KR, Elston JS, Williams A, Dunne E, Hyman NM, (1999). Do the same genes predispose to Gilles de la Tourette syndrome and dystonia? Report of a new family and review of the literature. *Mov Disord*, **14**, 826–31.

Niehaus DJ, Emsley RA, Brink P, Stein DJ (2000). Stereotypies: prevalence and association with compulsive and impulsive symptoms in college students. *Psychopathology*, **33**, 31–5.

Nokelainen P, Flint J (2002). Genetic effects on human cognition: lessons from the study of mental retardation syndrome. *J Neurol Neurosurg Psychiatry*, **72**, 287–96.

Novak MA (2003). Self-injurious behavior in rhesus monkeys: new insights into its etiology, physiology, and treatment. *Am J Primatol*, **59**, 3–19.

Obeso JA, Rothwell JC, Marsden CD (1982). The neurophysiology of Tourette syndrome. *Adv Neurol*, **35**, 105–14.

Ondo WG, Vuong KD, Jankovic J (2002). Exploring the relationship between Parkinson disease and restless legs syndrome. *Arch Neurol*, **59**, 421–4.

Owley T (2002). The pharmacological treatment of autistic spectrum disorders. *CNS Spectr*, **7**, 663–9.

Percy AK (2002). Rett syndrome: current status and new vistas. *Neurol Clin N Am*, **20**, 1125–41.

Peterson BS (2001). Neuroimaging studies of Tourette syndrome: a decade of progress. *Adv Neurol*, **85**, 179–96.

Rampoldi L, Dobson-Stone C, Rubio JP, Danek A, Chalmers RM, Wood NW, *et al.* (2001) A conserved sorting-associated protein is mutant in chorea-acanthocytosis. *Nat Genet*, **28**, 119–20.

Research Units on Pediatric Psychopharmacology Autism Network (2002). Risperidone in children with autism and serious behavioral problems. *N Engl J Med*, **347**, 314–21.

Ringman JM, Jankovic J (2000). Occurrence of tics in Asperger's syndrome and autistic disorder. *J Child Neurol*, **15**, 394–400.

Robertson MM (2000). Tourette syndrome, associated conditions and the complexities of treatment. *Brain*, **123**, 425–62.

Rosa AL, Jankovic J, Ashizawa T (2003). Screening for mutations in the MECP2 (Rett syndrome) gene in Gilles de la Tourette syndrome. *Arch Neurol*, **60**, 502–3.

Rosario-Campos MC, Leckman JF, Mercadante MT, Mercadante MT, Shavitt RG, Prado HS, *et al.* (2003). Adults with early-onset obsessive–compulsive disorder. *Am J Psychiatry*, **158**, 1899–1903.

Rothenberger A, Kostanecka T, Kinkelbur J, Cohrs S, Woerner W, Hajak G, (2001). Sleep and Tourette syndrome. *Adv Neurol*, **85**, 245–60.

Sallee FR, Kurlan R, Goetz CG, Singer H, Scahill L, Law G, *et al.* (2000). Ziprasidone treatment of children and adolescents with Tourette's syndrome: a pilot study. *J Am Acad Child Adolesc Psychiatry*, **39**, 292–9.

Sato S, Hashimoto T, Nakamura A, Ikeda S (2001). Stereotyped stepping associated with lesions in the bilateral medial frontoparietal cortices. *Neurology*, **51**, 711–13.

Schroeder SR, Oster-Granite ML, Berkson G, Bodfish JW, Breese GR, Cataldo MF, *et al.* (2001). Self-injurious behavior: gene–brain–behavior relationships. *Ment Retard Dev Disabil Res Rev*, **7**, 3–12.

Serrien DJ, Nirkko AC, Loher TJ, Lovblad KO, Burgunder JM, Weisendanger M, (2002). Movement control of manipulative taks in patients with Gilles de la Tourette syndrome. *Brain*, **125**, 290–300.

Snider LA, Swedo SE (2000). Pediatric obsessive–compulsive disorder. *JAMA*, **284**, 3104–6.

Stacy M, Cardoso F, and Jankovic J (1993). Tardive stereotypy and other movement disorders in tardive dyskinesia. *Neurology*, **43**, 937–41.

Stein DJ (2002). Obsessive–compulsive disorder. *Lancet*, **360**, 397–405.

Stern E, Silbersweig DA, Chee K-Y, Holmes A, Robertson MM, Trimble M, *et al.* (2000). A functional neuroanatomy of tics in Tourette syndrome. *Arch Gen Psychiatry*, **57**, 741–8.

Stober G, Seelow D, Ruschendorf F, Ekici A, Beckmann H, Reis A (2002). Periodic catatonia: confirmation of linkage to chromosome 15 and further evidence for genetic heterogeneity. *Hum Genet*, **111**, 323–30.

Stone L, Jankovic J (1991). The coexistence of tics and dystonia. *Arch Neurol*, **48**, 862–5.

Thompson CL, Reid A (2002). Behavioural symptoms among people with severe and profound intellectual disabilities: a 26-year follow-up study. *Br J Psychiatry*, **181**, 67–71.

Ueno S, Maruki Y, Nakamura M, Tomemori Y, Kamae K, Tanabe H, *et al.* (2001). The gene encoding a newly discovered protein, chorein, is mutated in chorea-acanthocytosis. *Nat Genet*, **28**, 121–2.

Vandewalle V, Van Der Linden C, Groenegen HJ, Caemaert J (1999). Stereotactic treatment of Gilles de la Tourette syndrome by high frequency stimulation of thalamus. *Lancet*, **353**, 724.

Yeargin-Allsopp M, Rice C, Karapurkar T, Doernberg N, Boyle C, Murphy C (2003). Prevalence of autism in a US metropolitan area. *JAMA*, **289**, 49–55.

Chapter 22

Psychogenic motor disorders

Tamara Pringsheim, Robert Chen, and
Anthony Lang

Background

Psychogenic motor disorders make up a small percentage of referrals seen by neurologists and movement disorder specialists, but present a real diagnostic and treatment challenge. Psychogenic motor disorders are disorders for which no known organic syndrome can explain the symptoms experienced by the patient, and which appear clinically to have significant psychiatric or psychological contributing or causative factors. Psychogenic motor disorders encompass a variety of disorders of motor function, such as paralysis, gait disturbance, dystonia, tremor, myoclonus, and parkinsonism. The recognition that motor disorders can be caused by psychiatric disturbances dates back to the nineteenth century; however, an understanding of the neurophysiological basis of these disorders is only now evolving. In contrast with previous reviews of psychogenic motor disorders (Marjama *et al.* 1995; Williams *et al.* 1995; Gálvez-Jiménez and Lang 1997), it is not our intention to summarize all the clinical aspects of these conditions. Instead, we will limit our discussion to the epidemiology, diagnosis, psychopathology, neuroimaging, electrophysiological testing, prognosis, and treatment of psychogenic motor disorders.

Epidemiology

Medically unexplained symptoms are common in neurological and medical practice. Between 20% and 33% of patients seen by neurologists have symptoms that are poorly explained by identifiable organic disease, despite appropriate and exhaustive investigation (Ron 1994; Carson *et al.* 2000). When looking specifically at the type of presenting symptom, motor disorders make up a smaller subset of psychogenic disorders seen. A study conducted at the University of Munich Neurological Clinic, covering all patients admitted between 1985 and 1987, revealed that 405 of 4470 (9%) consecutive neurological in-patients presenting with typical neurological symptoms were found to have a psychogenic rather than a neurological dysfunction as the primary cause of admission. Pain of psychogenic origin was the most frequent symptom, accounting for 2.1% of patients admitted, with psychogenic motor disorders, such as paresis, gait disturbance, and tremor, making up the second-largest group of psychogenic disorders at 1.8% (Lempert *et al.* 1990).

Table 22.1 Combined data on psychogenic movement disorders seen at Columbia-Presbyterian Medical Center, Toronto Western Hospital, Cleveland Clinic Florida, and Albany Clinic[a]

Disorder	Columbia(%)	Toronto(%)	Cleveland (%)	Albany(%)	Total(%)
Dystonia	82 (53)	34 (20)	14 (25)	6 (21)	136 (33)
Tremor	21 (13)	52 (30)	18 (32)	15 (54)	106 (26)
Myoclonus	11 (7)	34 (20)	4 (7)	4 (14)	53 (13)
parkinsonism	3 (2)	14 (8)	0	2 (7)	19 (5)
Gait disorder	14 (9)	7 (4)	1 (2)	0	22 (5)
Blepharospasm/ facial movements	4 (2)	0	4 (7)	1 (4)	9 (2)
Tics	2 (1.3)	0	2 (3.6)	0	4 (1)
Stiff person	1 (0.6)	0	0	0	1 (0.2)
Other	14 (9)	30 (18)	13 (23)	1 (4)	58 (14)
Total	152	171	56	28	407

[a] Columbia Presbyterian Medical Center (Williams *et al.* 1995) listed all types of PMD; Toronto Western Hospital (A. E. Lang, personal observations) listed only predominant PMD; Cleveland Clinic Florida (N. Gálvez Jiménez, personal observations) listed only the predominant PMD 1998–2002; Albany Clinic (Factor *et al.* 1995).

Combined data on psychogenic movement disorders seen at Columbia Presbyterian Medical Centre (Williams *et al.* 1995), the Toronto Western Hospital (unpublished data), Cleveland Clinic Florida (unpublished data), and Albany Medical College (Factor *et al.* 1995) are presented in Table 22.1. Dystonia makes up the largest subgroup, accounting for 33% of psychogenic movement disorders seen at these clinics. This is mostly due to the large number of psychogenic dystonia cases seen at Columbia Presbyterian Medical Centre, which during the time these data were collected served as a Dystonia Medical Research Foundation centre of excellence and therefore probably had a strong referral bias. Tremor was the most frequent psychogenic movement disorder seen in the other three centres, and accounts for 26% of patients in the combined series. Myoclonus was seen in 13% of patients, with the remainder of patients suffering from psychogenic parkinsonism, disorders of gait, blepharospasm or other facial movements, tics, stiff person syndrome, or other movement disorders.

Diagnosis

The diagnosis of psychogenic motor disorders is made on phenomenological grounds by an experienced neurologist, although neuroimaging and electrophysiological testing are developing a complementary role, which will be discussed further. Skilful observation and examination of the patient by an experienced clinician will reveal inconsistencies suggestive of a psychogenic origin of the patient's symptoms. Tables 22.2 and 22.3 provide lists of important historical and clinical clues to the diagnosis of a psychogenic

Table 22.2 Historical clues suggesting a psychogenic movement disorder

Abrupt onset

Minor trauma (litigation or compensation are frequently present)

Static course

Purely paroxysmal (exclude other paroxysmal dyskinesias) or paroxysmal worsening

Spontaneous remissions/cures

Multiple somatizations/undiagnosed conditions

Other psychiatric illness

Employed in allied health professions (infrequent)

Clear secondary gain (often not apparent)

Adapted from Gálvez-Jiménez and Lang 1997.

Table 22.3 General examination clues suggesting a psychogenic movement disorder

Movement incongruous with organic movement disorders

   Mixed (often bizarre) movement disorders

   Paroxysmal attacks (including pseudoseizures)

   Precipitated paroxysms (often suggestible/startle)

Movement inconsistent

   Over time variability

   Selective disabilities (exclude task-specific movement disorders)

   Distraction reduces or resolves (caution: tics, akathisia)

   Attention increases

   Complex repetitive motor tasks entrain (especially in the case of tremor)

Response to placebo with suggestion

   Worsening/improving (may trigger or relieve movement with unusual or non-physiological interventions such as trigger points on the body, tuning fork)

Refuses videotaping (infrequent; might suggest malingering)

False weakness

False sensory complaints

Deliberate slowness of movements

Adapted from Gálvez-Jiménez and Lang 1997.

movement disorder. Importantly, none of these are definitive and many of these features may also be seen in organic movement disorders.

Fahn and Williams developed a classification system for psychogenic movement disorders (Williams *et al*. 1995). Originally developed for the diagnosis of psychogenic dystonia, it is now used in the classification of psychogenic movement disorders of all

Table 22.4 Fahn–Williams classification system for psychogenic movement disorders

Documented features[a]	Clinically established features[a]	Probable features (classified into three categories of patient)	Possible features
Movement disorder is persistently relieved by psychotherapy, psychological suggestion, or administration of placebos	Movement disorder is inconsistent over time or is incongruent with the clinical presentation of an organic movement disorder	Movements are inconsistent or incongruent with an organic disorder, but no other features exist to support a psychogenic origin	Obvious psychiatric disturbance present in a patient with abnormal movements that are consistent and congruent with an organic movement disorder
Absence of symptoms when unaware of being observed	Supportive evidence is provided by presence of other physical signs that are definitely psychogenic (e.g. false weakness, non-anatomical sensory loss), multiple somatizations, or an obvious psychiatric disturbance	Abnormal movements are consistent and congruent with an organic disorder, but physical signs are present that are definitely psychogenic[b] Movements are consistent and congruent with an organic movement disorder, but multiple somatizations are present[b]	Supportive evidence includes inappropriate affect, discrepancy between the movement disorder and the reported disability, and the presence of secondary gain

[a] Documented and clinically established groups could be combined as clinically definite.

[b] These features are not uncommon in patients with organic movement disorders. We would not support using these criteria to give a diagnosis of a 'probable psychogenic movement disorder'.

Source: Williams *et al.* 1995.

types. This classification system allows the neurologist to categorize the degree of diagnostic certainty as documented, clinically established, probable, or possible. Table 22.4 outlines the features of each diagnostic category. The authors of the classification system suggest combining the categories of documented and clinically established to form a category of clinically definite, as both categories imply a definite diagnosis. Tables 22.5–22.9 list features which help to distinguish psychogenic from organic disorders for four of the more common types of psychogenic movement disorders seen (dystonia, tremor, myoclonus, and parkinsonism) and for psychogenic paralysis.

Psychopathology

The *Diagnostic and Statistical Manual of Mental Disorders* (American Psychiatric Association 1994) considers patients with a psychogenic motor disorder to have a diagnosis of conversion disorder, motor subtype (see criteria for conversion disorder in

Table 22.5 Features suggestive of psychogenic dystonia

Onset with resting dystonia
Adult onset leg involvement common
Often fixed spasm
Rapid progression and spread to maximum disability early in the course
Dystonic movements inconsistent over time
No geste antagoniste
Selective disabilities or abilities inconsistent with fixed spasms
Painful (often with pronounced tenderness to touch and exaggeration with passive movement)
No improvement after sleep
Attempted voluntary movement to command in the opposite direction of the dystonic posturing may activate antagonists with little apparent action in agonist muscles
Paroxysmal dystonia (isolated or mixed with persistent dystonia) and/or other paroxysmal movements
Other psychogenic movement disorders
Other non-organic neurological features
Precipitant common
Remissions: spontaneous or with non-physiological treatments
No family history

Source: Lang 1995.

Table 22.6 Clinical features of psychogenic tremor

Abrupt onset
Rapid evolution
Spontaneous remission, with later relapses in another site
Distractibility
Variability of tremor in terms of frequency, direction, amplitude, or involved site
Entrainment: change of the original tremor frequency to match the frequency of a requested repetitive task in another limb
Same amplitude of tremor at rest, with postural maintenance and action
Suggestibility/increase with attention
Coactivation of antagonist muscles of the tremulous joint
Amplitude increases with weighting of involved limb

Source: Kim *et al.* 1999; Deuschl *et al.* 1998.

Table 22.7 Features of psychogenic myoclonus

Inconsistent character of the movement amplitude, frequency, and distribution with typical organic myoclonus
Associated psychogenic symptomatology
Marked reduction of the myoclonus with distraction
Exacerbation or relief with placebo and suggestion
Spontaneous periods of remission
Acute onset and sudden resolution
Evidence of underlying psychopathology

Source: Monday and Jankovic 1993.

Table 22.8 Features suggesting psychogenic parkinsonism

Abrupt onset
Static course, maximum disability early
Dominant side most affected
Tremor of equal amplitude at rest, with postural maintenance (no delay in onset of tremor after taking up new position) and action; reduces with distraction/concentration, and increases with attention
'Voluntary' resistance to passive movement; may decrease with distraction/'activation' maneuvers in contrast with the usual increase with true rigidity
Absence of cogwheeling
'Bradykinesia': no true fatiguing, marked slowness
Atypical gait, arm held stiffly at side, antalgic if pain associated
Extreme or bizarre responses to minimal displacement on testing of postural stability
False weakness, non-anatomic sensory loss
Presence of psychiatric features
Pending litigation or compensation

Source: Lang *et al.* 1995.

Table 22.10). Conversion disorder falls into the broader category of somatoform disorders. Primary or secondary gain, or both, underlie symptom production. Primary gain refers to the conversion of psychological distress into physical symptoms. Secondary gain refers to external factors that may be influenced by the symptom development. Clinical studies have confirmed that the primary psychiatric diagnosis in 75%–100% of patients with psychogenic motor disorders is conversion, with the remaining patients suffering from somatization disorder, factitious disorder, and malingering (Williams *et al.* 1995; Feinstein *et al.* 2001).

Table 22.9 Features suggestive of psychogenic paralysis

Inconsistent findings
No adjustment between physical and functional findings
Absence of muscle atrophy, contractures, bed sores
Jerky sharp movements
Slow-motion movements
Normal muscle tone
Normal reflexes
Flexor plantar responses
Simultaneous contraction of agonist and antagonist muscles
Absence of autonomic dysfunction; full sphincter control

Source: Heruti *et al.* 2002.

Table 22.10 DSM IV Criteria for Conversion Disorder

A	One or more symptoms or deficits affecting voluntary motor or sensory function that suggest a neurological or other general medical condition
B	Psychological factors are judged to be associated with the symptom or deficit because initiation or exacerbation of the symptom or deficit is preceded by conflicts or other stressors
C	The symptom or deficit is not intentionally produced or feigned (as in Factitious Disorder or Malingering)
D	The symptom or deficit cannot, after appropriate investigation, be fully explained by a general medical condition, or by the direct effects of a substance, or as a culturally sanctioned behaviour or experience
E	The symptom or deficit causes clinically significant distress or impairment in social, occupational, or other important areas of functioning or warrants medical evaluation
F	The symptom or deficit is not limited to pain or sexual dysfunction, does not occur exclusively during the course of Somatization Disorder, and is not better accounted for by another medical disorder

Source: American Psychiatric Association 1994.

Comorbid axis 1 (clinical disorders) diagnoses are common in patients with psychogenic motor disorders, occurring in 33–100% of newly diagnosed patients (Williams *et al.* 1995; Binzer and Eisemann 1998; Crimlisk *et al.* 1998; Feinstein *et al.* 2001). Affective disorders are most common (31–80%), followed by anxiety disorders (15–50%). Personality disorders are also frequent in this patient population, occurring in 42–67% of patients studied and including histrionic, dependent, borderline, and mixed personality disorders. Only one of 30 patients in one study (Binzer and Eisemann 1998) was identified to have experienced childhood sexual abuse, in contrast with earlier studies which have suggested a relationship between conversion disorders and sexual abuse (Chu *et al.* 1990). The importance of sexual abuse to conversion may depend on the clinical manifestation of the conversion symptoms, as there appears to be a clear association between sexual abuse in childhood and pseudoseizures (Krumholz and Niedermeyer 1983). Proper diagnosis and treatment of these varied underlying psychiatric problems may aid the resolution of psychogenic motor disorders.

Role of neuroimaging and electrodiagnostic testing

Neuroimaging

In recent years, neuroimaging with positron emission tomography (PET) and single-photon emision computed tomography (SPECT), and electrophysiological testing with electroencephalography (EEG), electromyography (EMG), and evoked potentials, have had an increasing role in the evaluation and diagnosis of psychogenic motor disorders, and, perhaps more importantly, in advancing our understanding of the neurophysiology behind these disorders.

The first report on brain metabolism in a patient with psychogenic left-sided paralysis and paraesthesia appeared in 1995 (Tiihonen *et al.* 1995). SPECT studies were performed during electrical stimulation of the left median nerve before and after resolution of the patient's symptoms. Prior to recovery, there was increased perfusion in the right frontal lobe ($+$ 7.2% compared with the left side) and hypoperfusion in the right parietal region ($-$ 7.5% compared with the left side). After recovery, the perfusion in the right parietal region was 6% greater than in the left side, as expected during stimulation of the left median nerve. The authors concluded that psychogenic paraesthesia may be associated with the simultaneous activation of frontal inhibitory areas and inhibition of the somatosensory cortex. They suggest that distressing psychological events may alter the neurophysiology of the human brain in a specific way, and trigger symptoms of motor or sensory dysfunction through activation or inhibition of critical areas of the brain.

Further understanding of neurophysiology of psychogenic paralysis comes from the work of Marshall *et al.* (1997), who measured changes in regional cerebral blood flow (rCBF) in a woman with long-standing left-sided paralysis due to motor conversion disorder. Brain activity was recorded when the patient (a) prepared to move and (b) tried to move her paralyzed (left) leg, and when she (a) prepared to move and (b) did move her good (right) leg. The areas activated when the patient moved her right leg included (as expected) the dorsolateral prefrontal cortex bilaterally, and left lateral premotor areas, left primary sensorimotor cortex, bilateral secondary somatosensory areas (inferior parietal cortex), and the vermis and cerebellar hemispheres bilaterally. As predicted, preparation to move the right leg activated a subset of these areas, including the dorsolateral prefrontal cortex bilaterally, right lateral premotor and bilateral inferior parietal cortex, and the vermis and cerebellar hemispheres, but not the left primary sensorimotor cortex. Preparation to move the (paralyzed) left leg activated the left lateral premotor cortex and the cerebellar hemispheres bilaterally, indicating the patient's readiness to move the paralyzed leg. Attempting to move the paralyzed leg led to activation of movement-related areas including the left dorsolateral prefrontal cortex and the cerebellar hemispheres bilaterally, but no activation of the right premotor areas or the right primary sensorimotor cortex. Instead, the right anterior cingulate was significantly activated during this condition. Cingulate activation was confirmed when the attempt to move the left leg was compared with preparation to move the left leg. In addition, this latter comparison revealed significant activation of right orbitofrontal cortex. The authors propose that the anterior cingulate and orbitofrontal cortex actively inhibited movement of the left leg despite dorsolateral prefrontal cortex activation and downstream activation of the cerebellum. They propose that the orbitofrontal cortex may be the distal source of unconscious inhibition, while the anterior cingulate, which mediates emotion and action, is the proximal instrument that disconnects premotor/prefrontal areas from primary motor cortex. The authors speculate that in the absence of functional or structural pathology, it is a disturbance of the will to move that triggers the hemiparalysis via pathological activation of the orbitofrontal and cingulate cortex.

The same research group performed the same experimental design using PET to analyze cerebral blood flow in a patient with hypnotically induced paralysis of the left leg (Halligan *et al.* 2000). Hypnotic paralysis activated similar brain areas to those of motor conversion disorder. The authors believe that the anterior cingulate and orbitofrontal cortex activations probably represent the neural activity responsible for inhibiting the patient's voluntary attempt to move the left leg, or that these activations could represent the management of mental dissonance produced when the suggestion of paralysis of the left limb conflicts with the explicit instruction to move it. This may also apply to patients with motor conversion disorder.

PET studies comparing patients with conversion paralysis with patients who feign paralysis have suggested the important role of the left dorsolateral prefrontal cortex and its involvement in voluntary chosen action (Spence *et al.* 2000). Comparing brain activations during movement of the left hand in patients with conversion paralysis versus controls and feigners showed that conversion patients exhibited relative hypoactivity of the left dorsolateral prefrontal cortex. The authors hypothesize that the selective dysfunction of the dorsolateral prefrontal cortex in patients with conversion involves the higher components of volition, and that a disorder of volition may be present in such patients.

Vuilleumier *et al.* (2001) measured rCBF changes associated with unilateral hysterical sensorimotor loss using SPECT. Cerebral activation was measured at rest and during bilateral vibration of both affected and unaffected limbs, which is known to elicit widespread activity in both sensory and motor areas. Brain activations were compared when the patient's conversion deficit was present, and a few weeks later when it had resolved. Significant differences in cerebral activation were observed between the presence and absence of conversion deficits in patients whose symptoms had resolved on follow-up scanning. When patients were experiencing their neurological deficits, rCBF during vibration was decreased in the contralateral thalamus, caudate, and putamen compared with when the deficit had resolved, while it was increased in the ipsilateral somatosensory and premotor cortex. Lower activation of the contralateral caudate during conversion symptoms predicted poor recovery at follow-up. The authors conclude that conversion paralysis may involve a functional disorder in stria-tothalamocortical circuits controlling sensorimotor function and voluntary motor behaviour, and that the basal ganglia may be particularly well situated to modulate motor processes based on emotional and situational cues from the limbic system. Decreased activity in the basal ganglia–thalamic circuits might set the motor system in a functional state characterized by impaired motor readiness and initiation, resulting in abnormal voluntary behaviour.

There have been no neuroimaging studies evaluating psychogenic hyperkinetic motor disorders. One major confound is the non-specific effects of the ongoing motor activity on widespread sensory and motor brain regions. The work of Eidelberg and coworkers in their studies of patients with idiopathic torsion dystonia (Eidelberg *et al.* 1998) and essential blepharospasm (Hutchinson *et al.* 2001) might suggest novel approaches to the study of psychogenic movement disorders. These authors imaged seven non-manifesting and 10 clinically affected DYT1 carriers, and 14 normal controls, using 2-[fluorine-18]fluoro-2-deoxy-D-glucose PET (FDG-PET). By studying asymptomatic DYT1 carriers, the authors were able to detect an abnormal neural network that was specifically related to genotype without the confound of functional abnormalities resulting from the presence of involuntary movement. Studying affected DYT1 carriers (in whom involuntary movements were suppressed by sleep) in a sleep state also allowed observation of the primary functional abnormality in brain metabolism in these patients without the secondary effects of movement. Such a technique could be applied to patients with psychogenic movement disorders. Comparison should be made with organic counterparts for the specific psychogenic movement disorder as well as normal controls feigning the same type of movements.

Neurophysiological studies

Both motor and somatosensory evoked potentials may aid in confirming a diagnosis of psychogenic paralysis. Motor evoked potentials can be used to confirm the physiological integrity of the motor system. Cantello *et al.* (2001) found that the use of motor evoked potentials enabled the diagnosis of psychogenic paraplegia to be made 50% earlier than prior to application of this technique. Somatosensory evoked potentials can also confirm the integrity of the sensory system in a patient with complaints of sensorimotor dysfunction (Haghighi and Meyer 2001).

EMG has been useful in the evaluation of movement disorders, including myoclonus, tremor, and dystonia, and can be of help in distinguishing psychogenic from organic disorders. Thompson *et al.* (1992) used EMG in five patients presenting with stimulus-sensitive jerks and appeared at initial clinical assessment to have reflex myoclonus or a pathological startle syndrome. EMG activity was recorded from clinically affected muscles, and the latency and variability of the responses were measured. Patients were compared with nine normal subjects who were requested to imitate a generalized jerk involving the neck, elbow, and ankle flexion in response to stimulation. Several electrophysiological features of the jerks in the patients suggested that they were not due to myoclonus or exaggerated startle response. The latency to onset of jerking after stimulation was long (within voluntary reaction time) and variable from trial to trial. The jerks were produced by EMG bursts of long duration and there was a variable order of muscle recruitment. The stimulus-induced responses tended to habituate with repeated presentation of stimuli as in the normal startle response. These features help to distinguish such responses from cortical and brainstem reflex myoclonus, both of which consist of short-duration EMG bursts at short and reproducible latencies following effective stimuli, and exhibit characteristic and stereotyped orders of muscle recruitment without significant habituation. Furthermore, the stimulus-induced jerking recorded in the five patients closely resembled the movements of normal volunteers responding in reaction time tasks to the same stimuli. The similarities included the onset latencies and the variable pattern of muscle recruitment. As the jerks exhibited by these patients were indistinguishable from voluntary reactions, the authors suggest that they were also 'voluntary' in origin.

EMG and accelerometry can be helpful in the diagnosis of psychogenic tremor. As discussed by Brown and Thompson (2001), the most important electrophysiological signs of psychogenic tremor relate to the difficulty in voluntarily maintaining two or more unrelated rhythms in different body parts. The presence of frequency dissociation is strongly supportive of organic tremor. Both frequency dissociation and entrainability can be confirmed by polymyography and time-frequency and pure frequency domain measures.

Comparison of EMG activity in patients with idiopathic torticollis with controls matching the head posture or imitating tremulous torticollis has provided information regarding the pattern of rhythmic drive to the muscles of the neck which may be useful in differentiating organic from psychogenic torticollis (Tijssen *et al.* 2000). EMG activity in the sternocleidomastoid and splenius capitis muscles of patients and controls were analyzed in the frequency and time domains. Control subjects showed a significant peak in the autospectrum of splenius capitis EMG at 10–12 Hz, which was absent in all patients with torticollis. Patients with torticollis had evidence of a 4–7 Hz drive to the splenius capitis and sternocleidomastoid that was absent in coherence spectra from controls. The activity in the sternocleidomastoid and splenius capitis was in phase in patients but not in controls. These EMG features could prove useful in differentiating organic from psychogenic dystonia.

The presence of the *Bereitschaftspotential* (premovement potential) preceding myoclonic movements can help distinguish psychogenic from organic myoclonus (Terada *et al.* 1995). The technique of jerk-locked back-averaging (i.e. back-averaging of EEG time-locked to the EMG onset of jerks) can be used to detect the slow positive potential, beginning about 1 s prior to movement. Self-initiated voluntary movements are preceded by the *Bereitschaftspotential*, but they are absent in organic spontaneous myoclonus. Terada and coworkers demonstrated a slow negative EEG shift corresponding to the *Bereitschaftspotential* in the central region, starting 0.7–2.1 s before the onset of the myoclonic jerk in five patients with psychogenic myoclonus. Therefore the authors concluded that the jerks in these patients were generated through the mechanisms common to those underlying voluntary movement. Thus the absence of a *Bereitschaftspotential* prior to a spontaneous abnormal movement suggests that the nature of the movement is involuntary, or organic. However, there are situations in which voluntary movements are not preceded by a *Bereitschaftspotential*. For example, the *Bereitschaftspotential* is absent or shortened when voluntary movements occur in response to an external stimulus, such as turning the head to the direction of a loud sound. Of 11 patients with Tourette syndrome in two independent studies, eight did not have a normal *Bereitschaftspotential* prior to spontaneous tics (Obeso *et al.* 1981; Karp *et al.* 1996). Tics are often appreciated as a wilful action in response to an internally generated stimulus (Lang 1991). Therefore, the presence of a *Bereitschaftspotential* in advance of a hyperkinetic movement does not always indicate that the movement is psychogenic. The subjective experience of the patient may be very helpful in this case; tic patients most often appreciate a volitional or purposeful component of the movement (Lang 1991), while patients with psychogenic movements regularly deny this experience.

A variety of electrophysiological features have been defined in patients with organic forms of dystonia. It would be logical to evaluate these in patients with psychogenic dystonia. However, most studies have not assessed the effects of simply maintaining the muscles of the body in question tonically contracted for prolonged periods (in a dystonic-like posture). Therefore it is unclear whether the electrophysiological features described in dystonia are a primary feature of the disorder or simply secondary to the abnormal postures (in which case they would be of little help in differentiating psychogenic from non-psychogenic dystonias). For example, abnormalities of recurrent spinal inhibition are widely described in patients with dystonia. However, similar findings may be evident in normal individuals purposely maintaining those limbs in a dystonic-like posture (K Bhatia, personal communication).

Prognosis and treatment

The prognosis of psychogenic motor disorders is most favourable in patients with a shorter duration of symptoms prior to diagnosis. This is most convincing when contrasting the remission rates in the follow-up study by Binzer and Kullgren (1998) with those of other studies. Binzer and Kullgren prospectively studied 30 patients with motor conversion disorder for 2–5 years after diagnosis, but only included patients with an original symptom duration not exceeding 3 months prior to diagnosis and treatment. All of the original 30 patients participated in the follow-up study: 19 (63%) patients had complete remission of initial symptoms, eight (27%) were improved, and three (10%) were unchanged or worse. Of the 19 patients with total recovery, 16 were already symptom free 6 months after diagnosis. None of the patients was rediagnosed with a neurological disorder.

Remission rates have not been nearly as favourable in other follow-up studies where the mean duration to the establishment of the diagnosis of psychogenic motor disorder ranged from 18 months to 2 years (Williams *et al.* 1995; Crimlisk *et al.* 1998). Rates of complete recovery ranged from 25% to 28%, with the remaining patients reporting only partial to no improvement.

Several factors have been identified with a good outcome, including symptoms present for less than 1 year at admission to hospital, a sudden onset of symptoms, a psychiatric diagnosis indicated by the schedule for affective disorders and schizophrenia that coincided with the unexplained motor symptoms (reinforcing the importance of screening for affective and anxiety disorders in these patients), and a change in marital status during the follow-up period (Crimlisk *et al.* 1998; Feinstein *et al.* 2001). Factors associated with a poor outcome include the presence of a personality disorder, a greater number of axis 1 diagnoses, concomitant somatic disease at symptom onset, a longer duration of symptoms, a higher Beck's Hopelessness Scale score, receipt of financial benefits at the time of admission to hospital, and pending litigation (Binzer and Kullgren 1998; Crimlisk *et al.* 1998; Feinstein *et al.* 2001).

After the diagnosis of a psychogenic motor disorder has been established as clinically definite by an experienced neurologist, a coordinated treatment approach is essential, especially given the poor prognosis of these disorders. Clinicians at the Columbia Presbyterian Medical Centre recommend admitting the patient to hospital if there is doubt about the diagnosis, or resistance from the patient in accepting a diagnosis of a psychogenic cause for the motor disorder (Williams *et al.* 1995). Necessary and reasonable tests should be performed to reassure the patient and the clinician that no organic basis for the symptoms has been overlooked. Placebo and suggestion can be used to exacerbate movements or relieve them, and may provide further diagnostic information. Psychiatric consultation should be obtained early to try and identify coexisting psychopathology and psychosocial stressors which may be contributing to the clinical picture. The diagnosis of a psychogenic movement disorder should be given to the patient while he or she is in hospital, and in the presence of both the neurologist and psychiatrist. A face-saving interpretation of the pathophysiology of the disorder is recommended, emphasizing the mind–body interaction and the unconscious origin of symptom production. Appropriate treatment using a combination of psychotherapy, physiotherapy, and psychopharmacological treatment as necessary should be instituted in hospital. However, as stated, despite this approach the prognosis in these patients is often rather poor.

Conclusion

Psychogenic motor disorders are not an uncommon problem faced by the practising neurologist. These disorders cause considerable disability to patients, and impact on the economy due to the cost of medical care and loss of employment. While the recognition of these disorders by clinicians has improved considerably with the development of new imaging and electrophysiological tests to aid clinical examination, the pathogenesis of these disorders remains poorly understood. The prognosis is also poor, especially in patients in whom the diagnosis of a psychogenic cause is delayed. Therefore there is great need for future research in this area to help further our understanding of the cause of psychogenic motor disorders, with the hope of improving the treatment of this difficult clinical problem.

References

American Psychiatric Association (1994). *Diagnostic and Statistical Manual of Mental Disorders*, 4th edn. Washington, DC: American Psychiatric Association.

Binzer M, Eisemann M (1998). Childhood experiences and personality traits in patients with motor conversion symptoms. *Acta Psychiatr Scand*, **98**, 288–95.

Binzer M, Kullgren G (1998). Motor conversion disorder: a prospective 2 to 5 year follow-up study. *Psychosomatics*, **39**, 519–27.

Brown P, Thompson PD (2001). Electrophysiologic aids to the diagnosis of psychogenic jerks, spasms and tremor. *Mov Disord*, **16**, 595–9.

Cantello R, Boccagni C, Comi C, Civardi C, Monaco F (2001). Diagnosis of psychogenic paralysis: the role of motor evoked potentials. *J Neurol*, **248**, 889–97.

Carson AJ, Ringbauer B, Stone J, McKenzie L, Warlow C, Sharpe M (2000). Do medically unexplained symptoms matter? A prospective cohort study of 300 new referrals to neurology outpatient clinics. *J Neurol Neurosurg Psychiatry*, **68**, 207–10.

Chu JA, Dill DL (1990). Dissociative symptoms in relation to childhood physical and sexual abuse histories. *Compr Psychiatry*, **147**, 887–92.

Crimlisk HL, Bhatia K, Cope H, David A, Marsden CD, Ron MA (1998). Slater revisited: 6 year follow up study of patients with medically unexplained motor symptoms. *BMJ*, **316**, 582–6.

Deuschl G, Koster B, Lucking CH, Scheidt C (1998). Diagnosis and pathophysiologic aspects of psychogenic tremor. *Mov Disord*, **13**, 294–302.

Eidelberg D, Moeller J, Antonini A, Kazumata K, Nakamura T, Dhawan V, *et al.* (1998). Functional brain networks in DYT1 dystonia. *Ann Neurol*, **44**, 303–12.

Factor SA, Podskalny GD, Molho ES (1995). Psychogenic movement disorders: frequency, clinical profile and characteristics. *J Neurol Neurosurg Psychiatry*, **59**, 406–12.

Feinstein A, Stergiopoulos V, Fine J, Lang AE (2001). Psychiatric outcome in patients with a psychogenic movement disorder. *Neuropsychiatry Neuropsychol Behav Neurol*, **14**, 169–76.

Gálvez-Jiménez N, Lang AE (1997). Psychogenic movement disorders. In RL Watts, WC Koller, (ed.) *Movement Disorders. Neurologic Principles and Practice*, pp. 715–32. New York: McGraw-Hill.

Haghighi SS, Meyer S (2001). Psychogenic paraplegia in a patient with normal electrophysiologic findings. *Spinal Cord*, **39**, 664–7.

Halligan PW, Athwal BS, Oakley DA, Frackowiak RSJ (2000). Imaging hypnotic paralysis: implications for conversion hysteria. *Lancet*, **355**, 986.

Heruti RJ, Reznik J, Adunski A, Levy A, Weingarden H, Ohry A (2002). Conversion motor paralysis disorder: analysis of 34 consecutive referrals. *Spinal Cord*, **40**, 335–40.

Hutchinson M, Nakamura T, Moeller JR, Antonini A, Belakhlef A, Dhawan V, *et al.* (2000). The metabolic topography of essential blepharospasm. *Neurology*, **55**, 673–7.

Karp BI, Porter S, Toro C, Hallet M (1996). Simple motor tics may be preceded by a premotor potential. *J Neurol Neurosurg Psychiatry*, **61**, 103–6.

Kim YJ, Pakiam ASI, Lang AE (1999). Historical and clinical features of psychogenic tremor: a review of 70 cases. *Can J Neurol Sci*, **26**, 190–5.

Krumholz A, Niedermeyer E (1983). Psychogenic seizures: a clinical study with follow-up data. *Neurology*, **33**, 498–502.

Lang AE (1991). Patient perception of tics and other movement disorders. *Neurology*, **41**, 223–8.

Lang AE (1995). Psychogenic dystonia: a review of 18 cases. *Can J Neurol Sci*, **22**, 136–43.

Lang AE, Koller WC, Fahn S (1995). Psychogenic parkinsonism. *Arch Neurol*, **52**, 802–10.

Lempert T, Dietrich M, Huppert D, Brandt T (1990). Psychogenic disorders in neurology: frequency and clinical spectrum. *Acta Neurol Scand*, **82**, 335–40.

Marjama J, Troster AI, Koller WC (1995). Psychogenicmovement disorders. *Neurol Clin*, **13**, 283–97.

Marshall JC, Halligan PW, Fink GR, Wade DT, Frackowiak RSJ (1997). The functional anatomy of hysterical paralysis. *Cognition*, **64**, B1–8.

Monday K, Jankovic J (1993). Psychogenic myoclonus. *Neurology*, **43**, 349–52.

Obeso JA, Rothwell JC, Marsden CD (1981). Simple tics in Gilles de la Tourette's syndrome are not prefaced by a normal premovement EEG potential. *J Neurol Neurosurg Psychiatry*, **44**, 735–8.

Ron M (1994). Somatization in neurological practice. *J Neurol Neurosurg Psychiatry*, **57**, 1161–4.

Spence SA, Crimlisk HL, Cope H, Ron MA, Grasby PM (2000). Discrete neurophysiological correlates in prefrontal cortex during hysterical and feigned disorder of movement. *Lancet*, **355**, 1243.

Terada K, Ikeda A, Van Ness PC, Nagamine T, Kaji R, Kimura J, *et al.* (1995). Presence of *Bereitschaftspotential* preceding psychogenic myoclonus: clinical application of jerk-locked back averaging. *J Neurol Neurosurg Psychiatry*, **58**, 745–7.

Thompson PD, Colebatch JG, Brown P, Rothwell JC, Day BL, Obeso JA, *et al.* (1992). Voluntary stimulus-sensitive jerks and jumps mimicking myoclonus or pathological startle syndromes. *Mov Disord*, **7**, 257–62.

Tiihonen J, Kuikka J, Viinamaki H, Lehtonen J, Partanen J (1995). Altered cerebral blood flow during hysterical paresthesia. *Biol Psychiatry*, **37**, 134–5.

Tijssen MAJ, Marsden JF, Brown P (2000). Frequency analysis of EMG activity in patients with idiopathic torticollis. *Brain*, **123**, 677–86.

Vuilleumier P, Chicherio C, Assal F, Schwartz S, Slosman D, Landis T (2001). Functional neuroanatomical correlates of hysterical sensorimotor loss. *Brain*, **124**, 1077–90.

Williams DT, Ford B, Fahn S (1995). Phenomenology and psychopathology related to psychogenic movement disorders. *Adv Neurol*, **65**, 231–57.

Chapter 23

Frontostriatal circuits and disorders of goal-directed actions

Facundo Manes and Ramón Leiguarda

The basal ganglia receive inputs from a wide variety of neocortical domains that subserve not only motor but also sensory, limbic, and associative functions (Parent and Hazrati 1995a,b). Therefore the basal ganglia process information associated with higher functions accompanying motor behaviour including learning, memory, attention, motivation, emotion, and volitional behaviour (Evarts and Wise 1984; Rolls 1994; Saper 1996; Schultz *et al.* 2000). The main driving force of the basal ganglia is the frontal cortex. The frontostriatal projections are organized in multiple parallel reverberating circuits which appear to maintain many of the physiological and behavioural properties of the cortical areas that they subserve (Alexander *et al.* 1986). Therefore, this circuitry subserves many of the motor, cognitive, emotional, and motivated functions involved in goal-directed behaviour. Thus goal-directed behaviour is understood as a set of related processes by which an internal state (derived from an internal or external event) is translated, through action, into the attainment of a goal (Brown and Pluck 2000). Damage to diverse circuit structures (i.e. basal ganglia, thalamus, frontal lobes) may cause similar abnormalities in planned motivated motor behaviour (Cummings 1993). Moreover, patients with major psychiatric diseases such as schizophrenia, obsessive–compulsive disorders, depression, and mania exhibit a spectrum of disorders of goal-directed actions, such as apathy, agitation, catatonic behaviour, compulsions, perseverative motor behaviour, and imitative response tendencies, which are strikingly similar from the phenomenological viewpoint to those observed in patients with frontal lobe and basal ganglion damage.

Therefore, the frontostriatal circuits seem to provide a unifying framework integrating the sensorimotor, cognitive, and limbic elements of a variety of higher-order motor disorders associated with several disparate neurological and psychiatric illnesses. In this chapter, we begin by describing the anatomofunctional organization of corticostriatal circuits and how such organization is ideally suited to mediate goal-directed behaviours. Then we will describe the major clinical features of the motivational and cognitive motor disorders ascribed to dysfunction of these circuits in both neurological and psychiatric conditions. Thus we hope to provide possible answers to the following questions.

1 What specific aspects of this circuitry contribute to component processes in complex goal-directed action?

2 How do symptoms such as apathy, obsessions, and perseverations relate to disruption of one or several corticostrial circuits?

3 Can we somehow provide a unifying account for the disorders in planned and motivated motor behaviour following frontostriatal dysfunction?

Anatomofunctional organization of frontostriatal circuits

Anatomy of the corticostriatal circuits

Actions represent purposeful goal-directed behaviour, which usually involves movements. Goal-directed actions are intentional (willed) or automatic, routine, or stereotyped (see Chapter 9).

The entire frontal cortex is often considered the 'motor cortex' in the broadest sense, in that it is devoted to action, be it expression of emotion, motivation, logical reasoning, or skeletal movements (Fuster 1997). The connectional organization of the frontal cortex makes up a hierarchy in which a cascade of pathways, from prefrontal through premotor regions, ultimately terminates in areas that mediate motor expression (see Chapter 1). This hierarchy of organization is reflected in the corticostriatal projections (Passingham 1993).

The striatum receives information from virtually all cortical domains subserving motor, sensory, associative, and limbic functions (Parent and Hazrati 1995a,b). Alexander *et al.* (1986) suggested that, rather than serving as a funnel for information from widespread cortical areas, the basal ganglia actually participate in multiple parallel circuits with different regions of the frontal lobe. According to these authors, the frontostriatal projections would be anatomically and functionally organized in five parallel and segregated circuits, originating in the motor, oculomotor, dorsolateral prefrontal, lateral orbitofrontal, and anterior cingulate cortices and projecting to specific parts of the striatum which, via connections with the globus pallidus internus (GPi) and substantia nigra pars reticulata (SNr), sends its outputs through specific thalamic nuclei back to the frontal lobe (Fig. 23.1). Within each of the corticostriatal circuits there would be two pathways: a) a direct pathway which selects the most appropriate response (actions/movements); and b) an indirect pathway which suppresses unwanted responses (actions/movements). These pathways converge on a subset of GPi/SNr neurons which in turn disinhibit or inhibit a corresponding subset of thalamic neurons. The excitatory output from the thalamic neurons converges on the same group of frontal neurons as that where the striatal afferents originate in a highly segregated manner (Fig. 23.2). Many of the same cortical areas that reach the striatum also project to the subthalamic nucleus (STN), constituting a subthalamic path (Alexander *et al.* 1986; Alexander and Crutcher 1990; DeLong 1990). Middleton and Strick (2000a,b) have further proposed broadening the original five-circuit scheme to include seven

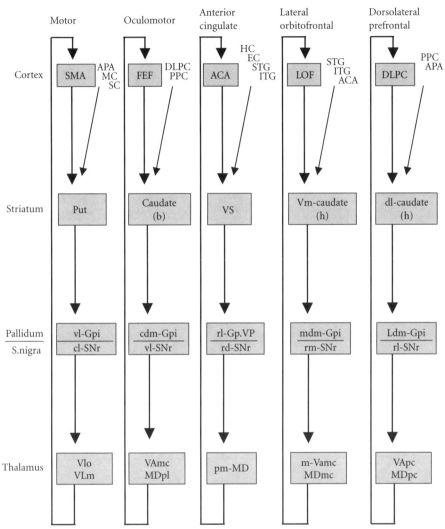

Fig. 23.1 The frontostriatal circuits:motor, oculomotor, anterior cingulate, orbitofrontal, and dorsolateral. Abbreviations: ACA, anterior cingulate; APA, arcuate premotor area; caudate (b), body; caudate (h), head; DLPC, dorsolateral prefrontal cortex; EC, entorhinal cortex, FEF, frontal eye fields; GPi, internal segment of the globus pallidus; HC, hippocampal cortex; ITG, inferior temporal gyrus; LOF, lateral orbitofrontal cortex; MC, motor cortex; MDpl, medialis dorsalis pars paralamellaris; MDmc, medialis dorsalis pars magnocellularis; MDpc, medialis dorsalis pars parvocellularis; PPC, posterior parietal cortex; SC, sensory cortex; SNr, substantia nigra pars reticulata; STG, superior temporal gyrus; VAmc, ventralis anterior pars magnocellularis; VApc, ventralis anterior pars parvocellularis; VLm, ventralis lateralis pars medialis; Vlo, ventralis lateralis pars oralis; VP, ventral pallidum; VS, ventral striatum; cl-, caudolateral; cdm-, caudal dorsomedial; dl-, dorsolateral; l-, lateral; ldm-, lateral dorsomedial; m-, medial; mdm-, medial dorsomedial; pm, posteromedial; rd-, rostrodorsal; rl-, rostrolateral; rm-, rostromedial; vm-, ventromedial; vl-, ventrolateral. Reproduced from Alexander *et al.* (1986). *Annu Rev Neurosci*, **9**, 357–81.

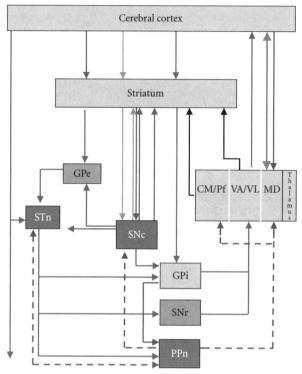

Fig. 23.2 Schematic view of the classic model of corticostriatal circuitry (red) with the direct pathway to the GPi and the indirect pathway through the GPe and STn to the GPi. The subthalamic path is also shown in red. The striosomal path (cortex–striatum–SNc–striatum) is shown in green. The corticothalamic reciprocal and non-reciprocal projections are shown in pink and violet, respectively. The striatal–nigrostriatal projections are simplified and are shown in blue. The efferent and afferent projections to and from the PPN are shown in broken violet lines. Explanations are given in the text. Abbreviations: GPe, external segment of the globus pallidus; GPi, internal segment of the globus pallidus; SNr, substantia nigra pars reticulata; SNc, substantia nigra pars compacta; STn, subthalamic nucleus; CM/Pf, centromedian parafascicular complex; VA, ventralis anterior; VL, ventralis lateralis; MD, medialis dorsalis; PPn, pedunculopontis nucleus.

general categories of circuits: motor (skeletomotor), oculomotor, dorsolateral prefrontal, lateral orbitofrontal, medial orbitofrontal, cingulate, and inferotemporal-posterior parietal. By virtue of their reciprocal connections with posterior cortical areas, the basal ganglia would influence a wider range of behaviour than that proposed by Alexander *et al.* (1986), in which the basal ganglion inputs from posterior cortical areas are integrated in basal ganglion circuits and ultimately influenced regions of the frontal lobe. Joel and Weiner (1994) challenged the segregated organization of the corticostriatal circuits; they suggested that thalamic projections synapse not only in the frontal area which was the source of the cortical input to the striatal subregion (closed circuit), but also in a different frontal area which innervates a different striatal subregion, thus forming an open pathway. This open interconnected principle would also govern the organization of the indirect pathways, one of which would terminate in the same subregion as the direct pathway (closed indirect pathway), whereas another one would terminate in a subregion distinct from the direct pathways (open indirect pathways). The connections of the striatum with the dopaminergic system follows a similar anatomical organization. The split circuit scheme would allow either integrated or segregated processing of information within as well as between different basal ganglion-thalamus-cortical circuits (Joel and Weiner 1994; Joel 2001; Yelnik 2002).

Moreover, while striatal afferents from motor and higher association cortices target neurons in the striatal matrix, inputs from many orbitofrontal and temporal limbic cortical regions target regions of the striatum called patches or striosoms; whose cells do not participate in the same types of circuitry as do neurons in the striatal matrix. The substantia nigra pars compacta (SNc) region which receives the **striosomal path** (cortex-striatum-SNc) sends widespread projections to the striatum, which may represent a route for the basal ganglia to integrate information about primary reward and behavioural states received from orbitofrontal and temporolimbic cortices, with modality specific information being processed in the cortical-basal ganglion (striatal matrix) circuits, thus making up another open-loop component of basal ganglion circuitry (Fig. 23.2) (Middleton and Strick (2000 a,b). The specific organization of the **striatonigral-striatal pathway** allows ventral striatal regions to influence more dorsal striatal regions via spiralling projections, thus providing another route through which motivation (reward) can influence cognitive functions and cognition can influence motor functions (Haber *et al.* 2000) (Fig. 23.2).

Cross-talk between circuits can also occur through the corticothalamo-cortical pathway. The corticothalamic projections possess two components: a reciprocal component in which the cortical area receiving the thalamic input projects back to the same thalamic area, and a non-reciprocal component in which a given cortical area projects to a region of thalamus but fails to receive its output. In addition, thalamic relay nuclei, such as VA/VL that carry basal ganglion output to motor and premotor areas, also project to the striatum. The flow of information in corticothalamic pathways also seems to be from limbic and cognitive areas into the premotor and motor regions of the thalamus. Therefore the information that the thalamic relay nuclei convey to the cortex is not only affected by the parallel pathway through the basal ganglia, but is also modified by the non-reciprocal thalamic pathway, resulting in an integrating feedforward processing that facilitates information transfer from one cortical area to another, similar to the mechanism through which the primary sensory cortex can influence higher cortical association areas (McFarland and Haber 2002) (Fig. 23.2).

Control of goal-directed actions: distinct roles of the corticostriatal circuits

Goal-directed actions have been hypothesized to be triggered in several ways: by environmental stimuli, including verbal and social information, by drives and emotions, and by intention to act (Joel and Weiner 2000).

Externally triggered actions that require neither motor preparation nor decision-making about the precise timing only activate part of the motor circuit, namely the sensorimotor cortex and the putamen, as well as the insular cortex (Jahanshahi *et al.* 1995). Regular rate externally triggered actions, which engage motor preparation but involve no decision-making about initiation time, activate components of the 'motor' as well as the anterior cingulate circuits, including the supplementary motor area (SMA), the premotor cortex, the anterior cingulate, and the inferior parietal cortex, as well as the sensorimotor cortex, putamen, and insular cortex (Jahanshahi *et al.* 1995; Deiber *et al.* 1996).

The orbital and medial prefrontal cortex (OMPFC) is involved in linking primary reward with motivational and emotional features and is thought to play a key role in the development of reward-guided behaviour (Damasio 1994; Rolls 1996; Schultz 2000; Schultz *et al.* 2000). The OMPFC projects to the ventromedial regions of the striatum, including the ventromedial regions of the caudate, putamen, and nucleus accumbens. The ventral striatum has efferent connections with the ventral and rostro-lateral GP and the rostrodorsal SNr. Pallidal and nigral efferents project to the MD and VA thalamic nucleus as well as to the ventral tegmental area, habenula, hypothalamus, and amygdala; MD thalamic neurons project back to the OMPFC. The 'limbic striatum' also receives projections from limbic regions, including the amygdala, hippocampus, and related cortical regions, and from association cortices, such as the inferior and superior temporal gyri. Thus the OMPFC appears to function as a sensory–visceromotor link, critical for the guidance of reward-related behaviour and mood setting; it is densely connected with the dorsolateral prefrontal cortex (DLPFC) (Öngür and Price 2000). Furthermore, several structures within the orbitofrontal–striatal–midbrain–dopamine circuit are related to specific aspects of reward, such as prediction and expectation, which thus seem to represent the neuronal substrates of reward during learning and established behavioural performance; access to central representations of reward may be used for neural control of goal-directed actions (Schultz *et al.* 2000). According to Elliott *et al.* (2000), it might be suggested that the medial orbitofrontal striatal circuits play a specific role in monitoring the reward values of stimuli and responses, so that reward value may be used to choose appropriate actions in a flexible and purposeful manner, particularly in novel and uncertain situations. In turn, the lateral orbitofrontal circuit could be preferentially involved when the selected action requires the suppression of previously rewarded responses.

Intention to act is encoded mainly in the frontal lobe. Neurophysiological and neuroimaging studies have shown that the dorsal (motor) anterior cingulate gyrus together with the neighbouring SMA are involved in the intentional effort to carry out an action. The anterior cingulate gyrus in particular would subserve the function of an interface between the limbic system and neocortex that translate motivation, emotion, and volition into action (Paus *et al.* 1998). The internal process whereby a subject generates actions based on the will to do so activates a frontal network, in addition to the parietal association cortex, insula, and precuneus, comprising the DLPFC, pre-SMA, and anterior cingulate gyrus (Frith *et al.* 1991; Jahanshahi *et al.* 1995). The lateral prefrontal cortex lies at the top of the hierarchy of information processing; it plays a crucial role in every aspect of the cognitive processes required for behavioural planning and action organization: processing and integration of perceived or memorized information, associative learning, behavioural selection/decision-making, and behavioural guidance (Tanji and Hoshi 2001). Hence it is in a unique position to integrate information about motivational factors, external context, targets of actions, and success of the response for the conscious development and monitoring of goal-directed actions (Passingham and Toni 2001). The DLPFC projects primarily to the dorsolateral head of the caudate nucleus, which connects to the dorsomedial GPi and rostral SN. Pallidal and nigral projections travel through the VA and MD thalamic nuclei back to the lateral prefrontal region, thus forming the dorsolateral frontostriatal circuit.

The lateral aspects of the prefrontal cortex, together with the premotor cortex, are engaged in the integration of external information; accordingly, both code 'what to do' in relation to cue–response associations. Ventral prefrontal activation appears to be enhanced when subjects are required to adapt learned stimulus–response associations to new circumstances (Passingham and Toni 2001). On the other hand, medial frontal areas, particularly the pre-SMA and the anterior cingulate gyrus, are engaged during the selection and internal generation of actions (Deiber *et al.* 1991; Ballard *et al.* 1997). Unlike the prefrontal cortex, the pre-SMA receives no information from posterior association cortices. Thus it has been proposed that the medial control system renders the onset of action possible only when external contingencies and motivation factors are favourable (Rizzolatti *et al.* 1998). A recent functional magnetic resonance imaging (fMRI) study further dissociates the role of the medial and lateral prefrontal striatal circuits in planning; the anterior cingulate/anterior medial prefrontal-ventral striatal circuit would subserve the ability to carry out predictive action plans, whereas the lateral/polar prefrontal-dorsolateral striatal circuit would process contingent action plans, i.e. it would dynamically adjust the sequential structure of ongoing plans to new environmental demands (Koechlin *et al.* 2000).

The ability to select between possible actions in a given situation is central to human behaviour. Successful motor behaviour requires not only the selection of the appropriate action ('what to do'), but also the precise time to do it (timing adjustment or 'when to do it'). Response selection and timing adjustment are processed by parallel and converging systems involving several brain structures including DLPFC, pre-SMA, rostral cingulate motor area (CMA), lateral premotor cortex and parietal association cortex, as well as the basal ganglia and cerebellum (Sakai *et al.* 2000). The contribution of the cingulate gyrus and the frontal and parietal regions to response selection seems to be dissociable. Rostral CMA, connected with the pre-SMA, seems specifically involved in movement selection based on rewards (see above). Whereas both the prefrontal and parietal regions are thought to be involved in responses on the basis of learned stimulus–response associations, the PFC would be more active when the selection of competing responses is required. Thus the PFC is particularly active in selecting the appropriate response as well as in ignoring distractions and inhibiting inappropriate ones (behavioural inhibition). Response inhibition in the GO–NOGO task consistently activates the pre-SMA, ventrolateral PFC (VLPFC), anterior cingulate gyrus, dorsal premotor cortex, and intraparietal cortex. Whereas the VLPFC could be related to the generation of the stop message in the GO–NOGO task, the anterior cingulate gyrus would be active in situations of high response competition (Casey *et al.* 1997; Garavan *et al.* 1999; Braver *et al.* 2001; Watanabe *et al.* 2002). Functional brain imaging studies have shown that perseveration of competing motor memories reactivates neural circuits (DLPC–putamen) that participate in acquiring that memory, whereas the inhibitory control of competing motor memory causes activation of VLPC–caudate (Shadmehr and Holcomb 1999). The caudate nucleus has been considered as a gate that moderates response choice by selectively inhibiting competing input from the cortex (Mink 1996). The activation of the DLPC during inhibition of prepotent or imitative response tendencies (Brass *et al.* 2001) highlights its supervisory role in those conditions which engender conflict (Shallice and Burgess 1996). It may be further speculated that the DLPFC monitors conflicts between intention and sensory feedback, while the VLPFC deals with conflicts between sensory modalities (e.g. vision and proprioception) (Fink *et al.* 1999). This concept would be in line with models that posit a hierarchical relationship between the DLPFC and VLPFC in executive processes such that the latter guides active on-line maintenance of the retrieved representations from posterior cortices, whereas the former would operate on the product of the ventral region; it would monitor and select goal-relevant representations being maintained by the VLPFC (D'Esposito *et al.* 1998; Rowe *et al.* 2000; Wagner *et al.* 2001).

Impairment of goal-directed actions in frontal-lobe- and basal-ganglion-damaged patients and psychiatric illnesses

From akinesia and apathy to akinetic mutism and catatonia

Akinesia

Akinesia is defined as inability or difficulty in initiating a movement in the absence of a corticospinal or motor unit lesion; whereas the term bradykinesia refers to slowness of movement. Akinesia is a cardinal feature of many basal ganglion disorders, in particular

Parkinson's disease, and may be observed in patients with frontomedial cortex damage (Dick *et al.* 1986; Haussermann *et al.* 2001). In experimental and functional imaging studies, akinesia has been correlated with underactivity of the 'motor' frontostriatal subcircuit involving the SMA; such dysfunction is reversed, as is the early part of the *Bereitschaftspotential* (premovement potential), with dopamine agonist drugs, pallidotomy, and STN stimulation (Berardelli *et al.* 2001; Haslinger *et al.* 2001; Escola *et al.* 2003).

Apathy

Apathy (from the Greek *pathos*, lack of passion) is characterized as follows: lack of initiative, effort, and productivity (decreased drive and motivation); lack of responsiveness towards positive and negative events, ineffectiveness, and emotional flattening (affect and emotion impoverishment); and lack of interest, concern, and insight into one's own situation (cognitive involvement) (Marin 1991; Andersson *et al.* 1999). Abulia (from the Greek *abulia*, lack or weakness of will) has been equated with 'psychic akinesia' (Bhatia and Marsden 1994). Apathy and abulia may, at first, appear to be difficult to dissociate. Marin (1991) suggested that apathy has validity as a symptom, a syndrome, or a behavioural dimension, and introduced the term apathy and 'disorders of diminished motivation', which to be properly diagnosed must include 'simultaneous diminution in the overt behavioural, cognitive and emotional concomitants of goal-directed behaviour'; nevertheless, motivational deficits are the core aspects of apathy.

Apathy as a pure motivational deficit is considered to be mainly due to disruption of the anterior cingulate–striatal circuit (Cummings 1993). Apathy is common in Parkinson's disease, Huntington's disease, and Alzheimer's disease, and is very frequent in progressive supranuclear palsy and frontotemporal dementia (Litvan *et al.* 1998). In Parkinson's disease, akinesia and apathy, i.e. the motor and motivational deficits in goal-oriented actions, can be loosely coupled; a severely akinetic patient may be well motivated, whereas a severely apathetic one may show mild akinesia (Marin 1991). Furthermore, we have found that apathy can be observed associated with depression, but also independent of the latter in patients with Parkinson's disease; in fact, negative thoughts about the self and the future are absent in apathy (Starkstein *et al.* 1992; Starkstein and Manes 2000). Abulia has been found to be the most common behavioural disorder in patients with basal ganglion lesions in general (Bhatia and Marsden 1994) and with caudate infarctions in particular (Caplan *et al.* 1990). Striatal and, more specifically, globus pallidus and thalamic lesions usually involve several circuits simultaneously, thus causing mixed behavioural syndromes. In these cases, clinical manifestations reflect the involvement of other frontosubcortical circuits besides the anterior cingulate circuit, such as the orbitofrontal and dorsolateral prefrontal circuits. Patients with psychic akinesia due to pallidal lesions, which some authors liken to abulia, exhibit emotional disturbances and executive dysfunction in addition to loss of drive and motivation (Starkstein *et al.* 1989; Merello *et al.* 2001).

Bilateral focal damage to the globus pallidus as a result of carbon monoxide intoxication (Laplane *et al.* 1984; Starkstein *et al.* 1989), manganese intoxication (Mena *et al.* 1967), haemorrhages (Strub 1989), and posteroventral pallidotomy (Merello *et al.* 2001) are liable to cause prominent apathy, withdrawal, and loss of interest, as well as impaired memory and executive functions. Patients with bilateral lesions of the medial dorsal and ventral anterior thalamic nuclei, which receive projections from the dorsolateral prefrontal, orbitofrontal, and anterior cingulate circuits, may exhibit apathy and withdrawal together with abnormalities of recent memory and executive function including set-shifting, word-list generation, and serial motor behaviour, although some patients appear irritable and disinhibited (Gentilini *et al.* 1987; Stuss *et al.* 1988; Sandson *et al.* 1991). Bilateral lesions restricted to the rostroventral globus pallidus, nucleus accumbens, and septal nuclei have been described as causing reduced spontaneous activity, lack of initiative, apathy, and withdrawal, similar to but less severe than the clinical picture of akinetic mutism, together with memory impairment and confabulation but without executive deficits (Phillips *et al.* 1987).

As mentioned above, apathy and diminished initiative are the cardinal manifestations of the medial frontal–anterior cingulate gyrus syndrome (Cummings 1993). However, apathy has also been described in patients with dorsolateral prefrontal damage (Stuss and Benson 1984) as well as in those with orbitofrontal involvement due to vascular pathology or tumours (Hunter *et al.* 1968; Logue *et al.* 1968; Bogousslavsky and Regli 1990).

The orbitofrontal syndrome features prominent disinhibition and irritability, but also lability, euphoria, and poor social judgement. Some patients may have alterations in interest, initiative, and conscientiousness, and on occasion they show imitation and utilization behaviour. Similar personality changes are observed in the early stages of Huntington's disease, when involvement of the medial caudate regions receiving projections from the orbitofrontal and anterior cingulate circuits predominates, and in neuroacanthocytosis, a disorder primarily affecting the caudate nucleus. Bilateral pallidal damage (Mena *et al.* 1967) and bilateral medial thalamic infarctions (Gentilini *et al.* 1987) may cause 'frontal-lobe' type personality and behavioural disinhibition, including utilization behaviour (Eslinger *et al.* 1991).

Therefore, and as described before, the limbic-ventrostriatopallidal and related pathways such as the striato-nigrostriatal and cortico-thalamocortical circuits are crucially involved in the translation of motivation into action. The ventral tegmental area (VTA) provides dopamine-mediated input to the ventral striatum and other limbic structures, as well as to the prefrontal cortex via the mesolimbic and mesocortical systems. Cortical dopamine release modulates descending corticostriatal fibres, potentially influencing the activity of many striato-thalamocortical circuits. Another modulating influence may be exerted through the output from the ventral striatum, which diffusely projects to the SNc and from there extensively affects the frontal cortex. Furthermore, cholinergic neurotransmitter dysfunction due to involvement of the pedunculopontine nucleus may also contribute to the development of apathy in some diseases such as progressive supranuclear palsy and Alzheimer's disease. The pedunculopontine nucleus may act as another 'integrator' of motor with motivational or limbic information (Davidson and Irwin 1999). These findings explain why motivational deficits may improve to some extent under dopamine agonist therapy (Powell *et al.* 1996).

Overall, motivational and affective components of apathy and abulia seem to be mediated by the anterior cingulate and orbitofrontal circuits; the latter also exert a local influence on motivational aspects of behaviour (Elliott *et al.* 2000). We would suggest in addition that the difference between apathy (lack of passion) and abulia (lack of will) lies in the presence of cognitive manifestations in the latter (e.g. lack of interest and concern), reflecting involvement of the dorsolateral prefrontal circuit, since the concept of willed action is linked to attention, conscious awareness, and intentionality, which are particularly represented in the dorsolateral prefrontal cortex (Stephan *et al.* 2003). Thus abulia could be qualitatively distinct from apathy, rather than being a more severe form, whereas akinetic mutism, but not abulia, would then be a severe form of apathy.

Akinetic mutism

Akinetic mutism refers to a state in which the patient, although seemingly awake, remains mute and motionless (Cairns *et al.* 1941). Only the eyes dart in the direction of moving objects; despite the lack of movements there are hardly any signs indicative of damage to the descending motor pathways. Instead 'frontal release signs', such as grasping or sucking, may be present. Patients are profoundly apathetic, entirely lack initiative and attention, display no emotion even when in pain, and are indifferent even to their hazardous circumstances. Even though patients fail to speak and move spontaneously, they may answer questions monosyllabically or show partial, delayed, or hesitant verbal and motor responses. They are incontinent and eat and drink only if fed. Akinetic mutism is most often associated with bilateral anterior cingulate cortex and adjacent frontal cortical lesions, as well as with lesions involving the medial forebrain bundle, anterior hypothalamus, ventral striatum, ventral globus pallidus, and medial thalamus. The most devastating injury is a bilateral loss of basal–mesial cortical tissue, after which little further recovery develops (Barris and Schuman 1953; Lavy 1959; Klee 1961; Messert *et al.* 1966). More posteriorly located lesions involving anterior midbrain or mesodiencephalic junctions cause a syndrome resembling akinetic mutism, but patients usually appear asleep most of the time and have oculomotor abnormalities (Segarra 1971). 'Hyperkinetic mutism', a condition in which patients are apathetic and mute but with bilateral hyperkinesias, has been described with multiple subcortical and cortical infarcts (Inbody and Jankovic 1986).

The common denominator of all akinetic mute states can be related to the disruption of corticostriatopallidal–thalamocortical circuits that originate in the anterior cingulate and SMA, either directly or indirectly (Mega and Cummings 1994). Akinetic mutism resulting from thalamic injury is likely to reflect the unique role of the thalamic nuclei, including the nucleus reticularis, in gating the corticostriatal circuits (Groenewegen and Berendse 1994) and specific long-range cortico-cortical interactions. Isolated injury to the periaqueductal grey region has also been described in experimental models of akinetic mutism. Selective injury to the medial forebrain bundle removes a strong dopaminergic modulation of medial frontal lobe structures; such loss of modulation is reversible, and can be corrected by giving patients dopaminergic agonists (Ross and Stewart 1981; Fleet *et al.* 1987). However, when lesions include the areas where ascending forebrain dopaminergic fibres terminate (e.g. cingulate, orbitofrontal, and septal areas), there is no improvement with such medication (Devinsky *et al.* 1987). The most typical cases of akinetic mutism are those caused by bilateral lesions of the anterior cingulate cortex and the SMA. When only the bilateral anterior cingulate cortex is involved, there is profound apathy but neither akinesia nor mutism. Thus the preservation of motor activity is mainly related to the sparing of the SMA and caudal cingulate motor area (area 23), which are reciprocally interconnected (Laplane *et al.* 1981).

Catatonia

In 1843, the French psychiatrist Baillarger described a delusional syndrome in alienated patients occurring in a state of stupor, with fixed gaze, a facial expression of frozen astonishment, muteness, and indifference, which he termed '*melancholia avec stupeur*'. However, it was the German psychopathologist Kahlbaum who, in 1874, defined '*vesania katatonica*', a condition 'in which the patient remains completely mute and motionless, with a staring expression, the gaze fixed into space, with an apparent complete loss of will, no reaction to sensory stimuli, on occasion with the symptoms of waxy flexibility fully developed, as in catalepsy'. Later, Wernicke (1900) suggested the term '*motilitatpsychose*' to emphasize the relationship of the disorder to a likely dysfunction of a 'psychomotor path', leading to akinesia, parakinesis, or hyperkinesis. Whereas Kahlbaum and Wernicke placed catatonia within the range of affective disorders, Kraepelin (1920) regarded it as a type of schizophrenia.

Catatonia refers to a wide range of motor signs which can be divided into those that occur spontaneously and those that appear during examination or interview (Hamilton 1976). Abnormal spontaneous movements and postures include stereotypies, mannerisms, staring, iteration, bizarre postures, stupor (complete unresponsiveness), and catatonic furor (short periods of excitement and agitation). Whereas mannerisms are goal-directed activities performed in a bizarre or exaggerated way (e.g. unusual ways of eating, smoking, etc.), stereotypies refer to movements carried out in a uniform manner and are not regarded as goal-directed behaviours (see Chapter 21) (Marsden *et al.* 1975). On examination a diverse array of motor and behavioural abnormalities are disclosed, which can be subdivided into those related to automatic or involuntary obedience, and those exhibiting oppositional behaviours. The former include echophenomena (echolalia and echopraxia), waxy flexibility (plastic increased tone with a tendency to maintain unusual postures induced by the clinician), *mitgehen* (patients are propelled by the light touch of the examiner), and *mitmachen* (abnormal cooperation and passivity with slow return of the limbs from an induced to a resting posture), as well as speech-prompted responses, i.e. immediately answering a question with an unrelated or bizarre reply (Hamilton 1976). Oppositional catatonic behaviour may include negativism, aversion, mutism, and *gegenhalten* or paratonia (increased muscle tone with further tensing up when the examiner attempts to move the joint).

The aetiology of idiopathic catatonia is as yet unknown. Primary catatonia is associated with mania, depression, and schizophrenia. Roughly 10% of patients with acute psychiatric illness exhibit a cluster of motor signs that are identified as the syndrome of catatonia (Fink and Taylor 2001). Periodic catatonia is a variant of bipolar illness in which the clinical course is characterized by alternating catatonic stupor and catatonic furor (Gjessing 1974). Malignant catatonia is a severe catatonic syndrome of rather sudden onset, associated with autonomic dysfunction (i.e. fever, tachycardia, hypertension); it may prove fatal unless treatment is not promptly instituted. Catatonia secondary to organic disease may be observed with pathological processes affecting the frontal lobes (i.e. traumatic contusions, ruptured cerebral artery aneurysms, neoplasm), the limbic system (e.g. herpes encephalitis, subacute sclerosing panencephalitis), basal ganglia (e.g. postencephalitic parkinsonism, bilateral globus pallidus lesions), and diencephalic structures (e.g. Wernicke's encephalopathy, thalamotomy, neoplasm). Catatonia has also been described with metabolic and systemic disorders, such as hepatic encephalopathy, diabetic ketoacidosis, hypercalcaemia, systemic lupus erythematosus, and as adverse reactions to many drugs, including neuroleptic malignant syndrome (NMS) and neuroleptic-induced catatonia, and toxic serotonine syndrome (TSS) which is precipitated by selective serotonine-reuptake inhibitors or monoamine oxidase inhibitors (Gelenberg 1976; Fink and Taylor 2001).

It has been debated whether NMS and TSS are variants of catatonia (Fink and Taylor 2001), or whether they are different entities with distinct pathophysiological mechanisms which, nevertheless, strongly overlap with one another (Northoff 2002). Akinesia, muscle rigidity, hyperthermia, autonomic instability, and altered consciousness are the hallmarks of NMS, whereas posturing and staring, affective symptoms, and behavioural abnormalities (i.e. negativism, echophenomena) are uncommon or absent (Northoff 1997). Dysfunction of the nigrostriatal and anterio-infundibular dopaminergic systems characterizes NMS. Dopamine agonists, such as apomorphine, together with dantrolene provide the main treatment for this syndrome. Therefore NMS has been mainly regarded as a subcortical motor syndrome due to dysregulation of the striato-frontal motor circuit, although other neurotransmitter systems (i.e. serotoninergic, gabaergic) may also be involved (Fink and Taylor 2001).

The exact functional status of the dopaminergic system in catatonia is still unclear. [^{18}F] Dopa positron emission tomography (PET) studies in two catatonic patients failed to disclose any major abnormalities in the striatum (Northoff 2002), and we could not find any therapeutic effect of apomorphine in acute catatonia patients (Starkstein *et al.* 1996), although changes in plasma levels of homovainillic acid, a dopamine metabolite, have been described (Northoff *et al.* 1996). While there is some indirect evidence for involvement of the glutamatergic and serotoninergic systems in catatonia, the basic neurotransmitter dysfunction seems to be mostly gabaergic. Lower GABA-A receptor binding and altered right–left relations have been found in orbitofrontal, posterior parietal, and sensorimotor cortices. Furthermore, the late readiness potential, which appears to be modulated by GABA, is delayed in catatonic patients. These findings are in agreement with functional imaging studies revealing decreased perfusion or activation in medial and lateral orbitofrontal cortices, lateral prefrontal cortex, and posterior parietal and premotor–motor cortices. While behavioural and affective catatonic manifestations correlated significantly with reduced lateral and medial orbitofrontal cortical activity, respectively, motor symptoms were more closely related to parietal and premotor–motor activity. Moreover, prefrontal connectivity between orbitofrontal and premotor–motor cortex was shown to be abnormal in catatonia. Accordingly, catatonia has been regarded as a cortical psychomotor syndrome, in full agreement with Kahlbaum's original description (reviewed by Northoff 2002). Dysfunction of the direct connections between the medial orbitofrontal cortex and the brainstem nuclei could explain negative emotional processing, whereas defective motor behavioural inhibition, either internally generated (i.e. perseveration, stereotypies) or externally induced (i.e. echophenomena), as well as abnormal initiation and termination of movements and postures (akinesia, perseveration, abnormal spatial position), can also be readily ascribed to disruption of distinct frontostriatal circuits. Moreover, Northoff (2002) has suggested the term 'motor anosognosia' to label the unawareness of abnormal posture inhibition in catatonia patients, and attributed it to right posterior parietal dysfunction.

Lastly, clinical resemblances between catatonia and NMS may be accounted for by functional overlaps between 'top-down' and 'bottom-up' modulation, respectively, reflecting interaction between the prefrontal cortex and basal ganglia (Northoff 2002).

Obsessions, compulsions, and perseverations

Obsessions are recurrent and persistent thoughts, images or impulses, such as aggressive acts, ideas of filth, or sexual activity, which are experienced as intrusive and cause anxiety and distress. **Compulsions** are repetitive stereotyped involuntary acts or rituals typically involving cleaning, checking, touching, avoiding, and repetition of specific activities (American Psychiatric Association 1987). In turn, perseveration is the inappropriate persistent repetition or continuance of activity.

Obsessive–compulsive disorder (OCD) is a heterogeneous psychopathological entity including at least three main subtypes: a familial type related to tic disorders, a familial type unrelated to tics, and a non-familial type (Pauls *et al.* 1995). Recently, a new subtype of OCD associated with group A β-haemolytic streptococcal infections (GABHS) has been described and referred to as a paediatric autoimmune neuropsychiatric disorder (PANDAS) associated with GABHS (Swedo *et al.* 1998).

There is close association between obsessive–compulsive behaviour (OCB) and neurological disorder, in particular with basal ganglion pathology; they often occur in post-encephalitic parkinsonism and Tourette syndrome, and may be observed in Parkinson's disease, parkinsonism due to manganese toxicity, Huntington's and Sydenham's choreas, and Meige's syndrome, as well as with focal basal ganglion lesions (Schilder 1938; Mena *et al.* 1967; Eldridge *et al.* 1977; Jankovic and Ford 1983; Laplane *et al.* 1989). Obsessions and compulsions may also be associated with epileptogenic lesions located in the temporal and frontal cortices or in the anterior cingulate gyrus (Ward 1988; Levin and Duchowny 1991; Kroll and Drummond 1993) and observed in frontotemporal dementia (Mendez *et al.* 1997), following rupture of an anterior communicating aneurysm or traumatic brain injury (McKeon *et al.* 1984), or with more focal lesions involving frontal and temporal structures (Berthier *et al.* 1996a).

Schilder (1938) discerned 'organic' signs, such as facial rigidity, arm flexor rigidity, tremor, urge to talk, and propulsive speech features, in about one-third of cases of obsessional patients lacking any history suggestive of encephalitis.

Rachman (1974) described what he termed 'primary obsessional slowness' in OCD patients who showed severe slowness in carrying out their ordinary day-by-day activities, such as washing, dressing, or eating. Later, Hymas *et al.* (1991) studied 11 cases with obsessional slowness gleaned from 59 OCD patients, who were found to exhibit severe motor abnormalities much more frequently than OCD patients who failed to display slowness. Motor slowness was mainly due to difficulty in initiating goal-directed actions and in suppressing intrusive and perseverative behaviour; it was preceded or interrupted by hesitation. As well as deficits in simple movement initiation, they displayed difficulty in shifting between and sequencing diverse patterns of movements and in performing more than one movement simultaneously. More complex action sequences, such as dressing, were disintegrated. Their goal-directed behaviour was commonly disrupted by perseveration of unwanted movements, and some patients also manifested perseveration of hand movements elicited during examination.

While some patients showed environmental avoidance, in others there was repetitive touching of diverse body parts and increased contact with the environment. Visual checking or searching behaviour was common, and distractibility to visual and auditory stimuli was found on occasion. A striking feature was their inability to use verbal functions to guide or modify motor behaviour. This deficit can be disclosed by means of the three-step hand sequence test, whereby the patient is requested to recite aloud the words 'fist', 'slap', and 'side', while simultaneously placing the hand through the same sequence of positions. The feeling of action incompleteness was a frequent manifestation, as some patients experienced doubts, indecision, counting to themselves, perfectionism, and ruminations. Echopraxia, i.e. the unsolicited imitation of movements and gestures made by the examiner, was observed at times.

In addition to the above findings, the 11 patients with obsessional slowness displayed more 'elementary motor deficits' including decreased or increased blinking, positive glabellar tap, mild cogwheel rigidity, speech abnormalities (e.g. pressure of speech), lip curling, mirror movements of the contralateral hand when performing rapid alternating pronation–supination movements, 'mannerisms' and 'tic-like' movements, and gait anomalies. Some of these additional abnormal neurological findings were also observed in the non-slow group of patients with OCD.

Berthier *et al.* (1996a) studied 13 patients with OCD associated with brain lesions and compared them with 25 patients with idiopathic OCD. They found a considerable phenomenological overlap among both groups of patients and a similar pattern of neuropsychological deficits. Acquired OCD patients usually exhibit motor and phonic tics and had lesions involving exclusively temporal, frontal, and cingulate cortices and basal ganglion structures.

PET and single-photon emission tomography (SPET) studies in patients with OCD have disclosed aberrant hyperactivity within corticostriatal circuits involving mainly orbitofrontal, premotor, and cingulate cortices, with normal or increased activity in the caudate nucleus (Sawle *et al.* 1991; Baxter 1992). Furthermore, abnormal activity within these circuits usually decreases after successful behavioural therapy or pharmacologic treatments (McGuire 1995). Rauch *et al.* (1994) have proposed that the ventral frontostriatal circuit (projections from the anterior and lateral orbitofrontal cortex via the ventral caudate nucleus) specifically mediates obsessive manifestations. Paediatric OCD patients show increased volume of the anterior cingulate gyrus and medial thalamic regions (Rosenberg and Keshevan 1998; Gilbert *et al.* 2000) and proton magnetic resonance spectroscopy has identified functional neurochemical marker abnormalities in the medial thalamus (Fitzgerald *et al.* 2000).

The development of OCD in patients with temporal epileptogenic or non-epileptogenic lesions may be due to either disruption of amygdalohippocampal ventral striatal connections or long-term changes in pathways linking the hippocampus and parahippocampus with the DLPF and orbitofrontal cortices (Berthier *et al.* 1996a).

Finally, it has been suggested that the basal ganglia are essential for the development of automatic or semi-automatic behaviours that underlie habits in everyday life (Salmon and Butters 1995; Graybiel 1998). To form a habit, it may be necessary to 'chunk' together movements, complex acts or sequences, or cognitive acts by means of developing novel neural firing patterns that represent the motor action sequence, or that at least release the action sequences when triggered by an external or internal stimulus (Graybiel 1998). If habits are coordinated ensembles of thoughts and actions, then tics, stereotypies, and compulsions may be regarded as those prewired bits of behaviour that are available to be assembled into habits. If the release of such thoughts and actions is related to striatal dysfunction, they might represent abnormally released, and possibly abnormally 'chunked', activity patterns of corticobasal ganglion loop function (Leckman and Riddle 2000).

Over the years, a number of taxonomies have been used to classify **perseverations**, and several theories have been proposed to explain the mechanisms underlying this phenomenon. Nevertheless, there are essentially two forms of motor perseveration: the continuous repetition of an action even though the task is completed, and the impairment in switching from one action to another. The two forms of perseveration have been termed, respectively, 'clonic' and 'tonic' by Liepmann (1905), 'efferent motor' and 'cortical' by Luria (1965), 'compulsive repetition' and 'impairment of switching' by Freeman and Gathercole (1966), and 'continuous' and 'stuck-in-set' by Sandson and Albert (1984). Patients with 'clonic', 'efferent motor', 'compulsive repetition', or 'continuous' perseveration stick out their tongues repetitively instead of once as requested, keep drawing circles one on top of another when asked to draw a single circle, and/or continue to draw loops when asked to draw only three. Patients with 'tonic', 'cortical', 'impairment of switching', or 'stuck-in-set' perseveration draw a square when asked to do so, but when they are later asked to draw a triangle they again draw a complete or partial square; subsequently, when asked to draw a circle, patients again draw elements of a square. This may lead to the observation of fragments of several motor sequences combined in a single behaviour. Thus the analysis of patients' graphomotor performance (drawing) is the most valuable and practical task for eliciting and differentiating among different forms of perseveration.

Lesion studies of both animals and humans commonly view motor perseverations as a feature of frontal lobe (Luria 1965; Stuss *et al.* 1983) or frontosubcortical damage (Sandson and Albert 1984). Whereas 'efferent motor' or 'continuous' perseveration have been attributed to dorsolateral prefrontal pathology (Stuss *et al.* 1983) and prefrontal and subcortical damage (Luria 1965), 'cortical' or 'stuck-in-set' perseveration has been ascribed to mesial frontal lesions (Luria 1965) and frontosubcortical mesolimbic damage (Sandson and Albert 1984).

Finally, a third form of perseveration, named 'intentional' (Liepmann 1905) and 'recurrent' (Sandson and Albert 1984), consists of the inappropriate repetition of a previous response after an intervening response or stimulus, and has been attributed to left temporoparietal involvement (Sandson and Albert 1984).

Goldberg and Tucker (1979) have demonstrated that perseverations are ubiquitous, affecting virtually every domain of cognition and behaviour regardless of the sensory modality and the output involved. In contrast, patients with lesions outside the frontal lobe may show perseverations which are usually limited to a specific sensory modality or type of behaviour and directly related to the site of the lesion. These authors showed that perseverations in patients with frontal pathology affect multiple levels of cognitive control that are implicit in any single behaviour. They studied 19 post-operative patients with frontal lesions and found two types of perseverations: hyperkinesia-like motor perseverations (Luria's efferent perseverations) or lower-order motor perseverations, and higher-order perseverations which include not only the cortical type of Luria's perseverations, but also other subtypes which would reflect deficits at higher levels of a cognitive hierarchy (i.e. generic spatial characteristics and semantic categories) that satisfies these requirements.

Agitation, irritability, aggression, and self-injurious behaviour

The term **psychomotor agitation** denotes excessive motor activity associated with the feeling of inner tension (Salloway and Cummings 1994), while **irritability** is defined as a feeling state characterized by reduced control of the temper, which usually results in irritable verbal or behavioural outbursts (Snaith and Taylor 1985). It has been hypothesized that hyperactive behaviour (i.e. agitation, irritation, euphoria) in Huntington's disease and Tourette syndrome results from an excitatory subcortical output through the frontomedial and orbitofrontal circuits to the pallidum, thalamus, and cortex, which may occur with the concomitant excitatory stimulation of the motor cortices, leading to either chorea or tics (Litvan *et al.* 1998; Kulisevsky *et al.* 2001). Functional imaging studies support this view since they have demonstrated reduced metabolic rates in basal ganglia (putamen and caudate in Huntington's disease and ventral striatum in Tourette syndrome) that coexist with normal or increased metabolism in various cortical regions (Antonini *et al.* 1996; Eidelberg *et al.* 1997; Andrews and Brooks 1998). Even aggressiveness in Huntington's disease has been considered part of the frontal lobe syndrome (Rosenblat and Leroi 2000). Davidson *et al.* (2000) suggested that impulsive aggression and violence reflect abnormalities in the motion regulation circuitry of the brain (individuals are unable to regulate negative affects and respond appropriately to the anticipated consequences of their behaviour) made up by the orbitofrontal circuit and interconnected structures including other prefrontal territories, the anterior cingulate gyrus, the amygdala, and the ventral striatum.

Whereas hypoactive behaviour (e.g. apathy) is associated mainly with hypokinetic movement disorders (i.e. Parkinson's disease, progressive nuclear palsy), hyperactive behaviour (e.g. agitation) is particularly observed in hyperkinetic movement disorders such as Huntington's disease, Sydenham's chorea, and Tourette syndrome (Litvan *et al.* 1998; Kulisevsky *et al.* 2001), and also in fluctuating patients with Parkinson's disease, in whom agitated, even manic, states may develop together with dyskinesias during ON periods (Menza *et al.* 1990).

Patients with Tourette syndrome frequently develop **self-injurious behaviour** in association with echo- and coprophenomena as well as comorbid general psychopathology (Robertson *et al.* 1989). Self-injuries, such as self-attempted strangulation, eye injuries, and pulling out the tongue, may initially occur in response to external provocative stimuli (e.g. stressful visual scenes), although thereafter the abnormal motor behaviour is automatically executed in the absence of intrusive thoughts or mental images, which has led to the suggestion that it is generated in subcortical structures (Lang *et al.* 1994; Berthier *et al.* 1996b). In fact, increased metabolic activity in the caudate, thalamus, anterior cingulate gyrus, and mesial frontal cortex, which resolved after limbic leucotomy, has been described in a Tourette syndrome patient with compulsion to harm himself and obsessional slowness (Sawle *et al.* 1993). Autonomous self-aggressive activity has also been described in patients with epileptogenic foci or destructive lesions in the mesial frontal lobe (Waterman *et al.* 1987; Banks *et al.* 1989).

Action-sequencing deficits

Patients with **dysexecutive syndrome** due to dorsolateral prefrontal lesions exhibit deficits in higher-order cognitive abilities, including focused and sustained attention, working memory, problem-solving, decision-making, and planning and regulation of adaptive goal-directed behaviour (Manes *et al.* 2002), which may result in severe disorganization of action control. They are unable to plan novel actions and to use verbal functions to guide motor activity. This deficit is evident in the daily behaviour of the patient, who performs incorrectly despite clear instructions, and during examination, where the patient is unable to use verbal cues to guide the three-step hand sequence ('fist', 'slap', and 'side') or to perform alternating and reciprocal programmes (Luria 1965; Stuss and Benson 1984). Patients may develop motor perseveration or motor impersistence and may have a severe action-sequencing deficit (Sirigu *et al.* 1995; Zanini *et al.* 2002).

Frontal lobe damage can cause impairment in action processing at both the schema type action and script levels, but not at the motor schema level. The terms frontal apraxia (Luria 1966) or action disorganization syndrome (Humphreys and Forde 1998) refer to the derangement of schema-type actions with frequent errors such as step omissions, anticipations, utilizations, and perseverations which affect the correct planning of a routine action sequence like 'prepare coffee' (Duncan *et al.* 1996; Schwartz *et al.* 1991, 1998; Humphreys and Forde 1998). This type of action-sequencing deficit has been described with large lesions involving the frontal lobe and on occasion extending beyond its boundaries. However, patients with prefrontal cortex lesions are characteristically affected at a higher level of cognitive control in the processing of the temporal structure of script actions (Sirigu *et al.* 1995; Zanini *et al.* 2002).

While cognitive planning and spatial working memory deficits are core features of Parkinson's disease (Owen *et al.* 1992; Gabrieli 1996), severe cognitive motor disorders such as those observed in frontal-lobe-damaged patients are absent. However, bilateral lesions at the output level of the frontostriatal circuits (e.g. globus pallidus), produced either naturally or surgically, may cause marked motivational and cognitive–motor disorders (Laplane *et al.* 1989; Stuss *et al.* 1989; Trepanier *et al.* 2000; Merello *et al.* 2001). In addition to psychic akinesia (see above), patients may develop environmental dependence and imitative and utilization behaviour, as described by Lhermitte *et al.* (1986) in patients with bilateral orbitofrontal lesions (see Chapter 20).

Lesions involving the rostral and dorsomedial regions of the GPi produce the most severe cognitive–motor impairment, consistent with the fact that these GPi regions contain neurons that project to prefrontal areas 46 and 9 (Middleton and Strick 2000a,b).

We studied two patients with Parkinson's disease refractory to medical treatment and severe drug-induced dyskinesias who underwent bilateral pallidotomy (C. Abeleira *et al.*, Unpublished data). Both patients developed apathy and marked speech and swallowing difficulties. They were oriented in time and place, and language was normal in both patients although memory was mildly affected. Executive functions were severely impaired. Although both patients exhibited temporospatial errors when pantomiming transitive gestures to verbal command, neither showed any type of praxic errors either during gesture imitation or when using single tools/objects. Performance on multiple object use task (MOT) was normal in both patients. However, both showed impaired performance when asked to arrange in the correct sequence a set of photographs each depicting one of the same five everyday actions produced in the MOT task. Furthermore, both scored far below normal when requested to order five script-type actions, using pictures and verbal descriptions, in the correct temporal sequence. Thus both patients exhibited action-sequencing deficits similar to those presented by frontal patients (Zanini *et al.* 2002), consistent with disruption of the dorsolateral prefrontal striatal circuit.

Conclusions

Cognitive and motivated motor behavioural deficits observed in various neurological and psychiatric conditions may be interpreted as manifestations of a common underlying dysfunction of a 'goal-directed behavioural system' centred around the frontostriatal circuitry, but working and interacting with posterior brain systems and cerebrocerebellar networks. Future anatomical, functional neuroimaging, and more refined clinical studies will lead to a deeper insight into the processes, representations, and their interactions involved in the wide spectrum of behaviour that comprises goal-directed actions, as well as their disorders.

References

Alexander GE, Crutcher MD (1990). Functional architecture of basal ganglia circuits: neural substrates of parallel processing. *Trends Neurosci*, **13**, 266–71.

Alexander GE, Delong MP, Strick PL (1986). Parallel organizations of functionally segregated circuit linking basal ganglia and cortex. *Annu Rev Neurosci*, **9**, 357–81.

American Psychiatric Association (1987). *Diagnostic and Statistical Manual of Mental Disorders*, 3rd edn, revised. Washington, DC: American Psychiatric Association.

Andersson S, Krogstad JM, Finset A (1999). Apathy and depressed mood in acquired brain damage: relationship to lesion localization and psychophysiological reactivity. *Psychol Med*, **29**, 447–56.

Andrews TC, Brooks DJ (1998). Advances in the understanding of early Huntington's disease using the functional imaging techniques of PET and SPET. *Mol Med Today*, **4**, 532–9.

Antonini A, Leenders KL, Spiegel R, Meier D, Vontobel P, Weigall-Weber M, *et al.* (1996). Striatal glucose metabolism and dopamine D2 receptor binding in asymptomatic gene carriers and patients with Huntington's disease. *Brain*, **119**, 2085–95.

Baillarger JG (1843). De l'etal désigné chez les aliénés sous le nom de stupidité. In *Recherches sur les Maladies Mentales*. Paris: Masson.

Ballard DH, Hayhoe MM, Pook PK, Rao RP (1997). Deictic codes for the embodiment of cognition. *Behav Brain Sci*, **20**, 723–67.

Banks G, Short P, Martínez AJ, Latchaw R, Ratcliff G, Boller F (1989) Alien hand syndrome: clinical and post mortem findings. *Arch Neurol*, **46**, 456–9.

Barris RW, Schuman HR (1953). Bilateral anterior cingulate gyrus lesions; syndrome of the anterior cingulate gyri. *Neurology*, **3**, 44–52.

Baxter LR (1992). Neuroimaging studies of obsessive–compulsive disorder. *Psychiatr Clin North Am*, **15**, 871–84.

Berardelli A, Rothwell JC, Thompson PD, Hallett M (2001). Pathophysiology of bradykinesia in Parkinson's disease. *Brain*, **124**, 2131–46.

Berthier M, Kulisevsky J, Gironell A, Heras J (1996a). Obsessive–compulsive disorder associated with brain lesions: clinical phenomenology, cognitive function, and anatomic correlates. *Neurology*, **47**, 353–61.

Berthier M, Campos V, Kulisevsky J (1996b). Echopraxia and self-injurious behavior in Tourette's syndrome. A case report. *Neuropsychiatry Neuropsychol Behav Neurol*, **9**, 280–3.

Bhatia KP, Marsden CD (1994). The behavioural and motor consequences of focal lesions of the basal ganglia in man. *Brain*, **117**, 859–76.

Bogousslavsky J, Regli F (1990). Capsular genu syndrome. *Neurology*, **40**, 1499–1502.

Brass M, Zyssef S, von Cramon DI (2001). The inhibition of iniciative response tendencies. *Neuroimage*, **14**, 1416–23.

Braver TS, Barch DM, Gray JR, Molfese DL, Snyder A (2001). Anterior cingulate cortex and response conflict: effects of frequency, inhibition and errors. *Cereb Cortex*, **11**, 825–36.

Brown R, Pluck G (2000). Negative symptoms: the 'pathology' of motivation and goal-directed behaviour. *Trends Neurosci*, **23**, 412–17.

Cairns H, Oldfield RC, Pennybacker JB, Whitteridge D (1941). Akinetic mutism with an epermoid cyst of the third ventricle. *Brain*, **75**, 109–46.

Caplan LR, Schmahmann JD, Kase CS, Feldmann E, Baquis G, Greenberg JP, *et al.* (1990). Caudate infarcts. *Arch Neurol*, **47**, 133–43.

Casey BJ, Castellanos FX, Giedd JN, Marsh WL, Hamburger SD, Schubert AB, *et al.* (1997). Implication of right frontostriatal circuitry in response inhibition and attention-deficit/hyperactivity disorder. *J Am Acad Child Adolesc Psychiatry*, **36**, 374–83.

Cummings JL (1993). Frontal-subcortical circuits and human behavior. *Arch Neurol*, **50**, 873–80.

Damasio AR (1994). *Descartes' Error*. New York: Putnam.

Davidson RJ, Irwin W (1999). The functional neuroanatomy of emotion and affective style. *Trends Cogn Sci*, **3**, 11–21.

Davidson R, Putnam K, Larson C (2000). Dysfunction in the neural circuitry of emotion regulation—a possible prelude to violence. *Science*, **289**, 591–4.

Deiber MP, Passingham RE, Colebatch JG, Friston KJ, Nixon PD, Frackowiak RS (1991). Cortical areas and the selection of movement: a study with positron emission tomography. *Exp Brain Res*, **84**, 393–402.

Deiber MP, Ibanez V, Sadato N, Hallett M (1996). Cerebral structures participating in motor preparation in humans: a positron emission tomography study. *J Neurophysiol*, **75**, 233–47.

DeLong MR (1990). Primate models of movement disorders of basal ganglia origin. *Trends Neurosci*, **13**, 281–5.

D'Esposito M, Ballard D, Aguirre GK, Zarahn E (1998). Human prefrontal cortex is not specific for working memory: a functional MRI study. *Neuroimage*, **8**, 274–82.

Devinsky O, Lemann W, Evans AC, Moeller JR, Rottenberg DA (1987). Akinetic mutism in a bone marrow transplant recipient following total-body irradiation and amphotericin B chemoprophylaxis. A positron emission tomographic and neuropathologic study. *Arch Neurol*, **44**, 414–17.

Dick JP, Rothwell JC, Berardelli A, Thompson PD, Gioux M, Benecke R, *et al.* (1986). Associated postural adjustments in Parkinson's disease. *J Neurol Neurosurg Psychiatry*, **49**, 1378–85.

Duncan J, Emslie H, Williams P, Johnson R, Freer C (1996). Intelligence and the frontal lobe: the organization of goal-directed behavior. *Cogn Psychol*, **30**, 257–303.

Eidelberg D, Moeller JR, Antonini A, Kazumata K, Dhawan V, Budman C, *et al.* (1997). The metabolic anatomy of Tourette's syndrome. *Neurology*, **48**, 927–34.

Eldridge R, Sweet R, Lake R, Ziegler M, Shapiro AK (1977). Gilles de la Tourette's syndrome: clinical, genetic, psychologic, and biochemical aspects in 21 selected families. *Neurology*, **27**, 115–24.

Elliott R, Dolan R, Frith C. (2000). Dissociable functions in the medial and lateral orbitofrontal cortex: evidence from human neuroimaging studies. *Cereb Cortex*, **10**, 308–17.

Escola L, Michelet T, Macia F, Guehl D, Bioulac B, Burbaud P (2003). Disruption of information processing in the supplementary motor area of the MPTP-treated monkey: a clue to the pathophysiology of akinesia? *Brain*, **126**, 95–114.

Eslinger PJ, Warner GC, Grattan LM, Easton JD (1991). 'Frontal lobe' utilization behavior associated with paramedian thalamic infarction. *Neurology*, **41**, 450–2.

Evarts EV, Wise SP (1984). Basal ganglia outputs and motor control. *Ciba Found Symp*, **107**, 83–102.

Fink GR, Marshall JC, Halligan PW, Frith CD, Driver J, Frackowiak RS, *et al.* (1999). The neural consequences of conflict between intention and the senses. *Brain*, **122**, 497–512.

Fink M, Taylor MA (2001). The many varieties of catatonia. *Eur Arch Psychiatry Clin Neurosci*, **251** (Suppl 1), 1/8–13.

Fitzgerald KD, Moore GJ, Paulson LD, Stewart CM, Rosenberg DR (2000). Proton spectroscopic imaging of the thalamus in treatment-naive pediatric obsessive compulsive disorder. *Biol Psychol*, **47**, 174–82.

Fleet WS, Valenstein E, Watson RT, Heilman KM (1987). Dopamine agonist therapy for neglect in humans. *Neurology*, **37**, 1765–70.

Freeman T, Gathercole CE (1966). Perseveration—the clinical symptoms—in chronic schizophrenia and organic dementia. *Br J Psychiatry*, **112**, 27–32.

Frith CD, Friston K, Liddle PF, Frackowiak RS (1991). Willed action and the prefrontal cortex in man: a study with PET. *Proc R Soc Lond B Biol Sci*, **244**, 241–6.

Fuster JM (1997). *The Prefrontal Cortex*. New York: Raven Press.

Gabrieli JD (1996). Memory systems analyses of mnemonic disorders in aging and age-related diseases. *Proc Natl Acad Sci USA*, **93**, 13534–40.

Garavan H, Ross TJ, Stein EA (1999). Right hemispheric dominance of inhibitory control: an event-related functional MRI study. *Proc Natl Acad Sci USA*, **96**, 8301–6.

Gelenberg AJ (1976). The catatonia syndrome. *Lancet*, i, 1339–40.

Gentilini M, De Renzi E, Crisi G (1987). Bilateral paramedian thalamic artery infarcts: report of eight cases. *J Neurol Neurosurg Psychiatry*, **50**, 900–9.

Gilbert AR, Moore GJ, Keshavan MS, Paulson LD, Narula V, MacMaster PP, *et al.* (2000). Decrease in thalamic volumes of pediatric patients with obsessive–compulsive disorder who are taking paroxetine. *Arch Gen Psychiatry*, **57**, 449–56.

Gjessing LR (1974). A review of periodic catatonia. *Biol Psychiatry*, **8**, 23–45.

Goldberg E, Tucker D (1979). Motor perseverations and the levels of encoding a visual form. *J Clin Neuropsychol*, **4**, 273–88.

Graybiel AM (1998). The basal ganglia and chunking of action repertoires. *Neurobiol Learn Mem*, **70**, 119–36.

Groenewegen HJ, Berendse HW (1994). The specificity of the 'nonspecific' midline and intralaminar thalamic nuclei. *Trends Neurosci*, **17**, 52–7.

Haber SN, Fudge JL, McFarland NR (2000). Stritonigrostriatal pathways in primates form an ascending spiral from the shell to the dorsolateral striatum. *J Neurosci*, **20**, 2369–82.

Hamilton M (1976). *Fish's Schizophrenia*, 2nd edn. Bristol: John Wright.

Haslinger B, Erhard P, Kampfe N, Boecker M, Rummery E, Schwaiger M, *et al.* (2001). Event-related functional magnetic resonance imaging in Parkinson's disease before and after levodopa. *Brain*, **124**, 558–70.

Haussermann P, Wilhelm T, Keinath S, Stolze C, Conrad B, Ceballos-Baumann A (2001). Primary central nervous system lymphoma in the SMA presenting as rapidly progressive parkinsonism. *Mov Disord*, **16**, 962–5.

Humphreys GW, Forde EME (1998). Disordered action schema and action disorganization syndrome. *Cogn Neuropsychol*, **15**, 771–811.

Hunter R, Blackwood W, Bull J (1968). Three cases of frontal meningiomas presenting psychiatrically. *BMJ*, **114**, 137–60.

Hymas N, Lees A, Bolton D, Epps K, Head D (1991). The neurology of obsessional slowness. *Brain*, **114**, 2203–33.

Inbody S, Jankovic J (1986). Hyperkinetic mutism: bilateral ballism and basal ganglia calcification. *Neurology*, **36**, 825–7.

Jahanshahi M, Jenkins IH, Brown RG, Marsden CD, Passingham RE, Brooks DJ (1995). Self-initiated versus externally triggered movements. I. An investigation using measurement of regional cerebral blood flow with PET and movement-related potentials in normal and Parkinson's disease subjects. *Brain*, **118**, 913–33.

Jankovic J, Ford J (1983). Blepharospasm and orofacial-cervical dystonia: clinical and pharmacological findings in 100 patients. *Ann Neurol*, **13**, 402–11.

Joel D (2001). Open interconnected model of basal ganglia-thalamocortical circuitry and its relevance to the clinical syndrome of Huntington's disease. *Mov Disord*, **16**, 407–23.

Joel D, Weiner I (1994). The organization of the basal ganglia-thalamocortical circuits: open interconnected rather than closed segregated. *Neuroscience*, **63**, 363–79.

Joel D, Weiner I (2000). The connections of the dopaminergic system with the striatum in rats and primates: an analysis with respect to the functional and compartmental organization of the striatum. *Neuroscience*, **96**, 451–74.

Kahlbaum KL (1874). *Die Katatonie oder das Spannungsirreseins*. Berlin: Hirschwald.

Klee A (1961). Akinetic mutism: review of the literature and report of a case. *J Nerv Ment Dis*, **133**, 536–53.

Koechlin E, Corrado G, Pietrini P, Grafman J (2000). Dissociating the role of the medial and lateral anterior prefrontal cortex in human planning. *Proc Natl Acad Sci USA*, **97**, 7651–6.

Kraepelin E (1920). Die Erscheinungsformen des Irreseins. *Z Gesamte Neurol Psychiatrie*, **62**, 1–30.

Kroll L, Drummond LM (1993). Temporal lobe epilepsy and obsessive–compulsive symptoms. *J Nerv Ment Dis*, **181**, 457–8.

Kulisevsky J, Litvan I, Berthier ML, Pascual-Sedano B, Paulsen JS, Cummings JL (2001). Neuropsychiatric assessment of Gilles de la Tourette patients: comparative study with other hyperkinetic and hypokinetic movement disorders. *Mov Disord*, **16**, 1098–104.

Lang A, Consky E, Sandor P (1994). 'Signing tics'—insights into the pathophysiology of symptoms in Tourette's syndrome. *Ann Neurol*, **33**, 212–15.

Laplane D, Degos JD, Baulac M, Gray F (1981). Bilateral infarction of the anterior cingulate gyri and of the fornices. Report of a case. *J Neurol Sci*, **51**, 289–300.

Laplane D, Baulac M, Widlocher D, Dubois B (1984). Pure psychic akinesia with bilateral lesions of basal ganglia. *J Neurol Neurosurg Psychiatry*, **47**(4), 377–85.

Laplane D, Levasseur M, Pillon B, Dubois B, Baulac M, Mazoyer B, *et al.* (1989). Obsessive–compulsive and other behavioral changes with bilateral basal ganglia lesions. A neuropsychological, magnetic resonance imaging and positron tomography study. *Brain*, **112**, 699–725.

Lavy S (1959). Akinetic mutism in a case of craniopharyngioma. *Psychiatr Neurol (Basel)*, **138**, 369–74.

Leckman JF, Riddle MA (2000). Tourette's syndrome: when habit-forming systems form habits of their own? *Neuron*, **28**, 349–54.

Levin B, Duchowny M (1991). Childhood obsessive–compulsive disorder and cingulated epilepsy. *Biol Psychiatry*, **30**, 1049–55.

Lhermitte F, Pillon B, Serdarn M (1986). Human anatomy and the frontal lobes. Part I: Initation and utilization behaviour: a neuropsychological tendency of 75 patients. *Ann Neurol*, **19**, 326–34.

Liepmann HL (1905). *Die perseveration. Veber Storungen des Handelns bei Gehirnkrauber.* Berlin: Karger.

Litvan I, Paulsen JS, Mega MS, Cummings JL (1998). Neuropsychiatric behavioral assessment of patients with hyperkinetic and hypokinetic movement disorders. *Arch Neurol*, **55**, 1313–19. Erratum: *Arch Neurol*, **55**, 1591.

Logue V, Durward M, Pratt RT, Piercy M, Nixon WL (1968). The quality of survival after rupture of an anterior cerebral aneurysm. *Br J Psychiatry*, **114**, 137–60.

Luria AR (1965). Two kinds of motor persseveration in massive injury of the frontal lobes. *Brain*, **88**, 1–9.

Luria AR (1966). *Higher Cortical Functions in Man.* London: Tavistock Press.

McFarland NR, Haber SN (2002). Thalamic relay nuclei of the basal ganglia form both reciprocal and nonreciprocal cortical connections, linking multiple frontal cortical areas. *J Neurosci*, **22**, 8117–32.

McGuire PK (1995). The brain in obsessive–compulsive disorder. *J Neurol Neurosurg Psychiatry*, **59**, 457–9.

McKeon J, McGuffin P, Robinson P (1984). Obsessive–compulsive neurosis following head injury. A report of four cases. *Br J Psychiatry*, **144**, 190–2.

Manes F, Sahakian B, Clark L, Rogers R, Antoun A, Aitken M, *et al.* (2002). Decision-making processes following damage to the prefrontal cortex. *Brain*, **125**, 624–39.

Marin RS (1991). Apathy: a neuropsychiatric syndrome. *J Neuropsychiatry Clin Neurosci*, **3**, 243–54.

Marsden CD, Tarsy D, Baldessarini RJ (1975). Spontaneous and drug-induced movement disorders in psychiatry patients. In DF Benson, D Blumer, (ed.) *Psychiatric Aspects of Neurological Disease*, pp. 219–65. New York: Grune & Stratton.

Mega MS, Cummings JL (1994). Frontal–subcortical circuits and neuropsychiatric disorders. *J Neuropsychiatry Clin Neurosci*, **6**, 358–70.

Mena I, Marin O, Fuenzalida S, Cotzias GC (1967). Chronic manganese poisoning. Clinical picture and manganese turnover. *Neurology*, **17**, 128–36.

Mendez MF, Perryman KM, Miller BL, Swartz JR, Cummings JL (1997). Compulsive behaviors as presenting symptoms of frontotemporal dementia. *J Geriatr Psychiatry Neurol*, **10**, 154–7.

Menza MA, Sage J, Marshall E, Cody R, Duvoisin R (1990). Mood changes and 'on–off' phenomena in Parkinson's disease. *Mov Disord*, **5**, 148–51.

Merello M, Starkstein S, Nouzeilles MI, Kuzis G, Leiguarda R (2001). Bilateral pallidotomy for treatment of Parkinsons's disease induced corticobulbar syndrome and psychic akinesia avoidable by globus pallidus lesion combined with contralateral stimulation. *J Neurol Neurosurg Psychiatry*, **71**, 611–14.

Messert B, Henke TK, Langheim W (1966). Syndrome of akinetic mutism associated with obstructive hydrocephalus. *Neurology*, **16**, 635–49.

Middleton FA, Strick PL (2000a). Basal ganglia and cerebellar loops: motor and cognitive circuits. *Brain Res Brain Res Rev*, **31**, 236–50.

Middleton FA, Strick PL (2000b). A revised neuroanatomy of frontal subcortical circuits. In DG Lichter, JL Cummings, (ed.) *Frontal Subcortical Circuits in Psychiatric and Neurological Disorders*, pp. 44–58. New York: Guilford Press.

Mink JW (1996). The basal ganglia: focused selection and inhibition of competing motor programs. *Progr Neurobiol*, **50**, 381–425.

Northoff G (1997). *Catatonia—A Psychomotor Syndrome.* Stuttgart: Enke.

Northoff G (2002). Catatonia and neuroleptic malignant syndrome: psychopathology and pathophysiology. *J Neural Transm*, **109**, 1453–67.

Northoff G, Demisch L, Wenke J, Pflug B (1996). Plasma homovanillic acid concentrations in catatonia. *Biol Psychiatry*, **39**, 436–43.

Öngür D, Price JL (2000). The organization of networks within the orbital and medial prefrontal cortex of rats, monkeys and humans. *Cereb Cortex*, **10**, 206–19.

Owen AM, James M, Leigh PN, Summers BA, Marsden CD, Quinn NP, *et al.* (1992). Fronto-striatal cognitive deficits at different stages of Parkinson's disease. *Brain*, **115**, 1727–51.

Parent A, Hazrati LN (1995a). Functional anatomy of the basal ganglia. I. The cortico-basal ganglio-thalamo-cortical loop. *Brain Res Rev*, **20**, 91–127.

Parent A, Hazrati LN (1995b). Functional anatomy of the basal ganglia. II. The place of subthalamic nucleus and external pallidum basal ganglia circuitry. *Brain Res Rev*, **20**, 128–54.

Passingham R (1993). *The Frontal Lobes and Voluntary Action.* Oxford: Oxford University Press.

Passingham RE, Toni I (2001). Contrasting the dorsal and ventral visual systems: guidance of movement versus decision making. *Neuroimage*, **14**, S125–31.

Pauls DL, Alsobrook JP, Goodman W, Rasmussen S, Leckman JF (1995) A family study of obsessive–compulsive disorder. *Am J Psychiatry*, **152**, 76–84.

Paus T, Koski L, Caramanos Z, Westbury C (1998). Regional differences in the effects of task difficulty and motor output on blood flow response in the human anterior cingulate cortex: a review of 107 PET activation studies. *NeuroReport*, **9**, R37–47.

Phillips S, Sangalang V, Stern G (1987). Basal forebrain infection, a clinico-pathologic correlation. *Arch Neurol*, **49**, 1134–8.

Powell JH, al-Adawi S, Morgan J, Greenwood RJ (1996). Motivational deficits after brain injury: effects of bromocriptine in 11 patients. *J Neurol Neurosurg Psychiatry*, **60**, 416–21.

Rachman S (1974). Primary obsessional slowness. *Behav Res Ther*, **12**, 9–18.

Rauch SL, Jenike MA, Alpert NM (1994). Regional cerebral blood flow measured during symptom provocation in obsessive compulsive disorder using oxygen ^{15}O-labeled carbon dioxide and positron emission tomography. *Arch Gen Psychiatry*, **51**, 62–70.

Rizzolatti G, Luppino G, Matelli M (1998). The organization of the cortical motor system: new concepts. *Electroencephalogr Clin Neurophysiol*, **106**, 283–96.

Robertson MM, Trimble MR, Lees AJ (1989). Self-injurious behaviour and the Gilles de la Tourette syndrome: a clinical study and review of the literature. *Psychol Med*, **19**, 611–25.

Rolls ET (1994). Neurophysiology and cognitive functions of the striatum. *Rev Neurol (Paris)*, **150**, 648–60.

Rolls ET (1996). The orbitofrontal cortex. *Philos Trans R Soc Lond B Biol Sci*, **351**, 1433–44.

Rosenberg DR, Keshavan MS (1998). Toward a neurodevelopmental model of obsessive compulsive disorder. *Biol Psychiatry*, **43**, 623–40.

Rosenblatt A, Leroi I (2000). The neuropsychiatry of Huntington's disease and basal ganglia disorders. *Psychosomatics*, **41**, 24–30.

Ross ED, Stewart RM (1981). Akinetic mutism from hypothalamic damage: successful treatment with dopamine agonists. *Neurology*, **31**, 1435–9.

Rowe JB, Toni I, Josephs O, Frackowiak RS, Passingham RE (2000). The prefrontal cortex: response selection or maintenance within working memory? *Science*, **288**, 1656–60.

Sakai ST, Stepniewska I, Qi HX, Kaas JH (2000). Pallidal and cerebellar afferents to pre-supplementary motor area thalamocortical neurons in the owl monkey: a multiple labeling study. *J Comp Neurol*, **417**, 164–80.

Salloway S, Cummings J (1994). Subcortical disease and neuropsychiatric illness. *J Neuropsychiatry Clin Neurosci*, **6**, 93–9.

Salmon DP, Butters N (1995). Neurobiology of skill and habit learning. *Curr Opin Neurobiol*, **5**, 184–90.

Sandson J, Albert ML (1984). Varieties of perseveration. *Neuropsychologia*, **22**, 715–32.

Sandson TA, Daffner KR, Carvalho PA, Mesulam MM (1991). Frontal lobe dysfunction following infarction of the left-sided medial thalamus. *Arch Neurol*, **48**, 1300–3.

Saper CB (1996). Role of the cerebral cortex and striatum in emotional motor response. *Progr Brain Res*, **107**, 537–50.

Sawle GV, Lees AJ, Hymas NF, Lees AJ, Frackowiak RSJ (1991). Obsessional slowness: functional studies with positron emission tomography. *Brain*, **114**, 2191–202.

Sawle GV, Lees AJ, Hymas NF, Brooks DJ, Frackowiak RS (1993). The metabolic effects of limbic leucotomy in Gilles de la Tourette syndrome. *J Neurol Neurosurg Psychiatry*, **56**, 1016–19.

Schilder P (1938). The organic background of obsession and compulsion. *Am J Psychiatry*, **94**, 1397–416.

Schultz W (2000). Multiple reward signals in the brain. *Nat Rev Neurosci*, **1**, 199–207.

Schultz W, Tremblay L, Hollerman JR (2000). Reward processing in primate orbitofrontal cortex and basal ganglia. *Cereb Cortex*, **10**, 272–83.

Schwartz MF, Reeds ES, Montgomery HW, Palmer C, Mayer NH (1991). The quantitative description of action disorgnization after brain damage. *Cogn Neuropsychol*, **8**, 341–414.

Schwartz MF, Montgomery MW, Buxbaum LJ, Lee SS, Carew TG, Coslett HB, *et al.* (1998). Naturalistic action impairment in clsoed head injury. *Neuropsychology*, **12** (1). 13–28.

Segarra JH (1971). After image test with polarized light. *Ann Ocul (Paris)*, **204**, 981–8.

Shadmehr R, Holcomb HH (1999). Inhibitory control of competing motor memories. *Exp Brain Res*, **126**, 235–51.

Shallice T, Burgess P (1996). Response suppression, initiation and strategy use following frontal lobe lesions. *Neuropsychologia*, **34**, 263–72.

Sirigu A, Zalla T, Pillon B, Grafman J, Agid Y, Dubois B (1995). Selective impairments in managerial knowledge following pre-frontal cortex damage. *Cortex*, **31**, 301–16.

Snaith RP, Taylor CM (1985). Irritability: definition, assessment and associated factors. *Br J Psychiatry*, **147**, 127–36.

Starkstein SE, Manes F (2000). Apathy and depression following stroke. *CNS Spectr*, **5**, 43–50.

Starkstein S, Berthier M, Leiguarda R (1989). Psychic akinesia following bilateral pallidal lesions. *Int J Psychiatry Med*, **19**, 155–64.

Starkstein SE, Mayberg HS, Preziosi TJ, Andrezejewski P, Leiguarda R, Robinson RG (1992). Reliability validity and clinical correlates of apathy in Parkinson's disease. *J Neuropsychiatry Clin Neurosci*, **4**, 134–9.

Starkstein S, Petracca G, Teson A, Merello M, Leiguarda R (1996). Catatonia in depression: prevalence, clinical correlates and validation of a scale. *J Neurol Neurosurg Psychiatry*, **60**, 326–32.

Stephan KE, Marshall JC, Friston KJ, Rowe JB, Ritzl A, Zilles K, *et al.* (2003). Lateralized cognitive processes and lateralized task control in the human brain. *Science*, **301**, 384–6.

Strub RL (1989). Frontal lobe syndrome in a patient with bilateral globus pallidus lesions. *Arch Neurol*, **46**, 1024–7.

Stuss DT, Benson DF (1984). Neuropsychological studies of the frontal lobes. *Psychol Bull*, **95**, 3–28.

Stuss DT, Benson DF, Kaplan EF, Weir WS, Naeser MA, Lieberman I, *et al.* (1983). The involvement of orbitofrontal cerebrum in cognitive tasks. *Neuropsychologia*, **21**, 235–48.

Stuss DT, Guberman A, Nelson R, Larochelle S (1988). The neuropsychology of paramedian thalamic infarction. *Brain Cogn*, **8**, 348–78.

Stuss DT, Stethem LL, Hugenholtz H, Picton T, Pivik J, Richard MT (1989). Reaction time after head injury: fatigue, divided and focused attention, and consistency of performance. *J Neurol Neurosurg Psychiatry*, **52**, 742–8.

Swedo SE, Leonard HL, Garvey M, Mittleman B, Allen AJ, Perlmutter S, *et al.* (1998). Pediatric autoimmune neuropsychiatric disorders associated with streptococcal infections: clinical description of the first 50 cases. *Am J Psychiatry*, **155**, 264–71. Erratum: *Am J Psychiatry*, **155**, 578.

Tanji J, Hoshi E (2001). Behavioral planning in the prefrontal cortex. *Curr Opin Neurobiol*, **11**, 164–70.

Trepanier L, Kumar R, Lozano A, Lang A, Saint-Cyr JA (2000). Neuropsychological outcome of neurosurgical therapies in Parkinson's disease: a comparison of GPi Pallidotomy and deep brain stimulation of GPi or STN. *Brain Cogn*, **42**, 324–47.

Wagner AD, Maril A, Bjork RA, Schacter DL (2001). Prefrontal contributions to executive control: fMRI evidence for functional distinctions within lateral Prefrontal cortex. *Neuroimage*, **14**, 1337–47.

Ward C (1988). Transient feelings of compulsion caused by hemispheric lesions: three cases. *J Neurol Neurosurg Psychiatry*, **51**, 266–8.

Watanabe J, Sugiura M, Sato K, Sato Y, Maeda Y, Matsue Y, *et al.* (2002). The human prefrontal and parietal association cortices are involved in NO-GO performances: an event-related fMRI study. *Neuroimage*, **17**, 1207–16.

Waterman K, Purves SJ, Kosaka B (1987). An epileptic syndrome caused by mesial frontal lobe seizure foci. *Neurology*, **37**, 577–82.

Wernicke C (1900). *Grundriss der Psychiatrie*. Leipzig: Thieme.

Yelnik J (2002). Functional anatomy of the basal ganglia. *Mov Disord*, **17**, S15–21.

Zanini S, Rumiati R, Shallice T (2002). Action sequencing deficit following frontal lobe lesion. *Neurocase*, **8**, 88–99.

Chapter 24

Delusions of control: a disorder of forward models of the motor system

Sarah-Jayne Blakemore

Summary

How do we know that our own actions belong to us? How are we able to distinguish self-generated sensory events from those that arise externally? In this chapter I evaluate one class of symptoms associated with schizophrenia that are characterized by a confusion between the self and other: a delusion of control. It has been proposed that this symptom arises because of a failure in the mechanism by which the predicted consequences of self-produced actions are derived from an internal forward model. I shall review psychophysical and neuroimaging studies that have investigated how we recognize the consequences of our own actions, and why patients with delusions of control confuse self-produced and externally produced actions and sensations. Studies investigating the failure of this 'self-monitoring' mechanism in patients with delusions of control will be discussed in the context of the hypothesis that overactivity in the parietal cortex and the cerebellum contribute to the misattribution of an action to an external source.

Introduction

> My fingers pick up the pen, but I don't control them. What they do is nothing to do with me.
> (Mellors 1970)

Delusions of alien control are symptoms associated with schizophrenia in which people misattribute self-generated actions to an external source (Schneider 1959). The actions in question can be mundane, such as picking up a cup or combing one's hair. Auditory hallucinations are common in schizophrenia, and normally consist of hearing spoken speech or voices (Johnstone 1991). Both delusions of alien and auditory hallucinations are included as 'first-rank' features in schizophrenia (Schneider 1959).

Normally, we can readily detect whether a movement is self-generated or externally caused. When I make an arm movement, I know that the movement is my own and do not confuse it with a passive arm movement; similarly, I can distinguish self-generated touch from external tactile stimulation and know when a voice is my own and when it belongs to someone else. It has been proposed that an internal predictor, or forward model, uses information about intentions to enable this distinction between self-generated and externally generated sensory events (Wolpert *et al.* 1995, 2001; Miall and Wolpert 1996; see also Chapter 9, this volume). Forward models use an 'efference copy' of the motor command (von Holst 1954) to make a prediction of the consequences of the motor act. A forward dynamic model makes predictions about the next state of the system and compares this with the desired state. A forward output model makes predictions about the sensory consequences of the movement, and compares this with the actual sensory consequences of a movement (Fig. 24.1). This comparison can be used to cancel the sensory effect of the motor act, attenuating it perceptually compared with identical stimulation that is externally produced.

This predictive system is useful because it can be used to filter incoming sensory signals, picking out sensory information caused externally, such as touch produced by an external object or agent, and distinguishing it from sensory stimulation that occurs

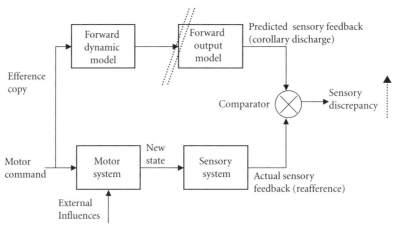

Fig. 24.1 The forward model of motor control as proposed by Miall *et al.* (1993). A forward dynamic model predicts the consequences of motor commands and these are compared with the desired state. The forward output model makes a prediction of the sensory consequences of motor commands, which is compared with the actual consequences of movement (reafference). Discrepancies resulting from this comparison can be used to cancel reafferent inputs and to distinguish self-produced and externally produced signals. The dashed lines indicate the proposed underlying disorder leading to delusions of control, and a possible mechanism by which hypnotic suggestion can alter the experience of a self-produced movement. In both delusions of control and hypnotic suggestion the subject can formulate the action appropriate to his or her intention and the action is successfully performed. The forward output model is dysfunctional such that it cannot make an accurate prediction of the sensory consequences of the movement based on the efference copy. This might be because the efference copy signals do not reach the forward output model, or that the forward output model cannot make accurate predictions based on the efference copy it receives. This results in a high level of sensory discrepancy (indicated by the dashed arrow) and no cancellation of the reafference, so that the (self-produced) movement feels externally produced.

as a necessary consequence of self-produced motion. An impairment in such a predictive system could cause a lack of attenuation of the sensory consequences of self-produced actions, which would therefore be indistinguishable from externally generated sensations. This would result in the interpretation of one's own movements as being externally caused—a delusion of alien control (Frith 1992; Frith *et al.* 2000).

Perception of the sensory consequences of actions

Evidence suggests that the sensory consequences of some self-generated movements are perceived differently from an identical sensory input when it is externally generated. An example of such differential perception is the phenomenon that people cannot tickle themselves (Weiskrantz *et al.* 1971). It has been argued that efference copy produced in parallel with the motor command underlies this phenomenon. To investigate this proposal, we asked participants to rate the sensation of a tactile stimulus on the palm of their hand, and examined the perceptual effects of altering the correspondence between self-generated movement and its sensory (tactile) consequences.

A robotic interface was employed to produce the delays and trajectory rotations. Participants moved a robotic arm with their left hand and this movement caused a second foam-tipped robotic arm to move across their right palm. Thus motion of the left hand determined the tactile stimulus on the right palm. By using this robotic interface so that the tactile stimulus could be delivered under remote control by the participant, delays of 100, 200, and 300 ms were introduced between the movement of the left hand and the tactile stimulus on the right palm. In a further condition trajectory rotations of 30°, 60°, and 90° were introduced between the direction of the left hand movement and the direction of the tactile stimulus on the right palm. Under all delays and trajectory rotations the left hand made the same sinusoidal movements and the right hand experienced the tactile stimulus. Only the temporal or spatial correspondence between the movement of the left hand and the sensory effect on the right palm was altered. The result of increasing the delay or trajectory rotation is that the sensory stimulus no longer corresponds to that which would be normally expected based on the efference copy produced in parallel with the motor command. Therefore as the delay or trajectory rotation increases, the sensory prediction becomes less accurate.

The results demonstrated that participants rated the self-produced tactile sensation as being significantly less tickly, intense, and pleasant than an identical stimulus produced by the robot (Blakemore *et al.* 1999a). Furthermore, participants reported a progressive increase in the tickly rating as the delay was increased between zero and 200 ms and as the trajectory rotation was increased between zero and 90°. These results support the hypothesis that the perceptual attenuation of self-produced tactile stimulation is due to precise sensory predictions. As the sensory feedback deviates from the prediction of the forward model (by increasing the delay or trajectory rotation), the sensory discrepancy between the predicted and actual sensory feedback increases, which leads to a decrease in the amount of sensory attenuation.

Behavioural evidence for problems of self-monitoring in schizophrenia

People with delusions of control feel as if their intentions are being monitored and their actions made for them by some external force. This could arise if there were an impairment of either the prediction or the comparison process of the forward model (Frith *et al.* 2000). For example, if the comparison process were impaired and always produced a high level of sensory discrepancy despite the accuracy of the sensory prediction, then self-produced sensations would be associated with high levels of sensory discrepancy despite being accurately predicted. In this way, self-produced stimulation could be interpreted as being externally produced.

To test the hypothesis that delusions of control and auditory hallucinations occur due to a defect in self-monitoring, we investigated whether individuals with auditory hallucinations and/or passivity experiences are abnormally aware of the sensory consequences of their own movements. Individuals with a diagnosis of schizophrenia, bipolar affective disorder, and depression were divided into two groups on the basis of the presence or absence of auditory hallucinations and/or passivity experiences. These patient groups and a group of age-matched healthy control participants were asked to rate the perception of a tactile sensation (a piece of soft foam) on the palm of their left hand. The tactile stimulation was either self-produced by movement of the participant's right hand or externally produced by the experimenter.

The results demonstrated that healthy control participants and participants with neither auditory hallucinations nor passivity symptoms experienced self-produced stimuli as less intense, tickly, and pleasant than identical externally produced tactile stimuli. In contrast, participants with these symptoms did not show a decrease in their perceptual ratings for tactile stimuli produced by themselves as compared with those produced by the experimenter (Blakemore *et al.* 2000). Figure 24.2 shows the difference between the ratings for self-produced and externally produced tactile stimulation for the three participant groups. These results support the proposal that auditory hallucinations and passivity experiences are associated with an abnormality in the forward-model mechanism that normally allows us to distinguish self-produced from externally produced sensations. It is possible that the neural system associated with this mechanism, or part of it, operates abnormally in people with such symptoms.

The physiological basis of the perceptual modulation of self-produced sensory stimuli

Neurophysiological data demonstrate that neuronal responses in the somatosensory cortex are attenuated by self-generated movement. Active touch is attenuated in the primary somatosensory cortex of animals (Chapman 1994) compared with passive and external touch of an identical tactile stimulus. It is possible that this

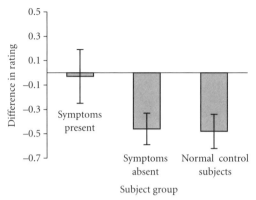

Fig. 24.2 Graph showing the mean (tickly, pleasant, and intense combined) perceptual rating difference between self-produced and externally produced tactile stimulation conditions for the three participant groups: patients with auditory hallucinations and/or passivity, patients without these symptoms, and normal controls. There was no significant difference between the perceptual ratings in the two conditions for participants with auditory hallucinations and/or passivity; hence the mean rating difference was close to zero. In contrast, there was a significant difference between the perceptual ratings in the two conditions for patients without these symptoms and in normal control participants; both groups rated self-produced stimulation as less tickly, intense, and pleasant than externally produced stimulation.

movement-induced somatosensory attenuation is the physiological correlate of the decreased sensation associated with self-produced tactile stimuli in humans. In order for somatosensory cortex activity to be attenuated to self-produced sensory stimuli, these stimuli need to be predicted accurately. The cerebellum is a possible site for a forward model of the motor apparatus that provides predictions of the sensory consequences of motor commands. This proposal has been supported by computational data (Miall *et al.* 1993; Wolpert *et al.* 1998), neurophysiological data (Simpson *et al.* 1995), and functional neuroimaging data (Imamizu *et al.* 2000).

To investigate the hypothesis that the somatosensory cortex and the cerebellum are involved in modulating the sensation of a self-produced tactile stimulation, we used functional magnetic resonance imaging (fMRI) to examine the neural basis of self-produced versus externally produced tactile stimuli in humans (Blakemore *et al.* 1998). Healthy participants were scanned while a tactile stimulation device allowed a tactile stimulus (a piece of soft foam) to be applied to the participant's left palm. The touch stimulus was produced either by the participant's right hand or by the experimenter.

The results showed an increase in activity of the secondary somatosensory cortex (SII) and the anterior cingulate cortex (ACC) when participants experienced an externally produced tactile stimulus relative to a self-produced tactile stimulus. The reduction in activity in these areas to self-produced tactile stimulation might be the physiological correlate of the reduced perception associated with this type of stimulation. The activity in the ACC in particular may have been related to the increased tickliness and pleasantness of externally produced compared with self-produced tactile stimuli. Previous studies have implicated this area in affective behaviour and positive reinforcement (Vogt and Gabriel 1993). Alternatively, the activity in ACC might be related to the requirement to monitor the sensations that the participants were experiencing (Lane *et al.* 1997; Frith and Frith 2003).

While the decrease in activity in SII and ACC might underlie the reduced perception of self-produced tactile stimuli, the pattern of brain activity in the cerebellum suggests that this area is the source of the SII and ACC modulation. In SII and ACC, activity was attenuated by all movement; these areas were equally activated by movement that did and that did not result in tactile stimulation. In contrast, the right anterior cerebellar cortex was selectively deactivated by self-produced movement that resulted in a tactile stimulus, but not by movement alone, and was significantly activated by externally produced tactile stimulation. This pattern suggests that the cerebellum distinguishes between movements depending on their specific sensory consequences.

A second experiment supported the proposal that the cerebellum distinguishes between movements depending on their specific sensory consequences (Blakemore *et al.* 2001). In this experiment participants were scanned using positron emission tomography (PET) while generating a tactile stimulus on the palm of their hand, as before. This time, however, the tactile stimulation was produced under remote control via a robotic interface. Participants moved a robotic arm with their left hand and this movement caused a second foam-tipped robotic arm to move across their right palm. By using this robotic interface so that the tactile stimulus could be delivered under remote control by the participant, delays of zero, 100, 200, and 300 ms were introduced between the movement of the left hand and the tactile stimulus on the right palm. Under all delays the left hand made the same movements and the right hand experienced the tactile stimulus. Only the temporal correspondence between the movement of the left hand and the sensory effect on the right palm was altered. The assumption behind this design was that as the delay increases, the forward-model prediction becomes less accurate and the sensory discrepancy between the predicted and actual sensory feedback from movement increases. Blood flow in the right cerebellar cortex significantly correlated with delay. This suggests that activity in this region increases as the actual feedback from movement deviates from the predicted sensory feedback. On the basis of these results, we proposed that the cerebellum is involved in signalling discrepancies between the predicted and actual consequences of action.

The role of the parietal cortex in the distinction between the self and the other

There is accumulating evidence that, in addition to the cerebellum, the parietal cortex is involved in distinguishing self-produced actions and actions generated by others.

Activity in the parietal operculum (secondary somatosensory cortex) is attenuated during self-initiated movements compared with passive movements (Weiller *et al.* 1996), and, as discussed in the previous section, during self-produced compared with external sensory stimulation (Blakemore *et al.* 1998).

There is evidence from neurological patients that the parietal cortex plays a role in the distinction between the self and the other. Patients with left parietal lesions tend to confuse the ownership of hand movements when they are shown someone else's hand making movements similar to those that they are making themselves (Sirigu *et al.* 1999; see also Chapter 19, this volume). A recent case study reported a patient with a right hemisphere lesion in which the white matter underlying the cortex, including the parietal operculum, had been damaged. This patient suffered from the delusional belief that her left limb belonged to her niece (Bottini *et al.* 2002).

Parietal lesions impair the ability to use mental motor imagery, a process believed to involve an internal model of action. Parietal patients are unable to predict the time necessary to perform finger movements and visually guided pointing gestures using their imagination. Normally, imagined and executed movement times are highly correlated, with Fitts' law accounting equally well for both types of movement (Decety and Jeannerod 1995; Sirigu *et al.* 1995). This was found to be true for a patient with motor cortex damage, whereas in patients with parietal lesions actual movement execution was modulated by target size but motor imagery was not (Sirigu *et al.* 1996). More recently, using similar tasks, a patient with a right temporoparietal lesion was tested on his ability to imagine and perform visually guided hand movements. It was found that, unlike his performance for visually guided actions, there was no relationship between accuracy and speed for imagined movements (Danckert *et al.* 2002).

Functional neuroimaging studies have also demonstrated that the parietal cortex is involved in the distinction between self and other. The right inferior parietal cortex is activated when subjects simulate actions from someone else's perspective but not from their own (Ruby and Decety 2001). This region is activated when subjects observe their own actions being imitated by someone else compared with when they imitate someone else's action (Decety *et al.* 2002). The inferior parietal cortex is differentially activated according to whether subjects attend to someone else's actions or to their own (Farrer and Frith 2002) and whether they lead or follow another person's actions (Chaminade and Decety 2002).

Delusions of control and the cerebellum and parietal cortex

Overactivity of the parietal cortex appears to contribute to the feeling that active movements are externally controlled in delusions of alien control (Spence *et al.* 1997). In this PET study, patients with delusions of control were scanned while they performed a simple motor task in which they were required to move a joystick in one of four directions, chosen at random. This 'willed action' task was compared with a similar task in which the joystick movements were paced. The patients with delusions of control showed overactivity in the superior parietal cortex and the cerebellum relative to normal controls and to patients who did not have delusions of control. Normally, activity in the parietal cortex is more typical of passive than active movements. Thus, at the experiential level, when the patient makes an active movement it can feel like a passive movement. It is this feeling that leads to the belief about alien control. Further support for this suggestion came from the finding that parietal activity had returned to 'normal' levels when, some months later, the same patients who were scanned in the initial study and whose symptoms had now subsided were rescanned performing the same task.

Inducing delusions of control in the normal brain

Further evidence that overactivity of the parietal cortex and cerebellum are involved in generating the feeling that a movement is externally produced comes from a recent study in which experiences of alien control were induced in healthy control subjects (Blakemore *et al.* 2003). In this study, hypnosis was used as a cognitive tool to create delusions of alien control in normal healthy subjects. 'Ideomotor movement' is a frequently demonstrated hypnotic phenomenon in which self-produced actions are attributed to an external source (Heap and Aravind 2002). A typical example involves suggesting to the hypnotized subject that their arm is being raised upwards passively by an external device, such as a helium balloon attached to their wrist. This suggestion causes highly hypnotizable subjects to produce an appropriate movement. Despite generating the movement themselves, subjects describe the raising and lowering of their arm as being involuntary and typically claim that it was caused by the helium balloon.

In our study, PET was used to scan highly hypnotizable subjects during a similar 'alien control' experience. In an Active Movement condition subjects were instructed to move their left arm up and down, which they correctly attributed to themselves. In another condition (the Deluded Passive Movement condition), subjects were told that their left arm would be moved up and down by the pulley, but in fact the pulley did not move and resulting arm movements were self-generated. This suggestion induced the subjects, who were all highly hypnotizable according to the Harvard Hypnotizability Scale (Shor and Orne 1962), to move their arms up and down in the suggested manner. However, crucially, subjects misattributed this movement to the pulley. All conditions were performed while subjects were hypnotized. Thus movements in the Active Movement and Deluded Passive conditions were identical; subjects made the same self-generated arm movements in both conditions. The only difference between these two conditions was the source to which the movement was attributed.

Using this paradigm we were able to compare brain activation during active movements that are correctly attributed to the self with identical active movements that are misattributed to an external source. The results demonstrated that the cerebellum and parietal operculum were differentially activated depending on whether an active movement was experienced as truly active or as passive. Parietal-opercular and cerebellar activity was significantly higher and more widespread in the Deluded Passive condition, in which movements were misattributed to an external source, than in the Active Movement condition, in which identical movements were correctly attributed to the self.

In terms of the forward model (Fig. 24.1), which is believed to be stored in the cerebellum (Miall *et al*. 1993; Imamizu *et al*. 2000), the abnormality in the Deluded Passive condition might lie in the forward output model, and not the forward dynamic model. The forward dynamic model compares the estimated state with the desired state, and the results of this comparison are used to adjust motor commands in order to optimize motor control and learning. Subjects produced the same smooth arm movements in the Deluded Passive and Active Movement conditions. Therefore the motor system appears to be functioning normally in terms of motor control in the Deluded Passive condition. In contrast, the forward output model compares the predicted consequences of motor commands with the actual consequences of movement (reafference), and discrepancies resulting from this comparison can be used to cancel reafferent inputs and to distinguish self-produced and externally produced sensory signals.

We have tentatively suggested that hypnotic suggestion in the Deluded Passive condition prevents the motor intentions from reaching the forward output model. In this case the forward output model would no longer be able to make an accurate prediction of the sensory consequences of the movement. This would lead to a discrepancy between predicted and actual sensory feedback, which would result in no attenuation of the sensory feedback, making the (self-produced) movement feel externally produced. If the cerebellum signals sensory discrepancies between predicted sensory feedback of movements and their actual sensory consequences (Andersson and Armstrong 1985; Blakemore *et al*. 2001), increased cerebellar activation would be expected in the Deluded Passive condition.

According to evidence from the patient and neuroimaging studies described above, the parietal cortex appears to be involved in inducing the feeling that an action or sensory event is external. Activity in the parietal cortex seems to be required for an arm movement to feel as if it is externally generated. The inferior parietal lobe is the direct target of output from the cerebellum (Clower *et al*. 2001) and parietal-opercular cortex activity can be influenced by cerebellar activity (Blakemore *et al*. 1999b). In the Deluded Passive condition, if the cerebellum signals a discrepancy between predicted and actual sensory feedback, then no parietal-opercular attenuation would occur, which is what normally happens during externally produced sensory stimulation.

There is an alternative, or additional, explanation for the parietal activity in the Deluded Passive condition. It is well established that attention to a particular sensory modality or feature increases activity in the brain region that processes that feature even in the absence of a sensory signal (Driver and Frith 2000). It has also been suggested that hypnotic suggestion, by focusing attention, can produce increased activity in specific brain areas, which causes a modulation of sensory experience (Rainville *et al.* 1997). Rainville and coworkers have shown that the hypnotic suggestion to increase or decrease the affective components of constantly applied experimental pain are accompanied by a modulation of activity in the anterior cingulate cortex, an area previously shown to be involved in the experience of pain. Activity in this region increased as the experience of pain increased in response to suggestion, even though the painful stimulus itself did not change. It is possible that, in our study, subjects' attention is more highly focused on the sensations associated with passive movement in the Deluded Passive condition than in the Active Movement condition. This increased attention produces activation in brain regions that process such sensations (the parietal operculum). It is the activation in this region that causes the movement to feel external.

A similar mechanism may underlie the disorder leading to delusions of control in schizophrenia and other clinical conditions. In particular, it has been proposed that delusions of control are caused by an impairment in the forward-model system that predicts the sensory consequences of one's own actions (Frith *et al.* 2000). This could cause a lack of attenuation of the sensory consequences of self-produced actions, which would therefore be indistinguishable from externally generated sensations, hence causing a confusion between the self and the other (Frith 1992; Frith *et al.* 2000). A similar theory that attempts to account for delusions of control posits that these symptoms reflect a disruption of the cognitive processes that normally produce a sense of agency or volitional control (Jeannerod 1999; see also Chapter 9, this volume). Jeannerod has suggested that conscious judgement about a movement requires a different form of representation from that needed for unconscious comparisons of predictions and outcomes within the motor system. Specifically, conscious judgements about movements require 'third-person' information, while control of movement depends upon private 'first-person' information. On this basis Jeannerod proposes that patients with delusions of control fail to monitor the third-person signals that enable them to make judgements about their own actions. On the other hand, Spence (1996) has suggested that the problem underlying delusions of control has to do with the timing of awareness. The awareness of the actual outcome of the movement precedes the awareness of the predicted outcome, which is contrary to the normal experience of our own agency.

The ability to distinguish between active and passive movements is an important part of a 'who' system, which allows one to link an action with its cause (Georgieff and Jeannerod 1998). The data reviewed in this chapter suggest that overactivation of a cerebellar-parietal network during self-generated actions is associated with the misattribution of those actions to an external source. Overactivity of the parietal cortex and cerebellum occurs during self-generated movements in patients with delusions of alien control, and subsides when the same patients are in remission (Spence *et al.* 1997). It is possible that malfunctioning in this network, leading to overactivity, produces the feeling of 'otherness' associated with self-produced movements in delusions of alien control.

Acknowledgement

The support of the Wellcome Trust UK is gratefully acknowledged. The work described in this Chapter was carried out with C. Frith and D. Wolpert.

References

Andersson G, Armstrong DM (1985). Climbing fibre input to b zone Purkinje cells during locomotor perturbation in the cat. *Neurosci Lett Suppl*, **22**, S27.

Blakemore S-J, Wolpert DM, Frith CD (1998). Central cancellation of self-produced tickle sensation. *Nat Neurosci*, **1**, 635–40.

Blakemore S-J, Frith CD, Wolpert DW (1999a). Spatiotemporal prediction modulates the perception of self-produced stimuli. *J Cogn Neurosci*, **11**, 551–9.

Blakemore S-J, Wolpert DM, Frith CD (1999b). The cerebellum contributes to somatosensory cortical activity during self-produced tactile stimulation. *Neuroimage*, **10**, 448–59.

Blakemore S-J, Smith J, Steel R, Johnstone E, Frith CD (2000). The perception of self-produced sensory stimuli in patients with auditory hallucinations and passivity experiences: evidence for a breakdown in self-monitoring. *Psychol Med*, **30**, 1131–9.

Blakemore S-J, Frith CD, Wolpert DW (2001). The cerebellum is involved in predicting the sensory consequences of action. *NeuroReport*, **12**, 1879–85.

Blakemore S-J, Oakley DA, Frith CD (2003). Delusions of alien control in the normal brain. *Neuropsychologia*, **41**(8), 1058–67.

Bottini G, Bisiach E, Sterzi R, Vallar G (2002). Feeling touches in someone else's hand. *NeuroReport*, **13**, 249–52.

Chaminade T, Decety J (2002). Leader or follower? Involvement of the inferior parietal lobule in agency. *NeuroReport*, **13**, 1975–8.

Chapman CE (1994). Active versus passive touch: factors influencing the transmission of somatosensory signals to primary somatosensory cortex. *Can J Physiol Pharmacol*, **72**, 558–70.

Clower DM, West RA, Lynch JC, Strick PL (2001). The inferior parietal lobule is the target of output from the superior colliculus, hippocampus, and cerebellum. *J Neurosci*, **21**, 6283–91.

Danckert J, Ferber S, Doherty T, Steinmetz H, Nicolle D, Goodale MA (2002). Selective, non-lateralized impairment of motor imagery following right parietal damage. *Neurocase*, **8**, 194–204.

Decety J, Jeannerod M (1995). Mentally simulated movements in virtual reality: does Fitts's law hold in motor imagery? *Behav Brain Res*, **14**, 127–34.

Decety J, Chaminade T, Grezes J, Meltzoff AN (2002). A PET exploration of the neural mechanisms involved in reciprocal imitation. *Neuroimage*, **15**, 265–72.

Driver J, Frith C (2000). Shifting baselines in attention research. *Nat Rev Neurosci*, **1**, 147–8.

Farrer C, Frith CD (2002). Experiencing oneself vs another person as being the cause of an action: the neural correlates of the experience of agency. *Neuroimage*, **15**, 596–603.

Frith CD (1992). *The Cognitive Neuropsychology of Schizophrenia*. Hove, UK: Lawrence Erlbaum.

Frith U, Frith C (2003). Development and neurophysiology of mentalizing. *Proc R Soc Lond Biol Sci*, **358**, 459–73.

Frith CD, Blakemore S-J, Wolpert DM (2000). Abnormalities in the awareness and control of action. *Philos Trans R Soc Lond Biol Sci*, **355**, 1771–88.

Georgieff N, Jeannerod M (1998). Beyond consciousness of external reality. A 'Who' system for consciousness of action and self-consciousness. *Conscious Cogn*, **7**, 465–77.

Heap M, Aravind KK (2002). *Hartland's Medical and Dental Hypnosis*, 4th edn. Edinburgh: Churchill Livingston.

Imamizu H, Miyauchi S, Tamada T, Sasaki Y, Takino R, Putz B, *et al.* (2000). Human cerebellar activity reflecting an acquired internal model of a new tool. *Nature*, **403**, 192–5.

Jeannerod M (1999). To act or not to act: perspectives on the representation of actions. *Q J Exp Psychol A*, **52**, 981–1020.

Johnstone EC (1991). Defining characteristics of schizophrenia. *Br J Psychiatry Suppl*, **13**, 5–6.

Lane RD, Fink GR, Chua PM, Dolan RJ (1997). Neural activation during selective attention to subjective emotional responses. *NeuroReport*, **8**, 3969–72.

Mellors CS (1970). First-rank symptoms of schizophrenia. *Br J Psychiatry*, **117**, 15–23.

Miall RC, Weir DJ, Wolpert DM, Stein JF (1993). Is the cerebellum a Smith predictor? *J Mot Behav*, **25**, 203–16.

Miall RC, Wolpert DM (1996). Forward models for physiological motor control. *Neural Netw*, **9**, 1265–79.

Rainville P, Duncan GH, Price DD, Carrier B, Bushnell MC (1997). Pain affect encoded in human anterior cingulate but not somatosensory cortex. *Science*, **277**, 968–71.

Ruby P, Decety J (2001). Effect of subjective perspective taking during simulation of action: a PET investigation of agency. *Nat Neurosci*, **4**, 546–50.

Schneider K (1959). *Clinical Psychopathology* New York: Grune & Stratton.

Shor RE, Orne EC (1962). *Harvard Group Scale of Hypnotic Susceptibility*. Palo Alto, CA: Consulting Psychologists Press.

Simpson JL, Wylie DR, De Zeeuw CI (1995). On climbing fiber signals and their consequence(s) *Behav Brain Sci*, **19**, 384.

Sirigu A, Cohen L, Duhamel JR, Pillon B, Dubois B, Agid Y, *et al.* (1995). Congruent unilateral impairments for real and imagined hand movements. *NeuroReport*, **6**, 997–1001.

Sirigu A, Duhamel JR, Cohen L, Pillon B, Dubois B, Agid Y (1996). The mental representation of hand movements after parietal cortex damage. *Science*, **273**, 1564–8.

Sirigu A, Daprati E, Pradat-Diehl P, Franck N, Jeannerod M (1999). Perception of self-generated movement following left parietal lesion. *Brain*, **122**, 1867–74.

Spence SA (1996). Free will in the light of neuropsychiatry. *Philos Psychiatry Psychol*, **3**, 75–90.

Spence SA, Brooks DJ, Hirsch SR, Liddle PF, Meehan J, Grasby PM (1997). A PET study of voluntary movement in schizophrenic patients experiencing passivity phenomena (delusions of alien control). *Brain*, **120**, 1997–2011.

Vogt BA, Gabriel M (ed.) (1993). *Neurobiology of Cingulate Cortex and Limbic Thalamus*. Boston, MA: Birkauser.

von Holst E (1954). Relations between the central nervous system and the peripheral organs. *Br J Anim Behav*, **2**, 89–94.

Weiller C, Juptner M, Fellows S, Rijntjes M, Leonhardt G, Kiebel S, *et al.* (1996). Brain representation of active and passive movements. *Neuroimage*, **4**, 105–10.

Weiskrantz L, Elliot J, Darlington C (1971). Preliminary observations of tickling oneself. *Nature*, **230**, 598–9.

Wolpert DM, Ghahramani Z, Jordan MI (1995). An internal model for sensorimotor integration. *Science*, **269**, 1880–2.

Wolpert DM, Miall RC, Kawato M (1998). Internal models in the cerebellum. *Trends Cogn Sci*, **2**, 338–47.

Wolpert DM, Ghahramani Z, Flanagan R (2001). Perspectives and problems in motor learning. *Trends Cogn Sci*, **5**, 487–94.

Chapter 25

Cortical plasticity and motor disorders

Pablo A. Celnik and Leonardo G. Cohen

Introduction

The view of the central nervous system as rigidly organized has been replaced by a more dynamic conception that emphasizes its ability to change. This paradigm shift took place over several decades and has led, in the last few years, to a tighter connection between basic scientists working in animal models of plasticity and clinicians interested in the application of principles of plasticity to the treatment of human disease. Influential studies leading the way of this new trend included those of Hubel and Wiesel (1965), who showed that visual experience during the early life of kittens has a profound impact in shaping the responsiveness of individual cortical neurons, the discovery of nerve growth factor in the adult mammal brain (Levi-Montalcini and Angeletti 1968), and the characterization of long-term potentiation and depression (Bliss and Gardner 1973; Douglas and Goddard 1975; Lynch *et al.* 1977). Research that stimulated the application of some of these principles in behavioral settings in adult human and non-human primates included that of Merzenich (Merzenich *et al.* 1983, 1984; Merzenich 1988), Kaas (Kaas *et al.* 1990; Kaas 1991), Pons (Pons *et al.* 1991; Pons 1996), Donoghue (Donoghue JP and Sanes 1987, 1988; Donoghue *et al.* 1990, 1996), and Nudo (Nudo *et al.* 1996a,b, 1990). These studies inspired a wave of research in human laboratories across the world that attempted to apply these principles to clinical settings. In this way, researchers demonstrated, using non-invasive techniques, that the human central nervous system has the ability to adapt to new environmental requirements or lesions and that the mechanisms underlying some of these changes may be similar to those described in animal models. Research in these areas has already moved from the realm of experimentation in primates or normal human volunteers to clinical settings that address conditions like stroke and dystonia. The purpose of this chapter is to review this work and its relevance to the understanding of the mechanisms underlying motor disorders and to highlight rational strategies to promote recovery of motor function in neurorehabilitation.

Mechanisms of plasticity

It is now known that the central nervous system can reorganize in a variety of ways. Mechanisms underlying this reorganization include unmasking of silent synapses, and forming new connections, such as collateral sprouting. Neurons in the cerebral cortex have extensive anatomical connections with other neurons. The strength of these connections varies, but a portion of the total anatomical network is often physiologically 'inactive'. The main inhibitory neurotransmitter in the cerebral cortex, GABA, is thought to play a fundamental role in the regulation of inhibition and excitation in these cortical networks. Unmasking refers to the process by which a cortical region or anatomical connection that was previously silent becomes disinhibited (Jacobs and Donoghue 1991). This process takes place in the absence of obvious anatomical rewiring and may become evident within minutes (Brasil-Neto *et al.* 1992, 1993). Another mechanism of plasticity is change in synaptic strength, as seen in long-term potentiation (LTP) and long-term depression (LTD) (Douglas and Goddard 1975; Lynch *et al.* 1977). LTP and LTD are thought to underlie a variety of plastic processes, including learning and memory in the intact central nervous system and recovery of function after brain lesions, as in stroke (Bear and Malenka 1994), and have been documented in different areas of the adult central nervous system, including the motor cortex (Hess and Donoghue 1994). LTP and LTD develop over longer time periods relative to unmasking (Bear and Malenka 1994). The establishment of new anatomical connections, or sprouting, requires longer periods of time. These mechanisms may underlie practice-dependent improvements in motor learning, memory, and activity-dependent plasticity in human health and disease (Nudo *et al.* 1996, 2001).

Studies of cortical plasticity in animal models

Basic science studies, such as those described above, have substantially advanced our understanding of the mechanisms of plasticity and metaplasticity (Abraham and Bear 1996; Fischer *et al.* 1997). These mechanisms are thought to operate in multiple areas of human cognition, such as learning and memory, and in functional recovery from lesions in the central nervous system, as in stroke (Buonomano and Merzenich 1998). Although these findings may have direct implications for the ways in which human diseases are treated, relatively few efforts have been invested in research that translates these advances in the basic science domain to the formulation of new rational strategies for promoting recovery of function in humans (Taub *et al.* 2002).

Animal studies over the last two decades demonstrated that the cerebral cortex experiences constant remodeling and that these changes are shaped by experience. Representations of skin regions (Kalaska and Pomeranz 1979; Merzenich *et al.* 1983, 1984; Pons *et al.* 1991), cochlea (Robertson and Irvine 1989), and retina (Wall and Kaas 1986; Wall 1988; Kaas *et al.* 1990; Chino *et al.* 1992) reorganize after deafferentation. In general, cortical representations near the deafferented one take over the cortical sites deprived of inputs. In the somatosensory system, cortical reorganization has been detected after interruption and reconnection of peripheral nerves (Wall *et al.* 1986), after crossing the connections between two peripheral nerves, after fusion of fingers (Allard *et al.* 1991), after moving islands of skin to new locations across the hand (Merzenich *et al.* 1988), and after operant conditioning, such as discrimination of surface roughness (Guic *et al.* 1993), maintenance of finger contact pressure for several seconds for food reward (Jenkins *et al.* 1990), and discrimination of vibratory frequencies (Recanzone *et al.* 1992a,b,c,d).

In the motor system, cortical reorganization has been detected following nerve transection (Donoghue and Sanes 1987, 1988; Donoghue *et al.* 1990, Sanes *et al.* 1990), modified limb positions (Sanes *et al.* 1992), repetitive stimulation (Nudo *et al.* 1990), focal lesions in the motor cortex (Nudo *et al.* 1996), practice with a small-object-retrieval task (Nudo *et al.* 1996), and training in a target-reaching task (Aizawa *et al.* 1991; Mitz *et al.* 1991).

Role of somatosensory input on cortical reorganization

Somatosensory input is required for motor learning (Bastian 1887; Pearson 2000) and for recovery of function after cortical lesions, as in stroke (Johansson *et al.* 1993; Powell *et al.* 1999; Wong *et al.* 1999; Conforto *et al.* 2002). Recent studies have documented in detail reorganizational changes associated with deafferentation, as well as somatosensory stimulation.

Chronic deafferentation in the form of amputation leads to enhanced cortical motor outputs targeting the muscles immediately proximal to the stump (Cohen *et al.* 1991; Fuhr *et al.* 1992; Chen *et al.* 1997; Karl *et al.* 2001). Interestingly, cortical reorganization after amputation appears to be more prominent in patients with phantom limb pain (Karl *et al.* 2001). Acute limb deafferentation induced by ischemic nerve block (INB) also has profound effects on the organization of the intact human motor cortex. Studies in healthy volunteers using transcranial magnetic stimulation (TMS) demonstrated that acute deafferentation results in bilateral cortical reorganization. In TMS, a strong electric current is passed through a copper coil and elicits a magnetic field that passes through the scalp and skull, resulting in currents delivered over target neural structures (Cohen *et al.* 1990). Acute deafferentation of the hand results, within minutes, in increased cortical excitability of the representation of muscles immediately proximal to the deafferented level (upper arm) (Brasil-Neto *et al.* 1992, 1993). This change has been interpreted as consistent with the idea that hand deafferentation leads to disinhibition of the cortical representation of the upper arm. Further, administration of the GABAergic agent lorazepam blocked this effect, suggesting that GABAergic neurotransmission is a mechanism operating in this form of plasticity (Werhahn *et al.* 2002a), a view consistent with the findings of Jacobs (Jacobs and Donoghue 1991). Additional evidence pointing to the role of GABA comes from a study by Levy *et al.* (2002) using magnetic resonance spectroscopy. The authors demonstrated a rapid decrease in GABA levels in the deafferented sensorimotor cortex during acute hand deafferentation.

Ziemann *et al.* (2002) demonstrated that it is possible to upregulate the deafferentation-dependent increase in excitability of the upper-arm representation by TMS application to the upper-arm representation of the motor cortex. Conversely, stimulation of the hand or the face representation blocks this effect. Therefore the picture emerging from these experiments is one of a dynamic interaction between body part representations in the human motor cortex. Acute hand deafferentation leads to enhanced excitability of the nearby upper-arm representation that is upregulated by TMS of the upper-arm representation, downregulated by TMS of the face or hand representations, and influenced by GABAergic neurotransmission.

Interestingly, acute limb deafferentation appears to influence activity in both cerebral hemispheres (Sadato *et al.* 1995). Werhahn *et al.* (2002a) found that acute deafferentation of one hand results in a transient increase in corticomotor excitability targeting the non-deafferented hand (Fig. 25.1 (a), (b)). This effect was reversed by the GABAergic agent lorazepam. The mechanisms underlying the effects of acute deafferentation on motor cortex excitability are likely to include unmasking of preexisting anatomical connections. Those underlying the effects of chronic deafferentation could involve establishment of new anatomical connections. Finally, Werhahn *et al.* (2002b) addressed the behavioral consequence of acute limb deafferentation by showing that right-hand anesthesia resulted in rapid improvements in tactile spatial acuity and changes in cortical processing for the left hand (Fig. 25.1 (c), (d)).

On the other side of the spectrum of deafferentation is somatosensory stimulation. Stefan *et al.* (2000) showed that peripheral nerve stimulation applied in synchrony with TMS of the contralateral motor cortex induced an increment in motor cortical excitability, as demonstrated by larger motor evoked potential (MEP) amplitudes. This effect developed rapidly, persisted for approximately 30–60 min, and had topographic specificity. Similarly, prolonged peripheral nerve stimulation of the ulnar nerve induced an increase of excitability of the cortical representation of the first dorsal interosseus and abductor digiti minimi muscles, but not of the median nerve-innervated muscles (Ridding *et al.* 2001; Kaelin-Lang *et al.* 2002). F-wave and transcranial electric stimulation studies failed to reveal any subcortical changes, suggesting a cortical origin of this plastic phenomenon. Interestingly, application of this strategy of stimulating peripheral nerves to patients with stroke led to an improvement in functional measures of motor performance, such as pinch muscle strength (Conforto *et al.* 2002). Hamdy *et al.* (1998) found that stimulation of the pharyngeal muscles results in an increased excitability of the cortical area representing the pharynx, but not the esophagus. In patients with chronic stroke, this form of cortical reorganization correlated with clinical improvement of dysphagia (Fraser *et al.* 2002). These findings suggest a link between motor cortical excitability and motor function.

Plasticity in the human motor cortex associated with motor training

Previous studies have demonstrated that motor training leads to reorganizational changes in the motor cortex in animals and humans (Karni *et al.* 1995; Pascual-Leone

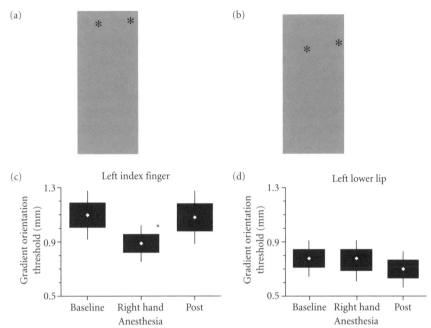

Fig. 25.1 The behavioral and physiological effects of right-hand anesthesia by ischaemic nerve block (INB). In the anesthesized hand, note an MEP amplitude decrement in the first dorsal interosseus (FDI) below the INB (motor block) (A) and an MEP amplitude increase in the biceps brachii immediately proximal to the tourniquet (B). On the other hand, MEP amplitudes from FDI in the non-anesthesized hand increased significantly (A). Therefore anesthesia of one hand results in increased motor cortical excitability targeting homologous muscles in the non-anesthesized hand. In a separate experiment, right-hand anesthesia led to a decrease (improvement) in thresholds for a grating orientation task performed with the left index finger (C) in the absence of changes in the lip (D). Modified from Werhahn *et al.* (2002). *Brain*, **125**, 1402–13, and Werhahn *et al.* (2002). *Nat Neurosci*, **5**, 936–8.

et al. 1995; Nudo *et al.* 1996b; Shadmehr and Holcomb 1997; Classen *et al.* 1998; Muellbacher *et al.* 2001). For example, performance of simple repetitive finger motions leads to use-dependent plasticity that encodes the kinematic details of the practised movements (Classen *et al.* 1998) (Fig. 25.2).

Mechanisms operating in this form of plasticity include *N*-methyl-D-aspartate (NMDA), muscarinic, and GABAergic neurotransmission (Butefisch *et al.* 2000; Sawaki *et al.* 2002a). Modulation of noradrenergic neurotransmission appears to be the mechanism by which dextroamphetamine accelerates the development and prolongs the duration of this form of plasticity (Butefisch *et al.* 2002; Sawaki *et al.* 2002b). Preliminary evidence appears to indicate that this drug could enhance use-dependent plasticity in patients with chronic stroke (Sawaki *et al.* 2003). These experiments are only samples of studies done in many laboratories over the world that emphasize the role of motor training in cortical reorganization. This concept triggered a new emphasis

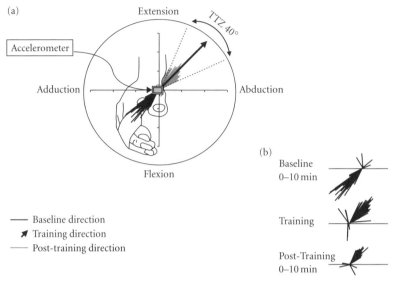

Fig. 25.2 The figure represents the results of one subject who underwent training-induced use-dependent plasticity. (a) The direction of TMS-evoked or voluntary movement was obtained from the first-peak acceleration of movement, measured by a two-dimensional accelerometer mounted on the proximal phalanx of the thumb. At baseline, TMS evoked predominantly flexion and adduction thumb movements. Training movements (60 trials, 10 min) were performed in a direction approximately opposite to baseline (arrow). Post-training, the direction of TMS-evoked thumb movements changed from the baseline direction to the trained direction. The mean training direction is at the center of the training target zone (TTZ). TMS-induced movement (60 trials, 10 min) directions after training largely fell within the TTZ, close to a 180° change from baseline direction. (b) Schematic diagram of directional changes of first-peak-acceleration vector of movements evoked by TMS before, during, and after training. Before training (baseline direction), TMS evoked predominantly flexion and adduction thumb movements. Training consisted of repetitive stereotyped brisk thumb movements in a extension and abduction direction. In post-training, the direction of TMS-evoked thumb movements changed from the baseline direction to the trained direction. Modified from Butefisch *et al.* (2002). *Ann Neurol*, **51**, 59–68, and Sawaki *et al.* (2002). *Neurology*, **59**, 1262–4.

on attempting to apply these principles to enhance recovery of function after motor disorders such as stroke and dystonia.

Influence of principles of plasticity on rehabilitative strategies used for the treatment of motor disorders

Stroke

Stroke is defined as an 'acute neurologic dysfunction of vascular origin with symptoms and signs corresponding to the involvement of focal areas of the brain' (World Health Organization 1989). Between 73% and 88% of first-time ischemic strokes result in an acute sensorimotor contralateral hemiparesis (Tangeman *et al.* 1990; Winstein *et al.* 1999). Approximately 3 million American stroke survivors have different degrees of residual neurological impairment (American Heart Association 1998). The economic burden of disability from stroke has been estimated to be $30 billion in health care costs and lost productivity this year. The main purpose of motor rehabilitation is to enhance spontaneous recovery of function, but the results from standard interventions have been only moderately successful.

Chronic stroke

Motor training can contribute to recovery of motor function in the paretic hand of chronic stroke patients. One of the most recent demonstrations has been the use of constraint-induced movement therapy, a rehabilitative technique that focuses on increasing the 'amount of use' in the paretic arm (Ostendorf and Wolf 1981; Wolf *et al.* 1989; Taub *et al.* 1993, 1999; Kopp *et al.* 1999; Kunkel *et al.* 1999; Miltner *et al.* 1999). In this technique, patients with chronic stroke are instructed to perform a training plan focused on practice of motor tasks with the paretic hand while the use of the intact hand is restricted, usually during waking hours. The neural substrates underlying the beneficial effect of training are incompletely understood but may include reorganization within the primary motor cortex (Liepert *et al.* 1998). A multicenter NINDS-funded study is currently under way to determine whether this strategy can be successfully applied in the subacute stage that follows the ictal event.

One of the overall purposes of research in this field is the development of rational strategies to enhance the effects of motor training. A recent study proposed that selective deafferentation of the paretic upper arm of chronic stroke patients could enhance the beneficial effects of motor training and improve hand function (Muellbacher *et al.* 2002). The proposal is based on an extensive body of research that previously characterized plastic changes associated with ischemic nerve block (Brasil-Neto *et al.* 1992, 2002a; Werhahn *et al.* 2002b; Ziemann *et al.* 1997, 1998a,b). In this study, the investigators applied a local anesthetic to the upper trunk of the brachial plexus of the paretic arm, inducing anesthesia and weakness of the proximal arm but sparing the distal limb. This intervention led to enhanced motor function in the paretic hand and increased motor cortical excitability.

Another strategy thought to have beneficial effects on motor function is somatosensory stimulation. In one study, eight chronic patients were exposed in a randomized crossover experiment to either median nerve electrical stimulation or placebo stimulation to determine changes in pinch strength. After 2 hrs of nerve stimulation, pinch strength increased in a manner proportional to the intensity of the stimulation. Interestingly, two patients reported that they could write better and hold objects and play cards more accurately, a perception that lasted for approximately 24 hrs (Conforto *et al.* 2002). These preliminary results raise the hypothesis of a potentially promising role of this intervention in patients with chronic stroke.

The neural substrates underlying recovery of motor function after stroke are incompletely understood. However, recent studies have started to explore this issue in some detail. For example, Weiller *et al.* (1993) studied patients who recovered hand function after discrete lesions of the posterior internal capsule using positron emission tomography (PET). They found that hand movements activated cortical areas extending laterally to the face representation, suggesting that the hand representation shifts toward the face area. However, this phenomenon was not observed in patients with lesions of the anterior limb of the internal capsule. Because fibers that travel to the face muscles are more anterior in the internal capsule than in those going to the arm and leg (Hardy *et al.* 1979), posterior lesions would have spared them and left them available for reorganization. These data, together with those of Muellbacher *et al.* (2002), suggest that representational plasticity in the primary motor cortex could contribute to functional recovery.

Another possible mechanism contributing to recovery of motor function after chronic stroke is the involvement of non-primary motor areas. For example, the dorsal premotor cortex (Johansen-Berg *et al.* 2002) and the ventral premotor cortex (Frost *et al.* 2003), functional subdivisions of the motor cortex with direct corticomotoneuronal connections, appear to participate in the recovery process. It is also possible that the intact hemisphere contributes to functional recovery, particularly in patients with more impairment (Palmer *et al.* 1992; Caramia *et al.* 1996; Turton *et al.* 1996).

Studies using TMS were also performed to determine the role of the intact motor cortex in functional recovery from stroke. Palmer *et al.* (1992) studied nine stroke-recovered patients but found no evidence that the ipsilateral corticospinal track was involved in the recovery of function. In another study, 21 stroke survivors were followed from the onset of stroke up to 12 months. Those who had MEPs in the paretic hand at the onset of the study had the most prominent improvement of motor function, whereas nine other patients who had ipsilateral MEPs had poorer recovery (Turton *et al.* 1996).

Subacute stroke

In the subacute stage following cortical lesions in animal models and stroke in humans, it has been proposed that prior administration of amphetamine can enhance the effects of motor training. In the late 1970s, researchers determined that a decline in brain catecholamines follows experimental stroke (Robinson *et al.* 1975). This finding led to the hypothesis that manipulation of neurotransmitters might be useful in treating patients with stroke (McDowell 1991). A number of animal studies were done addressing the role of amphetamines in recovery from brain lesions. In the first such study, Clark *et al.* (1975) showed that amphetamine could improve motivation, mobility, and self-care in patients with stroke. In the second study, Lipper and Tuchman (1976) showed that amphetamine improved orientation and recall in patients with post-traumatic brain injury. Animal studies showed widespread changes in brain content of neurotransmitters and a decrease of cerebral metabolism in areas indirectly involved in cerebral injury (Robinson *et al.* 1975). Some of the abnormalities described in these two experiments remitted within 1 month following the injury.

Soon, amphetamine became one of the most extensively studied drugs thought to facilitate recovery after focal brain injury in animals (Feeney *et al.* 1993; Goldstein 1993). It was found that following lesions in the primary sensorimotor cortex, locomotor deficits improve in 2–3 weeks in the absence of any treatment. Amphetamine given during the first 2 weeks after the injury accelerated functional recovery. When given as a single dose in rats (Feeney *et al.* 1982) or as multiple doses alternated over 4 days in cats (Hovda and Feeney 1984), amphetamine reduced the time of recovery. Improvement in beam walking started within hours of the first dose.

Some experiments made clear that amphetamine in the presence of physical restraint does not work as well (Feeney *et al.* 1982). In fact, rats that were physically restrained during the week after injury recovered less rapidly, despite receiving adequate amphetamine treatment. In contrast, rats given repeated exposure to beam walking improved more rapidly with amphetamine. These results indicate that both amphetamine and motor experience are crucial for faster recovery. Therefore when amphetamine is administered during a critical time period following a cortical lesion and coupled with use of the affected body parts, it can enhance and speed motor recovery (Feeney *et al.* 1982; Hovda and Feeney 1984; Sutton *et al.* 1989; Goldstein and Davis 1990).

Similar findings have been reported with reference to recovery of depth perception. Cats with bilateral occipital cortex ablation lose depth perception but not visual acuity, which recovers after injury (Feeney and Hovda 1985). If animals are given amphetamine after surgery, they will recover depth perception. This recovered function persists after treatment is completed and is believed to be permanent. However, if the animal is placed in the dark after surgery, function does not recover, despite treatment with amphetamines (Hovda *et al.* 1989). These experiments with occipital cortex ablation indicate that pairing of amphetamine and experience produce permanent recovery of depth perception. It appears that in both occipital and motor cortex, amphetamine 'requires' use or experience for functional recovery to occur.

Available data suggest that amphetamine modifies recovery through its effects on central norepinephrine (Goldstein 1993). For example, the facilitation of recovery by amphetamine has been mimicked by infusions of norepinephrine, but not dopamine, in the brain 24 hrs after injury (Boyeson and Feeney 1990; Boyeson *et al.* 1994). It has been hypothesized that enhancement of recovery results from the alleviation of injury-induced metabolic depression of structures remote from, but connected to, the site of injury (Feeney *et al.* 1985; Feeney 1991). The locus ceruleus axonal projections bifurcate, and the same neuron (originating in the locus ceruleus) sends projections to the ipsilateral sensorimotor cortex and to both cerebellar hemispheres. Because of this unique anatomy of noradrenergic forebrain projections, injury of locus ceruleus axon terminals in the sensorimotor cortex could influence the amount of norepinephrine released in areas remote from the injury, such as the cerebellum. It has been proposed that this neurochemical disbalance in the cerebellum results in decreased output from the deep cerebellar nuclei to rubrospinal, reticulospinal, and vestibulospinal tracts, leading to motor deficits (Boyeson *et al.* 1993, 1994).

Rats with sensorimotor cortex injury and ipsilateral locus ceruleus injury do not recover promptly, but if norepinephrine is infused in the contralateral cerebellum, they recover beam-walking ability in 6 hrs. Norepinephrine appears to be responsible for the accelerated recovery of function from hemiparesis (McDowell 1991). If this interpretation were true, one would expect that administration of pharmacologic agents that block the effects of norepinephrine would have a deleterious effect on the process of recovery of function. This is indeed the case with haloperidol (Feeney *et al.* 1982), diazepam (Schallert *et al.* 1986), clonidine (Goldstein and Davis 1990), prazosin, phenytoin (Brailowsky *et al.* 1986), and phenobarbital. In contrast, agents that enhance the effects of norepinephrine, such as yohimbine, accelerate recovery (Feeney and Sutton 1987). Infusion of GABA, an inhibitory neurotransmitter in the sensorimotor cortex, produces similar motor deficits to the ones described above (Brailowsky *et al.* 1986). Interestingly, if a norepinephrine antagonist is given to a rat after cortical injury and recovery, the motor deficit does return (Brailowsky and Knight 1987). In summary, these experiments in rats indicate that amphetamine plus use accelerates the process of natural recovery following lesions in the sensorimotor cortex and that norepinephrine is probably involved in mediating this effect.

Are the animal studies described here relevant to humans? In the late1970s, researchers reported that hemiplegic patients who received a single dose of amphetamine administered 45 min before intensive physical therapy scored 40% better on motor tests than patients on placebo for at least 24 hrs (Crisostomo *et al.* 1988). The authors studied a total of eight patients (with acute onset of focal neurologic deficit within 10 days of commencing the study) in a double-blind configuration in which four patients received a single dose of amphetamine (10 mg) and four received placebo. They found that the treated patients experienced improvement in motor function, as measured by the Fugl–Meyer scale (although two showed almost no effect), while the control group (placebo) did not. This line of research remained inactive during the 1980s.

In the early 1990s, two papers reported beneficial effects of amphetamine on recovery from aphasia (Walker-Batson D *et al.* 1990, 1992). A more recent report (Walker-Batson D *et al.* 1995) studied 10 patients with hemiplegia (with acute onset of neurologic deficits between 16 and 30 days of starting the study). They received a 10 mg dose of amphetamine or a placebo every fourth day for 10 sessions, paired with physical therapy. In this study, the primary investigator, the neurologist, and the nurse following the patients were unblinded. All other participants in the study were blinded as to the drug/placebo assignment. The dependent measure was also the Fugl–Meyer scale. The target treatment increased the rate and extent of motor recovery. Differences between the two groups began to emerge by session 2, and the level of recovery was maintained at the 12-month follow-up evaluation. Whereas Crisostomo *et al.* (1988) treated patients within 10 days of the ictal episode, this study drew on patients within 30 days of the ictal episode (Walker-Batson *et al.* 1995), extending the 'therapeutic window' of the intervention. Additionally, the authors administered amphetamine every fourth day for a total of 10 doses. Physical therapy and drug administration were timed to parallel the peak period of drug action (Feeney and Sutton 1987). Another study (Borucki *et al.* 1992) included patients 30 days after the stroke and did not standardize the time interval after drug administration before initiation of physical therapy or the the length or intensity of physical therapy. The drug administration plan included continuous dosage for 17 days. It used the same dependent variable (Fugl–Meyer scale) and did not find significant differences in recovery between target and placebo groups.

Tentative conclusions raised by these studies are that (i) the known therapeutic window for this type of treatment is up to 30 days, (ii) multiple sessions of drug and physical therapy (drug-PT) administration appear to provide further therapeutic benefit than single sessions, and (iii) beneficial effects in the target versus the control group lasted for at least 12 months, suggesting that prolonged drug administration is not necessary. The number of drug-PT administrations needed for optimal level of recovery remains unknown. The failure of the trial performed by Borucki *et al.* (1992) to achieve success could also be attributed to the daily administration of the drug. Because amphetamine is a potent releaser of neurotransmitters, continuous administration could deplete the stores of the neurotransmitter system (particularly norepinephrine) required for recovery to take place. A multicenter NINDS funded study is under way to determine the validity of this approach.

Dystonia

Dystonia is a syndrome characterized by involuntary sustained muscle contractions of agonist and antagonist muscles, causing twisting movements and abnormal postures (Hallett 1998). Writer's cramp is a focal action dystonia characterized by dystonic symptoms superimposed on voluntary movement. It is usually task specific, occurring only with writing, typing, playing certain musical instruments (guitar, piano), engaging in specific sports (golf, darts, or sports that involve throwing), or performing activities that involve repetitive hand movements (Chen and Hallett 1998).

Focal hand dystonia may be associated with sensory dysfunction (Hallett 1995). Animal studies performed on owl monkeys showed that long-term training in consistent grip opening and closing resulted in dystonic symptoms. Electrophysiological mapping demonstrated a breakdown of normally separated finger representations in the somatosensory cortex and an enlargement of receptive fields (Byl *et al.* 1996a). Similarly, studies in patients with focal hand dystonia have shown abnormalities of the homuncular representation in the somatosensory cortex (Bara-Jimenez *et al.* 1998;

Elbert *et al.* 1998; Byl *et al.* 2000). Sensorimotor integration may be abnormal in these patients (Odergren *et al.* 1996), and graphesthesia, stereagnosia (Byl *et al.* 1996b), and perception of tonic vibration reflex and movement (Grunewald of *et al.* 1997). It has been proposed that this condition is also associated with difficulties on interpreting sensory information before and during voluntary movement (Murase *et al.* 2000). Decreased tactile spatial acuity and localization (Bara-Jimenez *et al.* 2000a) and abnormal temporal discrimination of somatosensory stimuli (Bara-Jimenez *et al.* 2000b; Sanger *et al.* 2001) have also been reported.

Because somatosensory perception is important for motor control, these findings raised the hypothesis of a cause–effect link between abnormalities in somatosensory cortical representations and dystonia. It was proposed that training-dependent reorganization of the somatosensory homunculus could improve dystonic symptoms (Byl *et al.* 1996a; Byl and Melnick 1997; Chen and Hallett 1998). Zeuner *et al.* (2002) trained patients with focal hand dystonia and normal match volunteers to read Braille as a strategy to decrease the overlap in finger representations in these patients (Sterr *et al.* 1998a,b, 1999). A training period of 8 weeks resulted in improvement in spatial tactile acuity that correlated with an improvement in dystonic symptoms (Zeuner *et al.* 2002). In another study, Candia *et al.* (2002) worked with a group of musicians with focal hand dystonia. These researchers reported immobilization of the non-dystonic fingers of the hand in association with practice of finger motor sequences using the dystonic fingers. It was reported that the guitar and piano players (eight subjects) experienced a significant reduction of dystonic symptoms. However, the three wind players did not show significant improvements. The authors suggested that this lack of response might be related to different types of coordination required between mouth and fingers, different use of the fingers to hold the instruments and maintain constant pressure, or the nature of the fingering required to play these instruments. Although more information is required to draw firm conclusions, these studies represent examples of strategies that use principles of plasticity to plan interventions geared to improve dystonia.

Conclusions

Basic and clinical studies over the last decade have demonstrated that the adult motor cortex experiences substantial reorganization in response to motor training and manipulation of somatosensory input, and that these changes often have important behavioral implications. New strategies described in this chapter have been developed to improve motor function in patients with motor disorders, including stroke and dystonia.

References

Abraham WC, Bear MF (1996). Metaplasticity: the plasticity of synaptic plasticity. *Trends Cogn Sci* 1996; **9**, 126–30.

Aizawa H, Inase M, Mushiake H, Shima K, Tanji J (1991). Reorganization of activity in the supplementary motor area associated with motor learning and functional recovery. *Exp Brain Res*, **84**, 668–71.

Allard T, Clark SA, Jenkins WM, Merzenich MM (1991). Reorganization of somatosensory area 3b representations in adult owl monkeys after digital syndactyly. *J Neurophysiol*, **66**, 1048–58.

American Heart Association. (1998). *1998 and Stroke Statistical Update*. Dallas, TX: AHA.

Bara-Jimenez W, Catalan MJ, Hallett M, Gerloff C (1998). Abnormal somatosensory homunculus in dystonia of the hand. *Ann Neurol* 1998; 44: 828–31.

Bara-Jimenez W, Shelton, Hallett M (2000b). Spatial discrimination is abnormal in focal hand dystonia. *Neurology*, **55**, 1869–73.

Bara-Jimenez W, Shelton P, Sanger TD, Hallett M (2000b). Sensory discrimination capabilities in patients with focal hand dystonia. *Ann Neurol*, **47**, 377–80.

Bastian H (1887). The 'muscular sense'; its nature and cortical localisation. *Brain*, **10**, 1–137.

Bear MF, Malenka R (1994). Synaptic plasticity: LTP and LTD. *Curr Opin Neurobiol*, **4**, 389–99.

Bliss TV, Gardner MA (1973). Long-lasting potentiation of synaptic transmission in the dentate area of the unanaesthetized rabbit following stimulation of the perforant path. *J Physiol (Lond)*, **232**, 357–74.

Borucki SJ, Langberg J, Reding M (1992). The effect of dextroamphetamine on motor recovery after stroke. *Neurology*, **42**, 329.

Boyeson MG, Feeney D (1990). Intraventricular norepinephrine facilitates motor recovery following sensorimotor cortex injury. *Pharmacol Biochem Behav*, **35**, 497–501.

Boyeson MG, Krobert KA, Scherer PJ, Grade C (1993). Reinstatement of motor deficits in brain injured animals: the role of cerebellar norepinephrine. *Restor Neurol Neurosci*, **5**, 283–90.

Boyeson MG, Jones JL, Harmon R (1994). Sparing of motor function after cortical injury. A new perspective on underlying mechanisms. *Arch Neurol*, **51**, 405–14.

Brailowsky S, Knight RT, Efron R (1986). Phenytoin increases the severity of cortical hemiplegia in rats. *Brain Res*, **376**, 71–7.

Brailowsky S, Knight R (1987). Recovery from GABA-mediated hemiplegia in young and aged rats: effects of catecholaminergic manipulations. *Neurobiol Aging*, **8**, 441–7.

Brasil-Neto JP, Cohen LG, Pascual-Leone A, Jabir FK, Wall RT, Hallett M (1992). Rapid reversible modulation of human motor outputs after transient deafferentation of the forearm: a study with transcranial magnetic stimulation. *Neurology*, **42**, 1302–6.

Brasil-Neto JP, Valls-Solé J, Pascual-Leone A, Cammarota A, Amassian VE, Cracco R, *et al.* (1993). Rapid modulation of human cortical motor outputs following ischemic nerve block. *Brain*, **116**, 511–25.

Buonomano DV, Merzenich MM (1998). Cortical plasticity: from synapses to maps. *Annu Rev Neurosci* 1998; **21**, 149–186.

Butefisch CM, Davis BC, Wise SP, Sawaki L, Kopyler L, Classen J, *et al.* (2000). Mechanisms of use-dependent plasticity in the human motor cortex. *Proc Natl Acad Sci USA*, **97**, 3661–5.

Butefisch CM, Davis BC, Sawaki L, Waldvogel D, Classen J, Kopylev L, *et al.* (2002). Modulation of use-dependent plasticity by D-amphetamine. *Ann Neurol*, **51**, 59–68.

Byl NN, Melnick M (1997). The neural consequences of repetition: clinical implications of a learning hypothesis. *J Hand Ther*, **10**, 160–74.

Byl NN, Merzenich MM, Jenkins W (1996a). A primate genesis model of focal dystonia and repetitive strain injury: I. Learning induced dedifferentiation of the representation of the hand in the primary somatosensory cortex in adult monkeys. *Neurology*, **47**, 508–20.

Byl N, Wilson F, Merzenich M, Melnick M, Scott P, Oakes A, *et al.* (1996b). Sensory dysfunction associated with repetitive strain injuries of tendinitis and focal hand dystonia: a comparative study. *J Orthop Sports Phys Ther*, **23**, 234–44.

Byl NN, McKenzie A, Nagarajan S (2000). Differences in somatosensory hand organization in a healthy flutist and a flutist with focal hand dystonia: a case report. *J Hand Ther*, **13**, 302–9.

Candia V, Schafer T, Taub E, Rau H, Altenmuller E, Rockstroh B, *et al.* (2002). Sensory motor retuning: a behavioral treatment for focal hand dystonia of pianists and guitarists. *Arch Phys Med Rehabil*, **83**, 1342–8.

Caramia MD, Iani C, Bernardi G (1996). Cerebral plasticity after stroke as revealed by ipsilateral responses to magnetic stimulation. *NeuroReport*, **7**, 1756–60.

Chen R, Hallett M (1998). Focal dystonia and repetitive motion disorders. *Clinical Orthop Relat Res*, **351**, 102–6.

Chen R, Corwell, B, Hallett, M, Cohen LG (1997). Mechanisms involved in motor reorganization following lower limb amputation. *Neurology*, **48**: A345.

Chino Y, Kaas JH, Smith E, Langston AL, Cheng H (1992). Rapid reorganization of cortical maps in adult cats following restricted deafferentation in retina. *Vision Res*, **32**, 789–96.

Clark AN, Mankikar GD, Gray I (1975). Diogenes syndrome. A clinical study of gross neglect in old age. *Lancet*, **i**, 366–8.

Classen J, Liepert J, Wise SP, Hallett M, Cohen L (1998). Rapid plasticity of human cortical movement representation induced by practice. *J Neurophysiol*, **79**, 1117–23.

Cohen LG, Roth BJ, Nilsson J, Dang N, Panizza M, Bandinelli S, *et al.* (1990). Effects of coil design on delivery of focal magnetic stimulation. Technical considerations. *Electroencephalogr Clin Neurophysiol*, **75**, 350–7.

Cohen L, Bandinelli S, Findley TW, Hallett M (1991). Motor reorganization after upper limb amputation in man. A study with focal magnetic stimulation. *Brain*, **114**, 615–27.

Conforto AB, Kaelin-Lang A, Cohen L (2002). Increase in hand muscle strength of stroke patients after somatosensory stimulation. *Ann Neurol*, **51**, 122–5.

Crisostomo EA, Duncan PW, Propst M, Dawson DV, Davis J (1988). Evidence that amphetamine with physical therapy promotes recovery of motor function in stroke patients. *Ann Neurol*, **23**, 94–7.

Donoghue JP, Sanes J (1987). Peripheral nerve injury in developing rats reorganizes representation pattern in motor cortex. *Proc Natl Acad Sci USA*, **84**, 1123–6.

Donoghue JP, Sanes JN (1988). Organization of adult motor cortex representation patterns following neonatal forelimb nerve injury in rats. *J Neurosci*, **8**, 3221–32.

Donoghue JP Hess G, Sanes JN (1996). *Substrates and Mechanisms for Learning in Motor Cortex*. Cambridge, MA: MIT Press.

Donoghue JP, Suner S, Sanes JN (1990). Dynamic organization of primary motor cortex output to target muscles in adult rats. II. Rapid reorganization following motor nerve lesions. *Exp Brain Res*, **79**, 492–503.

Douglas RM, Goddard G (1975). Long-term potentiation of the perforant path-granule cell synapse in the rat hippocampus. *Brain Res*, **86**, 205–15.

Elbert T, Candia V, Altenmuller E (1998). Alteration of digital representations in somatosensory cortex in focal hand dystonia. *NeuroReport*, **9**, 3571–5.

Feeney D (1991). Pharmacological modulation of recovery after brain injury. A reconsideration of diaschisis. *Neurol Rehabil*, **5**, 113–28.

Feeney DM, Hovda D (1985) Reinstatement of binocular depth perception by amphetamine and visual experience after visual cortex ablation. *Brain Res* **342**, 352–356.

Feeney DM, Sutton R (1987). Pharmacotherapy for recovery of function after brain injury. *CRC Crit Rev Neurobiol*, **3**, 135–97.

Feeney DM, Gonzalez A, Law W (1982). Amphetamine, haloperidol, and experience interact to affect rate of recovery after motor cortex injury. *Science*, **217**, 855–7.

Feeney DM, Sutton RL, Boyeson MG, Hovda DA, Dail W (1985). The locus coeruleus and cerebral metabolis: recovery of function after cortical injury. *Physiol Psychol*, **13**, 197–203.

Feeney DM, Weisend MP, Kline A (1993). Noradrenergic pharmacotherapy, intracerebral infusion and adrenal transplantation promote functional recovery after cortical damage. *J Neural Transplant Plast* 1993; **4**, 199–213.

Fischer TM, Blazis DE, Priver NA, Carew TJ (1997). Metaplasticity at identified inhibitory synapses in aplysia. *Nature*, **389**, 860–5.

Fraser C, Power M, Hamdy S, Rothwell J, Hobday D, Hollander I, *et al.* (2002). Driving plasticity in human adult motor cortex is associated with improved motor function after brain injury. *Neuron*, **34**, 831–40.

Frost SB, Barbay S, Friel KM, Plautz EJ, Nudo RJ (2003). Reorganization of remote cortical regions after ischemic brain injury: a potential substrate for stroke recovery. *J Neurophysiol*, **89**, 3205–14.

Fuhr P, Cohen LG, Dang N, Findley TW, Haghighi S, Oro J, *et al.* (1992). Physiological analysis of motor reorganization following lower limb amputation. *Electroencephalogr Clin Neurophysiol*, **85**, 53–60.

Goldstein L (1993). Basic and clinical studies of pharmacologic effects on recovery from brain injury. *J Neural Transplant Plast*, **4**, 175–92.

Goldstein LB, Davis J (1990). Clonidine impairs recovery of beam-walking after a sensorimotor cortex lesion in the rat. *Brain Res*, **508**, 305–9.

Grunewald RA, Yoneda Y, Shipman JM, Sagar H (1997). Idiopathic focal dystonia: a disorder of muscle spindle afferent processing? *Brain*, **120**, 2179–85.

Guic E, Rodriguez E, Caviedes P, Merzenich M (1993). Use-dependent reorganization of the barrel field in adult rats. *Abstr Soc Neurosci*, **19**, 163.

Hallett M (1995). Is dystonia a sensory disorder? *Ann Neurol*, **38**, 139–40.

Hallett M (1998). The neurophysiology of dystonia. *Arch Neurol*, **55**, 601–3.

Hamdy S, Rothwell JC, Aziz Q, Singh KD, Thompson D (1998). Long-term reorganization of human motor cortex driven by short-term sensory stimulation. *Nat Neurosci*, **1**, 64–8.

Hardy TL, Bertrand G, Thompson C (1979). The position and orgnaization of motor fibers in the internal capsule found during sterotactic surgery. *Appl Neurophysiol*, **42**, 160–170.

Hess G, Donoghue J (1994). Long-term potentiation of horizontal connections provides a mechanism to reorganize cortical motor maps. *J Neurophysiol*, **71**, 2543–7.

Hovda DA, Feeney D (1984). Amphetamine and experience promote recovery of locomotor function after unilateral frontal cortex injury in the cat. *Brain Res*, **298**, 358–61.

Hovda DA, Sutton RL, Feeney D (1989). Amphetamine-induced recovery of visual cliff performance after bilateral visual cortex ablation in cats: measurements of depth perception thresholds. *Behav Neurosci*, **103**, 574–84.

Hubel DH, Wiesel T (1965). Binocular interaction in striate cortex of kittens raised with artificial squint. *J Neurophysiol*, **28**, 1041–59.

Jacobs KM, Donoghue JP (1991). Reshaping the cortical motor map by unmasking latent intracortical connections. *Science*, **251**, 944–7.

Jenkins WM, Merzenich MM, Ochs MT, Allard T, Guic-Robles EJ (1990). Functional reorganization of primary somatosensory cortex in adult owl monkeys after behaviorally controlled tactile stimulation. *J Neurophysiol*, **63**, 82–104.

Johansen-Berg H, Rushworth MF, Bogdanovic MD, Kischka U, Wimalaratna S, Matthews PM (2002). The role of ipsilateral premotor cortex in hand movement after stroke. *Proc Natl Acad Sci USA*, **99**, 14518–23.

Johansson K, Lindgren I, Widner H, Wiklund I, Johansson B (1993). Can sensory stimulation improve the functional outcome in stroke patients? *Neurology*, **43**, 2189–92.

Kaas J (1991). Plasticity of sensory and motor maps in adult mammals. *Annu Rev Neurosci*, **14**, 137–67.

Kaas JH, Krubitzer LA, Chino YM, Langston AL, Polley EH, Blair N (1990). Reorganization of retinotopic cortical maps in adult mammals after lesions of the retina. *Science*, **248**, 229–31.

Kaelin-Lang A, Luft AR, Sawaki L, Burstein AH, Sohn YH, Cohen LG (2002). Modulation of human corticomotor excitability by somatosensory input. *J Physiol (Lond)*, **540**, 623–33.

Kalaska J, Pomeranz B (1979). Chronic paw denervation causes an age-dependent appearance of novel responses from forearm in 'paw cortex' of kittens and adult cats. *J Neurophysiol*, **42**, 618–33.

Karl A, Birbaumer N, Lutzenberger W, Cohen LG, Flor H (2001). Reorganization of motor and somatosensory cortex in upper extremity amputees with phantom limb pain. *J Neurosci*, **21**, 3609–18.

Karni A, Meyer G, Jezzard P, Adams MM, Turner R, Ungerleider LG (1995). Functional MRI evidence for adult motor cortex plasticity during motor skill learning. *Nature*, **377**, 155–8.

Kopp B, Kunkel A, Muhlnickel W, Villringer K, Taub E, Flor H (1999). Plasticity in the motor system related to therapy-induced improvement of movement after stroke. *NeuroReport*, **17**, 807–10.

Kunkel A, Kopp B, Muller G, Villringer K, Villringer A, Taub E, *et al.* (1999). Constraint-induced movement therapy for motor recovery in chronic stroke patients. *Arch Phys Med Rehabil*, **80**, 624–8.

Levi-Montalcini R, Angeletti PU (1968). Nerve growth factor. *Physiol Rev*, **48**, 534–69.

Levy LM, Ziemann U, Chen R, Cohen LG (2002). Rapid modulation of GABA in sensorimotor cortex induced by acute deafferentation. *Ann Neurol*, **52**, 755–61.

Liepert J, Miltner WHR, Bauder H, Sommer M, Dettmers C, Taub E, *et al.* (1998). Motor cortex plasticity during constraint-induced movement therapy in stroke patients. *Neurosci Lett*, **250**, 5–8.

Lipper S, Tuchman M (1976). Treatment of chronic post-traumatic organic brain syndrome with dextroamphetamine: first reported case. *J Nerv Ment Dis*, **162**, 366–71.

Lynch GS, Dunwiddie T, Gribkoff V (1977). Heterosynaptic depression: a postsynaptic correlate of long-term potentiation. *Nature*, **266**, 737–9.

McDowell F (1991). Activation of rehabilitation. *Arzneimittelforschung*, **41**, 355–9.

Merzenich MM, Kaas JH, Wall JT, Sur M, Nelson RJ, Felleman DJ (1983). Progression of change following median nerve section in the cortical representation of the hand in areas 3b and 1 in adult owl and squirrel monkeys. *Neuroscience*, **10**, 639–65.

Merzenich MM, Nelson RJ, Stryker MP, Cynder MS, Shoppmann A, Zook JM (1984). Somatosensory cortical map changes following digit amputation in adult monkeys. *J Comp Neurol*, **224**, 591–605.

Merzenich MM, Recantone G, Jenkins WM, Allard TT, Nudo RJ (1988). Cortical representational plasticity. In: PW Rakic, S Singer, (ed.) *Neurobiology of Neocortex*, pp. 41–67. New York: Wiley.

Miltner WH, Bauder H, Sommer M, Dettmers C, Taub E (1999). Effects of constraint-induced movement therapy on patients with chronic motor deficits after stroke: a replication. *Stroke*, **30**, 586–92.

Mitz AR, Godschalk M, Wise SP (1991). Learning-dependent neuronal activity in the premotor cortex: activity during the acquisition of conditional motor associations. *J Neurosci*, **11**, 1855–72.

Muellbacher W, Ziemann U, Boroojerdi B, Cohen L, Hallett M (2001). Role of the human motor cortex in rapid motor learning. *Exp Brain Res*, **136**, 431–8.

Muellbacher W, Richards C, Ziemann U, Wittenberg G, Weltz D, Boroojerdi B, *et al.* (2002). Improving hand function in chronic stroke. *Arch Neurol*, **59**, 1278–82.

Murase N, Kaji R, Shimazu H, Katayama-Hirota M, Ikeda A, Kohara N, *et al.* (2000). Abnormal premovement gating of somatosensory input in writer's cramp. *Brain*, **123**, 1813–29.

Nudo JR, Wise BM, SiFuentes FS, Milliken G (1996a). Neural substrates for the effects of rehabilitative training on motor recovery after ischemic infarct. *Science*, **272**, 1791–4.

Nudo RJ, Milliken GW, Jenkins WM, Merzenich MM (1996b). Use-dependent alterations of movement representations in primary motor cortex of adult squirrel monkeys. *J Neurosci*, **16**, 785–807.

Nudo RJ, Jenkins WM, Merzenich MM (1990). Repetitive microstimulation alters the cortical representation of movements in adult rats. *Somatosens Mot Res*, **7**, 463–83.

Nudo RJ, Plautz EJ, Frost S (2001). Role of adaptive plasticity in recovery of function after damage to motor cortex. *Muscle Nerve*, **24**, 1000–19.

Odergren T, Iwasaki N, Borg J, Forssberg H (1996). Impaired sensory motor integration during grasping in writer's cramp. *Brain*, **119**, 569–83.

Ostendorf CG, Wolf S (1981). Effect of forced use of the upper extremity of a hemiplegic patient on changes in function. A single-case design. *Phys Ther*, **61**, 1022–8.

Palmer E, Ashby P, Hajek VE (1992). Ipsilateral fast corticospinal pathways do not account for recovery in stroke. *Ann Neurol*, **32**, 519–25.

Pascual-Leone A, Nguyet D, Cohen LG, Brasil NJ, Cammarota A, Hallett M (1995). Modulation of muscle responses evoked by transcranial magnetic stimulation during the acquisition of new fine motor skills. *J Neurophysiol*, **74**, 1037–45.

Pearson K (2000). Motor systems. *Curr Opin Neurobiol*, **10**, 649–54.

Pons T (1996). Novel sensations in the congenitally blind. *Nature*, **380**, 479–80.

Pons TP, Garraghty PE, Ommaya AK, Kaas JH, Taub E, Mishkin M (1991). Massive cortical reorganization after sensory deafferentation in adult macaques. *Science*, **252**, 1857–60.

Powell J, Pandyan AD, Granat M, Cameron M, Stott D (1999). Electrical stimulation of wrist extensors in poststroke hemiplegia. *Stroke*, **30**, 1384–9.

Recanzone GH, Jenkins WM, Hradek GT, Merzenich, MM (1992a). Progressive improvement in discriminative abilities in adult owl monkeys performing a tactile frequency discrimination task. *J Neurophysiol*, **67**, 1015–30.

Recanzone GH, Merzenich MM, Jenkins WM, Grajski KA, Dinse HR (1992b). Topographic reorganization of the hand representation in cortical area 3b owl monkeys trained in a frequency-discrimination task. *J Neurophysiol*, **67**, 1031–56.

Recanzone GH, Merzenich MM, Jenkins WM (1992c). Frequency discrimination training engaging a restricted skin surface results in an emergence of a cutaneous response zone in cortical area 3a. *J Neurophysiol*, **67**, 1057–70.

Recanzone GH, Merzenich MM, Schreiner CE (1992d). Changes in the distributed temporal response properties of SI cortical neurons reflect improvements in performance on a temporally based tactile discrimination task. *J Neurophysiol*, **67**, 1071–91.

Ridding MC, McKay DR, Thompson PD, Miles TS (2001). Changes in corticomotor representations induced by prolonged peripheral nerve stimulation in humans. *Clin Neurophysiol*, **112**, 1461–9.

Robertson D, Irvine D (1989). Plasticity of frequency organization in auditory cortex of guinea pigs with partial unilateral deafness. *J Comp Neurol*, **282**, 456–71.

Robinson RG, Shoemaker WJ, Schlumpf M, Valk T, Bloom F (1975). Effect of experimental cerebral infarction in rat brain on catecholamines and behaviour. *Nature*, **255**, 332–4.

Sadato N, Zeffiro TA, Campbell G, Konishi J, Shibasaki H, Hallett M (1995). Regional cerebral blood flow changes in motor cortical areas after transient anesthesia of the forearm. *Ann Neurol*, **37**, 74–81.

Sanes JN, Suner S, Donoghue JP (1990). Dynamic organization of primary motor cortex output to target muscles in adult rats. I. Long-term patterns of reorganization following motor or mixed peripheral nerve lesions. *Exp Brain Res*, **79**, 479–91.

Sanes JN, Wang J, Donoghue JP (1992). Immediate and delayed changes of rat motor cortical output representation with new forelimb configurations. *Cereb Cortex*, **2**, 141–52.

Sanger TD, Tarsy D, Pascual-Leone A (2001). Abnormalities of spatial and temporal sensory discrimination in writer's cramp. *Mov Disord*, **16**, 94–9.

Sawaki L, Boroojerdi B, Kaelin-Lang A, Burstein AH, Butefisch CM, Kopylev L, *et al.* (2002a). Cholinergic influences on use-dependent plasticity. *J Neurophysiol*, **87**, 166–71.

Sawaki L, Cohen LG, Classen J, Davis BC, Butefisch CM (2002b). Enhancement of use-dependent plasticity by D-amphetamine. *Neurology*, **59**, 1262–4.

Sawaki L, Wu C, Stefan K, Yaseen Z, Cohen L (2003). Training-dependent encoding of a motor memory in patients with chronic stroke (Abstract). *Neurology*.

Schallert T, Hernandez TD, Barth T (1986). Recovery of function after brain damage: severe and chronic disruption by diazepam. *Brain Res*, **379**, 104–11.

Shadmehr R, Holcomb H (1997). Neural correlates of motor memory consolidation. *Science*, **277**, 821–5.

Stefan K, Kunesch E, Cohen LG, Benecke R, Classen J (2000). Induction of plasticity in the human motor cortex by paired associative stimulation. *Brain*, **123**, 572–84.

Sterr A, Muller MM, Elbert T, Rockstroh B, Pantev C, Taub E (1998a). Changed perceptions in Braille readers. *Nature*, **391**, 134–5.

Sterr A, Muller MM, Elbert T, Rockstroh B, Pantev C, Taub E (1998b). Perceptual correlates of changes in cortical representation of fingers in blind multifinger Braille readers. *J Neurosci*, **18**, 4417–23.

Sterr A, Muller M, Elbert T, Rockstroh B, Taub E (1999). Development of cortical reorganization in the somatosensory cortex of adult Braille students. *Electroencephalogr Clin Neurophysiol Suppl*, **49**, 292–8.

Sutton RL, Hovda DA, Feeney D (1989). Amphetamine accelerates recovery of locomotor function following bilateral frontal cortex ablation in cats. *Behav Neurosci*, **103**, 837–41.

Tangeman PT, Banaitis DA, Williams A (1990). Rehabilitation of chronic stroke patients: changes in functional performance. *Arch Phys Med Rehabil*, **71**, 876–80.

Taub E, Miller NE, Novack TA, Cook EW, Fleming WC, Nepomuceno CS, *et al.* (1993). Technique to improve chronic motor deficit after stroke. *Arch Phys Med Rehabil*, **74**, 347–54.

Taub E, Uswatte G, Pidikiti R (1999). Constraint-induced movement therapy: a new family of techniques with broad application to physical rehabilitation—a clinical review. *J Rehabil Res Dev*, **36**, 237–51.

Taub E, Uswatte G, Elbert T (2002). New treatments in neurorehabilitation founded on basic research. *Nat Rev Neurosci*, **3**, 228–36.

Turton A, Wroe S, Trepte N, Fraser C, Lemon R (1996). Contralateral and ipsilateral EMG responses to transcranial magnetic stimulation during recovery of arm and hand function after stroke. *Electroencephalogr Clin Neurophysiol*, **101**, 316–28.

Walker-Batson D, Devous MD, Curtis S, Unwin H, Greenlee P (1990). Use of amphetamine to facilitate recovery from aphasia subsequent to stroke. *Clin Aphasiol*, **20**, 137–44.

Walker-Batson D, Unwin H, Curtis C (1992). Use of amphetamine in the treatment of aphasia. *Restor Neurol Neurosci*, **4**, 47–50.

Walker-Batson D, Smith P, Curtis S, Unwin H, Greenlee R (1995). Amphetamine paired with physical therapy accelerates motor recovery after stroke. Further evidence. *Stroke*, **26**, 2254–9.

Wall JT (1988). Development and maintenance of somatotopic maps of the skin: a mosaic hypothesis based on peripheral and central contiguities. *Brain Behav Evol*, **31**, 252–68.

Wall JT, Kaas J (1986). Long-term cortical consequences of reinnervation errors after nerve regeneration in monkeys. *Brain Res*, **372**, 400–4.

Wall JT, Kaas JH, Sur M, Nelson RJ, Felleman DJ, Merzenich M (1986). Functional reorganization in somatosensory cortical areas 3b and 1 of adult monkeys after median nerve repair: possible relationships to sensory recovery in humans. *J Neurosci*, **6**, 218–33.

Weiller C, Chollet F, Friston KJ, Wise RJ, Frackowiak RS (1992). Functional reorganization of the brain in recovery from striatocapsular infarction in man. *Ann Neurol*, **31**, 463–72.

Weiller C, Ramsay SC, Wise RJ, Friston KJ, Frackowiak RS (1993). Individual patterns of functional reorganization in the human cerebral cortex after capsular infarction. *Ann Neurol*, **33**, 181–9.

Werhahn KJ, Mortensen J, Kaelin-Lang A, Boroojerdi B, Cohen L (2002a). Cortical excitability changes induced by deafferentation of the contralateral hemisphere. *Brain*, **125**, 1402–13.

Werhahn KJ, Mortensen J, Van Boven R, Zeuner K, Cohen L (2002b). Enhanced tactile spatial acuity and cortical processing during acute hand deafferentation. *Nat Neurosci*, **5**, 936–8.

Winstein CJ, Merians AS, Sullivan K (1999). Motor learning after unilateral brain damage. *Neuropsychologia*, **37**, 975–87.

Wolf SL, Lecraw DE, Barton LA, Jann B (1989). Forced use of hemiplegic upper extremities to reverse the effect of learned nonuse among chronic stroke and head-injured patients. *Exp Neurol*, **104**, 125–32.

Wong AM, Su TY, Tang FT, Cheng PT, Liaw M (1999). Clinical trial of electrical acupuncture on hemiplegic stroke patients. *Am J Phys Med Rehabil*, **7**, 117–22.

World Health Organization (1989). Recommendations on stroke prevention, diagnosis and therapy: report of the WHO Task Force on Stroke and Other Cerebrovascular Disorders. *Stroke*, **20**, 1407–31.

Zeuner KE, Bara-Jimenez W, Noguchi PS, Goldstein SR, Dambrosia JM, Hallett M (2002). Sensory training for patients with focal hand dystonia. *Ann Neurol*, **51**, 593–8.

Ziemann U, Corwell B, Hallett M, Cohen L (1997). Modulation of plastic changes in human motor cortex after forearm ischemic nerve block. *Abstr Soc Neurosci*, **22**, 37.

Ziemann U, Corwell B, Cohen LG (1998a). Modulation of plasticity in human motor cortex after forearm ischemic nerve block. *J Neurosci*, **18**, 1115–23.

Ziemann U, Hallett M, Cohen LG (1998b). Mechanisms of deafferentation-induced plasticity in human motor cortex. *J Neurosci*, **18**, 7000–7.

Ziemann U, Wittenberg GF, Cohen L (2002). Stimulation-induced within-representation and across-representation plasticity in human motor cortex. *J Neurosci*, **22**, 5563–71.

Chapter 26

Perspectives in higher-order motor deficit rehabilitation. Which approach for which ecological result?

Yves Rossetti, Gilles Rode, and Georg Goldenberg

La notion même de geste se situe entre celle de contraction musculaire et celle de comportement, et l'on tend de façon répétitive à la réduire au premier ou au second de ces domaines, déniant ainsi sa spécificité, et situant la science des gestes ou bien dans ce détail de la mécanique musculaire, où l'unité de connaissance s'identifie à la contraction isolée d'un muscle, ou bien dans cette globalité de l'être-au-monde où tout doit s'envisager dans la totalité. (Hecaen and Lanteri-Laura 1983, p. 54)*

There is a wide variability of motor impairments. Motor deficits can result from the damage of pure motor, sensory, or cognitive systems, or from combinations of the three. While sensory deficits can be partially compensated by learning specific strategies to use the remaining senses, motor deficits due to lesion of the motor output areas and from cognitive functions linked to action planning or to space representation have strong debilitating consequences. As examples of these conditions, in this chapter we will discuss the methods used to rehabilitate some intrinsic or extrinsic motor disorders such as hemiplegia, apraxia, and those disorders resulting from misrepresentation of space. Because these pathologies have distinct origins and result from the impairment of separable levels of the organization of action, the methods proposed by recent research in rehabilitation can be very different. Nevertheless, it is interesting to consider these differences and to examine the rehabilitation techniques proposed for the corresponding disorders. Several crucial aspects of the rehabilitation procedure need to be considered: the generalization of the training, the duration of the therapeutic effects, and the level of action participating to the improvement. We will first review the current state of knowledge that is useful for developing or applying practical

---

* The very notion of gesture lies between that of muscular contraction and that of behaviour. One repeatedly tends to assimilate it to the former or to the latter, thereby denying its specificity and locating science of gesture either in this detail of muscular mechanics (where the knowledge unit is identified with an isolated muscular contraction) or in the wholeness of being-in-the-world (where everything must be envisaged in the totality).

techniques of rehabilitation. Then we shall classify the techniques and articulate their level of action to the anatomical and functional level of the physiopathological disturbances responsible for the deficit. These levels of action will be particularly examined with respect to the distinction between top-down and botton-up aproaches.

Hemiplegia

Ecological significance

The ecological significance of hemiplegia is obvious and does not require a detailed description here. Motor deficiency is the leading cause of disability following damage to the central nervous system, particularly in the case of middle cerebral artery stroke (Duncan *et al.* 1992). Other deficiencies such as sensory or cognitive impairments may be associated and worsen the severity of disability and consecutive disadvantage. Motor deficit remains the main target of rehabilitative interventions. Intensive rehabilitation interventions are being used more commonly in order to reduce long-term disability (Tallis 2000). The main question about these rehabilitation techniques is whether the observed improvements are attributable to spontaneous functional recovery or are due to specific cortical plasticity patterns. This functional question is further complicated by consideration of the brain activity markers of the improvements and their potential link with therapeutic interventions. In the present section we will focus on the recent interest in constraint-induced therapy and its anatomical correlates.

Neurophysiological significance

Motor recovery is a fairly well documented process. Classical studies reported that most of the spontaneous restitution of motor function occurs within the first 2 months after injury (Twitchell 1951; Van Buskirk 1954). However, the motor improvement may continue for up to a year, although to a lesser degree (Ahlsio *et al.* 1984; Kotila *et al.* 1984). Interestingly, functional motor recovery curves follow non-linear trends, at least at the individual level (Newman 1972; Partridge and Edwards 1988; Gray *et al.* 1990; Jones *et al.* 1990; Rode *et al.* 1996). The characteristic steps and plateaus observed may represent a staged process, reflecting the complexity of neurophysiological mechanisms involved in the recovery (Jeannerod 1988). Recovery from a motor deficit appears to be a complex multifactorial process. There is now increasing evidence that there is a relationship between the motor spontaneous recovery occuring after stroke and the cortical plasticity revealed by functional imaging (see also Chapter 25, this volume).

The advantage of elementary motor deficit (due to lesions in primary motor area) is that corresponding brain areas are best identified and described in both animal and human studies. Human brain imaging studies using activation positron emission tomography (PET) show that motor recovery is due in part to the extension of motor areas in the affected hemisphere, and in part to the recruitment of ipsilateral motor pathways (Chollet *et al.* 1991; Weiller *et al.* 1992). However, the exact pattern of change reported with movement of a recovered limb varies between studies; there is either a predominance of increased activity in the undamaged hemisphere (Chollet *et al.* 1991, 2000; Weiller *et al.* 1992; Caramia *et al.* 1996; Cramer *et al.* 1997; Honda *et al.* 1997; Cao *et al.* 1998), or changes in the extent (Cao *et al.* 1998) or location (Rossini *et al.* 1998; Pineiro *et al.* 2001) of activity in primary motor cortices (Netz *et al.* 1997) or other cortical networks. In particular, involvment of premotor (supplementary motor area) and parietal cortices (Pantano *et al.* 1996; Nelles *et al.* 1999, 2001), as well as the cerebellum and primary somatosensory cortices (Chollet 2000) have been described. The altered pattern of activation reflects the adaptive reorganization of the brain and the dynamic character of this reorganization.

Another crucial question is whether the spontaneous motor recovery can be boosted to improve the potential for recovering function and whether the improvement observed at the anatomical level can be correlated with the disability shown at the behavioural level. Results from experimental studies in monkeys argue for such a correlation. Nudo *et al.* (1996) carried out an innovative study using intracortical microstimulation in adult squirrel monkeys. An ischaemic infarct was produced surgically in the cortical area controlling the movements of one paw. It was shown that specific training of the more affected limb resulted in cortical reorganization. Specifically, the area surrounding the infarct, which would not normally be involved in control of the paw, began to participate in these movements. The results suggest that rehabilitative therapy prevents further shrinkage of hand area in the adjacent intact tissue, and that the surrounding intact tissue may become involved in the damaged function.

Top-down versus bottom-up processes

The classical approach to the rehabilitation of motor disorders consists of stimulating the use of the paretic arm during specific training sessions supervised by physiotherapists or occupational therapists, as well as encouragement to use this arm in everyday life. While some patients are particularly motivated to train the paretic arm actively in their daily life, others seem to rely mainly on their healthy arm and make little effort with their paretic arm. One theoretical approach to this question postulated that inhibiting the normal activity of brain areas which subserve activity of the healthy arm may enhance the development of cortical compensation mechanisms for the paretic arm.

The idea of a constraint-induced therapy relying on training the paretic arm and restraining the contralateral arm was initially proposed by Taub and colleagues (reviewed by Taub *et al.* 2002) This rehabilitation programme was proposed for patients with a chronic upper extremity hemiparesis. Patients received 14 days of constraint-induced therapy in which they agreed to wear a resting hand splint secured in a sling that prevented use of the non paretic upper extremity for 90% of waking hours. This arrangement obviously resulted in a major increase in the use of the paretic arm. In addition, during the 8 weekdays treatment period, the subjects received intensive daily training for 6 hrs in using the affected arm in a variety of tasks according to a behavioural technique termed 'shaping'. Control hemiparetic subjects were included. They were told that they had much greater movement of their affected limb than they were actually showing and were led through a series of passive movement exercises. The results showed a significant increase in the skill or quality of movement in the treated group, as measured by motor assessment test, and a much larger increase in real-world arm use over the 2 week period. Moreover, the treated group showed no decrease in real-world arm use when tested 2 years after the treatment, although the control subjects showed no change or even a decline in real-life arm use over the same period (Taub *et al*. 1993). The initial results with constraint-induced therapy have now been confirmed in other studies (Kunkel *et al*. 1999; Miltner *et al*. 1999; Sterr *et al*. 2002). It has been suggested that a direct repeated training of the paretic arm after stroke involves a long-term improvement of motor function. This improvement clearly differs from results obtained with classical rehabilitation techniques such as the Bobath method (De Pedro-Cuesta *et al*. 1992; Duncan 1997; Paci 2003). In the case of such low-level motor disorder, it is rather difficult to discuss the notion of top-down versus bottom-up rehabilitative approaches. However, we wish to suggest that the recently proposed constraint-induced therapy can be viewed as a bottom-up approach which can be contrasted with the classical top-down method consisting of intentional active stimulation of motor activity on the paretic side.

It is not our aim in this chapter to evaluate constraint-induced therapy. In fact, it is questionable whether passive movement (zero level) rather than conventional methods (stimulation) can be an appropriate control of constraint-induced therapy (stimulation plus ipsilateral inhibition). In any case, this approach confirms that active movements favour a functional recovery either by inhibiting spontaneous functional compensation or by stimulating the motor system through constant practice. In our view, constraint-induced therapy appears as a behavioural technique relying on a bottom-up approach, based on a commitment to perform actions with the paretic arm without questioning the manner of performing them. The aim is to establish a routine which will proceed automatically when the training is performed. In this sense, this technique clearly differs from classical rehabilitation techniques, which rely on a top-down approach. Indeed, in this situation patients have to relearn the type of movement that they must perform. The different phases of the movement (preparation, initiation, and execution) involve conscious participation by the patient. In the case of constraint-induced therapy it is rather the immediate situation of the patient that will stimulate (bottom up) the activation of motor activity in the free arm than a mediating strategy (top down) that will intentionally avoid or interrupt the spontaneous activation of the healthy arm.

Generalization of therapeutic gains

Even though interesting dissociations have been observed in the motor performance of individual patients between distinct levels of action control (Schenk *et al*. 1999), such rare dissociations have not been explored in terms of appropriate rehabilitation techniques.

In the case of hemiplegia due to a lesion of the pyramidal tract, improvements mainly deal with distinct anatomical territories rather than with distinct types of action. Therefore the main parameter for judging the generalization of a therapeutic gain on hemiplegia is the duration of the improvement.

It is interesting to note that the long-term improvement of motor function and generalization to performance of activity of daily living has mainly been reported with the bottom-up approach The treatment group demonstrated a significant increase in motor ability as measured by motor tests over the treatment, whereas the control patients showed no change in arm motor ability; moreover, the treatment group showed a very large increase in real-world arm use compared with the controls over the 2-week period and a further small advantage when tested 2 years after treatment (Taub et al. 1993). This long-term improvement of motor performances after constraint-induced therapy is associated with brain activity changes. Liepert et al. (2000) used transcranial magnetic stimulation (TMS) to map the extent of the motor output map in patients before and after constraint-induced therapy. They showed an enlargement in excitable cortex volume and a shift of the centre of the motor output area in the damaged hemisphere. When measured 4 weeks after the treatment, this area still remained significantly larger than before therapy. In a recent brain imaging study using functional magnetic resonance imaging (fMRI) Johansen-Berg et al. (2002) quantified neural changes associated with behavioural changes in a group of seven chronic stroke patients receiving constraint-induced therapy for hand function. The results showed that the extent of improvement in hand function after therapy varied access patients, and that therapy-induced improvements in hand function correlated with increases in fMRI activity in the premotor cortex and secondary somatosensory cortex contralateral to the affected hand, and in the superior posterior regions of the cerebellar hemispheres bilaterally. These therapy-induced changes do not seem to be related to the same brain activity changes which occur with spontaneous functional recovery. Increased activity in premotor and parietal cortices rather suggests an adaptive reorganization that mediates recovery.

Taken together, these results show that the relationship between the spontaneous motor recovery that occurs after brain damage and cortical plasticity can be manipulated in order to improve the potential for recovering function. In previous studies the improvement of motor performances has been demonstrated on a motor activity scale such as MAL (Taub et al. 1993; Liepert et al. 2000), motricity index, or grip strength (Johansen-Berg et al. 2002). An increase in speed or force of previously performed movements was noted, but the question of whether the movement repertoire of the patients was enlarged, as was found for trunk-restraint therapy of hemiparesis (Michaelsen et al. 2001), was not addressed. This may suggest that the changes induced by behavioural therapy are subsequent to the overcoming of the learned non-use. It is also possible that constraint-induced therapy favours the reduction of a motor neglect component associated with the primary motor deficit. This point has not yet been clarified because right- and left-brain-damaged patients were not distinguished in the published studies. Moreover the presence of associated cognitive deficiencies, such as neglect symptoms, apraxic motor extinction, or attentional disorders, was not indicated. It may be noteworthy that constraint-induced therapy puts constraints on patient selection: They must be able to attend 6 hrs of therapy per day and they must have some residual function in the paretic arm to follow the treatment programme. Nevertheless, the behavioural and brain activity changes after constraint-induced therapy should add to our understanding of rehabilitation-mediated recovery and stimulate the development of neurobiologically directed rehabilitation strategies.

Apraxia

The concept of 'apraxia' includes a number of disorders predominantly associated with left brain damage. It is questionable whether they can be subsumed into one unifying scheme (Liepmann 1908; Rothi *et al.* 1997), or whether they represent independent effects of left brain damage on different aspects of action planning and motor control (Goldenberg 2001, 2003). Traditionally, three domains of human action are considered for diagnosing apraxia: imitation of gestures, performance of meaningful gestures (mainly pantomime of object use) on command, and actual use of tools and objects. Use of tools and objects can refer to the isolated use of one tool with its object (e.g. hammering a nail, cutting a slice of bread) or to the performance of complex activities involving several tools and objects and requiring proper sequencing and coordination of a number of steps or actions (e.g. carrying out a household repair, preparing a meal) (see also Chapter 17, this volume).

Ecological significance of apraxia

Although highly interesting for the theoretical understanding of apraxia, disturbed imitation of gestures seems to have little impact on daily living. Communicative gestures, including pantomime of object use, can compensate for inadequate verbal expression in patients with aphasia. For these patients, the apraxic impairment of gesturing may be ecologically significant. Successful learning of meaningful gestures by such patients has been demonstrated (Code and Gaunt 1986; Coelho and Duffy 1990; Pilgrim and Humphreys 1994; Maher and Ochipa 1997; Smania *et al.* 2000). After training, the patients were able to produce the trained gestures on command, but it remained doubtful whether they used them in spontaneous communication, and whether training of a limited set of gestures helped them to recall or invent non-trained gestures when they needed them for communication.

The ecological significance of disturbed use of tools and objects appears obvious, but the correlation between errors in testing and coping with familiar activities outside the testing situation has been called into question (De Renzi 1990). Testing usually concentrates on the use of single tools and objects. Demonstration of their use is requested out of their habitual context and does not serve a purpose beyond this demonstration: Hammering does not result in fixing pieces together, and looking through binoculars does not enable the patient to see interesting distant objects. In contrast, activities of daily living (ADL) frequently require coordination of a number of actions with several tools and objects in order to achieve a purpose which lies beyond adequate tool use. The purpose of cooking is not the use of cooking utensils but the preparation of food. As a further difference, testing usually concentrates on the prototypical use of familiar tools and objects. In contrast, activities in the natural context sometimes involve unfamiliar or novel equipment, such as beverage or food containers which are difficult to open. Their use must be discovered by inference from structural properties or by trial and error.

The distinction between conventional testing of apraxia and 'naturalistic action' is borne out by their different sensitivities to brain damage. Whereas defective use of single tools and objects is bound to left brain damage and is always accompanied by other manifestations of apraxia (De Renzi *et al.* 1968; Goldenberg and Hagmann 1998b), problems with complex ADL requiring coordination of many chains of action have been documented in patients with right brain, diffuse, or frontal brain damage (Schwartz *et al.* 1998, 1999) who have no problems with the use of single tools and objects.

For patients with left brain damage, the search for correlations between impaired naturalistic action and conventional tests of apraxia has yielded conflicting results (Bjorneby and Reinvang 1985; Sundet *et al.* 1988; Walker and Lincoln 1991; Foundas *et al.* 1995; Buxbaum *et al.* 1998; Goldenberg and Hagmann 1998a; Poole 1998; Neimann *et al.* 2000; Goldenberg *et al.* 2001). Correlations between the isolated use of single tools and naturalistic action may be feigned by the parallel influence of size and severity of lesions on both activities, or conversely be masked by earlier recovery on the comparatively easy test of use of single familiar objects.

Studies of spontaneous recovery of apraxia have concentrated on imitation of gestures and performance of meaningful gestures, such as pantomiming object use, on command. On these tests only about half of the patients who were apraxic in the first week after a stroke are still apraxic after 3 months and only 20% after a year (Kertesz and Ferro 1984; Basso *et al.* 1987). Although some spontaneous recovery of tool use is likely, there are no data available on this issue. In a study of the efficacy of training of ADL in apraxic patients (Goldenberg and Hagmann 1998a), no spontaneous recovery of any of these complex activities was found during the first 2–3 months following stroke.

Regardless of whether they are sequelae of apraxia or not, problems with complex ADL are certainly ecologically significant and justify therapy. However, the uncertainty of their cognitive underpinning means that therapeutic attempts cannot be constructed on a firm theoretical base.

Top-down versus bottom-up approach

With respect to training of complex ADL, a top-down approach would be characterized by teaching the patients general principles of tool and object use which they can

Ecological significance of unilateral neglect

The presence of unilateral neglect worsens the severity of associated motor or sensory deficits, inducing many functionally debilitating effects on everyday life, and is responsible for poor functional recovery and ability to benefit from treatment (Halligan and Marshall 1989; Denes *et al.* 1982; Fullerton *et al.* 1986). For example, neglect patients can forget to read the left part of a journal or a book, omit to eat food from the left half of a plate, or forget to shave the left side of their face. Everyday activities are frequently perturbed in neglect patients and can be investigated by both self-rating and third-person rating (Bergego *et al.* 1994). Typical action deficits include distributing fruit only on the right side of an apple tart (Rossetti *et al.* 1999; Rode *et al.* 2003), exhibiting difficulties in finding their room when on the left side of the corridor and when driving a wheelchair (Rode *et al.* 2003), showing a biased postural balance (Rode *et al.* 1997), and slowing down actions directed to their left or hitting left-sided obstacles.

The history of neglect modulation by a specific intervention started with Diller and Weinberg (1977) 25 years ago. The study by Rubens (1985) renewed interest in rehabilitation methods for unilateral neglect and in both theoretical questions and experimental approaches. The experimental neuropsychology approach to unilateral neglect brought in clearer constraints for the precise quantification of the patients' performance and stimulated interest in focal or partial aspects of this syndrome. At this stage local interventions with the patients were shown to alleviate most of the symptoms of unilateral neglect (reviewed by Vallar 1997). More recently, the idea that specific learning could improve patients' performance has been reconsidered and incorporated to the physiological aspects of sensory stimulation (Kerkhoff 2000).

Top-down versus bottom-up approach

Many attempts have been made in the last 20 years to rehabilitate patients with neglect. Different approaches have been proposed relying mainly on passive physiological stimulations or active training(reviewed by Rossetti and Rode 2002). The main aim of these methods is to favour the reorientation of motor behaviour toward the neglect side, and the first difficulty is obtaining a generalization of effects at a functional level.

The various manifestations of unilateral neglect share one major feature: patients remain unaware of the deficit they exhibit, or at least fail to attend to these deficits fully consciously. This deficit in awareness is dramatically expressed in anosognosia and hemiasomatognosia (Bisiach *et al.* 1986). Therefore it is astonishing that the first methods proposed for the rehabilitation of neglect were based mainly on a voluntary orientation of attention to the left. This paradox was already underlined by Diller and Weinberg themselves:

> The first step in the treatment of hemi-inattention is to make the patient aware of the problem. This is particularly difficult in hemi-inattention since this failure in awareness appears to be at the heart of the patient's difficulty. (Diller and Weinberg 1977, p. 67)

It may indeed appear paradoxical to base a rehabilitation procedure on awareness and intention in patients with a deficit in consciousness. How can a sustained overt orientation to the left be obtained from individuals whose pathology is exactly to remain unable to attend to the left? These techniques have produced significant results, but are clearly exposed to several limitations. For example, rehabilitated patients may typically produce almost perfect performance on classical tests performed during a testing session and then hit the door when walking out of the room, i.e. their voluntary monitoring of attention can be activated in a specific context and does not apply as soon as more automatic control is required. Harvey and Milner (1999) have also shown that the training of visual scanning in unilateral neglect may improve line bisection, which requires a sustained voluntary orienting of attention, but not other tasks. To act on higher-level cognition in such a way as to bypass the impaired conscious awareness and intention, one should, at least in principle, find another entry route to space representation systems. The transformational theory proposed by Jeannerod and Biguer (1987) proposed that the transformation of the sensory input into the motor output is impaired in unilateral neglect. Thus this theoretical position proposes an alternative view to the classical top-down approach to neglect rehabilitation; peripheral sensory stimulations can be viewed as bottom-up tools to act on higher-level spatial cognition.

Different manifestations of neglect may be alleviated by sensory stimulation (vestibular, optokinetic, transcutaneous electrical, transcutaneous mechanical vibration, auditory). The first report of visual neglect improvement was given by Silberpfenning (1941) who applied a caloric vestibular stimulation to two patients suffering from a cerebral tumour. The stimulation led to a reduction of head and eye deviation and reduction of neglect dyslexia. These preliminary cases were confirmed later by Rubens (1985), who showed in 18 right-brain-damaged patients with neglect that a left cold caloric stimulation might improve left visual neglect, although a right stimulation might worsen the deficit. These exciting results showed that a cognitive deficit related to damage of the right hemisphere might be positively influenced by a physiological stimulation [for a review of the effects of vestibular stimulation, see Rode *et al.* (1998c) and Rossetti and Rode (2002)]. They were followed by numerous studies assessing the effects of other kinds of stimulation and the nature of the improved symptoms. Following the study by Rubens (1985) and the striking results obtained with caloric stimulation, many studies have replicated this result and extended its conclusions.

Several other types of sensory stimulation have been proposed and tested in patients. Many manifestations of neglect have been shown to be alleviated by sensory stimulation (vestibular, optokinetic, transcutaneous electrical, transcutaneous mechanical vibration, auditory) (reviewed by Vallar *et al.* 1997; Kerkhoff 2000; Rossetti and Rode 2002). The improvement has been mainly reported for extrapersonal neglect (classical neuropsychological testing), but many other aspects have been investigated, including personal neglect and sensory and motor deficits of the left hemibody associated with neglect or extinction. Even productive manifestations of unilateral neglect, such as anosognosia or somatoparaphrenia, can also be reduced by sensory stimulation (Rode *et al.* 1992). A transient improvement of force has also been observed in right-brain-damaged patients with unilateral neglect and hemiparesis (Rode *et al.* 1998). Positive effects were also reported on postural instability in right-brain-damaged patients with neglect (Rode *et al.* 1999). The second characteristic of effects reported through stimulation is their abrupt onset. In all studies the improvement was observed during or immediately after the stimulation. Unfortunately, however, a single application of these techniques produces positive effects lasting for only up to about 10–15 min, and then they vanish within minutes.

Another bottom-up approach that may have more sustained effects is to produce sensory adaptations which leave traces in the brain after the sensory manipulation is stopped. One interesting aspect of sensorimotor relationships is that they are highly susceptible to adaptive processes. Simple reaching behaviour can be adapted to dramatic changes of the relationship between the body and its environment. One very interesting correspondence between prism adaptation and spatial neglect is that prism adaptation can produce a shift in manual straight-ahead pointing in a direction opposite to the visual shift, just as has been described in some patients with spatial neglect (Jeannerod and Rossetti 1993; Redding *et al.* 2005). If a normal individual is exposed to right deviating prisms, he will exhibit a leftward deviation of his straight-ahead pointing, and the opposite is true for left-deviating prisms. When neglect patients were adapted to rightward visual shift produced by wedge prisms their straight ahead pointing was also shifted to the left (Rossetti *et al.* 1998; Pisella *et al.* 2002). Further investigations have shown that many aspects of unilateral neglect could be improved by a short session of prism adaptation (reviewed by Rossetti and Rode 2002; Rode *et al.* 2003). Classical neuropsychological tests of visuomotor (Rossetti *et al.* 1998; Farné *et al.* 2002; Pisella *et al.* 2002; McIntosh *et al.* 2002) or visuoverbal (Rossetti *et al.* 1998, Farné *et al.* 2002) neglect were improved for at least 24 hrs following a single adaptation session.

If one considers that both strategic and adaptive components of prism adaptation have been described (Redding and Wallace 1997; Redding *et al.* 2005), then one may question the idea that prism adaptation can be regarded as a pure bottom-up approach. However, an interesting observation allows this idea to be reinforced: none of the neglect patients we have examined so far (even when tested up to 28 years after the stroke) noticed anything special when wearing the prism goggles (Rossetti *et al.*, unpublished data; Calabria *et al.* 2004). This observation is in striking contrast with the obvious surprise spontaneously expressed by healthy subjects and partners of neglect patients, and thus strongly supporting the idea that prism adaptation in unilateral patients, unlike normal subjects, can be considered as involving only sensorimotor adaptation processes.

Generalization of therapeutic gains

It would seem logical that the effects of prism adaptation should be restricted to, or best for, visuomotor tasks, because they have more features in common with the visuomanual adaptation procedure (Redding *et al.* 2005). In the original study, we observed that the best improvement was observed for the Schenkenberg bisection test (all six patients markedly improved), whereas the weakest improvement was obtained for text reading (two of six patients markedly improved). Therefore many other tests of neglect were investigated (reviewed by Rossetti and Rode 2002; Rode *et al.* 2003).

Rode *et al.* (1999, 2001a) explored the effect of prism adaptation on visual imagery and found a clear-cut improvement in two patients who were initially unable to evoke cities on the western half of an internally generated map of France. This result strongly suggested that the after-effects of visuomanual adaptation cannot be considered to be restricted to visual and motor parameters (Rossetti *et al.* 1999). Farné *et al.* (2001) compared visuomotor tasks [including line and bell cancellation tests, and two subtests taken from the Behavioural Inattention Test (BIT) battery, namely letter cancellation and line bisection] with visuoverbal tasks (the visual scanning test, also taken from the BIT, requiring a verbal description of the objects depicted on a coloured picture, an object-naming task with 30 Snodgrass pictures of familiar objects intermingled with geometric shapes as distractors, and word and non-word reading) in six patients. They observed that the two groups of tasks followed a strictly parallel improvement which lasted for at least 24 hrs.

The fact that other sensory modalities can be improved [haptic circle centring (McIntosh *et al.* 2002), dichotic listening (Courtois-Jacquin *et al.* 2001), haptic object recognition (Toutounji *et al.* 2001), tactile extinction (Maravita *et al.* 2003)] and that several non-manual tasks (postural control, wheel-chair driving (Jacquin *et al.* 1998), imagery, verbal reports) were also improved demonstrate that the effects of prism adaptation are not restricted to visuomanual parameters as they are known to be in normal subjects. Recently, Berberovic *et al.* (2003) have shown that even a non-spatial and non-manual aspect of neglect could be improved, namely temporal order judgement. These results strongly suggest that adaptation to wedge prisms somehow affects the very core of unilateral neglect.

Recently, Zorzi *et al.* (2002) described a new feature of unilateral neglect. They used a simple test of mental number bisection where patients where requested to report where they saw the middle between two numbers (e.g. between 1 and 19). They found that, unlike controls, neglect patients exhibited a bias towards the larger number, as if their mental representation of the mental number line was distorted as is classically described for line bisection. Therefore we have investigated the effects of prism adaptation on this mental task without an explicit spatial component. We found that prism adaptation strongly improved the right-sided number bisecting bias in patients who bisected lines to the left (Rossetti *et al.* 2004). These results confirm the powerful bottom-up effects of prism adaptation.

More specifically in the motor domain, the visuomanual plasticity triggered by the visual shift produced effects on non-trained tasks (most of the tests used differed from the pointing task performed during prism exposure) as well as on non-manual tasks [postural control (Tilikete *et al.* 2001), wheelchair driving (Rode *et al.* 2003)]. In addition the intentional component of neglect, assessed by a task where the patients had to reach for a central ball and then throw it to the left or right side, can also be altered by adaptation (Rode *et al.* 2003). In an experimental condition aimed at investigating the effect of THE prism on the intentional control of action, patients where asked to grasp a centrally presented ball and then throw it to the left or the right. The kinematic analysis of the reach-to-grasp movement shows that neglect patients are overall slowed down when the secondary movement is directed to the left (Jacquin 2002). After a short prism adaptation session, this asymmetry was modified for several movement parameters (reaction time, movement time, peak velocity, time to peak velocity) (Rode *et al.* 2003). The pattern of result observed immediately after prism adaptation even showed the reverse pattern: reach movements were slower when the ball had to be sent to the right. This result demonstrates that the intentional control of action can be modified by prism adaptation.

Still at a motor level, there are several qualitative observations that prism adaptation can improve the motor behaviour of patients in everyday life (McIntosh *et al.* 2002). Quantification of everyday life activity also suggested that patients can be improved up for to a year (Parache *et al.* 2002).

One of the crucial questions raised by the observation of a strong and sustained improvement of hemispatial neglect by a single short adaptation session is whether this plastic effect is restricted to the acute phase of the deficit. In our original study, patients were tested between 3 weeks and 14 months post-stroke (Rossetti *et al.* 1998). We have now collected data on a group of patients who were exposed to the adaptation procedure between 5 and 28 years post-stroke and amazingly found the same amount of improvement.

Retention over time is the second main important characteristics of a rehabilitation method. The effects of a single session last much longer for prism adaptation (at least 2 hrs) than for other sensory stimulations (about 15 min). A group of patients showed a maintained improvement 24 hrs after the training session (Farné *et al.* 2002), whereas individual cases may exhibit long-lasting amelioration of neglect (McIntosh *et al.* 2002; Pisella *et al.* 2002).

Repetitive stimulation by sensory stimulation has been tested more recently. Frassinetti *et al.* (2002) reported that a group of patients who benefited from two prism adaptation sessions daily over 2 weeks (a total of 10 sessions) exhibited an improvement over 5 weeks after the end of the treatment. Schindler *et al.* (2002) also explored the effects of repetitive neck vibration and found a sustained improvement following an intensive daily programme. Obviously such studies should be undertaken to determine the optimal training frequency and duration as well as the optimal combination of techniques that can be used routinely for rehabilitation.

Influence of right brain damage

In contrast with apraxia (left sided lesions) and to hemplegia (either side), unilateral neglect is notoriously more severe and more resistant following a right-sided lesion. The question of whether the rehabilitation procedures used to improve neglect specifically act on the right hemisphere is questionable. First, recovery from neglect can be observed following a subsequent lesion of the left hemisphere. Secondly, the top-down approach to the rehabilitation of neglect may activate functional systems on either side. They may tend to inhibit some left-hemisphere functions but, as mentioned earlier, their effect does not generalize as much as with the bottom-up approaches. The effect of sensory stimulations clearly induces a stimulation of sensory input to the damaged right hemisphere. This effect has been considered to improve the functional balance between the two hemispheres (reviewed by Rossetti and Rode 2002), and a bilateral stimulation does not produce any improvement (Rode *et al.* 2002). The effect of prism adaptation is more difficult to evaluate in terms of hemisphere activation. While some brain imaging studies were interpreted as an argument that the posterior parietal cortex is involved in prism adaptation, patients with bilateral lesions of the posterior parietal cortex have been shown to adapt to prism at least as much as normal subjects (Pisella *et al.* 2003). In addition, the only lesion site that seems to disrupt prism adaptation is the olivopontocerebellar system (reviewed by Jeannerod and Rossetti 1993). The current most probable hypothesis about the effects of prism on neglect postulates that prism adaptation stimulates the cerebellum ipsilateral to the visual shift, which in turn inhibits the controlateral cortex (Pisella *et al.* 2003), as is the case with focal application of TMS (Fierro *et al.* 2000). A recent PET study of patients before and after adaptation confirms this hypotheis (Luauté *et al.* 2005). This hypothesis may also explain how leftward prism adaptation emulates mild neglect in healthy controls (Michel *et al.* 2003a,b). Whether prism adaptation specifically acts on neglect or on the right-hemisphere deficit may also be debated, as the postural balance of patients without neglect has been improved following prism adaptation (Tilikete *et al.* 2001).

Discussion

Three main motor disorders have been considered in the present review. Hemiplegia is a deficit of the motor production *per se*, while apraxia and unilateral neglect do not directly impair motor capacity. Rather, these two latter disorders affect higher levels of action organization, with an impairment of either action logic or analogical spatial representations, which produces strong disabilities in everyday life. Two main issues emerge from the confrontation of these three disorders. First, what is the level of action of the therapeutic interventions? Secondly, what is the impact of hemispheric specialization in terms of rehabilitation constraints?

Levels of action

Classical approaches to the rehabilitation of motor disorders have mainly focused on the conscious monitoring of the deficit in order to bypass its functional consequences. This typical top-down methodology has been widely used. The important attentional load inherent in conscious strategies is responsible for some limitations of their interest for everyday life situations. The present review has made it clear that bottom-up techniques of rehabilitation may produce better results than the traditional top-down methods. Their advantage is shown in terms of the duration of the therapeutic effects produced for all three rehabilitation techniques reviewed. In terms of generalization of the effects to non-trained tasks, the advantage of the bottom-up approach is obvious only for unilateral neglect. Several bottom-up approaches applied to unilateral neglect appear to produce more generalizable effects than the top-down approaches (Rode *et al.* 1998b; Rossetti and Rode 2002; Rode *et al.* 2003). The effects of bottom-up approaches for apraxia are apparently restricted to the trained tasks. However, it is questionable whether top-down approaches are successful at all, so that in sum bottom up appears to be more efficient than top down in rehabilitation of apraxia as well, although the duration of the improvement appears to be independent of this distinction. For example, a single application of sensory stimulation (e.g. caloric vestibular stimulation) may produce extremely generalizable effects although the benefit remains short lasting. The technique associating some kind of learning (at a physiological level) and a bottom-up principle (prism adaptation) appears to produce the optimal effect on the corresponding deficit (unilateral neglect). The interesting observation is that the primacy of the bottom-up approach appears independent of the higher (unilateral neglect) versus lower (hemiplegia) level of impairment considered. Rather, it may depend on the type of processing being impaired.

Mechanisms of action

In conventional nomenclature, restitution and compensation of functions are distinguished. While an authentic restitution can be expected in the case of the spontaneous recovery of transient strokes, a functional restitution may be obtained in the case of vicariant systems (Hecaen and Jeannerod 1979). 'Compensation' includes all mechanisms going around the basic deficit without restoring the basic function. While the training method proposed to improve patients with apraxia can be considered as going around the basic deficit of apraxia, the methods used for the other two pathologies may be viewed as inhibitory methods directed towards healthy remaining systems. It is obvious that blocking the movements of the healthy arm of patients with hemiplegia results in a direct inhibition of the sensory and motor areas linked to the motor activation of this arm. This sensory and motor 'deafferentation' technique has two types of consequences: first, it forces the paretic arm to work up to its maximal potential; secondly, it may reduce the activity of brain areas participating in its activity. This indirect inhibition of central structure appears to be beneficial for the recovery of both motor function and brain activity linked to the paretic arm. Along the same lines, the current interpretation of the therapeutic effects of prism adaptation on unilateral neglect is that such adaptation is responsible for an inhibition of central structures on the healthy side, which may in turn facilitate the recovery of the deficit observed on the side of the lesion (Rossetti and Rode 2002; Rode *et al.* 2003). If inhibition of the non-lesioned hemisphere appears to be a principle of efficient therapy for unilateral neglect, this does not appear to be the case for other neuropsychological deficits. Indeed, there are observations of recurrence of recovered aphasia after right brain damage (Cambier *et al.* 1982). Taken together, the strong differences between the outcome of rehabilitation techniques used in apraxia and unilateral neglect highlight the different neuronal and psychological mechanisms underlying the rehabilitation of different types of deficits.

Hemispheric specialization

Motor deficits are rarely the only symptom of cerebral lesions. This is particularly true of 'higher-level' disorders of motor control, apraxia, and hemi-neglect. Apraxia from left brain damage is virtually always accompanied by aphasia and hemi-neglect from right brain damage may be embedded in non-lateralized or even non-spatial deficits of attention (Husain and Rorden 2003). There are some anecdotal observations pointing to an influence of these hemisphere-specific symptoms on recovery and success of rehabilitation. For example, the inability of apraxic and aphasic patients to exploit insights into functional relationships, gained by comparisons between functionally similar and dissimilar objects or by drawing with a special emphasis on functionally relevant details, for improving their actual use of these objects has been ascribed to a loss of categorical or 'abstract' attitude associated with aphasia (Goldenberg *et al.* 2001). In contrast, there is the observation of patients with left-sided hemi-neglect who, after prism training, spontaneously enumerate towns on the left side of a map but now omit towns on the right side which they had mentioned before the training (Rode *et al.* 1998c). Possibly training had alleviated only the lateralized component of the attention disorder, resulting in a wider and more even spread of the still reduced general attentional capacity.

There may be differences in the ease of rehabilitation between patients with left and right brain damage beyond the influence of accompanying hemisphere-specific syndromes. One of the most striking development of recent years has been the demonstration of highly efficient bottom-up approaches to alleviation of hemi-neglect in patients with right brain damage. Not only do some of these procedures (e.g. prism adaptation) exert effects after very short exposure, they also display considerable generalization to non-trained tasks or tests (see above). We are not aware of similarly dramatic effects in the rehabilitation of the neuropsychological sequelae of left brain damage. Of course, there are many possible reasons for this discrepancy, the simplest being that corresponding methods have not yet been devised for the syndromes of left brain damage. Another likely possibility may be that the crucial difference is between hemi-neglect and other neuropsychological syndromes. If this was the case, bottom-up approaches should be equally efficient in right sided hemi-neglect from left-sided lesions. We have recently confirmed that this is the case in a patient with right neglect and no hemiplegia (Rode *et al.* in press). Another possibility, which is at present purely speculative, but may be worth being pursued further, is that the differential ease of rehabilitation may reflect basic differences between the neural architecture of both hemispheres. Right-hemisphere functions may be organized in neural networks with less distinct assignment of functions to circumscribed portions (Mesulam 1981; Buxhoeveden and Casanova 2000; Galuske *et al.* 2000; Rabinowicz *et al.* 2002). This feature of the neural architecture might facilitate plastic reorganization of the network for compensating the contribution of lost parts.

Possibly the ultimate key to the contrast between the comparatively easy amelioration of hemi-neglect and the difficulty of obtaining therapy effects for apraxia (and aphasia) may be the differential logic pertaining to the lesioned functions. It has been proposed for a long time that the right hemisphere is specialized for holistic processing of information while the left hemisphere is specialized for analytical processing. The fuzzier functions (e.g. space representation) predominant in the right hemisphere may appear easier to modulate than the logical functions (e.g. language, action grammar) predominant on the left side. While the ideomotor functions have to be established and maintained in a rigid form, representations of space have to adapt to multiple changes resulting from changes in perspective due to action. This distinction may correspond to differences in the microstructure of neuronal anatomy (e.g. size of functional units) between the hemispheres.

In conclusion, two points may be emphasized. First, the better ecological results of higher-order motor deficit rehabilitation seemed to be obtained from a bottom-up approach. In the treatments reviewed above—constraint-induced therapy, direct training for apraxia, and prism adaptation—the common factor is the central role attributed to action, particularly to the direct training imposed to the hemiparetic patient to use the paretic limb, to the apraxic patient to use tools and objects, and to the neglect patient to point quickly into peripersonal space. These neurobiologically directed rehabilitation strategies seem to refer to sensorimotor rather than to cognitive representations of action, probably relying on the involvement of subcortical structures such as basal ganglia, caudate, and cerebellum, implied in motor learning, automatism, and adaptation. Thus they underline the interest of non-cognitive (physiological) routes to the rehabilitation of cognitive disorders (Rossetti and Rode 2002). Secondly, the interesting question remains open: are the dimensions used in this chapter to classify the therapeutic approaches—top down versus bottom up, right versus left hemisphere, generalizable versus task-specific—orthogonal? It is most likely that these important dimensions of rehabilitation approaches are highly interdependent, though in very flexible ways.

References

Ahlsio B, Britton M, Murray V, Theorell T (1984). Disablement and quality of life after stroke. *Stroke*, **15**, 886–90.

Basso A, Capitani E, Della Sala S, Laiacona M, Spinnler H (1987). Recovery from ideomotor apraxia—a study on acute stroke patients. *Brain*, **110**, 747–60.

Berberovic N, Mattingley JB (2003). Effects of prismatic adaptation on judgements of spatial extent in peripersonal and extrapersonal space. *Neuropsychologia*, in press.

Bergego C, Bradat-Diehl P, Taillefer C, Migeot H (1994). Evaluation et rééducation de l'apraxie d'utilisation des objets. In D Le Gall, G Aubin, (ed.) *L'Apraxie*, pp. 214–23. Marseille: SOLAL.

Bisiach E, Vallar G, Peranin D, Papagno C, Berti A (1986). Unawareness of disease following lesions of the right hemisphere: anosognosia for hemiplagia and anosognosia for hemianopia. *Neuropsychologia*, **24**, 471–82.

Bjorneby ER, Reinvang ER (1985). Acquiring and maintaining selfcare skills after stroke. The predictive value of apraxia. *Scand J Rehabil Med*, **17**, 75–80.

Buxbaum LJ, Schwartz MF, Montgomery MW (1998). Ideational apraxia and naturalistic action, *Cogn Neuropsychol*, **15**, 617–44.

Buxhoeveden D, Casanova M (2000). Comparative lateralisation patterns in the language area of human, chimpenzee, and rhesus monkey brains. *Laterality*, **5**, 315–30.

Calabria M, Michel C, Honoré J, Pisella L, Rode G, Boisson D, *et al.* (2004). Prism adaptation and the lack of awareness in spatial neglect: a skin conductance study. Presented at the first congress of the European Neuropsychology Societies, Modena, Italy.

Cambier J, Elghozi D, Signoret J-L, Hénin D (1983). Contribution de l'hémisphère droit au language des aphasiques. Disparition de ce langage après lésion droite. *Rev Neurol (Paris)*, **139**, 55–63.

Cao Y, D'Olhaberriague L, Vikingstad EM, Levine SR, Welch KM (1998). Pilot study of functional MRI to assess cerebral activation of motor function after poststroke hemparesis. *Stroke*, **29**, 112–22.

Caramia MD, Iani C, Bernardi G (1996). Cerebral plasticity after stroke as revealed by ipsilateral responses to magnetic stimulation. *NeuroReport*, **7**, 1756–60.

Chollet F (2000). Plasticity of the adult human brain. In *Brain Mapping*, 621–38.

Chollet F, Di Piero V, Wise RJS, Brooks DJ, Dolan RJ, Frackowiak RSJ (1991). The functional anatomy of motor recovery after stroke in humans: a study with positron emission tomography. *Ann Neurol*, **29**, 63–71.

Code C, Gaunt C (1986). Treating severe speech and limb apraxia in a case of aphasia. *Br J Disord Commun*, **21**, 11–20.

Coelho CA, Duffy RJ (1990). Sign acquisition in two aphasic subjects with limb apraxia. *Aphasiology*, **4**, 1–8.

Courtois-Jacquin S, Rossetti Y, Rode G, Fischer C, Michel C, Allard C, *et al.* (2001). Effect of prism adaptation on auditory extinction: an attentional effect? Presented at the International Symponum: 'Neural control of space coding and action production'. Lyon, March 2001.

Cramer SC, Nelles G, Benson RR, Kaplan JD, Parker Ra, Kwong KK, *et al.* (1997). A functional MRI study of patients recovered from hemiparetic stroke. *Stroke*, **28**, 2518–27.

Denes G, Semenza C, Stoppa E, Lis A (1982). Unilateral spatial neglect and recovery from hemipligia. A follow-up study. *Brain*, **105**, 543–52.

De Pedro-Cuesta J, Widen-Holmquist L, Bach-y-Rita P (1992). Evaluation of stroke rehabilitation by randomized conrolled studies: a review. *Acta Neurol Scand* 1992 86:433–439.

De Renzi E (1990). Apraxia. In F Boller, J Grafman, (ed.) *Handbook of Clinical Neuropsychology* Vol 2, pp. 245–63. Amsterdam: Elsevier.

De Renzi E, Pieczuro A, Vignolo LA (1968). Ideational apraxia: a quantitative study. *Neuropsychologia*, **6**, 41–55.